Introduction to Audiologic Rehabilitation

SEVENTH EDITION

Introduction to Audiologic Rehabilitation

RONALD L. SCHOW
Idaho State University

MICHAEL A. NERBONNE
Central Michigan University

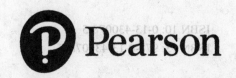 **Pearson**

330 Hudson Street, NY NY 10013

Editorial Director: Kevin Davis
Executive Portfolio Manager: Julie Peters
Managing Content Producer: Megan Moffo
Portfolio Management Assistant: Maria Feliberty
Executive Product Marketing Manager: Christopher Barry
Executive Field Marketing Manager: Krista Clark
Manufacturing Buyer: Deidra Smith
Cover Design: Carie Keller, Cenveo
Cover Art: Lisa Zador/Stockbyte/Getty Images
Editorial Production and Composition Services: Cenveo® Publisher Services
Full-Service Project Managers: Susan McNally, Kritika Kaushik
Text Font: New Aster LT Std

Library of Congress Cataloging-in-Publication Data

Names: Schow, Ronald L., editor. | Nerbonne, Michael A., editor.
Title: Introduction to audiologic rehabilitation / [edited by] Ronald L.
  Schow, Idaho State University, Michael A. Nerbonne, Central Michigan University.
Description: Seventh edition. | Boston : Pearson Education, Inc., [2017] |
  Includes bibliographical references and indexes.
Identifiers: LCCN 2017016701 | ISBN 9780134300788 (alk. paper)
Subjects: LCSH: Deaf—Rehabilitation. | Audiology.
Classification: LCC RF297 .I57 2017 | DDC 362.4/2—dc23 LC record available at
https://lccn.loc.gov/2017016701

2 18

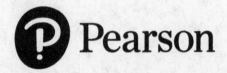 **Pearson**

ISBN 10:   0-13-430078-5
ISBN 13: 978-0-13-430078-8

Preface

Our introductory text first appeared in 1980 and has been used on college campuses for 37 years. It is with profound gratitude and pride that we now bring you the seventh edition.

During the years since 1980, we have watched cochlear implants move from their early beginnings in 1972 to become a major miracle for children born deaf and for others, including late-deafened adults. Traditional hearing aids also have shown tremendous advances during these years. They are more accepted and technologically more sophisticated, and they now enjoy wider usage among those with hearing loss, which has moved from 20 to 30 percent, a 50 percent improvement. However, both hearing aids and cochlear implants simply do not produce maximum benefit and satisfied users without a lot of support and technical help from hearing professionals.

Hearing assistive technology (HAT) devices as spurred by the miracle of the Internet, cell phones, and wireless technologies, and their associated software and hardware also present us with a vastly changed environment and are more easily used and accepted by those with hearing loss. HAT also requires professionals to provide strong support and encouragement.

Many of the 32 million persons with hearing loss in the United States and an estimated 10 percent of the worldwide population of more than 7 billion will not take advantage of these modern miracles until they learn of them and are shown how to find benefit by those using this book. This expertise by well-trained professionals is needed among adults and children.

Those who serve adults in private practice, medical settings, veterans clinics, and other settings are more skilled and available than ever before. Now that the baby-boom generation is beginning to reach retirement age, the proportion of the population with hearing loss is increasing dramatically such that even more older adults will need the help of rehabilitative audiologists in the coming years. The increasing numbers of the oldest old, including those with coexisting health issues, will place new demands on rehabilitation tailored to their needs and the needs of their caregivers in the context of new interprofessional team approaches.

Parent–infant professionals, school audiologists, speech-language pathologists, and a wide circle of other professionals help make referrals and marshal an important group to provide the support needed within families, preschools, and schools to help children benefit from these new developments.

During these years, with the emergence of the Au.D. in audiology, students in the university setting have been getting better and more extensive training than in the past. Students have also benefited increasingly from the support of professional associations that have provided guidelines and follow-up training after graduation to keep professionals up to date as new developments have rapidly emerged. The maturity of rehabilitative audiology is reflected in research that has given us higher-quality evidence of what interventions are effective. Client-centered and family-centered audiologic rehabilitation have advanced because of new procedures and developments based on evidence and more global multicultural understandings of the needs of those living with hearing loss.

We have been fortunate during these years to have worked with some amazing authors who have assisted in keeping this text current and relevant. We are immensely grateful to all of them, including those who have helped with this edition. They are thorough, have enviable expertise, and are among the best in our profession.

With their assistance, we have improved this new seventh edition by adding the following new features and changes:

- Our web design wizard, Jeff Brockett, has updated and improved the text website. Check it out at www.isu.edu/csed/audiology/rehab.
- Chapter 3 has been revised to focus on cochlear implants only.
- New learning outcomes have been added to each chapter.
- Updated information and references are included in all chapters.
- Updated websites also are provided in all chapters.
- New supplementary learning activities are provided in the chapters.
- Revised vestibular and tinnitus treatment sections are now placed in Chapter 10.
- New case studies have been added to Chapters 11 and 12.

Some of these improvements were made at the suggestion of a group of five reviewers whom we thank for their input: Stephanie Adamovich, University of Arizona; Lindsay M. Bondurant, Ph.D., Illinois State University; Demarcus Bush, Au.D., South Carolina State University; Julie L. Hazelbacker, Ohio State University; and Sarah Dawson Wainscott, Texas Woman's University.

We also thank our families and colleagues for their encouragement and enduring support as well as the universities that have sustained us all these years. They all have been truly remarkable to us throughout the nearly four decades that we have worked on this text.

Finally, we are pleased to have brought into our working group a set of new professionals for this edition. They will carry this text forward into the future as the two of us transition into another phase in our lives. These individuals will ensure that this text will continue to be a force in audiology for years to come.

Ron Schow
Mike Nerbonne

A website at http://www.isu.edu/csed/audiology/rehab/ has been updated to supplement and complement this edition. Not only has the content changed but all interactive files are now in a format that can be accessed on laptop, tablets and mobile phones. Some examples of content include: hearing loss simulation and classification, cloze procedure simulation, and a dB reference level activity. The laptop icon in the chapter margins indicates where related content is included on the website.

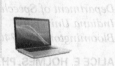

Contributors

GABRIEL A. BARGEN, PH.D.
Assistant Professor
Department of Communication Sciences and Disorders
Idaho State University Meridian Health Science Center
Meridian, ID 83642

KRISTINA M. BLAISER, PH.D.
Assistant Professor
Department of Communication Sciences and Disorders
Idaho State University Meridian Health Science Center
Meridian, ID 83642

JEFF E. BROCKETT, ED.D.
Associate Professor
Department of Communication Sciences and Disorders
Idaho State University
Pocatello, ID 83209

CATHERINE CRONIN CAROTTA, ED.D.
Associate Director
Center for Childhood Deafness
Boys Town National Research Hospital
Omaha, NE 68131

KRIS ENGLISH, PH.D.
Professor of Audiology
School of Speech-Language Pathology & Audiology
University of Akron
Akron, OH 44325

NICHOLAS M. HIPSKIND, PH.D.
Professor Emeritus of Audiology
Department of Speech and Hearing Sciences
Indiana University
Bloomington, IN 47401

ALICE E. HOLMES, PH.D.
Professor Emerita of Audiology
Department of Communicative Disorders
University of Florida Health Science Center
Gainesville, FL 32610

HOLLY S. KAPLAN, PH.D.
Clinical Professor
Department of Communication Sciences and Special
  Education
University of Georgia
Athens, GA 30602

MARY PAT MOELLER, PH.D.
Director
Center for Childhood Deafness
Boys Town National Research Hospital
Omaha, NE 68131

MICHAEL A. NERBONNE, PH.D.
Professor Emeritus of Audiology
Department of Communication Disorders
Central Michigan University
Mount Pleasant, MI 48859

M. KATHLEEN PICHORA-FULLER, PH.D.
Professor
Department of Psychology
University of Toronto Mississauga
Mississauga, ON L5L 1C6, Canada

CHRIS A. SANFORD, PH.D.
Associate Professor
Department of Communication Sciences and Disorders
Idaho State University
Pocatello, ID 83209

RONALD L. SCHOW, PH.D.
Professor Emeritus of Audiology
Department of Communication Sciences and Disorders
Idaho State University
Pocatello, ID 83209

MARY M. WHITAKER, AU.D.
Clinical Professor and Director of Audiology
Department of Communication Sciences and Disorders
Idaho State University
Pocatello, ID 83209

Contents

3

Cochlear Implants 69

Alice E. Holmes

4 Auditory Stimuli in Communication 93

Michael A. Nerbonne
Ronald L. Schow
Kristina M. Blaiser

5 Visual Stimuli in Communication 127

Nicholas M. Hipskind

8 Audiologic Rehabilitation Services in the School Setting   217

Kris English

9 Audiologic Rehabilitation for Children   247

Mary Pat Moeller
Ronald L. Schow
Mary M. Whitaker

10 Audiologic Rehabilitation across the Adult Life Span: Assessment and Management 307

M. Kathleen Pichora-Fuller
Ronald L. Schow

PART THREE: Implementing Audiologic Rehabilitation: Case Studies   393

11   Case Studies: Children   395

Mary Pat Moeller
Catherine Cronin Carotta

12 Case Studies: Adults and Elderly Adults 427

Michael A. Nerbonne
Jeff E. Brockett
Alice E. Holmes

part 1

Fundamentals of Audiologic Rehabilitation

Fundamentals
of Audiologic
Rehabilitation

Overview of Audiologic Rehabilitation

Ronald L. Schow, Michael A. Nerbonne, and Chris A. Sanford

CONTENTS

Visit the companion website when you see this icon to learn more about the topic nearby in the text.

Learning Outcomes

After reading this chapter, you will be able to

- Define audiologic rehabilitation and the primary goals associated with this process
- Be aware of the general estimates of hearing loss prevalence for children and adults in the United States and worldwide, and understand the difference between *deaf* and *hard of hearing*
- Understand environmental factors and personal factors in the way they influence hearing loss, based on the World Health Organization (WHO) model of functioning and disability. Give examples of each and compare them
- Explain how the suggested use of the terms *activity limitation* and *participation restriction* by WHO helps individuals properly understand the consequences of hearing loss
- Know the main professional associations and the importance of evidence-based practice and multicultural issues
- Describe the key components of the CORE and the CARE models and explain how these components influence audiologic rehabilitation
- Identify the variety of different health care providers who contribute to the coordination and implementation of audiologic rehabilitation
- List some of the recent technological advances that have led to improvements in audiologic rehabilitation

INTRODUCTION

Many individuals have had occasion to converse with someone who is deaf or hard of hearing. Unless the communication partners have alternative means of communicating (such as sign language) or the individual who is deaf or hard of hearing has received some type of assistance for his or her hearing difficulties, it may be a frustrating experience for both parties. When the person with hearing loss is a family member or close friend, we become aware that the emotional and social ramifications of this communication barrier can be substantial as well. Providing help to address all these hearing challenges is the focus of this book. While help is possible, it is often not utilized. This chapter gives an overview of this process, which is crucial for the welfare of persons who suffer from hearing loss and, in turn, for those who communicate with them.

Definitions and Synonyms

Simply stated, we may define *audiologic rehabilitation* as those professional processes performed in collaboration with a client who has hearing loss and the client's significant others to achieve better communication and minimize the resulting difficulties (American Speech-Language-Hearing Association [ASHA], 2001; Stephens & Kramer, 2010; World Health Organization [WHO], 2001).

> **Audiologic rehabilitation:** Professional processes performed in collaboration with a client who has hearing loss and the client's significant others to achieve better communication and minimize the resulting difficulties.

- The goal is to enhance the *activities* and *participation* of a person with hearing loss so as to improve his or her quality of life. Achieving adequate receptive and expressive communication is a major means of reaching this goal.
- The processes/procedures include the use of devices to minimize the hearing loss and teaching strategies and problem solving, which in combination assist the individual to overcome interpersonal, psychosocial, educational, and vocational difficulties resulting from the hearing loss.
- A clear objective is to involve family members or significant others to limit the negative effects on these relationships.
- Finally, it is important for the individual to accept and come to terms with any residual problems associated with hearing loss.
- Two important services that are closely related but distinct from the audiologic rehabilitation process are *medical intervention* and *education of the deaf*.

Several terms have been used to describe this helping process. *Audiologic habilitation* refers to remedial efforts with children having a hearing loss at birth since technically it is not possible to restore (rehabilitate) something that has never existed. *Audiologic rehabilitation*, then, refers to efforts designed to restore a lost state or function. In the interest of simplicity, the terms *habilitation* and *rehabilitation* are used interchangeably in this text, technicalities notwithstanding. Variations of the *audiologic rehabilitation* term include *auditory and aural rehabilitation*, *hearing rehabilitation*, and *rehabilitative audiology*. Terms used to refer to rehabilitative efforts with the very young child include *parent advising/counseling/tutoring* and *pediatric auditory habilitation*. *Educational* (or *school*) *audiology* is sometimes used to refer to auditory rehabilitative efforts performed in the school setting.

> Audiologic habilitation is sometimes used to refer to those efforts to assist children with hearing loss since we cannot rehabilitate something that was never there in the first place. Nevertheless, for simplicity's sake, audiologic rehabilitation (AR) is used throughout this text.

Providers of Audiologic Rehabilitation

Audiologic rehabilitation (AR), then, is referred to by different names and is performed in a number of different settings. All aspects of assisting the client and significant others in the audiologic rehabilitation process are not performed by one person. In fact, professionals from several different disciplines are often involved, including educators, psychologists, social workers, and rehabilitation counselors. Nevertheless, the audiologist in particular—and frequently the speech–language pathologist or the educator of the deaf—will assume a major AR role. These professionals provide overall coordination of the process or act as advocates for the person with hearing loss. Audiologic rehabilitation is not something we *do* to a person following a strict "doctor-knows-best" medical model. It is a process designed to counsel and work with persons who are deaf and hard of hearing so that they can actualize their own resources in order to meet their unique life situations. In addition, an individual's family, which could be defined as simply the individual alone or most often includes a partner, spouse, parent, or children, can be a valuable resource in the rehabilitation process (Ekberg, Meyer, Scarinci, Grenness, & Hickson, 2015). This so called family-centered care is generally thought to result in improved health outcomes, improved faithfulness to treatment recommendations, and increased satisfaction with medical services (Rathert, Wyrwich, & Boren, 2013). Therefore, inclusion of the family in the rehabilitative process should not be overlooked. This text has been written with the hope of orienting and preparing professionals as "counselors" or "advocates for better hearing" so that they can be effective participants in the problem-solving process.

Education Needs of Providers

There are multiple professionals involved in a rehabilitation team; most often, speech-language pathologists and/or audiologists lead the team. The entry-level degree for speech-language pathologists is the master's degree. From the audiologic perspective, there is now a well-established professional degree, the Doctorate in Audiology (Au.D.), that is the minimum educational requirement for those beginning work as audiologists. The major professional bodies for these professions include the American Speech-Language-Hearing Association (ASHA) and the American Academy of Audiology (AAA). These organizations, along with the Academy of Rehabilitative Audiology (ARA), all have position statements that emphasize the training needs of students so that they can be well prepared in both diagnostic and rehabilitative audiology. These statements generally have a list of relevant content areas in AR that should be incorporated into any program to ensure adequate preparation in rehabilitative audiology. These are available on a resource website (www.isu.edu/csed/audiology/rehab) that goes with this text (see AAA, ASHA, and ARA statements on competencies for AR).

Regardless of academic background, those from the different professions mentioned in the previous section who successfully perform AR must, like competent audiologists, possess an understanding of and familiarity with several areas of knowledge. These include (1) characteristics of hearing loss, (2) effect of hearing loss on persons, and (3) the previously noted competencies needed for providing audiologic rehabilitation. For purposes of the present treatment, it is assumed that other course work or study has brought the reader familiarity with the various forms of hearing loss as well as procedures used in the diagnostic measurement of hearing loss. These procedures, referred to as *diagnostic audiology*, serve as a preliminary step toward rehabilitative audiology. The task at hand, then, is to review briefly some characteristics of hearing loss, to explore the major consequences of such loss, and finally to discuss the methods and competencies needed to help with this condition.

To participate in AR, you need to know the characteristics of hearing loss, the effects of the loss, and the methods for remediation.

HEARING LOSS CHARACTERISTICS

Important characteristics of hearing loss as they relate to audiologic rehabilitation include (1) degree and configuration of loss, (2) time of onset, (3) type of loss, and (4) auditory speech recognition ability.

Degree of Hearing Loss and Configuration

One major aspect of hearing loss is the person's hearing sensitivity or degree of loss (see Table 1.1). The amount of loss will vary across the frequency range, leading to

TABLE 1.1 Degree of Hearing Loss Descriptions, Based on Pure Tone Findings

Degrees of Hearing Loss	PTA in dB Based on 0.5, 1, 2 k[a]Hz[b]	
	Children	Adults
Slight to Mild	21–40	26–40
Mild to Moderate	—	41–55
Moderate	—	56–70
Severe	—	71–90
Profound	—	91 plus

[a]k = 1000.

[b]The three frequencies of 0.5, 1, and 2 kHz routinely are used for interpreting audiograms and comparing to SRTs. Higher frequencies, including 3 kHz and 4 kHz, should be considered in hearing aid fitting decisions and compensation cases.

A reasonable estimate is that 10 percent of the population has hearing loss. In the United States, this includes about 32 million persons (as of 2017), but this counts only the most serious problems and not minor hearing difficulties.

different configurations or shapes of hearing loss on an audiogram, including the most common patterns of flat, sloping, and precipitous. (Practice in degree and configuration interpretation is provided on the website.) The categories of hearing loss include both the hard of hearing and the deaf. Persons with limited amounts of hearing loss are referred to as being *hard of hearing*. Those with an extensive loss of hearing are considered deaf. Generally, when hearing losses, measured by pure-tone average (PTA) or speech recognition threshold (SRT), are poorer than 80 to 90 dB Hearing Level (HL), a person is considered to be *audiometrically deaf*. However, deafness can also be described functionally as the inability to use hearing to any meaningful extent for the ordinary purposes of life, especially for verbal communication. This latter way of defining deafness is independent of the findings from audiometric test results.

The prevalence of hearing loss may be considered for all persons combined and for children and adults separately. In the United States, the prevalence of hearing loss is estimated to be from 14 million to 40 million, depending on whether conservative or liberal figures are used (Goldstein, 1984; Lin, Niparko, & Ferrucci, 2011; Schow, Mercaldo, & Smedley, 1996). These estimates vary depending on the definition of loss; the loss may be self-defined or involve different decibel fence levels, some as low as 15 dB HL, but most are higher, commonly 20 to 25 dB HL. Prevalence estimates increase to 48.1 million when individuals with a unilateral hearing loss are included (Lin et al., 2011). Authorities have suggested that a different definition of loss should be applied for children because in a younger person the consequences are greater for the same amount of loss. The prevalence of loss also varies depending on whether the conventional pure-tone average (500, 1000, 2000 Hz) is used or whether some additional upper frequencies (such as 3000 and 4000 Hz) are included. In this book, we recommend that different pure-tone average fences be used for children and adults at the "slight-to-mild" degree of loss level, although the degree designation is similar at most levels. In addition, we recommend that either 3000 or 4000 Hz be used in evaluating loss, although the usual three-frequency pure-tone average will typically be used in analyzing audiograms. Table 1.1 indicates that a hearing loss is found in children at a lower (better) decibel level than in adults; this is consistent with ASHA screening levels for schoolchildren that define normal hearing up to and including 20 dB HL (ASHA, 1997). A reasonable estimate from recent prevalence studies would be that at least 10 percent of the U.S. population has permanent, significant hearing loss. Using 10 percent as of 2017, this is approximately 32 million individuals in the United States and 737 million worldwide. Approximately one-third of 1 percent of the total

U.S. population is deaf (about 1 million). Thus, the remaining 31 million are in the hard of hearing group (Schow et al., 1996; U.S. Census Bureau, 2017). WHO uses about 5 percent and estimates that 360 million people worldwide have a disabling hearing loss, which is defined as hearing loss more severe than 40 dBHL in the better-hearing ear in adults and a hearing loss more severe than 30 dBHL in the better-hearing ear in children (WHO, 2015).

Children form a subpopulation of the total group of 32 million individuals with hearing loss. It is estimated that up to 3 million U.S. children are deaf and hard of hearing, and even more fit in this category if high-frequency and conductive losses

Audiometric Patterns of Hearing Loss Using Degree and Configuration

In rehabilitating adults, audiologists may use degree and configuration of loss to group those who are hard of hearing, thus focusing on the most common audiometric patterns. While a focus on the audiogram alone involves a simplification of the many variables discussed in this chapter, it nevertheless allows us to group persons in a useful way for treatment. One approach to hearing aid fitting proposed that nine common audiometric categories of flat, sloping, and precipitous configurations constitute the great bulk of all those who are usually fitted with hearing aids (McCandless, Sjursen, & Preeves, 2000). The data summarized here categorize loss, similar to this approach, and show a large sample of adult hearing losses (based on the better ear) involving 1200 persons. This sample shows eight exclusive groups of hearing loss: two flat (N = 286), two sloping (N = 248), two precipitous (N = 304), and two groups with loss only at 4000 Hz (N = 362). In the past, the two 4000 Hz loss groups were not often fitted with hearing aids, but this is done more often in recent times because the use of open fit hearing aids has become much more common. These eight categories constitute the bulk of hearing losses usually encountered by an average audiologist, but only six show the classic flat, sloping, or precipitous patterns that are most often amplified. For these six, when we look at the configuration (shape) of the loss between 1000 and the average of 2000 and 4000 Hz, almost equal-sized groups show a flat pattern, a sloping pattern, and a precipitous pattern (see Figure 1.1).

Flat 1 = 248*	Sloping 1 = 199*	Precipitous 1 = 250*	Total N = 838*
Flat 2 = 38*	Sloping 2 = 49*	Precipitous 2 = 54*	(*Six categories)

See Figure 1.1 and the resource website, where the reader may enter better-ear thresholds on any client for 1000, 2000, and 4000 Hz to categorize the loss into an exclusive audiometric pattern.

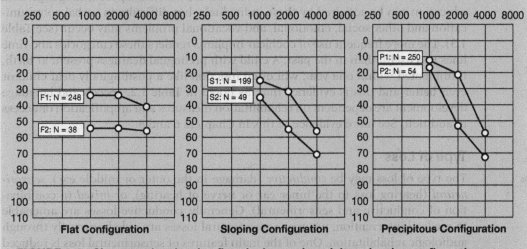

FIGURE 1.1   Six categories showing flat, sloping, and precipitous hearing configurations on 838 ears tested at health fairs.

Source: Based on Brockett and Schow (2001).

are included (Shepard, Davis, Gorga, & Stelmachowicz, 1981; see Chapter 9). Of these 3 million (2 million in school and 1 million younger), about 50,000 of school age are deaf (American Annals of the Deaf, 2005, 2011). As with children, most adults with hearing loss are considered to be hard of hearing, and only a small minority is deaf (Schow et al., 1996).

Degree (sensitivity), however, is only one of several important dimensions of a hearing loss. Even though it is often the first measure available and provides useful evidence of the impact of the loss, there are exceptions to this generalization. For example, some children with a profound loss of 90 dB HL outperform, in language and academic areas, average children who have a loss of only 70 dB HL.

Table 1.2 contains a description of deafness and hard of hearing categories in terms of typical hearing aspects, use of hearing, use of vision, language development, use of language, speech, and educational needs. Prevalence estimates are also shown.

Time of Onset

Most hard of hearing youngsters are thought to have hearing loss beginning early in life, but mild losses may not be detected, so prevalence data on young children are somewhat uncertain until school age (National Institute on Deafness and Other Communication Disorders, 2005). With youngsters who are deaf or have more severe hearing loss, the time when the loss is acquired and/or the progression of the loss will determine, in part, the extent to which normal speech and language will be present.

Severe hearing loss (deafness) may be divided into four categories (*prelingual, perilingual, postlingual, deafened*) depending on the person's age when the loss occurs (see Tables 1.2 and 1.3). *Prelingual deafness* refers to hearing loss present at birth or prior to the development of speech and language. The longer during the crucial language development years (up to age 5) that a person has normal hearing, the less chance there is that language development will be profoundly affected. This has led to a relatively new category of *perilingual deafness*, which has emerged to define the situation when deafness is acquired while developing a first language. *Postlingual deafness* means that loss occurs after about age 5; its overall effects are therefore usually less serious. However, even though language may be less affected, speech and education may be affected substantially (see Chapters 6 and 8). *Deafened* persons are those who lose hearing after their schooling is completed (i.e., sometime in their late teen years or thereafter). Normal speech, language, and education can be acquired by these individuals, but difficulty in verbal communication and other social, emotional, and vocational problems may occur (see Table 1.3). The more frequent use of cochlear implants renders these categories and time lines less useful than in the past. A child with prelingual deafness present at birth, if implanted within one year, will often function like a postlingually deaf child or even better and this is evidence that, as noted in Table 1.2, speech and language development are dependent on rehabilitation measures and amplification or access to audition. See more evidence of this in Chapters 6 and 8.

Type of Loss

The type of loss may be *conductive* (damage in the outer or middle ear), *sensorineural* (hearing loss in the inner ear or nerve of hearing), or *mixed* (a combination of conductive and sensorineural). Generally, conductive losses are amenable to medical intervention, whereas sensorineural losses are aided primarily through audiologic rehabilitation. One of the main features of sensorineural loss is reduced speech recognition. In addition, those with severe and profound sensorineural loss may obtain a cochlear implant (see Chapter 3). These three types of loss are the major ones, but there are a few other types. Functional losses have no organic basis and thresholds are often eventually found to be within normal limits. Two other

Cochlear implant recipients are increasingly avoiding the full effects from various kinds of deafness and are an exception to the general rule that sensorineural losses cannot be helped medically.

Most hearing losses are classified as conductive, sensorineural, or mixed.

TABLE 1.2 Categories and Characteristics of Hearing Loss

Characteristic	Hard of Hearing (31,000,000)[a]	CATEGORY OF DEAFNESS		
		Prelingual (115,000)[a]	Postlingual (230,000)[a]	Deafened (655,000)[a]
Hearing loss	*Sensitivity:* mild, moderate, or severe; *speech recognition:* fair to good (70–90%)	*Sensitivity:* severe or profound degree of loss; *speech recognition:* fair to poor		
Use (level) of hearing	Functional speech understanding (lead sense)	Functional speech understanding (lead sense)	Functional signal warning and environmental awareness (hearing minimized)	Functional signal warning and environmental awareness (hearing minimized)
Use of vision	Increased dependence	Increased dependence	Increased dependence	Normal
Language and speech development	Dependent on rehabilitation measures (e.g., amplification, audition via cochlear implant)	Dependent on rehabilitation and early intervention	Dependent on amplification/audition and school rehabilitation	Dependent on amplification/audition and school rehabilitation
Use of language	May be affected	Almost always affected	May be affected	Usually not affected
Use of speech	May be affected	Almost always affected	Usually affected	May be affected/dependent on audition
Educational needs	Some special education	Considerable special education	Some special education	Education complete

[a]U.S. prevalence data for these categories, based on Schow et al. (1996) and Davis (1994), incidence figures and current U.S. census (www.census.gov/popclock) accessed February 24, 2017).

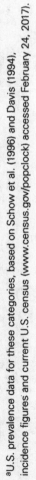

TABLE 1.3   Definitions of Hearing Loss

Persons with hearing loss have been historically divided into the following groups. In general, these are accurate, but early implantation of a cochlear implant and successful audiologic rehabilitation can alter outcomes.

Prelingually deaf persons were either born without hearing (congenitally deaf) or lost hearing before the development of speech and language: 3 to 5 years (adventitiously deaf). Both speech and language are affected to varying degrees. Some prelingually deaf persons communicate primarily through fingerspelling and signs, but others may primarily communicate via speech, particularly with early successful cochlear implantation and appropriate intervention.

Perilingual deaf persons contract deafness while acquiring a first language and may be considered a subset of prelingual.

Postlingually deaf persons are those who became profoundly deaf after the age of 5 to 10 years but had normal hearing long enough to establish fairly well developed speech and language patterns. While speech generally is affected (more for the 5- than for the 10-year-old), communication may be through speech, signs, fingerspelling, and writing. With successful early (after onset) cochlear implantation, speech may be quite understandable.

Deafened refers to those people who suffer hearing loss after completing their education, generally in their late teens or early twenties and upward. Such people usually have fairly comprehensible, nearly normal speech and language. They face problems of adjustment because of the late onset of their hearing loss. Cochlear implants are generally very effective for this group, particularly if implanted before any deprivation and subsequent neural degeneration.

Hard of hearing persons may have been born thus or subsequently experienced a partial loss of hearing. While they have acquired speech normally through hearing and communicate by speaking, speech may be affected to some extent; for example, the voice may be too soft or too loud. They understand others by speechreading, by using a hearing aid, or by asking the speaker to raise his or her voice or enunciate more distinctly.

Source: Adapted from Moores (2001) and Vernon and Andrews (1990).

forms of loss with tonal thresholds often within normal limits are *auditory processing disorders* (APD) and *hidden hearing loss*. AP disorders arise from the processing centers throughout the auditory system, while hidden hearing loss may be related to damage to the synaptic connections between the inner hair cells and cochlear nerve. In these two types of loss, the symptoms can be subtle. However, individuals may still suffer significant hearing difficulties and compromised speech perception abilities, especially in the presence of noise (Plack, Barker, & Prendergast, 2014). Treatment of these two conditions is not as well established as in purely conductive, sensorineural, and mixed losses.

Auditory Speech Recognition Ability

Auditory speech recognition or identification ability (clarity of hearing) is another important dimension of hearing loss. The terms *speech recognition*, *speech identification*, and *speech discrimination* will be used interchangeably throughout this text, and all are included under the general category of speech perception or comprehension (see Chapter 4). *Speech discrimination* has been used for many years to describe clarity of hearing as measured in typical word intelligibility tests, but *speech recognition* and *identification* have now replaced *discrimination* since they more precisely describe what is being measured. *Discrimination* technically implies only the ability involved in a same–different judgment, whereas *recognition* and *identification* indicate an ability to repeat or identify the stimulus. *Recognition* is commonly used by diagnostic audiologists, but *identification* meshes nicely with the nomenclature of audiologic rehabilitation procedures as discussed further in Chapter 4. All these terms will at times be used due to historical precedents and evolving nomenclature.

Speech recognition is typically measured by having the client repeat a list of 25 or 50 monosyllabic words and applying a percentage score for those words repeated correctly. The speech recognition ability for an individual who is hard of hearing typically is better than in a person who is deaf. In recent years, those who were deaf who have received a cochlear implant may function like a hard of hearing person. However, persons who are deaf without an implant are generally considered unable to comprehend conversational speech with hearing alone. Those who are hard of hearing can use their hearing to a significant extent for speech perception. Nevertheless, some minimal auditory recognition may be present in nonimplanted persons who are deaf even if verbal speech reception is limited since a person may use hearing for signal warning purposes or simply to maintain contact with the auditory environment (see Table 1.2). Auditory recognition ability can usually be predicted by degree of loss and also tends to get worse as the loss changes from flat to sloping to precipitous loss, but occasionally the expected relationship is not present.

In a person of advanced age, a mild degree of loss sometimes may be accompanied by very poor speech recognition. This sometimes is referred to as *phonemic regression* and is not unusual in hearing losses among elderly persons who evidence some degree of central degeneration. Disparity in degree of loss and speech recognition ability is also possible in a late cochlear implanted prelingually deaf adult where thresholds may be within normal limits but speech recognition is not achieved. In these cases, the implant augments speechreading and environmental awareness. Also in a reversed situation, a child may be considered deaf in terms of sensitivity but not in terms of auditory recognition or educational placement. Some children with a degree of loss that classifies them as audiometrically deaf (e.g., PTA = 90+ dB) may have unexpectedly good speech recognition. Thus, speech recognition also is an important variable in describing a hearing loss.

The degree of loss alone is not adequate to define whether a person is deaf or hard of hearing and to determine a rehabilitation plan. Many other factors, including time of onset and clarity of hearing (word recognition), must be considered.

CONSEQUENCES OF HEARING LOSS: PRIMARY AND SECONDARY

Communication Difficulties

The primary and most devastating effect of hearing loss is its impact on verbal (oral) communication. Children with severe to profound hearing loss who do not receive a cochlear implant do not generally develop speech and language normally because they are not exposed to the sounds of language in daily living. In a lesser degree of loss or if the loss occurs in adult years, the influence on speech and language expression tends to be less severe. Nevertheless, affected individuals still experience varying degrees of difficulty in receiving the auditory speech and environmental stimuli that allow us to communicate and interact with other humans and with our environment. For children, the choice of a communication (educational) system relates directly to this area of concern. If the educational setting and methods are chosen and implemented appropriately, according to the abilities of the child, the negative impact of the loss can be minimized. Secondary consequences and side effects of hearing loss include educational, vocational, psychological, and social implications (see Chapters 5 and 7 for a discussion of communication systems and their psychosocial implications).

Variable Hearing Disorder/Disability

A health condition, such as a hearing disorder, can be described by a classification system within WHO (2001, 2017), which standardizes terminology throughout the world. If hearing is not "functioning" normally, this is a disorder, and three dimensions are involved within this: (1) *impairment* or problems in body structure and function; (2) *activities*, in this case chiefly communication; and (3) *participation* within life situations. Besides these three dimensions, environmental and personal factors influence the disorder. This provides an excellent framework for the provision

The earlier WHO term *disability* has been changed to *activity limitation*. This refers to the primary consequence of hearing loss.

A new draft of the WHO manual is on the WHO (2017) website but is not considered final as of May, 2017. Only minor changes seem likely but the term "impairment" may be demphasized.

The earlier WHO term *handicap* has been changed to *participation restriction*. This refers to the secondary consequences of hearing loss, including restrictions in the social, emotional, educational, and vocational areas.

Disability and IQ are personal factors that influence the consequences from hearing loss.

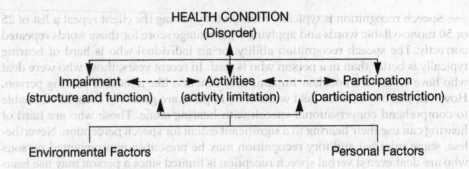

FIGURE 1.2 **Model of functioning and disability.**
Source: Adapted from WHO (2001), p. 18.

of audiologic rehabilitation, and these terms have been incorporated into the rehabilitation model discussed later in the chapter. *Activity* (especially communication) *limitations* can be thought of as the primary consequence of hearing loss, whereas *participation restrictions* involve secondary consequences of the loss that affect social, vocational, and other life situations (see Figure 1.2).

A useful method for measuring the activity limitations and participation restrictions is through self-reports of hearing, wherein persons make personal estimates about their hearing difficulties (Cox & Alexander 1995; Dillon et al., 1997; Ventry & Weinstein, 1982). This procedure has been applied with both children and adults. Both the person with hearing loss and significant others can be asked within the case history interview or may complete questionnaires independently to provide a more complete picture of the communication, psychosocial, and other effects from the loss (see Chapter 10; Schow & Smedley, 1990). Electronic versions of self-report can now be completed online and facilitate this process (Hodes, Schow, & Brockett, 2009).

In preparing to deal with the broad consequences of hearing loss, we must recognize that the impact of a hearing disorder will vary considerably depending on

When the eight categories of hearing loss are used, it is possible to develop profiles for *activity limitation* and *participation restriction* for each group using self-report. In this way, expectations for the consequences of hearing loss can be anticipated, and the measurement of rehabilitation success can be compared through the use of outcomes measures. Figure 1.3 shows the eight groupings when activity limitation and participation restriction self-report findings are compared. As can be seen, some hearing loss configuration categories, such as F2 (flat) and S2 (sloping), tend to produce more activity limitations and participation restrictions than other configuration categories (see Figure 1.1 for complete category definitions).

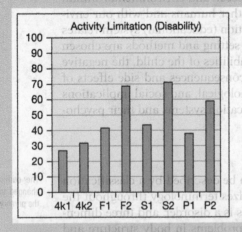
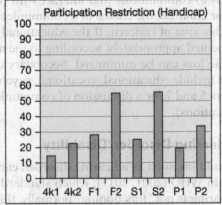

FIGURE 1.3 **Health fair self-report data.**
Source: Based on Brockett and Schow (2001).

a number of personal and environmental factors. Several of the most important personal factors were presented in Table 1.2. Although not included there, other variables are also important. For example, certain basic characteristics of the individual may have considerable impact on the primary consequences in verbal communication and the secondary effects in education, social, emotional, and vocational areas. The presence of other serious disabilities, such as blindness, physical limitations, or mental retardation, will complicate the situation. A person's native intelligence can also have a tremendous impact in conjunction with a hearing loss. Naturally, basic intelligence will vary from person to person regardless of whether he or she has hearing loss. However, Vernon (1968) reported on 50 years of research showing that, as a group, persons with hereditary deafness demonstrate a normal range of IQs as measured by performance scales. Whatever the native intellectual ability, it will influence the resultant primary and secondary consequences of hearing loss.

Environmental factors include barriers and facilitators that function within the environment that make things harder or easier for communication to occur.

REHABILITATIVE ALTERNATIVES

Little can be done to change basic, innate IQ or native abilities. Nevertheless, a number of AR procedures may have a profound effect on the personal and environmental factors relevant to hearing loss. For example, it is estimated that about 70 percent of Americans who have hearing loss are not using amplification (Abrams & Kihm, 2015; Kochkin et al., 2010). In addition, there are babies and young children who have hearing loss requiring amplification but whose losses have not been identified; schoolchildren whose aids are not in good condition; teenagers and young adults who, because of vanity or unfortunate experiences with hearing aids, are not getting the necessary help; adults and elderly individuals who have not acquired hearing aids because of pride or misinformation; and others whose instruments are not properly fitted or oriented to regular hearing aid use. Adults also have been found to be using many poorly functioning hearing aids (Schow, Maxwell, Crookston, & Newman, 1993). All of these cases represent a need for audiologic rehabilitation. Identifying those who need amplification, persuading them to obtain and use hearing aids or cochlear implants, adjusting them for maximum benefit, and orienting the new user to the instruments are all tasks in the province of AR that may reduce the negative effects of a hearing loss.

Audiologic rehabilitation also includes efforts to improve communication, as well as addressing a variety of other concerns for the person with hearing loss. Before discussing procedures and the current status of audiologic rehabilitation, however, a brief review of the history of AR is in order.

Historical Background

Although audiologic rehabilitative procedures are common today, they have not always been utilized for individuals with hearing loss. For centuries, it was assumed that prelingual deafness and the resultant language development delay and inability to learn were inevitable aspects of the hearing loss. The deaf were thought to be retarded, so for many years, no efforts were made to try to teach them. The first known teacher of persons with severe to profound hearing loss was Pedro Ponce de León of Spain, who in the mid- to late 1500s demonstrated that persons who are deaf can be taught to speak and are capable of learning. Other teachers, including Bonet and de Carrion in Spain and Bulwer in England, were active in the 1600s, and their methods gained some prominence. During the 1700s, Pereira (Pereire) introduced education of the deaf to France, and the Abbé de L'Epée founded a school there. Schools were also established by Thomas Braidwood in Great Britain and by Heinicke in Germany. De L'Epée employed fingerspelling and sign language in addition to speechreading, whereas Heinicke and Braidwood stressed oral speech.

Approximately 70 percent of Americans who have hearing loss are not using hearing aids.

Beginning in 1813, John Braidwood, a grandson of Thomas Braidwood, tried to establish this oral method in the United States, but he was unsuccessful because of his own ineptness and poor health. Thomas Gallaudet went to England in 1815 to learn the Braidwood oral method but was refused help because it was feared that he would interfere with John Braidwood's efforts. Consequently, Gallaudet learned de L'Epée's manual method in Paris through contact with Sicard and Laurent Clerc. He returned to the United States and opened his own successful school. (See additional details in Moores, 2001.)

The manual approach to teaching persons who were deaf remained the major force in the United States until the mid-1800s, when speechreading and oral methods were promoted and popularized by Horace Mann, Alexander Graham Bell, and others. The stress on the use of residual hearing had been suggested earlier, but it began to receive strong emphasis with the oral methods used during the 1700s and 1800s. Until electric amplification was developed in the early 1900s, the use of residual hearing required ear trumpets and *ad concham* (speaking directly in the ear) stimulation. More vigorous efforts in the use of residual hearing followed the introduction of electronic hearing aids in the 1920s (Berger, 1988).

Also in the early 1900s, between 1900 and 1930, several schools of lipreading were started and became quite prominent. Although these institutions were directed principally toward teaching adults with hearing loss how to speechread, considerable public recognition also was gained for this method of rehabilitating those with hearing loss. (*Speechreading* and *lipreading* will be used interchangeably in this text, although *speechreading* is the more technically accurate term; see Chapter 5 for details.)

Birth of Audiology.   During World War II, the need to rehabilitate servicemen with hearing loss resulted in the birth of the audiology profession. The cumulative effect of electronic amplification developments, adult lipreading courses, and the World War II hearing rehabilitation efforts gradually led to the recognition of audiologic rehabilitation as separate from education for persons who are deaf. Eventually, audiologists and speech-language pathologists were recognized as the professionals responsible for providing such services to adults, and soon it was also realized that these professionals could provide crucial help to youngsters who are deaf or hard of hearing.

In the military rehabilitation centers, a number of methods were developed to help those with hearing loss, including procedures for selecting hearing aids. Hearing aid orientation methods requiring up to three months of course work were developed. Considerable emphasis was also placed on speechreading and auditory training.

In the late 1940s and 1950s, as audiology moved into the private sector, the approach to hearing aids changed. Whereas hearing aids were freely dispensed in government facilities, in civilian life people bought amplification exclusively from hearing aid dealers. Methods evolved wherein audiologists would perform tests and recommend hearing aids but dealers would sell and service the instruments. Through the 1960s, audiologists thus had a limited role in hearing aid–related rehabilitation services, but starting in the 1970s, audiologists gradually became more involved in direct dispensing of hearing aids and currently provide about 74 percent of the direct service to hearing aid clients (Stika & Ross, 2011).

Infants.   Beginning in the 1960s, many audiologists recognized the need for early identification of hearing loss so that management could be initiated during the critical language development years. The incidence of hearing loss in newborns is about 3 per 1000 children (Centers for Disease Control and Prevention, 2010), a higher prevalence than for other disabilities screened routinely in the newborn. Efforts on many fronts, including advancements in screening and diagnostics and an emphasis on providing appropriate education for families and intervention for children identified with hearing loss, have resulted in the establishment of early hearing detection and intervention (EHDI) programs in all 50 states (White, 2014). With goals beyond the first steps of screening and identification, EHDI professionals work with

The name *audiology* was first used to describe this new profession in 1946. Raymond Carhart, who pioneered in the audiologic rehabilitation of World War II servicemen, not only helped name audiology but also started the first training program at Northwestern University in 1947.

families and children to help provide access to the most appropriate means and modes of communication so that the development of language can occur. Different communication options typically include either a manual-visual system (e.g., sign language) or an auditory-verbal/oral approach, often categorized as listening and spoken language therapy (Alberg, Wilson, & Roush, 2006) (see Chapter 6 for more information about these different communication options). Cochlear implantation, which began in the 1970s, was expanded in the 1980s for use in young children who are deaf, thus providing another important avenue for management of communication strategies in these youngsters (see Chapter 3). While challenges with screening and intervention still exists, such as a shortage of pediatric audiologists and early intervention specialists, great strides are being made to meet the goals of detection, diagnosis, and intervention before 6 months of age (see Chapter 6 for more details).

Children. School-age youngsters with hearing loss were also found to be in need of assistance. Many hard of hearing children are educated in the regular schools, and several studies since the 1960s have indicated that these children are not receiving the specialized support that they need. Even more recent reports indicate that these children are still falling behind, needing special education services or being underserved (Blair, Peterson, & Viehweg, 1985; Downs, Whitaker, & Schow, 2003; English & Church, 1999; Madell & Flexer, 2014). For example, Downs et al. (2003) found that in Idaho, there were only seven school districts with the services of audiologists. These districts identified and followed five times as many children with hearing loss as compared to seven similar-sized districts without an audiologist. The audiologist-served districts had 2.5 times more hearing aid users and 2.8 times more assistive device users. Unfortunately, only one-quarter of the children in the state were in districts with audiologists. Thus, rehabilitation for school-age youngsters is a priority, but there is an acute need for more educational audiologists or highly trained audiologic rehabilitation specialists and speech-language pathologists to serve this population.

Adults. Among adults, the needs for hearing rehabilitation are also apparent. Ries's (1994) data revealed that hearing problems are reported by 4 percent of the population from 25 to 34 years of age. This figure rises dramatically with age so that of those 75 years and older, 38 percent of the population report problems. In addition, Kochkin et al. (2010) estimate that there are now more than 8 million hearing aid users in this country, but most of those with hearing loss still do not own hearing

The incidence of hearing loss in newborns is approximately 3 per 1000.

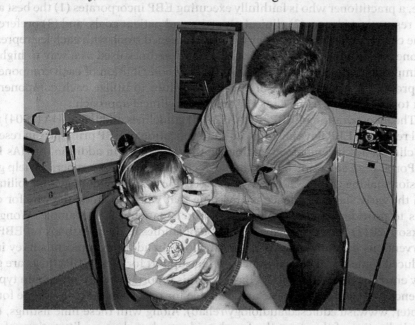

Basic screening is necessary to identify hard of hearing children. Unfortunately, many hard of hearing children are not receiving AR.

aids. Also, about one-fourth of the aids being used by adults have been shown to be in poor working condition (Schow et al., 1993).

Contemporary Issues

Professional Issues. Audiologists and speech-language pathologists now are widely recognized for the part they play in audiologic rehabilitation, which occurs through early intervention and the provision of services in schools and in adult and geriatric settings. The expanded role in rehabilitation for audiologists in particular has been encouraged within the three major national associations mentioned earlier in the chapter (ASHA, AAA, and ARA). Until 1979, ASHA's Code of Ethics prevented member audiologists from dispensing hearing aids, but after that, ASHA encouraged more audiology involvement. There are now a series of policy statements on rehabilitative audiology issued by special subcommittees that fully recognize the role of audiology (ASHA, 1997, 2001, 2006). Similar supportive statements on rehabilitation issues have emerged from another major professional organization for audiologists, the American Academy of Audiology (AAA, 1993, 2003, 2006), as well as the Joint Committee on Infant Hearing (2000). Other professional organizations also promote rehabilitation, including ARA, the Educational Audiology Association, the National Hearing Conservation Association, and the Military Audiology Association. In addition, the Americans with Disabilities Act (ADA) created an increased awareness of the need for hearing services (ADA, 1990). The text website (www.isu.edu/csed/audiology/rehab) can be accessed to study the previously mentioned documents and to locate other documents on professional issues, such as evidence-based practice, multicultural issues, and codes of ethics from ASHA and AAA.

Evidence-Based Practice. A trend in the health care arena—and in hearing rehabilitation as well—is the emphasis on evidence-based practice (EBP). For the beginning student, a thorough understanding of EBP can be challenging, so we have chosen in this introductory text to provide a brief description with the expectation that advanced courses will provide more complete coverage of this topic.

EBP simply means that in clinical practice, the methods chosen should be based on original research that measures treatment success on patients in the real world (Cox, 2005). More specifically, taken from the realms of evidence-based medicine, a practitioner who is faithfully executing EBP incorporates (1) the best available research evidence, (2) clinical expertise and patient goals, and (3) preferences in the care of patients. The imagery of a three-legged stool, with each leg representing one of the three components of EBP, is sometimes used as a way to highlight the importance of each component. While the contribution of each component is not proportional for all clinical questions, failure to utilize each component, at least to some degree, makes for an "unsteady" clinical approach.

The incorporation of EBP in AAA (2003) guidelines and the ASHA (2004) technical report on EBP have encouraged the application of EBP principles in research and clinical advancements in audiologic rehabilitation. In addition, ASHA's Practice Portal is an emerging tool available to clinicians and researchers to help guide decision making (ASHA, 2016). While a focus on EBP in audiologic rehabilitation is in the early stages, evidence is emerging that will help guide the way for clinicians to provide services and support to their patients. For example, Wong and Hickson (2012) have provided a collection of studies in their textbook on EBP and interventions for individuals with hearing loss. In addition, a recent survey in AR produced some evidence that indicates that support for these EBP efforts are gradually emerging (Johnson, 2012). Based on this report, there are nine main types of evidence we have in AR. (These are available for review on the text website for this chapter; www.isu.edu/csed/audiology/rehab). Along with these nine listings, there is an indication of the strength of such evidence, based on quality ratings of A, B, C, D, or I to VI quality rating (quality A or I is best).

Important professional organizations, such as ASHA and AAA, have provided guidelines and ethical codes in AR.

ADA, the Americans with Disabilities Act, has increased awareness and services in AR.

These EBP findings suggest most of the current evidence is associated with hearing aid–fitting issues, and most of this evidence is only at a B or II level. Also, most of this evidence, in fact, supports the conventional wisdom of past decades and the methods you will find in this text. It appears that considerably more will need to be done before we have EBP information uniformly at an A or I level. For those interested in a more in-depth treatment of EBP as applied to AR, the coverage by Johnson (2012) would be helpful.

Additional work by clinicians and academic clinical researchers will gradually help us refine clinical methods so that the procedures we are using and the methods found in texts will have efficacy (meaning positive outcomes in laboratory settings), effectiveness (meaning positive outcomes in the real world), and efficiency (meaning that some outcomes are better compared to competing methods). Issues of patient safety and cost-effectiveness also are subjects of EBP. At present, we can continue to use the best methods we have, including the methods described in this text but with an eye to always improving our efforts by attention to EBP.

EBP, evidence-based practice, involves using research to select the very best proven methods in AR.

Multicultural Issues. We live in a world of many different cultures and differences, including ethnicity, race, age, gender, sexual orientation, class, and religion. This simply means that there are a number of different subgroups that share a common characteristic. There are five common racial groups in the United States—White, Black/African American, Asian, American Indian/Alaska Native, or Native Hawaiian/Pacific Islander. Latinos or Hispanics may be of any race (U.S. Census Bureau, 2010). The largest minority group in the United States is Hispanic/Latino at 16 percent, followed by Black/African Americans at 13 percent and Asian Americans at 5 percent of the population. In the future, almost half of the U.S. population is expected to have linguistically and culturally diverse backgrounds. So there will eventually be a large portion of persons with communication disorders who may have limited proficiency with the dominant language or where some language besides English is spoken in their homes (U.S. Census Bureau, 2010). This helps to explain why the presence of discrimination, stereotyping, or prejudice can have an impact on the provision of our services. Prejudice is when we judge someone negatively without cause or rationale. It can be based on family or personal bias or stereotyping (simplistically defining a group). Racism, ageism, and sexism are all examples of prejudice. If we treat clients differently because of prejudice, this is considered discrimination. Our national associations have recommended that we avoid discrimination by recognizing that *every* client comes from a distinct culture influenced by gender, age, race, and the other cultural factors. In all our clinical interactions from the initial interview to our examinations, treatments, referrals, and recommendations, we should seek to avoid prejudice and discrimination. When this is achieved, we say that the clinician has attained cross-cultural competence. Such sensitivity requires a willingness to learn about and try to understand others who are different than we are. One particularly sensitive issue for someone in auditory rehabilitation is the need to acquire cultural sensitivity to the Deaf community where sometimes those in the communication sciences are seen as wanting (by devices such as cochlear implants) to eliminate Deaf culture.

Multicultural sensitivity and cross-cultural competence are needed in AR to avoid prejudice and discrimination toward our clients.

Current Status

A high percentage of audiologists are currently participating in rehabilitation activities related to hearing devices. The ASHA (2014) clinical focus practice patterns report shows that 76 percent of audiologists are involved in hearing aid dispensing, 80 percent provide fitting and orientation with assistive technology, and 87 percent counsel clients in communication strategies and realistic expectations. Smaller percentages are involved with cochlear implants (8%) and speechreading (6%). While these findings suggest a big change from the 1960s, there continues to be little change since the beginning of the past decade when Millington (2001) found that 79 percent

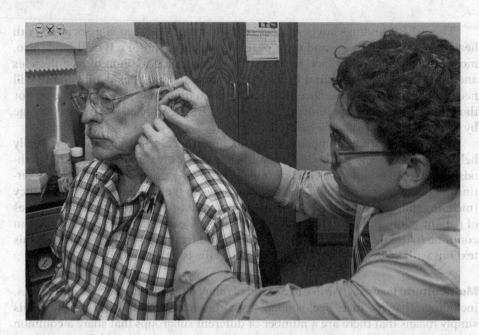

A major aspect of AR involves ensuring that hearing aids are working properly for the patient.

of ASHA audiologists were involved in direct dispensing of hearing aids, 81 percent were involved in hearing instrument orientation and rehabilitation counseling, and 12 to 23 percent reported being involved in speechreading and auditory training.

Despite these continuing patterns, during the past decade we have seen the emergence of several interesting and important new developments in audiologic rehabilitation. Perhaps the most important of these has been the technological advancement of feedback control in hearing aids, which has allowed for the use of more open-fit hearing aids (see Chapter 2). This has resulted in more persons with high-frequency losses being satisfactorily fitted than in the past and a major trend away from in-the-ear fittings to behind-the-ear fittings. This (and other reasons) has contributed to the use rate for hearing aids changing from 20 to 25 percent in the 2010 MarkeTrak VIII Survey (Kochkin et al., 2011) and now moving from 25 to 30 percent in the most recent survey (MarkeTrak IX) and even to 40 percent for individuals age 65 and above (Abrams & Kihm, 2015). In addition, cochlear implants, which have been around for several decades, have become more and more refined and effective. Furthermore, early identification of hearing loss at birth is so widespread throughout the United States that most deaf youngsters who are candidates for these implants are receiving them in many cases by 1 year of age. With proper parental and professional attention, these children are functioning now more like they are hard of hearing than deaf (see Chapters 6 and 9). Cochlear implants thus are now a major focus in audiologic rehabilitation for children and adults (see Chapter 3). Advances in phone and Internet technology also have led to interesting developments. For example, it is possible to obtain a phone application that allows an individual to self-screen hearing and, if failed, to immediately call a local hearing aid dispenser to arrange an appointment (see Chapter 10). Another computer software development is a 10-hour program called Listening and Communication Enhancement (LACE), which allows for the new hearing aid user to practice listening skills and thus improve the benefit received from the hearing aid. Other computer-based training programs, such as HearBuilder and LISN & Learn, are additional therapeutic approaches aimed at improving the individual's auditory capabilities. Additionally, new advances in outcome measures mean that it is now possible to measure hearing aid use time with a data tracker right within the hearing aid, to measure satisfaction and benefit via refined self-report tools, and to also measure benefit via real ear measures and other audiologic tests (see Chapter 10).

Technological advancements in hearing aids have helped the adult take-up rate increase from 20 to 30 percent.

Advances in phone and Internet technology are encouraging, but AR professionals need to apply our proven methods more consistently.

The progress in AR is very encouraging, as evident in the last two MarkeTrak surveys in terms of improved hearing aid use rate and technology. Further, the MarkeTrak findings have implications that support AR in that the use of hearing aids improves quality of life for users regularly (48%) or occasionally (40%). MarkeTrak IX findings show that users of hearing aids purchased in the past year had a 91 percent satisfaction rating, while users of hearing aids that were 6 or more years old had only a 74 percent satisfaction level. This goes along with the report from 51 percent of repeat users who consider their new aids to be "much better" than their first hearing aids. Hearing conversation in noise is the most difficult listening situation reported, but hearing aids reportedly allow their users to be 67 percent satisfied in this situation compared to 25 percent of nonusers with hearing loss. While satisfaction thus seems to be improved when hearing aids are used in noise and also because of better technology, in MarkeTrak VIII it was found that satisfaction is dependent on the level of AR implementation. Data from Kochkin et al. (2010) reinforce the need for everyone involved in hearing-related professional work to learn the methods found in this text and to apply them consistently. The Kochkin et al. study found that when we examine carefully those fitted with hearing aids and compare the most successfully fitted to the least successfully fitted, there are a few proven methods within the fitting protocol that will most influence success.

Mark Ross (2011), a longtime hearing aid user and audiologist, made a plea that we take the lessons from the Kochkin et al. research and redouble our efforts to strictly use the methods that have proven to be effective in audiologic rehabilitation. As Dr. Ross stated, "*Those people who are administered five of the specific tests in the protocol are much more likely to be satisfied users of hearing aids than those people who did not receive them.*" These five are listed in order of the largest to smallest differences between the successful users who received them and the unsuccessful users who did not receive them:

- Audiologic benefit measurement
- Self-report benefit measurement
- Loudness discomfort measures
- Real-ear (probe-tube microphone) measures
- Patient satisfaction measurement

Based on the Kochkin et al. study, it appears that fewer than 70 percent of the respondents recall receiving audiologic benefit and loudness discomfort tests; only about 40 percent of these clients received real-ear measures, and self-report benefit and satisfaction measures were obtained on only 20 percent. The implication of these findings is that the methods you will learn about in the chapters that follow have been proven effective. We urge you to learn and then use these methods consistently so that over time the take-up rate for hearing aids will improve even more and those with hearing loss will receive the assistance they need.

PROCEDURES IN AUDIOLOGIC REHABILITATION: AN AR MODEL—CORE AND CARE

This section describes important procedures and elements of audiologic rehabilitation in order to provide a framework for the remainder of this text.

The audiologic rehabilitation model used here emerged in 1980 when the first edition of this text appeared. It has been slightly revised with new editions of the text, based on the work of Goldstein and Stephens (1981) and other trends in audiology up to the present time (Stephens, 1996; Stephens & Kramer, 2010). In its current form, it is in harmony with the WHO (2001, 2017) International Classification of Functioning, Disability and Health. The model is intended to encompass all types and degrees of hearing loss as well as all age-groups.

Entry and discharge are considered peripheral to the central aspects of the model. The model consists of two major components: assessment and management. Each component has four divisions and associated subsections. The model is shown in Table 1.4 and Figure 1.4.

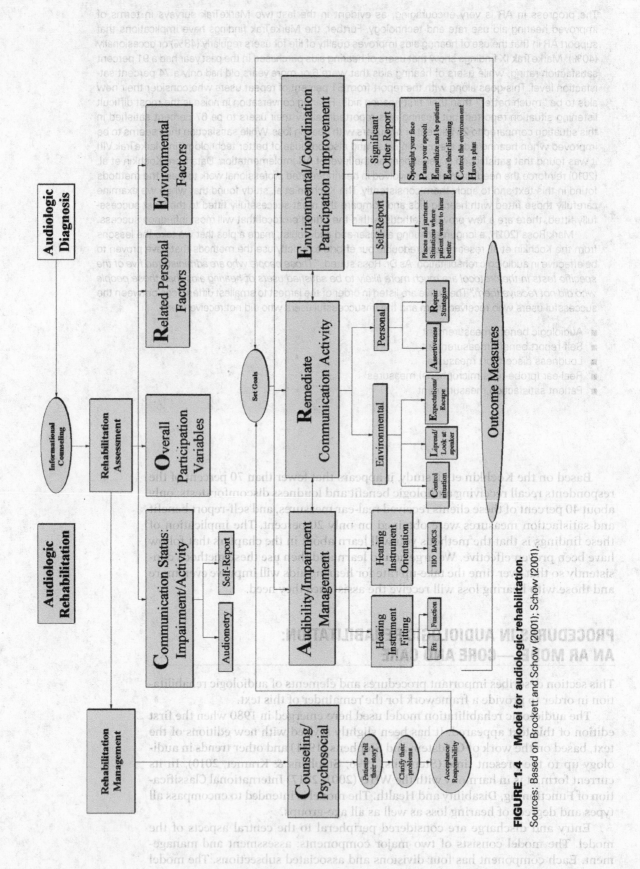

FIGURE 1.4 Model for audiologic rehabilitation.

Sources: Based on Brockett and Schow (2001); Schow (2001).

TABLE 1.4   Audiologic Rehabilitation Model Used in This Text

(Enter Through Diagnostic–Identification Process)

Assessment (CORE)	**C**ommunication status: Hearing loss and activity limitations	Auditory Visual Language Manual Communication self-report Previous rehabilitation Overall
	Overall participation variables	Psychological (emotional) Social Vocational Educational
	Related personal factors	Attitude types I, II, III, IV Personality IQ Age Race Gender
	Environmental factors	Services Systems Barriers Facilitators Acoustic conditions
Management (CARE)	**C**ounseling and psychosocial (modifying personal attitude)	Interpretation Information Counseling and guidance Acceptance Understanding Expectations and goals
	Audibility and amplification	Hearing aid fitting Cochlear implants Assistive devices Assistive listening Alerting and warning Tactile Communication Instruction and orientation
	Remediate communication activities	Tactics to control situation Philosophy based on realistic expectations Personal skill-building
	Environmental/coordination/participation improvement	Situation improvement Vocational Educational Social Communication partner Community context

(Discharge)

Note: This model is based on Goldstein and Stephens (1981), Stephens (1996), and the WHO (2001) terminology.

The CORE assessment issues help audiologists consider relevant factors that should be evaluated before treatment starts.

Rehabilitation Assessment Procedures

Following the initial auditory diagnostic tests that indicate the need for audiologic rehabilitation, it is necessary to perform more in-depth work-ups to determine the feasibility of various forms of audiologic rehabilitation. These assessment procedures should focus on **C**ommunication status, **O**verall participation variables, **R**elated personal factors, and **E**nvironmental factors (which are collectively abbreviated as CORE).

Communication Status. Within the area of *communication* status, which includes hearing loss and activity, both traditional audiometric tests and questionnaires may be used to assess auditory abilities and self-reported consequences of hearing loss. Visual abilities assessment should include a simple screening and measurement of speechreading abilities. Any evaluation of communication must also consider language because it is at the heart of verbal communication. If the patient understands a manual–gesture system, this needs to be evaluated, as does any prior treatment. Included in *overall communication* are combined sensory abilities, such as audiovisual and tactile–kinesthetic capacities. Both expressive and receptive communication skills should be considered.

Overall Participation Variables. Included in this area are participation aspects of hearing loss, including psychological, social, vocational, and educational factors. Social factors such as family and significant others, social class, and lifestyle are to be considered, according to the Goldstein and Stephens model. The vocational domain includes position, responsibility, and competence. In addition, the patient's level and form of education must be considered.

Related Personal Factors. These include the person's attitude, which is considered a crucial aspect of rehabilitation. Goldstein and Stephens (1981) suggested that rehabilitation candidates can be categorized into four types according to attitude. Type I candidates have a strongly positive attitude toward management and are thought to make up two-thirds to three-quarters of all patients. Most of the remaining candidates fit into Type II: Their expectations are essentially positive, but slight complications are present, such as hearing loss which is more challenging to fit with amplification. (Stephens and Kramer [2010] report that 90% of candidates have attitudes Type I or Type II). Persons with Type III attitudes are negative about rehabilitation but show some willingness to cooperate, and those in Type IV reject hearing aids and the rehabilitation process altogether. In the latter two categories, management cannot proceed in the usual fashion until some modification of attitude is achieved. (We consider it important to evaluate attitude prior to rehabilitation.) In the WHO (2001) system, personal factors listed also include age, race, gender, education, personality and character style, aptitude, other health conditions, fitness, lifestyle, habits, upbringing, coping styles (assertiveness), social background, profession, and past and current experiences.

Environmental Factors. These include individual aspects, services, and systems. The individual issues include the physical features of the environment as well as direct personal contacts. The services include social structures and services in the work environment, socially, communication-wise, and transportation-wise. Systems refer to laws, regulations, and rules, both formal and informal. Finally, the acoustic environmental conditions confronted by the person with hearing loss should be evaluated.

Management Procedures

CARE defines a management approach that includes four critical components of AR.

Once a thorough rehabilitation-oriented assessment has been completed, management efforts should be initiated. These may take the form of short- or long-term therapy and may involve individual or group sessions. The four aspects of management included here are those detailed in the previous editions of this book. They are also prominently featured in the Goldstein and Stephens model as well as in the WHO (2001) terminology. These include (1) **C**ounseling and psychosocial aspects, (2) **A**udibility or amplification aspects, (3) **R**emediation of communication activities, and (4) **E**nvironmental coordination/participation improvement (abbreviated as CARE).

Although all four management components are listed sequentially, they may occur simultaneously or in a duplicative and interactive fashion. For example, information about communication is generally introduced early in the counseling phase. However, additional information on how we hear, basics of speech acoustics, visible dimensions of speech, and how to maximize the use of conversational cues may be further emphasized later in the remediation of communication.

Counseling/Psychosocial. Counseling/psychosocial includes interpretation of audiologic findings to the client and other significant persons. In addition, pertinent information, counseling, and guidance are needed to help these individuals understand the educational, vocational, psychosocial, and communicative effects of hearing loss. Considerable understanding and support are necessary in dealing with children who are deaf and hard of hearing, their parents, adults of all ages with hearing loss, and their families. If the clinician is a good listener, in this process he or she will allow the clients to "tell their own story," and this will in turn help clients to clarify their problems, accept responsibility, and set appropriate goals. This process should bring acceptance and understanding of the conditions along with appropriate expectations for management. It is at this stage that good-attitude (Types I and II) patients must set goals to improve audibility with amplification, whereas clients with poor attitudes (Types III and IV), if not modified toward acceptance and understanding, may not be ready and will resist this type of goal.

Audibility Improvement Using Amplification and Other Devices

Amplification fitting. This phase is sometimes referred to as *Hearing Aid Evaluation,* but it needs to be broader in scope. Here we must consider all forms of amplification or audition, not just hearing aids. For example, cochlear implants, signal warning devices, and other assistive devices, such as telephone amplifiers, should be considered in this phase. In many cases, accurate fitting of these devices will go a considerable way toward resolution of the hearing problem. In most cases, the fitting of hearing devices should be followed by adjustment, modification, and alteration of the basic controls and coupler arrangement until satisfactory amplification is achieved. Effort should be made to ensure that no other amplification or audibility arrangements are substantially superior to the ones being used.

Hearing Instrument Orientation (HIO BASICS). Individuals need to learn about the purpose, function, and maintenance of hearing aids and other assistive devices used by themselves or their child or other family member to avoid misunderstanding and misuse. Amplification units are relatively complex, and this instruction must be given more emphasis than a five-minute explanation or a pamphlet.

Hearing instrument orientation (HIO), as defined throughout this text, includes basic instruction that should be given to help new hearing aid users. HIO basics are listed in detail in Chapter 2.

Remediate Communication Activity. The major impact of hearing loss lies in the area of communication activity. Communication deficits often manifest themselves in educational difficulties for children and in vocational difficulties for adults. In most cases, amplification is considered the most important tool in combating this problem, but some basic communication training and related strategies are recommended for all new amplification users. These involve both environmental and personal adjustments and may provide the basis for more extensive therapy if the client selects goals in this area.

Clear speech is an important communication strategy, as noted in Chapter 4.

Although a basic overview on communication issues is adequate in most cases of hearing aid fitting, cochlear implants require more extensive skill building wherein the patient learns methods to facilitate communication in conjunction with this new device. Speechreading and improvement of auditory listening strategies are included here, as are related speech and language rehabilitation efforts. Specific communication skills are identified in this phase of therapy, and then, through such things as assertiveness training and incorporation of anticipatory and repair strategies, clients may learn to cope better with communication challenges.

Environmental Coordination: Participation Improvement. Self-reports provide a useful method to help clients select a few situations (places and partners) wherein they would like to improve their hearing and communicating. With the therapist, they can identify strategies for improvement. Pre– and post–self-report measures can help determine the success of these efforts. Also, in this phase of treatment we include coordination with other sources of help. Disability is not an individual attribute but rather a collection of conditions, and many of these are created by the social and physical environment. It is a collective responsibility for all elements of society to help make necessary modifications. Although referrals in all areas are not usually necessary, they should be considered. Liaison among client, family, and other agencies is included, as are reassessment and modification of the intervention program.

Coordination and teamwork are useful concepts in audiologic rehabilitation. Particularly in the case of the youngster with hearing loss, many persons may work with or need to work with the child. The parents should be at the center of the rehabilitative process. Also, physicians, social workers, hearing aid dispensers, teachers, school psychologists, and other school personnel need to be coordinated to assist the child and family. For adults, much depends on the particular setting in which the rehabilitation occurs. Sometimes, physicians, psychologists, or social workers function in the same clinical setting. In these cases, involvement of another professional may occur naturally and easily. In other situations, the AR therapist can make referrals, when indicated, and encourage the adult to follow up. Sometimes, persons are resistant to obtaining medical care or seeing a rehabilitation counselor. Often, parents or adults resist social services, psychiatric assistance, or hearing aid devices. When a client refuses to accept advice, the audiologist must provide whatever insight and help possible, based on the audiologist's background and training, but must respect the rights of the client or the parents. Nevertheless, the audiologic rehabilitation process demands that referrals be made when indicated, and overall coordination within the relevant context is an important dimension that should not be neglected.

Additional clarification and details on this AR model can be found in Goldstein and Stephens (1981) and WHO (2001). A similar but slightly different approach can be seen in Stephens and Kramer (2010) and may provide additional insights for the interested clinician.

SETTINGS FOR AUDIOLOGIC REHABILITATION

Audiologic rehabilitation may be conducted in a variety of settings with children, adults, or the elderly who are either deaf or hard of hearing. A review of these settings may help to demonstrate the many applications of AR (see Table 1.5).

Children

Very young children with hearing loss and their parents may be recipients of early intervention efforts through home visits or clinic programs. Parent groups are also an important rehabilitation option. As children enter preschool and other school settings, audiologic rehabilitation takes on a supportive, coordinative function with

Self-report outcome measures have become a key element to help measure the communication improvement results of AR for different environments and situations (places and partners).

TABLE 1.5   Summary of Audiologic Rehabilitation Settings for Children, Adults, and Elderly Persons

Children	Adults	Elderly Adults
Early intervention	University and technical schools	(Most settings listed under Adults)
Preschool	Vocational rehabilitation	Community programs
Parent groups	Military-related facilities	Nursing homes and long-term care facilities
Regular classrooms	Ear, nose, and throat clinic–private practice	
School conservation program follow-up	Community, hospital, and university hearing clinics	
School resource rooms	Hearing instrument specialists and dispensers	
Residential school classrooms		

teachers of youngsters with hearing loss managing the classroom learning. Specifically, children in resource rooms, in residential deaf school classrooms, and in regular classrooms can be helped with amplification (both group and individual), communication therapy, and academic subjects. Important help and insights can also be given to the child's parents and teachers, and other professionals may be involved as needed. Hearing conservation follow-up for youngsters who fail traditional school screenings represents another type of rehabilitative work carried out with children.

Adults

Adult AR services are needed for individuals with long-standing hearing loss as well as for persons who acquire loss during adulthood. Such traumatic or progressive hearing disorders may be brought on by accident, heredity, disease, or noise.

Adults may be served in university or technical school settings, through vocational rehabilitation programs, in military-related facilities, in the office of an ear specialist, or in the private practice of an audiologist. In addition, many adults are served in community, hospital, or university hearing clinics or through hearing instrument specialists (previously referred to as hearing aid dealers). A variety of rehabilitative services may be provided in all these settings.

Elderly Adults

The vast majority of elderly clients are served through the conventional programs previously described for adults. A substantial proportion of clients seen in these settings for hearing aid evaluations and related services are 65 years of age or older.

The full array of hearing aid and communication rehabilitation services may be provided for the elderly in these clinics, including hearing aid evaluation, orientation, and group and individual therapy. Aside from conventional clinical service, rehabilitation may be provided to the elderly in community screening and rehabilitation programs in well-elderly clinics, retirement apartment houses, senior citizen centers, churches, and a variety of other places where senior citizens congregate. Nursing homes or long-term care facilities also provide opportunities for audiologic rehabilitation since so many residents in these settings have substantial hearing loss and are required to have hearing screening under Medicare law (Bebout, 1991). Nevertheless, rehabilitation personnel should be realistic and anticipate less

Elderly adults not served in traditional adult settings may receive AR services in community programs and long-term care facilities.

than 100 percent success with the elderly who are residents in health care facilities (Schow, 1992). Audiologic rehabilitation will be better accepted if it can be applied before persons enter such a facility.

Summary

Audiologic habilitation and rehabilitation involve a variety of assessment and management efforts for the person who is deaf or hard of hearing, coordinated by a professional with AR training. Audiologists and speech pathologists are the professionals at the center of these efforts, even though other professionals can and do play a significant supportive role. Recent developments in the past decade have been fostered by technological advances, such as open-fit hearing aids and cochlear implants, along with improved methods of outcome measurement and Internet software innovations. However, these new devices and methods must be used consistently if those with hearing loss are to be well served.

A model of rehabilitation has been presented here to provide a framework for assessment and management procedures in audiologic rehabilitation as described in the remaining chapters of this book. Professionals who intend to engage in AR must be familiar with the characteristics of hearing loss reviewed in this chapter if they are to perform effective rehabilitation.

Summary Points

- Audiologic rehabilitation (AR) is defined as those professional processes performed in collaboration with a client who has hearing loss and the client's significant others to achieve better communication and minimize the resulting difficulties. It does not include closely related medical intervention or the teaching of academics to the deaf.

- Audiologists are the chief providers of AR, but speech pathologists and teachers of the deaf also do a great deal of this work. In addition, other professionals, such as social workers and rehabilitation counselors, may provide key rehabilitative assistance to those with hearing loss.

- AR providers need some background in diagnostic audiology, and they need an understanding of hearing loss and its effect on both children and adults.

- Hearing loss can be defined in terms of degree of loss, time of onset, type of loss, and word recognition ability. Those with milder forms of hearing loss are called hard of hearing; those with extensive hearing loss who cannot use hearing for the ordinary purposes of life are considered deaf.

- The deaf may be divided into four groups: the prelingually deaf, who are born deaf or acquire it in the first five years of life; the perilingually deaf, who acquire deafness while acquiring a first language; the postlingually deaf, who acquire hearing loss after age 5 through the school years; and the deafened, who acquire hearing loss after their education is completed.

- The most serious and primary consequence of hearing loss is the effect on verbal (oral) communication, referred to as disability. The secondary consequences of hearing loss may be referred to as a handicap and includes social, emotional, educational, and vocational issues. WHO now suggests that communication *activity limitation* be used instead of *disability* and that we speak of *participation restriction* instead of *handicap*. In connection with these new terms, WHO also suggests that personal factors and environmental factors are key issues in the provision of AR hearing services. These terms and factors help us properly understand the consequences of hearing loss and provide the basis for a model of AR.

- Both children and adults are underserved, and many more should receive AR help. Only 30 percent of those who could be using hearing aids obtain them. Even those who have hearing aids can often be shown how to get more effective help from amplification and can benefit from other services to assist them in their communication breakdowns.

- The early history of AR is essentially the history of efforts to help the deaf, beginning in the 1500s. Audiology came into being as a profession in the mid-1940s in connection with World War II, and both audiologic diagnosis and AR are considered key elements within this profession.

- Beginning in the 1970s, audiologists became more involved in hearing aid fitting and in cochlear implants, and in the following decades until 2000, new developments, such as major advancements in cochlear implants and assistive listening devices, emerged to revolutionize audiologic rehabilitation. More recently, the increased use of open-fit hearing aids and software and Internet technology, along with improved outcome measures, have led to even more exciting advances in AR.

- Perhaps the most exciting aspect of audiologic rehabilitation is that beginning in the 1980s, a major portion of those who are born deaf are now acquiring cochlear implants and growing up with vastly improved, near normal language development.

- The model for AR includes assessment and management; rehabilitation assessment includes four elements defined by the acronym CORE. These elements include an assessment of **C**ommunication activity limitations and hearing loss through audiometry and self-report; **O**verall participation variables, including psychological, social, educational, and vocational factors; **R**elated personal factors; and **E**nvironmental factors.

- Management includes four elements also, and these are summarized by the acronym CARE. These elements include **C**ounseling, which includes an effort to help clients accept the hearing loss and set reasonable goals; **A**udibility improvement by using hearing aids and other devices; **R**emediation of communication; and **E**nvironmental coordination and participation goals.

- Children receive AR services in a variety of settings, including early intervention and school programs. Adults and elderly adults are usually served in settings that dispense hearing aids; these include private practice, medical or ear, nose, and throat offices, hearing aid specialists, military or Veterans Administration service centers, and community hearing clinics.

- The first eight chapters in this book are organized to provide an overview of the fundamentals in AR, including hearing aids (Chapter 2), cochlear implants (Chapter 3), auditory and visual stimuli (Chapters 4 and 5), speech and language issues (Chapter 6), psychosocial issues (Chapter 7), and school AR services (Chapter 8). Two chapters provide comprehensive explanations to illuminate AR for children (Chapter 9) and for adults (Chapter 10). Finally, two case study chapters illustrate how this work can be carried out with children (Chapter 11) and with adults (Chapter 12).

Supplementary Learning Activities

See www.isu.edu/csed/audiology/rehab to carry out these activities. We encourage you to use these to supplement your learning. Your instructor may give specific assignments that involve a particular activity.

1. Hearing Loss Simulations: Three digital audio samples are filtered to simulate normal hearing, a high-frequency hearing loss, and a low-frequency hearing loss and presented in this activity. Audiograms representing each hearing pattern are also displayed.

View the companion website to supplement your learning.

2. Hearing Loss Classification: To help understand the process of categorizing hearing loss in terms of type, degree, and configuration, this activity provides the learner with sample audiograms and asks you to categorize the loss in all three ways.

3. More Hearing Loss Classification: This activity is similar to the one above but in a different form.

4. Hearing Loss Configuration Profile: In this activity, you can enter dB levels at 1000, 2000, and 4000 Hz in the better ear, and the software will convert these into one of eight audiometric patterns considered hard of hearing. Deaf levels would be 80 or 90 dB or higher at these same frequencies. This activity allows the learner to see what type of communication difficulties would be experienced by hard of hearing persons with these different configurations.

5. In fitting hearing aids and measuring outcomes from amplification, it is important to understand the difference between dB SPL, dB HL, and dB SL. This activity on the website will help you learn how these dB levels relate to each other.

6. Review of studies to understand why children and adults need audiologic rehabilitation.

Recommended Reading

DeConde Johnson, C., & Seaton, J. B. (2011). *Educational audiology handbook.* Clifton Park, NY: Delmar Cengage Learning.

Gagne, J. P., & Jennings, M. B. (2000). Audiological rehabilitation intervention services for adults with acquired hearing impairment. In M. Valente, H. Hosford-Dunn, & R. Roesser (Eds.), *Audiology treatment.* New York: Thieme Medical Publishers.

Johnson, C. E. (2011). *Introduction to auditory rehabilitation: A contemporary issues approach.* Boston: Pearson.

Montano, J., & Spitzer, J. (2013). *Adult audiologic rehabilitation.* San Diego, CA: Plural.

Stephens, D., & Kramer, S. E. (2010). *Living with hearing difficulties: The process of enablement.* Chichester, UK: Wiley-Blackwell.

Tye Murray, N. (2015). *Foundations of aural rehabilitation* (4th ed.). Stamford, CT: Cengage Learning.

Recommended Websites

World Health Organization International Classification of functioning, disability, and health:
http://www.who.int/classifications/icf/en/

American Academy of Audiology:
http://www.audiology.org/publications/guidelines-and-standards

American Speech-Language-Hearing Association:
www.asha.org

References

Abrams H. B., & Kihm J. (2015). An introduction to MarkeTrak IX: A new baseline for the hearing aid market. *Hearing Review, 22*(6), 16.

Alberg, J., Wilson, K., & Roush, J. (2006). Statewide collaboration in the delivery of EHDI services. *The Volta Review, 106*(3), 259–274.

American Academy of Audiology. (1993). Audiology: Scope of practice. *Audiology Today, 5*(1), 16–17.

American Academy of Audiology. (2004). Pediatric Amplification Protocol. *Audiology Today, 16,* 46–53.

American Academy of Audiology. (2006). Guidelines for the Audiological Management of Adult Hearing Impairment. *Audiology Today, 18,* 32–36.

American Annals of the Deaf. (2005). Annual 2005 deaf program questionnaire. *American Annals of the Deaf, 150*(2), 77, 124–161.

American Annals of the Deaf. (2011). Annual 2011 deaf program questionnaire. *American Annals of the Deaf, 156*(2), 126–151.

American Speech-Language-Hearing Association. (1997). *Guidelines for audiologic screening.* Rockville, MD: Author.

American Speech-Language-Hearing Association. (2001). Knowledge and skills required for the practice of audiologic/aural rehabilitation. *ASHA desk reference* (Vol. 4, pp. 393–404). Rockville, MD: Author.

American Speech-Language-Hearing Association. (2006). *Preferred practice patterns for the profession of audiology.* Accessed August 3, 2016, from http://www.asha.org/policy/PP2006-00274

American Speech-Language-Hearing Association. (2014). *Audiology survey: Clinical focus patterns report.* Accessed December 21, 2016, from http://www.asha.org/uploadedFiles/2014-Audiology-Survey-Clinical-Focus-Patterns.pdf

American Speech-Language-Hearing Association. (2016). *The Practice Portal.* Accessed August 4, 2016, from http://www.asha.org/Practice-Portal

Americans with Disabilities Act. (1990). Public Law 101-336, 42 USC Sec. 12101. Equal opportunity for the disabled. Washington, DC: U.S. Government Printing Office.

Bebout, J. M. (1991). Long term care facilities: A new window of opportunity opens for hearing health care services. *Hearing Journal, 44*(11), 11–17.

Berger, K. W. (1988). History and development of hearing aids. In M. C. Pollack (Ed.), *Amplification for the hearing-impaired* (3rd ed., pp. 1–20). New York: Grune & Stratton.

Blair, J. C., Peterson, M., & Viehweg, S. H. (1985). The effects of mild hearing loss on academic performance among school-age children. *The Volta Review, 87,* 87–94.

Brockett, J., & Schow, R. L. (2001). Web site profiles common hearing loss patterns and outcome measures. *Hearing Journal, 54*(8), 20.

Centers for Disease Control and Prevention. (2010). Identifying infants with hearing loss—United States, 1999–2007. *Morbidity and Mortality Weekly Report, 59*(8), 220–223.

Cox, R.M. (2005). Evidence based practice in audiology. *Journal of the American Academy of Audiology, 16,* 408–09.

Cox, R., & Alexander, G. (1995). The abbreviated profile of hearing aid benefit. *Ear and Hearing, 16*(2), 176–186.

Davis, A. (1994). *Public health perspectives in audiology.* 22nd International Congress of Audiology. Halifax, NS, Canada: Author.

Dillon, H., James, A., & Ginis, J. (1997). Client Oriented Scale of Improvement (COSI) and its relationship to several other measures of benefit and satisfaction provided by hearing aids. *Journal of the American Academy of Audiology, 8,* 27–43.

Downs, S. K., Whitaker, M., & Schow, R. (2003). *Audiological services in school districts that do and do not have an audiologist.* Educational Audiology Summer Conference, St. Louis, MO.

Ekberg, K., Meyer, C., Scarinci, N., Grenness, C., & Hickson, L. (2015). Family member involvement in audiology appointments with older people with hearing impairment. *International Journal of Audiology, 54*(2), 70–76.

English, K., & Church, G. (1999). Unilateral hearing loss in children: An update for the 1990s. *Language, Speech and Hearing Services in Schools, 30,* 26–30.

Goldstein, D. P. (1984). Hearing impairment, hearing aids, and audiology. *ASHA, 25*(9), 24–38.

Goldstein, D. P., & Stephens, S. D. G. (1981). Audiological rehabilitation: Management model I. *Audiology, 20,* 432–452.

Hodes, M., Schow, R., & Brockett, J. (2009). New support for hearing aid outcome measures: The computerized SAC and SOAC. *Hearing Review, 16*(12), 26–36.

Johnson, C. E. (2012). *Introduction to auditory rehabilitation: A contemporary issues approach.* Boston: Allyn & Bacon.

Joint Committee on Infant Hearing. (2000). *Principles and guidelines for early hearing detection and intervention programs.* Year 2000 position statement from the Joint Committee on Infant Hearing. Accessed August 3, 2016, from http://www.jcih.org/posstatemts.htm

Kochkin, S., Beck, D. L., Christensen, L. A., Compton-Conley, C., Kricos, P. B., Fligor, B. J., et al. (2010). MarkeTrak VIII: The impact of the hearing healthcare professional on hearing aid user success. *Hearing Review, 17*(4), 12–34.

Lin, F. R., Niparko, J. K., & Ferrucci, L. (2011). Hearing loss prevalence in the United States. *Archives of Internal Medicine 171*(20), 1851–1853.

Madell, J., & Flexer, C. (2014). *Pediatric audiology: Diagnosis, technology and management.* New York: Thieme.

McCandless, G., Sjursen, W., & Preves, D. (2000). Satisfying patient needs with nine fixed acoustical prescription formats. *Hearing Journal, 53*(5), 42–50.

Millington, D. (2001). *Audiologic rehabilitation practices of ASHA audiologists: Survey 2000.* MS thesis, Idaho State University.

Moores, D. (2001). *Educating the deaf—Psychology, principles, practices* (5th ed.). Florence, KY: Cengage Learning.

National Institute on Deafness and Other Communication Disorders. (2005). *Statistical report: Prevalence of hearing loss in U.S. children, 2005.* Bethesda, MD: Author.

Plack, C. J., Barker, D., & Prendergast, G. (2014). Perceptual consequences of "hidden" hearing loss. *Trends in Hearing, 18*, 1–11.

Rathert, C., Wyrwich, M. D., & Boren, S. A. (2013). Patient-centered care and outcomes: A systematic review of the literature. *Medical Care Research and Review, 70*, 351–379.

Ries, P. W. (1994). *Prevalence and characteristics of persons with hearing trouble: United States, 1990–91.* National Center for Health Statistics. *Vital Health Statistics, 10*, 188.

Ross, M. (2011). *Dr. Ross on hearing loss: The hearing aid dispenser as the key factor in determining successful use of a hearing aid.* Accessed August 4, 2016, from www.hearingresearch.org/ross/hearing_aid_use/hearing_aid_dispenser_as_the_key_factoring_determining_successful_use_of_a_hearing_aid.php

Schow, R. L. (1992). Hearing assessment and treatment in nursing homes. *Hearing Instruments, 43*(7), 7–11.

Schow, R. L. (2001). A standardized AR battery for dispensers. *Hearing Journal, 54*(8), 10–20.

Schow, R. L., Maxwell, S., Crookston, G., & Newman, M. (1993). How well do adults take care of their hearing instruments? *Hearing Instruments, 44*(3), 16–20.

Schow, R. L., Mercaldo, D., & Smedley, T.C. (1996). *The Idaho hearing survey.* Pocatello: Idaho State University Press.

Schow, R. L., & Smedley, T.C. (1990). Self-assessment of hearing [Special issue]. *Ear and Hearing, 11*(5, Suppl.), 1–65.

Shepard, N., Davis, J., Gorga, M., & Stelmachowicz, P. (1981). Characteristics of hearing impaired children in the public schools: Part 1—Demographic data. *Journal of Speech and Hearing Disorders, 46*, 123–129.

Stephens, D. (1996). Hearing rehabilitation in a psychosocial framework. *Scandinavian Audiology, 25*(Suppl. 43), 57–66.

Stephens, D., & Kramer, S. E. (2010). *Living with hearing difficulties: The process of enablement.* West Sussex, UK: Wiley-Blackwell.

Stika, C. J., & Ross, M. (2011). *Hearing aid services and satisfaction: The consumer viewpoint.* Rehabilitation Engineering Research Center on Hearing Enhancement. Accessed August 3, 2016, from http://www.hearingresearch.org/ross/hearing_aid_use/hearing_aid_services_and_satisfaction_the_consumer_viewpoint.php

U.S. Census Bureau. (2010). *2010 census data.* Retrieved from http://www.census.gov/population/race/data/index.html

U.S. Census Bureau. (2017). *2017 census data.* Retrieved from http://www.census.gov/popclock

Ventry, I. M., & Weinstein, B. E. (1982). The hearing handicap inventory for the elderly: A new tool. *Ear and Hearing, 3*(3), 128–134.

Vernon, M. (1968). Fifty years of research on the intelligence of the deaf and hard of hearing: A survey of literature and discussion of implications. *Journal of Rehabilitation of the Deaf, 1*, 1–11.

Vernon, M., & Andrews, J. (1990). *The psychology of deafness*. White Plains, NY: Longman.

White, K. R. (2014). Newborn hearing screening. In J. Katz, L. Medwetsky, R. Burkard, & L. Hood (Eds.), *Handbook of clinical audiology* (7th ed.). (pp. 437–458). Philadelphia: Lippincott Williams & Wilkins.

Wong, L., & Hickson, L. (Eds.). (2012). *Evidence-based practice in audiology: Evaluating interventions for children and adults with hearing impairment*. San Diego, CA: Plural.

World Health Organization. (2001). *International classification of functioning, disability and health*. Geneva: Author.

World Health Organization. (2017). *International Classification of Functioning, Disability and Health (ICF)*. http://www.who.int/classifications/icf/en/ updated 10 May, 2017.

Hearing Aids and Hearing Assistive Technologies

Holly S. Kaplan, Alice E. Holmes

CONTENTS

Visit the companion website when you see this icon to learn more about the topic nearby in the text.

Learning Outcomes

After reading this chapter, you will be able to

- List the four basic components found in hearing aids
- Describe each of the following types of hearing aids: in-the-ear, behind-the-ear, completely-in-the-canal, and bone-anchored
- Define *acoustic feedback*
- Identify the three factors to consider when determining hearing aid candidacy
- Describe what gain, frequency response, and maximum output refer to regarding the electroacoustic properties of a hearing aid
- List nine elements that should be included in a hearing aid orientation with a new hearing aid user
- Define assistive listening devices (ALDs)
- Explain contralateral routing of the signal fittings
- Distinguish between frequency-modulated (FM), infrared, and audio-loop listening systems
- Explain closed captioning and its uses

INTRODUCTION

Hearing aids and assistive listening devices (ALDS)/hearing assistive technologies (HATS) are often the cornerstone of the audiologic rehabilitation program because they provide access to sound, oral language, and speech. Both are very aptly named, as they simply aid and assist the individual with hearing loss in being alerted to a fire alarm, understanding the quiet yoga instructor as she names the pose, or hearing birds singing while taking a morning walk. Hearing aids fitted appropriately and at an early age are an essential tool in the process of taking a severely hearing impaired baby with severe hearing loss from an early speech-language therapy client to an independent kindergarten student. The same instrument, again fitted appropriately, can help an elderly client maintain an independent lifestyle while enjoying hearing her family and friends.

In reading this chapter, one should understand that it is a brief overview of a complex topic. Hearing aids and ALDS/HATS as academic subjects are an accumulation of many topics, including acoustics, electronics, psychology, sociology, marketing, and a bit of history. Amplification is often covered in two or three semester-long classes and is a primary component of the clinical experience in audiology doctoral programs. Profit from selling hearing aids and ALDS/HATS is the foundation of most private practices in audiology and "keeps the lights on" in many audiology and speech-language clinics. Hearing aids are not miracle devices, but to many individuals with hearing loss, hearing aids are their passport to the world of sound. Both audiologists and speech-language pathologists involved in the (re)habilitation of individuals with hearing loss need to be aware of the importance of these devices to their clients and must serve as advocates of their use to not only individuals with hearing loss but also their medical care providers, their insurance companies, and their caregivers.

History of Amplification

Humans use hearing for safety, awareness of their surroundings, and effectively understanding the thoughts and emotions of other human beings. The need to hear well certainly predates our busy cell phone–connected world and probably started with early man cupping his hand to his ear in order to get the punch line of a joke while sitting around the fire in the cave. The natural basic gesture of cupping the hand to the ear is probably the oldest and certainly the longest-lasting "hearing aid," providing up to 12 dB of gain at 1000 Hz (Bauman, 2012; www.hearingaidmuseum.com). Other early devices include ear horns and ear trumpets, which were designed to have the individual speak into the belled end, channeling and using the resonance of the device to amplify the sound down into a narrow earpiece. The desire to make hearing loss and hearing aids less noticeable started early as horns and trumpets were designed to look like hair barrettes, walking sticks, handheld fans, or even the headrests of chairs. The user of the latter would simply lean into the hidden earpiece connected to the ear trumpet built into the chair in order to hear (Stephens & Goodwin, 1984). The Kenneth Berger Hearing Aid Museum and Archives at Kent State University has a large collection of hearing aids and listening devices from throughout the world and is well worth the visit for all audiology history buffs.

The manufacture of electronic instruments began in the 1800s; however, these cumbersome tabletop devices were not at all portable. One of the earliest personal devices, designed by Dr. Ferdinand Alt of Vienna (Pollack, 1988), appeared on the market around 1900. Alt's hearing aid consisted of a battery, a carbon microphone, and a magnetic earphone and worked best for individuals with milder hearing loss. Carbon microphone hearing aids were prevalent until the 1940s and advanced the ongoing pattern of making things smaller through reducing the size of the earpiece and more personalized by eventually using individualized earmolds to channel the sound into the ear. Body-worn vacuum tube instruments replaced carbon instruments and provided more gain for individuals with more severe hearing losses. The signal from vacuum tubes was also clearer, and the instruments were less susceptible to damage from dust and variations in signal due to humidity. Transistor technology, invented in 1947 by Bell Labs, revolutionized the hearing aid industry, with transistors completely overtaking vacuum hearing aids within a period of three years. Transistor-based hearing aids did not require a warm-up time and used much smaller batteries, making possible a small pocket-sized body aid with a simple cord leading to the ear-level receiver (Neuman, 1993).

Technology continued to improve with the dual goal of providing appropriate gain for a variety of losses while also making the instruments smaller. Transistor hearing aids could be placed in the frame of eyeglasses or in a simple behind-the-ear curved case, the first behind-the-ear hearing aids appearing in the 1950s. Both eyeglass aids and behind-the-ear instruments allowed efficient individual fitting of both ears (binaural amplification) and could provide enough gain for severe to profound losses. Eyeglass instruments were especially popular with the Veterans Administration, a primary national audiology service clinic. All-in-the-ear instruments were introduced in the 1960s and have evolved from larger full-shell instruments, filling the entire concha bowl, to very small, completely-in-the-canal instruments that sit deeply in the external meatus and require a removal filament to assist the wearer in pulling them out of the ear canal. The electronics of the instruments also evolved with smaller, more energy-efficient microphones, amplifiers, and receivers making smaller power source sizes (batteries) possible. Analog instruments, which are often compared to phonograph technology (as they use linear processing strategies without any digital conversion or manipulation of the auditory signal), were overtaken in the market by digital technology in the late 1980s and 1990s. Digital technology provides for rapid sound analysis and manipulation, multiple programs for various listening situations, and compatibility with a variety of other listening tools such as Bluetooth for the telephone and television with frequency-modulated (FM) auditory training systems for both classroom situations and noisy listening situations, such as restaurants. The hearing aid truly has come a long way from merely cupping the hand behind the ear; however, the simple goal of understanding the punch line while sitting around the campfire remains.

HEARING AID COMPONENTS

Although hearing aids are often advertised as miracle devices with amazing technological abilities, they really are small ear-sized public address systems. Hearing aids consist of the electronic parts shown in Figure 2.1.

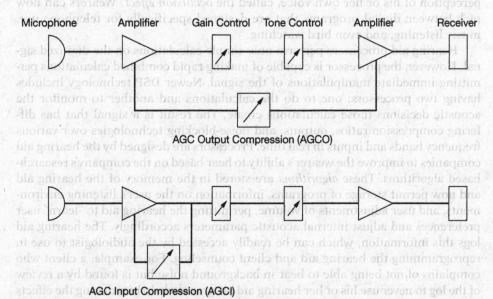

FIGURE 2.1 Schematic of basic hearing aid components.

Microphone

The microphone is a device that takes acoustic energy or sound pressure and changes, or *transduces*, it to electric energy. Hearing aid microphones are mere millimeters in size divided in half by a thin metal-coated layer called the diaphragm. The metal diaphragm permits electrical conduction. Parallel to the diaphragm is another metal plate coated with a polymer that can store electrical charge over time. When the diaphragm is moved by incoming sound pressure, the displacement creates a small voltage that transduces sound pressure to electricity. This current is so small that the microphone has an amplifier built into it to increase its strength and improve the frequency response of the microphone prior to sending the signal on in the hearing aid circuitry. The metal casing of the microphone protects it from electroacoustic interference, and the microphone port is often screened or partially covered to alleviate wind noise.

Many hearing aids are equipped with two microphones to improve directionality. *Omnidirectional* microphones are equally sensitive to sounds coming from all directions. *Directional* microphones permit varying sensitivity to sound coming from a given direction, usually greater sound from the front, or where most conversational partners are positioned. Directional microphones have been shown over time to improve signal (speech)-to-noise ratios, and improved signal-to-noise (SNR) ratios are known to improve the word-understanding ability of individuals with sensorineural hearing loss. Directionality can be achieved by having front and back microphones or by having two sound entry ports in one microphone. The reader seeking more in depth coverage of hearing aid technology is referred to Valente (2002).

Amplifier (Digital Processor)

After the electric signal leaves the microphone, it is converted into a digital code (by the analog-to-digital converter) for manipulation by the processor. The processor is where the signal is changed to approximate listening targets predetermined by the manufacturer based on the individual's hearing and is also where the manipulation and amplification of the signal takes place. Digital signal processing (DSP) has revolutionized hearing aid sound quality, presenting the audiologist with new ways to improve the lives of hearing aid wearers while also challenging the audiologist to keep up with the rapid changes in technology. DSP permits individualization of fittings in the office with the client's immediate input while also addressing age-old hearing aid problems, such as eliminating acoustic feedback (whistle or squeal), and improving speech understanding in the presence of background noise and reducing the deleterious effects on the individual's perception of his or her own voice, called the *occlusion effect*. Wearers can now pick between digital programs that are designed specifically for telephone use, music listening, and even bird watching.

Hearing aid processors perform only simple calculations on the digitized signal. However, the processor is capable of making rapid combined calculations permitting immediate manipulations of the signal. Newer DSP technology includes having two processors: one to do the calculations and another to monitor the acoustic decisions those calculations create. The result is a signal that has differing compression ratios, outputs, and noise-blocking technologies over various frequency bands and inputs in real time. Processors are designed by the hearing aid companies to improve the wearer's ability to hear based on the company's research-based algorithms. These *algorithms* are stored in the memory of the hearing aid and now permit storage of programs, information on the user's listening environments, and user adjustments of volume, permitting the hearing aid to "learn" user preferences and adjust internal acoustic parameters accordingly. The hearing aid logs this information, which can be readily accessed by the audiologist to use in reprogramming the hearing aid and client counseling. For example, a client who complains of not being able to hear in background noise but is found by a review of the log to never use his or her hearing aid program to help in reducing the effects of noise may need further counseling on when and how to use the program.

A transducer is a device that changes one form of energy to another. Microphones change acoustic energy to electrical, while speakers (or receivers, a hearing aid term hearkening to telephone technology terminology) change electrical energy to acoustical.

The occlusion effect can be simulated by sticking your fingers in your ears and talking.

Algorithms are formulas designed by using what we know about speech acoustics and hearing loss to alter the acoustical parameters of the input signal. In hearing aids, the principles behind the formulas are based on the individual's audiogram and have a primary goal of improving speech perception. These formulas have been developed by audiologists and hearing scientists. For example, the Berger, DSL, and NAL methods are used for all types of losses in a variety of cases. Hearing aid manufacturers include these formulas or proprietary formulas in their software for programming the instruments.

The next stage in the operation of the digital hearing aid is to change the processed digitized signal back to an analog electrical signal and amplify it using a Class D amplifier. Class D amplifiers are often integrated into the receiver and are efficient in battery use and produce very low distortion of the signal, even at high-intensity output levels. Newer instruments can send the digital signal to a digital transistor that transfers the signal directly to the receiver (direct digital drive).

Receiver

The receiver is another transducer that takes the amplified electrical signal and converts it back to an acoustic signal. Hearing aid receivers are also only millimeters in size; however, the larger the receiver, the greater its acoustic output and the better it is in using electrical power to achieve those outputs. A hearing aid receiver uses the amplified electrical signal to move a thin metal reed wrapped in a coil between two magnets. Differences in the current provided to the reed via the coil cause the reed to move. The reed's movement is transferred to the receiver diaphragm via a thin rod, with the movement creating the acoustic signal. Because balance between the coil, reed, magnets, drive rod, and diaphragm is critical to appropriate receiver function, receivers are designed to be shock resistant. Receivers are often subject to damage or blockage from cerumen, so clients must be instructed in proper care and cleaning of their hearing aids. Simple instructions, such as "sit down to take out your hearing aid, change batteries over a soft surface, replace the receiver cerumen filter often, and use the receiver cleaning tools provided, not a safety pin," can truly add years to the life of the hearing aid.

Batteries

Hearing aids require a power source usually in the form of a 1.4-volt single-cell zinc-air battery. In the past, the need for high levels of energy required large batteries, which prevented decreasing the size of the instrument. Due to improvements in the energy efficiency of the instruments, batteries have decreased in size to the point of making them difficult for some to handle. Batteries usually will last from one week to three weeks. However, battery life depends on the energy demands of the components of the specific instrument, size of the battery, hours of hearing aid use, and conservation efforts of the individual user. For example, individuals who open the battery door, breaking the contact when the aid is not in use, have better battery life. Battery specifications and packaging are standardized by the manufacturers, so size 13 batteries are always in orange wrapping, while size 10s are in yellow packaging. Batteries range in price depending on place of purchase, with large discount stores, online services, and other retailers selling them at around 30 cents to one dollar per battery. See Table 2.1 for more information about hearing aid batteries and battery use.

TABLE 2.1 Hearing Aid Battery Information

Battery life depends on hours of use and the current drain of the individual instrument. Typical battery life can vary from one day (cochlear implant) to three weeks (mild gain micro behind-the-ear worn for three to four hours daily).

Battery Size	Packaging Color	Voltage	Typical Instrument
5	Red	1.4	CIC, micro instruments
10	Yellow	1.4	RIC, CIC, micro-BTE
312	Brown	1.4	RIC, micro-BTE, ITE, Canals
13	Orange	1.4	BTE, ITE
675	Blue	1.4	High-power BTE, cochlear implant
AAA		1.5	Body aids
AA		1.6	Body aids, cochlear implants

Compared to batteries used in the past, battery life has been extended with zinc-air batteries.

Zinc-air batteries will last in the package for up to 18 months as long as the tab seal remains on the cell. Zinc-air batteries are activated by permitting air into small holes in the cell covered by the removable tab. Permitting air to enter the cell for a few minutes prior to using the battery is recommended by the manufacturers as a way to improve battery life. Although zinc-air batteries are more environmentally friendly than full mercury batteries, many zinc-air cells still contain trace amounts of mercury and should be recycled to prevent damage to the environment. Individuals should be encouraged to seek out and use batteries labeled as "Mercury Free."

Several hearing instrument manufacturers have developed hearing aids that use rechargeable batteries. Solar cells and solar-powered hearing aids also exist on a limited basis; however, the ease of use, poor stability of wireless signals with rechargeable batteries, and relative low cost of single-cell standard batteries currently preclude mass manufacturing or consumer interest in other energy sources.

HEARING AID STYLES

The term *hearing aid style* refers to the shape, size, and location of the instrument. Hearing aid styles appear to come in and out of fashion, but the general trend is for the aid to be smaller and less noticeable. Current analysis of hearing aid sales reveals that behind-the-ear receiver-in-the-canal instruments represent 46 percent of all new fittings, so they are the most popular style by far, outselling all in-the-ear and traditional behind-the-ear styles (Staab, 2015).

The head shadow effect is a reduction in sound intensity caused by the obstruction of the head that also creates changes in the frequency and phase of the sound picked up by the two ears. The brain stem uses the differences to localize the sound source. Individuals with asymmetric hearing loss often have difficulty localizing sound. The head shadow effect is more pronounced at frequencies above 1000 Hz. The head shadow in part explains why a hunter using a rifle will have more hearing loss in one ear than the other due to cocking his or her head when sighting the target. The effects of the head shadow on localization need to be considered whenever fitting an individual with only one amplification device and should be noted as a true benefit of binaural hearing and binaural fittings.

Behind-the-Ear

Behind-the-ear (BTE) devices are encased in plastic and curved to match their placement behind the pinna. The microphone(s) is/are placed at the top of the aid near the upper portion of the ear to take advantage of the *head shadow effect* and to approximate sound entry into the ear canal. In traditional BTE instruments, all of the electronic components are placed in the case. Amplified sound is transmitted from the receiver through the earhook to the earmold tubing and earmold. Refer to Figure 2.2 for examples of a BTE. The larger size of the device permits larger amplifiers and receivers to compensate for severe to profound losses. BTEs also permit easy access to volume and program control buttons, making them an excellent choice for infants, children, and adults with dexterity issues. BTEs are also often selected for children for economic reasons, as the less expensive earmold can be readily replaced as the child's ear grows.

The micro BTE is often called an open-fit or over-the-ear (OTE) instrument and uses a small earpiece instead of a conventional earmold, which allows the ear canal to remain relatively open, minimizing the "plugged ear" feeling. This, along with other advantages, has resulted in a major shift in interest among many hearing aid users in recent years from in-the-ear or in-the-canal styles to the open-fit type of BTE hearing aid. It also has attracted many first-time hearing aid users who otherwise might not have considered trying hearing aids at all. The popularity of open-fit BTE hearing aids certainly represents a significant event in recent audiologic rehabilitation activities.

FIGURE 2.2 Examples of the various styles of hearing aids.
Source: Courtesy of Widex Hearing Aids Incorporated.

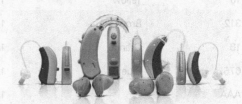

Receiver-in-the-Canal

Receiver-in-the-canal (RIC) BTE instruments are large enough to permit sophisticated microphone arrays and Bluetooth compatibility and dual computer chips while also being inconspicuous in using thin wire to connect the receiver hidden in the ear canal to a small BTE case for the microphone/DSP/amplifier/battery components. RICs are versatile instruments, as individuals with mild high-frequency losses can be fit, as can individuals with more severe hearing loss. RIC hearing aids take audiologists back to their early hearing science classes in remembering how low-frequency sound waves "bend" around obstacles and high-frequency sounds, such as the very important consonant sounds, bounce off obstructions. The RIC places the receiver/speaker in the ear canal near the tympanic membrane and avoids any acoustic impact from the hearing aid tubing by being connected by wire to the other instrument components. Wearers like the sound quality and "nearly invisible" appearance of the RIC, while audiologists appreciate the speed of being able to use standardized ear tips around the receiver to place the instrument in the ear canal. Individuals can be fit with tips and taught how to replace them as needed for the life of the hearing aid, or the audiologist can take the earmold impression for a custom tip as needed, for example, to reduce feedback or discomfort. The speaker/receiver can be easily replaced in-house, making costly and time-worrisome factory repairs happen less often. RIC instruments are being successfully marketed to baby boomers due to their convenience in fitting, sound quality, fashionable case colors/shapes, small size, and Bluetooth compatibility with cellular phones and other electronic devices.

In-the-Ear/In-the-Canal/Completely-in-the-Canal

All-in-the-ear instruments (see Figure 2.2) sit completely in the bowl of the ear, and the case or shell is usually custom molded to the individual. These instruments are named by amount of the concha bowl filled by the aid or placement in the ear canal. Hearing aids that fill the entire concha are referred to as in-the-ear (ITE) instruments, canal aids are smaller and fit in the canal (ITC), and completely-in-the-canal instruments (CIC) are barely visible with placement in the external ear canal. Electronics are in the case and can therefore be limited by the size of the ear and ear canal. Advantages of all-in-the-ear instruments include ease of management because the aid and shell are all in one piece and placement of the microphone is at the more natural level of the ear-canal opening. CIC instruments have the cosmetic advantage of being very difficult to see and the acoustic advantage of placement of the receiver near the tympanic membrane. The latter improves high-frequency reception with less chance for acoustic feedback or squeal. Receiver placement in the canal, however, can lead to increased repairs due to cerumen.

Individuals with mild to moderate hearing losses who use all-in-the-ear and CIC instruments often complain that their own voices are too loud or that they sound as if they are in a barrel. This perception, the *occlusion effect*, is caused by bone-conducted sound (from speaking or chewing reverberating in the ear canal), which is prevented from leaving the ear by the hearing aid. Occlusion can increase the intensity of low-frequency sounds by 20 dB.

Extended-Wear Hearing Aids

Another newer type of hearing aid, the Phonak Lyric, was specifically designed for individuals who want to hear better but are put off by the daily upkeep and care required by traditional hearing aids. This extended-wear instrument is placed deep in the canal (approximately 4 mm from the tympanic membrane) by the audiologist and remains in the canal for months at a time until the battery requires replacement. The individual can sleep, swim, and go about day-to-day activities with no need for battery changes or cleaning the hearing aid. The Lyric is sold on a one-year contract in the United States, which includes replacing the instrument as the battery dies. Phonak notes that the deep-seated nature of the hearing aid reduces the occlusion

In order to fit and to be discreet, hearing aids are small. Individuals with arthritis or poor feeling in their fingers may have difficulty changing batteries, manipulating controls, or placing the hearing aid in the ear. The audiologist must take time to ensure that the client can effectively use the instrument. Remote controls, deactivated volume controls, and removal posts can make the difference between successful use or a hearing aid returned for credit.

One downside to most hearing aids is the *occlusion effect*. Individuals with sloping hearing losses or mild to moderate hearing losses who use hearing aids often complain that their own voices are too loud or that they sound as if they are in a barrel. This perception, the occlusion effect, is caused when bone-conducted sound from speaking or chewing reverberating in the ear canal is prevented from leaving the ear via the ear canal opening by the hearing aid. Occlusion of the ear canal can increase the intensity of low-frequency sounds by 20 dB. One particular type of BTE fitting, the open-mold fitting, uses very thin tubing connected to an earmold that encircles the ear-canal opening with minimal obstruction. Open-mold fittings use the thin tubing to emphasize important high frequencies while leaving the ear canal as open as possible to avoid the occlusion effect (Kuk & Baekgaard, 2008).

effect, improves localization, and reduces the effects of wind noise for individuals who are deemed appropriate candidates. Hearing loss outside of the Lyric's fitting range (up to 60 dB Hearing Level [HL] in the low frequencies and 30 to 90 dB HL in the high frequencies), abnormalities of the external canal/tympanic membrane, and a desire to scuba dive or skydive are typical contraindications. Further limitations include individuals with diabetes, those who bruise easily, or those who have other medical issues impacting the ear, skin, or circulatory system. Many individuals worldwide are benefiting from deep-fitted extended wear instruments with over 42,000 fit as of July 2014 (Phonak Hearing Instruments, 2016).

Refer to Figure 2.2 for pictures of various styles of hearing aids.

THE EARMOLD

The earmold and earmold tubing connect the conventional BTE hearing aid to the ear while also serving as a sound conduit. Earmolds are made of a variety of plastics, each with positive and negative features. Lucite, a hard plastic material, is very durable but is prone to acoustic feedback or whistling/chiming with more gain. Vinyl is a softer material, which can be comfortable but is not as durable and discolors and/or shrinks with age. A variety of silicone materials are also available, providing a hypoallergenic alternative. Silicone can, however, hold moisture, making the earmold uncomfortable to wear in warmer weather. Silicone is also difficult to modify or file down in the office. Many audiologists use combination earmold materials, such as a silicone ear-canal portion with a Lucite concha bowl portion, to obtain the best features from both types of materials.

Earmolds are often vented for both acoustic reasons and patient comfort. A vent is a tunnel-like hole under the earmold tubing channel that permits air to flow in and out of the ear canal. Venting helps in relieving pressure, reducing the overamplification of low frequencies known as the occlusion effect. Venting also keeps the ear canal drier and cooler. Vents can be very large, essentially leaving the ear canal open, or pinpoint in diameter. Venting, however, makes the fitting more susceptible to *acoustic feedback* and must be used judiciously with fittings that require higher gain.

Earmold styles vary depending on the degree of hearing loss and needs of the client. Full-shell earmolds fill the concha bowl, providing a tighter seal against feedback. Skeleton earmolds ring the concha, leaving the bowl open. Canal style earmolds simply fill the canal. Because chewing and talking can push canal earmolds out of the canal, a canal lock or helix lock can hold the instrument in place. Both are essentially a footplate or flange off the canal earmold. Figure 2.3 shows examples of these three earmold styles, while Figure 2.4 features a shell-style earmold with venting added.

The earhook is a hard plastic "C"-shaped piece of tubing that is screwed onto the top of the BTE hearing aid case. Earhooks are often described by the degree of their "C" or crescent shape, specifically half-moon or quarter-moon earhooks. Earhooks also vary in size for pediatric or adult fittings. Dampers, which are mesh filters made

Acoustic feedback, or a "whistling" hearing aid, can be very irritating to the hearing aid user and others nearby. Feedback can be caused by hearing aid malfunction (internal) or due to the hearing aid microphone picking up the receiver's acoustic output of the hearing aid, resulting in a high-frequency chiming or whistling sound. Digital hearing aids have feedback controls built into their fitting algorithms, helping to prevent feedback.

FIGURE 2.3 Earmolds for BTE instruments (1: shell; 2, skeleton; 3: canal) can be made in a variety of colors and color swirls. Zebra stripes, school colors, and so on are all possible.
Source: Courtesy of Westone Laboratories, Inc.

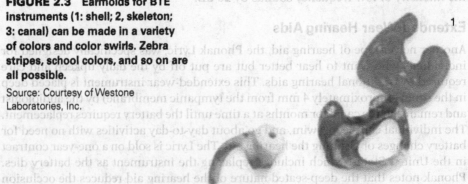

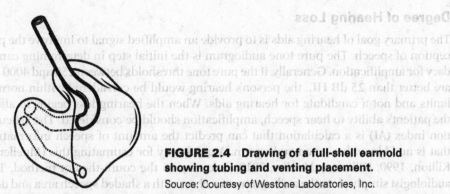

FIGURE 2.4 Drawing of a full-shell earmold showing tubing and venting placement.
Source: Courtesy of Westone Laboratories, Inc.

of plastic and metal, are often placed in the end of the earhook just prior to the attachment point of the hearing aid tubing. Placing a damper in an earhook smooths the frequency response of the hearing aid, reducing peaks of amplitude that can cause feedback. Dampers that reduce amplitude at 1000 Hz also reduce the upward spread of masking, leading to better word understanding in noisy listening situations (Cox & Gilmore, 1986). Dampers are labeled by how many ohms of resistance they provide.

Collectively, the earhook, tubing, and earmold are referred to as the "plumbing" of the BTE hearing aid system. As traditional plumbing connections impact the flow of water, changes in the tubing of the earmold and connectors can impact the flow of sound into the ear. Changes in the thickness, length, and diameter of the tubing impact the gain and frequency response of the sound from the hearing aid. Thicker tubing walls can aid in the prevention of feedback, increasing tubing length attenuates or reduces the gain, and increasing the end diameter creates a horn effect, permitting more high-frequency amplification. Tubing comes in standard sizes and can be bought either precut or in long strips.

The audiologist makes the casting for custom earmolds and all-in-the-ear hearing aid custom cases or shells using a silicone material with a hardening agent. A complete otoscopic check is the initial step in making an earmold, followed by placement of a stringed cotton or sponge dam in the canal. Otoscopy checks for any excess cerumen, bony overgrowth, or foreign body in the ear canal, while the dam serves as a stop for the silicone impression material. Impression material requires four to five minutes to set. After the impression is removed, the audiologist again checks the ear canal for any abrasion or remaining impression material. The casting of the ear is then sent to an earmold laboratory for production and setting of the tubing.

Newer open-fit and RIC instruments use premeasured tubing and tips, negating the need for an earmold impression and permitting more rapid fittings. Audiologists can have micro BTE instruments, tips, and tubing in stock and fit the instrument on the same day as the hearing evaluation.

WHO IS A HEARING AID CANDIDATE?

The recommendation of amplification must take into account a number of variables, including the person's hearing loss, communication disability (activity limitations and participation restrictions), and motivation (desire for quality of life). Hearing aids are appropriate for most individuals with hearing loss that cannot be medically corrected. These losses are sensorineural in nature (inner ear damage/nerve loss), although in some cases of conductive or mixed losses, such as otosclerosis, persons may receive assistance from intervention with hearing aids when the loss cannot be completely medically reversed or if they opt for amplification rather than surgery. Based on the evaluation of the patient, the audiologist must determine the need for a medical referral to a licensed physician. All youth up to 18 years of age who are being considered for hearing aids must have medical clearance from a physician prior to the fitting. Hearing aid sales are most often regulated by the state in which purchased; however, federal guidelines from the U.S. Food and Drug Administration (FDA) are also available.

Degree of Hearing Loss

The primary goal of hearing aids is to provide an amplified signal to improve the perception of speech. The pure tone audiogram is the initial step in determining candidacy for amplification. Generally, if the pure tone thresholds between 250 and 4000 Hz are better than 25 dB HL, the person's hearing would be considered within normal limits and not a candidate for hearing aids. When the hearing loss begins to affect the patient's ability to hear speech, amplification should be considered. The articulation index (AI) is a calculation that can predict the amount of speech information that is audible with a given audiogram. A quick way for estimating this (Mueller & Killion, 1990; Killion & Mueller, 2010) is known as the count-the-dot method. The audiologist simply plots the audiogram on a chart with a shaded speech area and dots representing the acoustical properties of conversational speech. By simply counting the dots above (softer than) the threshold line (the area the person cannot hear) and subtracting that from 100 percent, the estimated articulation index can be obtained. The higher the articulation index, the more of the speech signal is audible.

Degree of Communication Disability

Any person with a hearing loss can be considered for amplification devices, but hearing loss alone does not determine candidacy. The recommendation of amplification must take into account a number of variables, including the person's hearing loss, communication difficulties, hearing disability, activity restrictions, motivation, and quality of life. The hearing fitting process, therefore, must be preceded by a comprehensive hearing evaluation and needs assessment (see Chapters 1, 9, and 10). Self-report questionnaires can be very helpful in determining the needs of the patient (see Chapter 10).

Motivation to Use Amplification

Motivation is a key component to a successful amplification fitting. Patients must be aware of their hearing loss and acknowledge the disability and the participation restrictions created by the reality of the hearing loss before they become motivated to use amplification. Only 30 percent of individuals who report hearing problems seek professional help through the use of hearing aids (Abrams & Kihm, 2015). Reasons for this are many and can include factors such as denial ("My hearing loss is not that bad," "I can get along okay without them"), consumer issues ("I heard hearing aids do not work"), stigma ("Hearing aids will make me look old"), cost, cosmetic issues, other health issues, personality, and attitudes of others. The audiologist should provide the client with recommendations that will improve his or her quality of life, but the client will make the final decisions.

HEARING AID FITTING PROTOCOL

The American Academy of Audiology Guidelines for the Audiologic Management of Adult Hearing Impairment (Valente et al., 2008) list four critical areas to be addressed for every hearing aid fitting: selection, quality control, the fitting, and verification.

Selection

The recommendation for hearing aid style must be based on the gain and output needs for the hearing loss, audiogram configuration, the manipulation skills of the patient, the need for various features such as directional microphones, comfort, and patient preferences (cosmetic concerns, prior experience, etc.). In general, the more severe the hearing loss, the more gain is needed. BTE instruments can provide greater gain without acoustic feedback (whistling) than smaller ITE or ITC devices, whereas some ITE and ITC devices may be perceived as less visible. Open-fit BTE devices allow for low-frequency information to be delivered through the normal pathway while providing amplification to mid- and high frequencies through the hearing aid for patients with a moderate high-frequency loss and normal hearing in the low frequencies. These devices have been well received due to their small size and comfort.

In general, two hearing aids are better than one. Bilateral hearing aids can provide the listener better speech-understanding ability in noisy settings. Most patients are able to localize where sounds are coming from better with two hearing aids and will feel more balanced when fit bilaterally. A small number of individuals may not receive these benefits from two hearing aids and, in fact, may function more poorly with the second hearing aid. Persons with certain auditory processing difficulties, such as binaural inference, or with asymmetric hearing losses also may do better with one hearing aid. Sometimes, financial or cosmetic concerns also prevent patients from opting for two versus one hearing aid. In most cases, however, it is best to try two hearing aids first because the vast majority of patients are successful bilateral users.

Selection of the type of digital signal processing (DSP) is also important and should be based on the audiometric needs of the patient. The number of frequency bands or channels should be determined by the frequency shaping that is needed to provide the best audibility of the speech signal. Flatter-shaped audiograms with a similar loss across the speech frequencies may require fewer channels than those with sloping or unusual audiometric configurations.

Compression characteristics need to be considered based on the patient's *dynamic ranges*, which may vary by frequency. Persons with sensorineural hearing loss typically have recruitment. This means that they have smaller dynamic ranges and therefore need more gain or amplification for soft sounds and less gain or amplification for louder sounds. Compression circuitries enable the hearing aids to provide different levels of gain depending on the input. In most modern instruments, compression characteristics can be manipulated by channel. In order to appropriately select and fit compression DSP, some measure of dynamic range needs to be made. At a minimum, an estimate of the maximum comfort level (MCL) or uncomfortable loudness level (UCL) should be made preferably on at least two frequencies (500 and 2000 Hz). Another more complete approach would be to use loudness scaling.

Loudness scaling can be accomplished by measuring the patient's perceived hearing range between audiometric threshold and UCL, or threshold of discomfort (TD). This can be done at any frequency but should be completed at least at one low and one high frequency. The patient is typically provided a chart, such as the one shown in Table 2.2, and asked to rate the stimulus loudness using the provided categories. The audiologist then presents either pure tone or narrowband stimuli at various levels monaurally to the patient at each frequency to be tested. This can also be done using speech as the stimulus.

Dynamic range is the difference between the hearing aid user's pure tone or speech thresholds and his or her uncomfortable listening level. Many individuals with hearing loss have a reduced dynamic range as compared to individuals with normal hearing.

TABLE 2.2 Loudness Scaling Chart

Loudness Categories
7. Uncomfortably loud
6. Loud but okay
5. Comfortable, but slightly loud
4. Comfortable
3. Comfortable, but slightly soft
2. Soft
1. Very soft

(Cox, Alexander, Taylor, & Gray, 1997)

The telecoil setting on hearing aids uses a coil designed to pick up the electromagnetic signal from telephones or assistive devices, as compared to the microphone setting, which allows the hearing aid to pick up the acoustic signal. Prior to fitting, a visual inspection can ensure that the various features and physical parameters ordered are correct. The style and color of the hearing aid and earmold, the appropriate user controls, and so on need to be checked. In addition, a listening check of the hearing aids should be completed prior to fitting them on the patient using a specialized stethoscope. The audiologist can listen to the quality of the instrument to see if the user controls, such as volume, are working properly.

Directional microphones can help in some background noise situations. Many hearing aids also have digital noise reduction (DNR) circuitries that may provide greater comfort and sound quality. Digital feedback suppression (DFS) is also available on most instruments and helps prevent the hearing aid from whistling, which occurs when the sound from the receiver is picked up by the microphone and reamplified. This whistling is termed *acoustic feedback*.

Each of these features has various levels of technology and cost. Evidence-based practice must be used in deciding what features to provide for the patient. Audiologists need to systematically seek the highest level of evidence, whether it is from well-designed clinical trials or expert opinion, to provide what is best for the patient (Cox, 2005). Listening to a manufacturer's marketing claims without using evidence-based criteria could lead to providing unnecessary, higher-cost, and/or detrimental features for the patient. The advantages of each feature also must be based on the communication needs and financial and/or cosmetic concerns of each individual hearing aid consumer.

Quality Control

All hearing aids must undergo quality control measures prior to being fit on patients. The American National Standards Institute (ANSI, 2009) provides guidelines for testing the electroacoustic characteristics of hearing aids to ensure that the devices are providing what the manufacturers claim. The hearing aid performance specifications incorporate standard measures of gain, frequency response, compression, maximum output, distortion limits, directional microphone positioning, and *telecoil response*. Table 2.3 lists and defines some of the major measures that should be completed prior to any hearing aid fitting. Using ANSI standards allows the audiologist not only to know if the hearing aid is functioning as expected but also to be able to compare instruments across manufacturers in a uniform manner. The measurements can be done using a hearing aid analyzer that has a small test chamber and enables the audiologist to do input/output measures on the instruments.

TABLE 2.3   Examples of Measures Used for Electroacoustic Analysis of Hearing Aids

Measurement	Definition
Gain	The difference in dB between the input signal from the testing equipment and the output signal from the hearing aid. This can be completed with the hearing aid volume set to the user's level, set full on, or at a reference gain.
Frequency response curve	A graphic representation of the gain at each frequency. This is done by sweeping a test tone across the frequencies at a given input level.
Output sound pressure level 90 (OSPL90)	The dB SPL produced by the hearing aid with the gain control in the full-on position with an input of 90 dB SPL. This measurement is an indication of what the maximum power output of the hearing aid is. This information is important to ensure that the output is the hearing aid will not reach unsafe levels for the patient.
Harmonic distortion	A measurement of new frequencies generated by the hearing aid that are harmonics of the original signal. This is typically reported as a percent of the total output of the hearing aid.
Battery current	An indication of current battery consumption of the hearing aid
Equivalent input noise level	A reading of the overall internal noise of hearing aid.
Attack and release times	Measurements of the time it takes for the output to settle to the steady-state level after the input is changed from 55 to 90 dB and from 90 to 55 dB. This is a measurement of the time it takes for compression to turn on and off when the signal increases in volume.
Telephone magnetic field response	Provides the frequency response of the hearing aid in the telecoil position with an electromagnetic input.

The myriad ways that hearing aid companies first used to connect the hearing aid to the programming computer was one of the more frustrating aspects of the analog-to-digital conversion. Initially, all companies had a programming device with instrument-specific cords that could be plugged into the hearing aid either directly or through a programming boot. This cumbersome situation was soon replaced with a multicompany programming software platform called NOAH. Cords, hearing aid boots, and battery pills still abounded and seemed to many audiologists to reproduce or at least self-tangle in an embarrassing heap in the computer desk drawer. Clever audiologists invented cord organizers to deal with the confusion. Fortunately, the days of tangled hearing aid cords are coming to a close, as hearing aids are now using Bluetooth to connect to the computer for programming.

Fitting

The actual fitting of the hearing aids is both science and art. The audiogram provides information about the acuity loss at various frequencies, but it does not give any information about the comfortable dynamic range at the various frequencies or about the speech perception abilities of the individual when confronted with real-world listening situations.

Various methods have been developed to recommend the amount of gain and maximum power output of the instruments for a patient based on audiometric test measures. The two classifications of fitting methods are comparative and prescriptive. Comparative fitting protocols involve comparing different hearing aids or hearing aid characteristics by either self-report or audiometric measures. The comparative approach can be a lengthy procedure if done correctly and is rarely used for the initial fitting of the hearing aids in clinics today. Prescription methods, on the other hand, are formula based and recommend the gain and maximum power output based on audiometric information. They are designed to provide appropriate gain targets for maximum intelligibility or maximum comfort to the patient. The most common fitting formulas currently used are the National Acoustic Laboratory Nonlinear 1 and 2 procedures (NAL-NL1 and NAL-NL2) and the Desired Sensation Level (DSL) procedure, as well as manufacturers' proprietary formulas that are based on one of the above (Byrne, Dillon, Ching, Katsch, & Keidser, 2001; Scollie et al., 2010; Seewald, Moodie, & Scollie, 2005).

For the NAL-NL1 and NAL-NL2 procedures, first the audiogram is entered into the software along with information about the hearing aid selected, including the type (CIC, ITC, ITE, or BTE), number of compression channels, earmold style, and venting. The software then prescribes the gain and compression characteristic for that individual audiogram and hearing aid. The NAL formulas are designed to maximize speech intelligibility at their most comfortable loudness level (MCL) while keeping overall loudness level no greater than that perceived by persons with normal hearing. The NAL formulas assume that speech understanding is best with the same loudness perception across all frequencies. Equal loudness curves are the basis for this method. Average data from a large population of hearing aid users were used to develop these formulas. Their formulas are developed for both linear and wide dynamic range compression hearing aids and various modifications are made depending on the severity of the hearing loss.

The DSL-based prescription procedures attempt to make sounds comfortably loud across all hearing levels and all frequencies rather than equally loud. It was originally developed for use in pediatric cases but now is used in many clinics for adult patients also. The current program, DSL[i/o], uses an algorithm designed for wide dynamic range compression hearing aids. The hearing aid prescription provides output limiting targets that are appropriate for use with young children based on their age. A visual display of the targets is supplied by the software as an SPLogram, and an example is shown in Figure 2.5. This graph shows the hearing thresholds, maximum acceptable levels, and the recommended targets for the hearing aid in dB SPL.

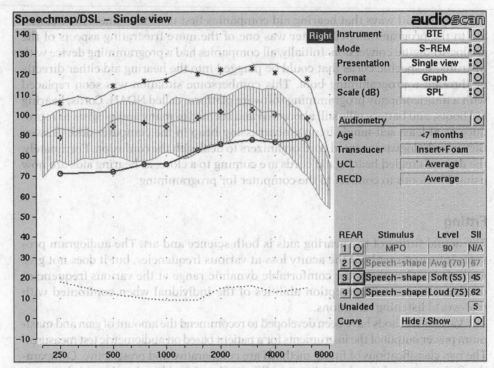

FIGURE 2.5 An example of an SPLogram used in the Desired Sensation Level (DSL) hearing aid fitting procedures. This graph shows the hearing thresholds, maximum acceptable levels, and the recommended targets for the hearing aid in dB SPL.

Source: Permission granted by the Child Amplification Laboratory, University of Western Ontario.

When using any prescriptive method, another obstacle we must overcome is the actual resonance of the ear canal and how that affects the output characteristics of the hearing aid at the eardrum. From basic physics, we know that when sound is put into a cavity, the length and volume of that space will change the frequency and gain characteristics of the signal. For the ANSI measurements, a 2-cc coupler is used to approximate the average adult ear-canal volume with an earmold in place. Most individuals do not have this exact volume in their ear canal. Young children tend to have much smaller ear canals, whereas older adults have larger ones. Just as sound changes when you put different water levels into a soda bottle and blow into it, the same thing happens with different ear-canal sizes. Someone with the smaller ear canal will have more gain in the high frequencies. Fortunately, we are able to measure this using a real-ear system, such as that shown in Figure 2.6. A real-ear system has a probe microphone (Figure 2.7). This thin tube is placed in the ear canal while sound is presented through a loudspeaker at various intensity levels. With the real-ear measurement system, we are able to measure the resonance of an unaided ear canal (real-ear unaided response [REUR]) along with a number of measurements with the hearing aid in place. These can be compared to the 2-cc coupler measurement to allow for correction factors within the formulas.

Any prescriptive formula is only the starting point for the programming of the hearing aids. Remember that these formulas are based on average patient data. Each person with a hearing loss has different needs, so modifications may be made to the hearing aid based on the feedback given by the patient or on speech intelligibility testing done with the hearing aids on. This is where the art of hearing aid fitting comes in. For example, the patient may report that sounds are hollow or that people seem to be speaking in a barrel when he or she is using hearing aids. In this case, the audiologist may want to decrease the amount of gain in the lower frequencies. Sometimes, patients may report that the amplified sound is tinny. Reduction of the high-frequency gain may help reduce this complaint. However, the audiologist must

The acclimatization process is a period of adjustment to a hearing aid, usually four to six weeks in duration after the initial fit.

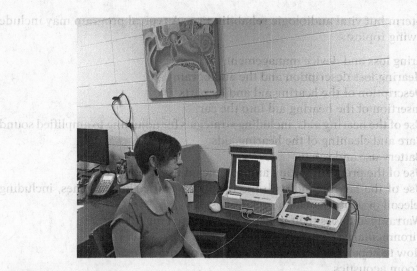

FIGURE 2.6 **A patient having real-ear measurements completed in connection with being fit with hearing aids.**
Source: Courtesy of University of Georgia Speech & Hearing Clinic

be aware that these modifications may reduce the speech-intelligibility improvements that the hearing aids are designed to give. The clinician performs a balancing act between perceived quality of the signal from the patient and improvements in his or her ability to understand speech. Often, new hearing aid users must get used to the new sound from the hearing aids. They must go through an adaptation period to adjust to the devices, often referred to as the *acclimatization process*. Many audiologists will make adjustments to the recommended formulas based on the patient's comments and will slowly provide more gain as the patient adapts to the new sound. This crucial adjustment period varies by the patient and can be immediate or last up to several months. Patients need to be seen for follow-up appointments to adjust the hearing aids appropriately as they become accustomed to wearing them.

Hearing Aid Orientation

No hearing aid ever helped anyone by sitting in a drawer, and the time spent teaching the new wearer and often his or her family how to use the instrument(s) is the key to successful use (Kemker, Goshorn, & Kaplan, 2015). For adult patients, orientation to the device can be done as part of the initial fitting or in individual or group hearing aid adjustment programs that usually consist of three or four sessions. In addition to learning about the hearing aids and how to use them, the hearing aid orientation (HAO) provides an opportunity to engage

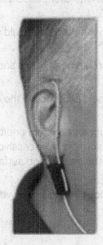

FIGURE 2.7 **Probe microphone for real-ear measurements.**
Source: Courtesy of Audioscan, Inc.

in short-term but vital audiologic rehabilitation. A typical program may include the following topics:

- Hearing loss and device management
  - Hearing loss description and the audiogram
  - Description of the hearing aid and its parts
  - Insertion of the hearing aid into the ear
  - Use of the hearing aids, including strategies for adjusting to amplified sound
  - Care and cleaning of the hearing aids
  - Battery use and safety
  - Use of the program setting and volume adjustment controls
  - Use of the hearing aid with the telephone and cellular phones, including telecoil or acoustic telephone settings
  - Warranty and loss/theft policies for the instrument
- Environmental issues
  - How to cope with noise and distance problems
  - Room acoustics
  - Factors that affect speechreading
- ALDs (as discussed below)
- Communication therapy
  - Assertiveness training
  - Coping strategies for communication breakdowns

Make clients and their families aware of ways to make communication easier. **CLEAR** and **SPEECH** (Schow, 2001) are handouts covering topics from making speechreading easier to assertiveness in communication.

An easy way to remember all of the topics that must be covered during a hearing aid orientation is the acronym HIO-BASICS, for Hearing Instrument Orientation Basics (Schow, 2001).

H = Hearing Expectations: Hearing aids are named well; they aid the individual in being able to hear better. They are not like eyeglasses, which usually make vision perfectly clear when worn. Adjustment to hearing aids can take months for some patients, and they need to know this time frame.

I = Instrument Operation: The patient must be able to turn the device on/off, change programs, adjust volume, and use a telephone. These tasks must be demonstrated by the audiologist and practiced by the wearer prior to leaving the office.

O = Occlusion Effect (OE): The client should talk with the hearing aids in his or her ears but turned off to determine if an occlusion effect is present. Many new digital instruments have electronic occlusion effect controls, and earmold modifications, such as increased venting or lengthening of the earmold canal, can also be used to minimize this problem.

B = Batteries: Discuss the battery type and size needed for the instrument, including places to purchase them, expected battery life, and the instrument's low-battery warning signal. The client should be able to place and remove a battery prior to leaving the appointment.

A = Acoustic Feedback: Demonstrate feedback and counsel the client as to when the aid should squeal and when it should not.

S = System Troubleshooting: Give a brief overview of how to fix common problems at home and point out the Troubleshooting Guide in the hearing aid's manual.

I = Insertion and Removal: Demonstrate the process and have the client insert and remove the device prior to leaving the office.

C = Cleaning and Maintenance: Demonstrate use of the wax cleaning tool and microphone/battery contact brushes. Note the importance of keeping the aid away from aerosol sprays, excessive heat, and water. Instruct in the use of dry aid kits and remind clients to change batteries over soft surfaces to prevent the aid from being dropped on a hard floor.

S = Service, Warranty, and Repairs: Explain the company and your clinic's policies regarding the warranty and what to do in case the aid is malfunctioning.

Both are wonderful to "hang on the refrigerator" for ready reference (see Chapter 10).

- At-home computer-based programs, such as Listening and Communication Enhancement (LACE), are convenient, as the client can schedule his or her time commitments. LACE is specifically designed for older adults and requires 30 minutes per day five days per week for one month. One study noted a 40 percent increase in word understanding in noise following use of LACE (Sweetow & Sabes, 2006).

Verification/Validation/Outcome Measures

Outcome measures that verify the acoustic parameters of the hearing aid as it is working in the ear and then validate that the patient's communication needs are being met are extremely important when doing any clinical procedure. We need the patient to verify hearing aid performance, to evaluate our own performance and fitting protocols, to determine the need for the continuation of services and the allocation of resources, to provide information to third-party payers regarding benefit, and finally to have a measurement of patient use, benefit, and satisfaction (Cox, et al, 2000).

Electroacoustic Outcome Measures. An important electroacoustic method for verification of the hearing aid electroacoustic performance is to use real-ear measurements with the hearing aid in the patient's ear. Table 2.4 has a listing of the various real-ear measurements that can be obtained with the patient. These measurements let us know what the output of the hearing aid is at the eardrum with various input levels. It is critical to know the response of the instrument at a normal conversational level and also with a loud input. If the gain of the hearing aid, combined with the ear canal *resonance*, is too loud with high-intensity inputs, the patient could be put at risk for additional noise-induced hearing loss when wearing the hearing aid. This is particularly critical with children who have small ear canals and much higher resonances within the system. Real-ear hearing aid verification needs to be completed at the time of fitting and during follow-up visits. Real-ear or probe microphone measurements are the main electroacoustic method of evaluating the performance of the hearing aid in the patient's ear.

Prior to the development of real-ear measurements, aided and unaided threshold measurements were performed to determine the functional gain of the hearing aid. Unfortunately, functional gain measurements can be unreliable and are incomplete since they tell the audiologist the gain of the instrument only at very soft input levels. They will not give any information on the functioning of the instrument at normal conversational or high input levels. Therefore, real-ear measurements are critical for appropriate hearing aid fitting and verification.

Audiologic Measures. The real-ear measurements tell us how the hearing aid is performing, but we also need measurements of how the patient is performing with

During the adjustment period, a 30- to 60-day return policy is required by most state licensure laws to allow patients to return their devices if they are not satisfied with them. Patients can receive a refund of the cost of the devices minus the professional fitting fee.

Resonance: The shape of the outer ear creates a resonating cavity that changes the frequency response characteristics of the incoming sound between 1500 and 3000 Hz. For smaller ear canals, this can significantly increase the sound pressure level at the eardrum.

TABLE 2.4   Listing of Common Real-Ear Measurements (REM)

Real-Ear Measurement	Measurement Made in Ear Canal
Real-Ear Unaided Response (REUR)	dB SPL in an open ear canal
Real-Ear Aided Response (REAR)	dB SPL with device in place and turned on
Real-Ear Occluded Response (REOR)	dB SPL with device in place and turned off
Real-Ear Saturation Response (RESR)	dB SPL at maximum output level for device
Real-Ear Insertion Gain (REIG) = difference between REAR and REUR	

TABLE 2.5 Examples of Audiometric Speech Perception Tests for Outcome Testing

Audiometric Speech Test	Quiet/Noise	Format	Developer (Year)
Central Institute for the Deaf (CID) W-22	Quiet	Monosyllabic words	Hirsch et al. (1952)
Northwestern University Auditory Test No. 6 (NU-6)	Quiet	Monosyllabic words	Tillman and Carhart (1966)
Hearing in Noise Test (HINT)	Noise	Sentences in broadband noise	Nilsson, Soli, and Sullivan (1994)
Quick Speech in Noise (QuickSIN)	Noise	Sentences in multitalker babble noise	Killion et al. (2004)
Words in Noise (WIN)	Noise	Words in multitalker babble noise	Wilson (2003)
Acceptable Noise Level (ANL)	Noise	Words in multitalker babble noise	Nabelek, Tucker, and Letowski (1991)

the hearing aids. This can be done using both audiologic and self-report measurements. Audiologic measurements include testing the patient with speech both in quiet and in noise in the sound booth. Comparisons can be made to the patient's unaided performance or performance with prior hearing aids. Using one of a number of commercially available taped evaluation measures (see Table 2.5), the audiologist can easily determine how the patient can perform with the hearing aids in a quiet or a noisy situation. The QuickSIN is one example of the type of test that can be used with adults (Killion, Niquette, Gudmundsen, Revit, & Banerjee, 2004). The patient listens and repeats 10 sentences that are presented in a noisy background. Each sentence is presented in a progressively louder background noise. The audiologist can then calculate the SNR that is needed to allow the patient to repeat 50 percent of the sentences correctly. The lower the SNR, the better the patient is performing in noise.

Self-Report Outcome Measurements. Beyond the electroacoustic and audiologic verification, the audiologist must also ascertain how the hearing aid user is doing in the real world when wearing the devices (Cox, et al, 2000). The clinician needs to find out how much the patient is using (*use*) the hearing aids, how much *benefit* he or she is perceiving, and how satisfied (*satisfaction*) the patient is with the devices. This can be done through an interview format that is documented in the patient records or through the use of self-report assessments. Examples of these tests can be found in Table 2.6. Each test has a different purpose. Some are designed to be given pre– and post–hearing aid fitting, others are only given after the hearing aid fitting, and others compare performance with previous hearing aids. For example, the International Outcome Inventory for Hearing Aids (IOI-HI; Cox & Alexander, 2001) is a seven-item questionnaire designed to be given after the patient has his or her hearing aids. It provides information on the amount of use, perceived benefit, residual activity limitations, residual participation restrictions, the impact on others, overall satisfaction, and quality of life. The IOI-HI is available in a number of languages and has normative data. Another commonly given test is the Abbreviated Profile of Hearing Aid Benefit (APHAB; Cox & Alexander, 1995). This test has four subtests that evaluate ease of communication, hearing abilities in background noise, reverberation, and aversiveness of the hearing aids. The APHAB can compare aided to unaided performance and between new and previous hearing aids.

TABLE 2.6   Examples of Self-Report Assessment Measures

Self-Report Assessment	Outcomes Measured	Developer (Year)
International Outcomes Inventory – Hearing Aids (IOI-HA)	Seven core communication outcomes in a seven-question scale	Cox et al. (2001)
Abbreviated Profile of Hearing Aid Benefit (APHAB)	Communication performance across four subscales	Cox and Alexander (1995)
Hearing Handicap Inventory for Elderly/Adults (HHIE/A)	Effects of hearing loss on two subscales; adult version has more occupational items	Newman et al. (1990); Ventry and Weinstein (1982)
Client Oriented Scale of Improvement (COSI)	Five patient-selected areas to improve with hearing aid use	Dillon, James, and Ginis (1997)
Glasgow Hearing Aid Benefit Profile (GHABP)	Alleviation of communication difficulty with hearing aids for eight situations (four patient selected)	Gatehouse (1999)
Self Assessment of Communication (SAC)	Measure of communication activity and psychosocial aspects of hearing loss (10 items)	Hodes, Schow, and Brockett (2009); Schow and Nerbonne (1982)
Significant Other Assessment of Communication (SOAC)	Measurement of the perceptions of the significant other in regard to the communication and psychosocial issues faced by the individual with hearing loss (10 items)	Hodes et al. (2009); Schow and Nerbonne, (1982)

PEDIATRIC FITTINGS

For pediatric fittings, a team approach is critical. Parents and family must be included at all levels in the process. Early identification is important so that the child may be fitted with hearing aids and be placed in an appropriate habilitation program as early as possible. Fortunately, with universal newborn screenings, many more infants with hearing loss are being identified within days of their birth. Intervention, including amplification, should be initiated immediately after the diagnosis of a hearing loss. In order to fit the hearing aids, the audiologist must use all audiologic results that are available. This may include results from auditory brainstem response (ABR), otoacoustic emissions (OAE), or behavioral testing. In a very young child, the use of auditory steady-state response (ASSR) testing can provide an objective measure of the child's auditory sensitivity with frequency specific information. These estimates of threshold can be put into one of the prescriptive approaches specifically developed for hearing aid selection with pediatric cases.

The use of real-ear analysis must be done in all pediatric fittings. Because the child's or infant's ear canal will have a much smaller volume than that of the 2-cc coupler, the ear-canal resonance will be very different. The audiologist must know what these differences are in order to protect the child from overamplification, which could give additional hearing loss from the hearing aids. The infant's real-ear responses can be done while the child is sleeping or in his or her parent's lap feeding. Real-ear measures must be repeated often as the child grows, as the shape and size of the ear canal are also changing. If children have been tested with real-ear measures since they were weeks old, they tend to tolerate the testing procedure even when they reach the more difficult behavioral periods that occur at around 2 years of age. In children who are identified later, the majority are tested using ABR or ASSR under sedation. This is an opportune time to also obtain some real-ear measurements of the unaided ear canal. These measurements can then be applied to the prescriptive formula being used. As stated earlier, the DSL prescriptive formulas were originally designed for use with children. They do include average ear canal resonance and dynamic range levels based on the child's age if for some reason real-ear measurements cannot be made. The DSL approach also uses data from the University of Ontario regarding the speech spectrum of children when deriving hearing aid targets. For the development of speech, it is critical that the child can hear the auditory feedback of his or her own voice; therefore, the DSL prescriptive formulas consider not only adult voices but also the child's own voice in its calculations.

Output-limiting compression is essential for protection of residual hearing for all hearing aids placed on children. Hearing aids with wide programming ranges are recommended for children because the instruments can be adjusted as needed as more is known about the hearing loss. It was once thought that directional microphones may be questionable for infants and toddlers because they may prevent some incidental learning when the child is playing on the floor or not looking in the direction where the sounds are originating. Research has shown that even the youngest hearing aid user can benefit from directional microphones, and they do not detract from awareness of environmental sounds and incidental speech and language learning (Ching et al., 2009).

One of the most difficult problems with hearing aids in infants and toddlers is appropriate earmold fitting. In the first few years of life, the ear canal is rapidly changing, and therefore the child can grow out of an earmold in weeks or months. The parents must be taught to check the fit of the earmolds on a daily basis so that they can schedule an appointment when replacement is needed. Soft materials are recommended for use in children because they provide better comfort and retention in the ear. Parents, therapists, day care workers, and teachers, along with anyone else working with the child, must be taught how to check the hearing aids, place the hearing aids in the child's ears, and work the controls.

Another issue that is sometimes a challenge when fitting hearing aids on a very young child is retention of the BTE devices on small ears. A number of retention devices have been designed to help with this issue. Clips that are designed to clip to the child's clothing and attach to the hearing aids via ribbons or cords can be very helpful. If the hearing aids fall out of the child's ear, the device will hang with the clip onto his or her clothing. Sweat bands or toupee or wig tape can be used to hold the hearing aids in place. Features such as smaller ear hooks, smaller devices, and color-coding options using red and blue to indicate which hearing aid goes in which ear can be very helpful. Tamper-resistant battery doors and volume control covers also are critical to prevent the child from opening the battery door and ingesting the battery or changing the controls of the hearing aid. Options for having the hearing aids function with other devices, such as the hearing assistive devices discussed in a later section, should also be considered in any pediatric fittings.

Extensive hearing aid orientations are needed for the parents and all significant others who work with the child. The audiologist needs to remember that these individuals are being overwhelmed with everything that they must deal with after identification of the hearing loss. Pediatric audiologists must show empathy and realize what stages of acceptance of the hearing loss the parents are in. Parents need to understand the importance of amplification for the speech and language development of their child with hearing loss. They also need to realize that the hearing aids are just tools and that the accompanying therapy is critical.

During the orientation, the parents and other caregivers need to be told the following:

- How to remove the hearing aids and work the controls
- How to troubleshoot the instruments
- How to do a listening check on the hearing aids
- How to care for and clean the instruments
- When the hearing aid should not be worn:
  - When the child has an outer ear infection or irritation in the canal
  - When there is a draining ear
  - Any time when the conventional hearing aid gets wet
  - When it is not working properly

The goal of a pediatric amplification fitting is to have the child wearing the hearing aids as much as possible as soon as possible. For the young child, a parent should be given a wearing schedule that gradually increases the amount of time the child wears the hearing aids. The parent or caregiver, not the child, should be in control of when the child wears the hearing aids. Parents need to be warned not to fall into a trap of taking the hearing aids out whenever the child is fussy. They should be encouraged to keep a diary of the wearing times and both the positive and the negative experiences they encounter as the child becomes accustomed to his or her amplification. This helps empower the parents to be contributing partners in their child's development and encourage the development of observational skills.

A typical wearing schedule that may be suggested for an infant would be as follows. During week 1, the parents should choose times when they are with the child in a controlled environment with not too many people and not too much noise. They should start with two to four wearing times of 15 to 30 minutes each day and increase the wearing times by 10 to 15 minutes every day. During the time the baby is wearing the instruments, parents should be doing enjoyable activities with the child. They should talk and talk and talk some more, keeping the experience positive. The parent should choose the time when to take the hearing aids out. Parents should also check for any canal irritation after they remove the devices. During the next two weeks, they should gradually increase the wearing times so that by the end of week 3, the child should be wearing his or her hearing aid during most waking hours. The child should see wearing the hearing aid as routine as putting on his or her shoes.

Audiologic follow-up needs to be done at least every three months during the first two years of hearing aid use. Earmold fitting should be checked more frequently because of the rapid growth of the outer ear (see Table 9.2). All audiologic follow-up should include behavioral audiometric evaluations, adjustment of the hearing aids based on updated audiologic information, electroacoustic evaluations both in the test box and on the ears, and earmold checks. Parent questionnaires also can provide important subjective information on how the child is doing. These include the Meaningful Auditory Integration Scale (MAIS; Robbins, Renshaw, & Berry, 2001), the Infant/Toddler Meaningful Auditory Integration Scale (IT-MAIS; Zimmerman-Phillips, Osberger, & Robbins, 1997), and the Early Listening Function test (ELF; Anderson, 2002). Audiologists also need to work closely with the speech-language pathologists and teachers of the hearing impaired who are involved with the children. They can provide important information on how the child is functioning outside the audiology clinic. Often, they may see instances where the child is not hearing as well with the hearing aid as he or she was in the past, indicating either malfunctioning instruments or changes in hearing. They can also provide good insight into how the child is adapting to amplification.

With universal newborn hearing screening, early identification has allowed pediatric audiologists to fit children with hearing aids within the first few weeks of life. Studies have shown that a child who receives intervention, including therapy and amplification, within the first six months of life is more likely to achieve normal speech and language development than a child who is identified later.

SPECIAL FITTINGS

Contralateral Routing of the Signal (CROS) Fittings

Individuals with unilateral hearing loss or extreme differences in the hearing threshold levels between ears have over time been difficult to successfully fit with amplification. The goal is to provide acoustic information from the poorer ear side to the better ear without interfering with the hearing in the better ear. One way to achieve this is through placing a microphone on the poor ear and routing the signal via a wire, FM, or Bluetooth technology to the other ear. If the good ear has normal hearing levels, the instrument on it would be a very mild gain amplifier/receiver with sound channeled

The head shadow effect occurs when sound is presented to one side of the head and has to travel through or around the head. It can reduce the overall intensity of the sound and filter the sound. A CROS hearing aid or bone-anchored implantable device can help reduce these issues (see the section "Bone-Anchored Devices").

via an open earmold. If the better ear has some hearing loss, then the device would have a microphone and provide appropriate gain for the loss in that ear, too. These devices are referred to as CROS, or contralateral routing of the signal (microphone only on the poorer ear, very mild gain to the normal ear), and Bi-CROS (microphone on both ears with more amplification provided to the better albeit impaired ear).

Bone-Conduction Hearing Aids

Another difficult fitting is the individual who cannot use standard hearing aid technology coupled with an earmold to hold the hearing aid in place. Individuals with chronic middle ear infections with effusion or individuals with atresia (absence of the ear canal) fall into the category of needing amplification that does not involve blocking or using the ear canal. These individuals still could have normal or near-normal cochlear function but have significant conductive losses requiring amplification provided directly to the cochlea usually through bone conduction. Bone-conduction hearing aids have the microphone and amplifier housed either in a BTE or a body aid attached with a metal headband to a bone vibrator on the mastoid. These instruments are usually very powerful, as they vibrate in response to sound input and must fit tightly to the mastoid, both of which can be uncomfortable for the wearer over time.

Bone-Anchored Devices

A more recent development in bone-conducted amplification is to surgically implant the titanium vibrator unit into the mastoid bone, coupling the unit through either

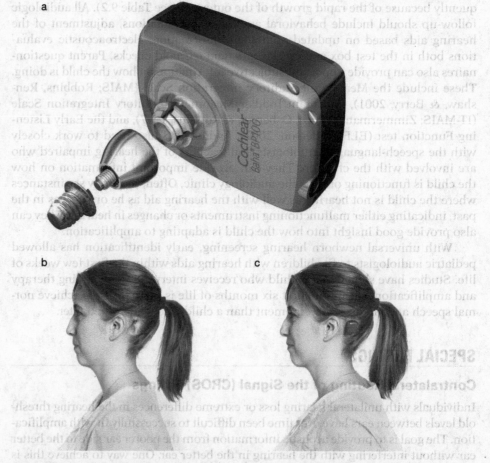

FIGURE 2.8 **The components of a bone anchored system are shown in Figure a. Figure b illustrates the abutment in the head, and Figure c shows the processor attached to the abutment.**
Source: Courtesy of Cochlear Americas, © 2011.

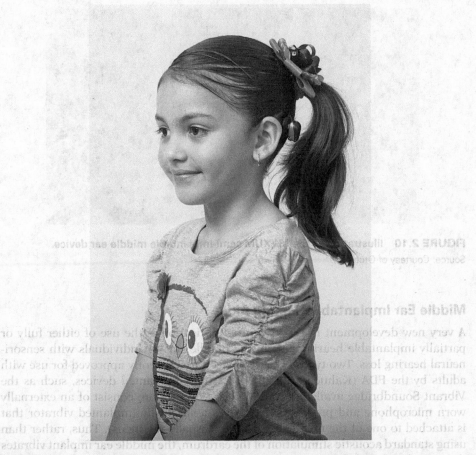

FIGURE 2.9   A child with a Baha 5 bone-anchored system, using a transcutaneous connection.
Source: Courtesy of Cochlear Americas, © 2016.

a transcutaneous (through the skin) connector (or abutment) to the microphone/amplifier device or a magnetic connection (Figures 2.8 and 2.9). If surgery to implant the vibrator is precluded due to health or age (birth to 5 years is not approved in the United States), the device can be held in place with a soft cloth headband. These bone-anchored hearing aids (BAHA) were introduced in Europe in 1977 and received initial FDA approval for use in conductive and mixed losses in 1999, for bilateral losses in 2001, and for unilateral losses in 2002. There are two major manufacturers of bone-anchored devices: The Oticon Pronto and the most popular device to date, Cochlear Americas' Baha (Figures 2.8 and 2.9; Christensen, Smith-Olinde, Kimberlain, Richter, & Dornhoffer, 2010). Bone-anchored devices have proven to be comfortable to wear and cosmetically appealing and provide an excellent amplification alternative for individuals with conductive losses who cannot use traditional hearing aids. Candidacy for bone-anchored devices has been expanded to include individuals with atresia/microtia/malformed pinna, unilateral deafness, chronic ear drainage, chronic irritation from earmolds, and feedback or poor overall loudness with a traditional hearing aid. A recent five-year retrospective study comparing the functional gain benefit of the Baha fit versus traditional bone-conduction instruments found the Baha to provide statistically significant improvement in functional gain across the speech frequencies as compared to traditional bone-conduction instruments for children with congenital atresia/microtia (Christensen et al., 2010).

The BAHA also has been used extensively in recent years as an option for cases with single-sided deafness. In this application, the BAHA provides stimulation from the poor ear to the good cochlea through the skull via bone-conduction stimulation.

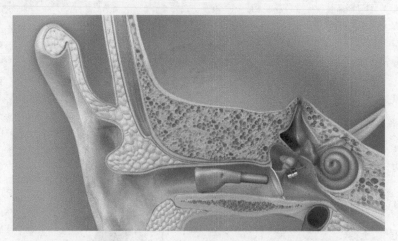

FIGURE 2.10 **Illustration of the MAXUM semi-implantable middle ear device.**
Source: Courtesy of Ototronix.

Middle Ear Implantable Hearing Aids

A very new development in the area of amplification is the use of either fully or partially implantable hearing aids in the middle ear for individuals with sensori-neural hearing loss. Two types of these devices are currently approved for use with adults by the FDA (Kahue et al., 2014). Partially implanted devices, such as the Vibrant Soundbridge available from MedEL Corporation, consist of an externally worn microphone and processor that drives a surgically implanted vibrator that is attached to one of the middle ear ossicles (usually the incus). Thus, rather than using standard acoustic stimulation of the eardrum, the middle ear implant vibrates the ossicular chain. These instruments avoid the problem of acoustic feedback and are helpful in individuals who cannot tolerate foreign bodies in their ear canal or for some other reason cannot wear a standard hearing aid.

The MAXUM System, available from Ototronixis (Figure 2.10), is another type of partially implanted device. It consists of a tiny rare-earth magnet implanted on the ossicular chain and a digital sound processor that is worn completely in the ear canal. Sounds are picked up by the microphone sound processor in the ear canal and transferred by electromagnetic energy across the eardrum to the MAXUM implant, which causes the ossicles to vibrate. The surgery can be performed under a local anesthetic and is done through the ear canal with no stitches required.

The Esteem middle ear implantable hearing aid was approved for use in adults in March 2010. The Esteem is the first fully implantable hearing aid for use in the United States. This device consists of a sensor that is attached to the ossicular chain and picks up vibrations from the eardrum, a sound processor that is implanted in the mastoid, and a driver that is attached to the stapes of the ossicular chain. A remote control is provided for the patient to change programs and volume and turn the instrument on and off. The instrument is powered by a battery in the sound processor. The estimated battery life is four and a half to nine years. At that point, the user must have surgery to change the battery. The developers of the Esteem have listed a number of possible advantages to their device, including invisibility, the ability to wear the device when swimming or at other times when a standard hearing aid could get wet, and the elimination of feedback and discomfort from wearing a standard hearing aid in the ear.

Currently, the cost of either a semi-implantable or fully implantable middle ear hearing aid is approximately $12,000 to $40,000 per ear, depending on the device. As with any surgery, there are risks. Patients must weigh the benefits and risks involved with such devices. With both types of devices, the surgeon (otolaryngologist) and the audiologist must work as a team for the patient to be a successful user. Very little published research is available on implantable hearing aids. Well-controlled evidence-based research is needed to show the advantages and disadvantages of these middle ear implantable devices compared to conventional amplification.

Surgical risks include temporary or permanent taste disturbances and facial paralysis due to close proximity to the VII cranial nerve. In addition, general surgical risks, such as those associated with anesthesia, need to be discussed with all candidates.

COCHLEAR AND BRAINSTEM IMPLANTS

Another important option for persons who do not receive significant benefit from traditional amplification is the use of cochlear implants. These devices are designed for individuals with severe to profound sensorineural hearing loss. Cochlear implants are surgically placed in the cochlea of the inner ear and stimulate the nerve ending for the VIII cranial or auditory nerve for the person to receive auditory stimulation. Brain stem implants are also an option for those individuals who do not have cochleae or functioning VIII nerves. These implants are placed on the cochlear nucleus, thereby bypassing the peripheral auditory system completely. Both implants are explained in depth in Chapter 3.

HEARING ASSISTIVE TECHNOLOGY, OR WHEN A HEARING AID MAY NOT BE ENOUGH

Although important personal amplification in the form of hearing aids should be viewed as the primary rehabilitative tool for most individuals with hearing loss, hearing assistive technology systems (HATS) can often be invaluable in helping the individual with hearing loss maintain independent function. HATS can improve the ability to listen/hear in background noise by reducing the distance to the microphone of the speaker, wake the client up by shaking the bed, or bark loudly when a car comes up the driveway! HATS work where hearing aids do not work well, and they provide the auditory information in ways (e.g., lights flashing, vibrotactile stimulation) that the person with hearing loss can use.

Types of Assistive Devices

HATS can be categorized by the area or space that needs to be covered, with large-area amplification systems specifically designed for auditoriums or individual devices designed for watching television. Devices can also be divided by purpose, such as

HATS or ALDs? What's the difference? HATS that help the individual with hearing in a specific situation, such as watching television, are often referred to as assistive listening devices (ALDs). The broader term, hearing assistive technologies (HATS), encompasses ALDs and devices for safety or alerting purposes.

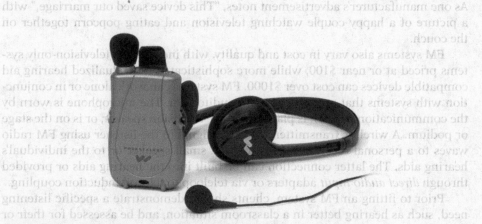

FIGURE 2.11 Hardwire personal amplifier system.
Source: Courtesy of Williams Sound LLC.

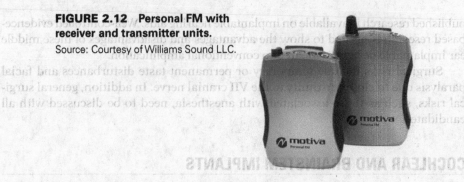

FIGURE 2.12 Personal FM with receiver and transmitter units.
Source: Courtesy of Williams Sound LLC.

safety or warning systems, telephone or television listening, or personal communication. HATS vary in their electronic sophistication, ranging from basic hardwire devices to sophisticated infrared systems designed for theaters or houses of worship.

Hardwire Devices. Hardwire devices are aptly named because they require a wire to connect the microphone to the amplifier and to the receiver/speaker in the individual's headset. These devices are small, with the microphone often being lapel style and the amplifier fitting into a pocket or easily clipped to the individual with hearing loss (see Figure 2.12 for an example of a simple hardwire device). The headsets vary with user preference, ranging from the larger foam "Walkman" style to earbuds. Hardwire devices work by electronically decreasing the distance from the speaker's mouth to the ear of the listener and thereby reduce background noise. These devices vary in quality but are relatively inexpensive and very durable, making them perfect for physicians' offices (reducing the need to "yell" at patients who cannot hear), in nursing homes where hearing aids may be easily lost, or as an inexpensive way to reduce road noise while conversing in a car. Hardwire devices are readily purchased through audiologists, online, or in electronics stores.

FM Sound Systems. Wireless frequency modulated (FM) sound systems operate in open space by sending radio waves from a transmitter to a receiver or speaker worn by or near the individual with hearing loss (see Figure 2.12). FM systems improve listening ability over distance and when in background noise by effectively reducing the distance of the speaker to the listener. FM works well in places of worship, meeting halls, concert halls, theaters, or schools while also working well in the comfort of the listener's den. Users have control over the gain, adjusting the entertainment system to their own comfortable listening level while their "normal" hearing companions are not overwhelmed or blasted out of the room by the volume. As one manufacturer's advertisement notes, "This device saved our marriage," with a picture of a happy couple watching television and eating popcorn together on the couch.

FM systems also vary in cost and quality, with inexpensive television-only systems priced at or near $100, while more sophisticated individualized hearing aid compatible devices can cost over $1000. FM systems can work alone or in conjunction with systems that are present in an auditorium. The microphone is worn by the communication partner, is placed near the television speaker, or is on the stage or podium. A wireless transmitter sends the signal to the listener using FM radio waves to a personal receiver headset or to a small speaker or to the individual's hearing aids. The latter connection can be built into the hearing aids or provided through *direct audio input* adapters or via teleloop to telecoil induction coupling.

Prior to fitting an FM system, clients should demonstrate a specific listening need, such as hearing better in a classroom situation, and be assessed for their or their caregiver's ability to use the device safely and effectively. The FM system must be compatible with their hearing aid system and undergo electroacoustic testing

Many hearing aids have a telecoil that allows for an electromagnetic field to transmit a signal to the hearing aid in a wireless manner. This can be very helpful for phone use as well as in a classroom or similar listening situation.

and real-ear measurements to verify its appropriateness. Validation measures or outcome measures must also be performed (see section to follow titled Verifying and Validating the Fitting of HATS.

Infrared Systems.   Infrared systems provide excellent sound quality by using the invisible infrared portion of the electromagnetic spectrum to transmit the signal from the microphone to headset receivers or any hearing aid equipped with a telecoil. Infrared systems and FM systems have overlapping purposes and places of use; however, infrared systems permit an unlimited number of receivers and contain the signal within a room, making them ideal for uses that require privacy, such as courtrooms. Infrared systems cannot be used in direct sunlight, as they are vulnerable to interference from natural lighting, and infrared signals will be blocked by pillars or columns.

Audio-Loop Systems.   An older but very cost-effective assistive listening device is the audio-loop system, a simple wire that surrounds the seating area. The talker's microphone signal is transmitted to the wire, creating an electrical current with a subsequent magnetic field that is picked up by the telecoil in the hearing aid. Audio loops can be permanently installed or moved from room to room as needed and operate using a universally hearing aid–accessible signal versus a specific FM radio signal. They do not require a specialized headset; rather, the hearing aid user simply accesses the signal through his or her own hearing aid. Currently, the American Academy of Audiology and other interested parties are advocating for increasing the awareness of and use of audio-loop systems through a public relations campaign: Loop America. This organization is promoting the use of loops in movie theaters, meeting rooms, and even drive-through lanes at banks and fast-food restaurants (Kricos, 2010).

Telephone Listening Devices.   Telephone conversation poses a unique challenge to individuals with hearing loss, as they must rely on a limited auditory signal with no visual input to communicate. Cellular telephones have only added to their telephone listening dilemma, as many conversations occur in the confusion of our noisy world. One of the simplest methods to improve landline telephone listening is to add an amplifier either built into the telephone handset or as an extra "line-in" unit that connects between the wall jack and the telephone. Portable amplifiers that snap onto the handset are also available for traveling.

Cellular telephones are really radios, and, as such, their signals are impacted by metal near them. The presence of a hearing aid on the ear of the user therefore can act as an antenna bringing the sound in or as a form of interference distorting the signal. The effective use of cellular telephones and hearing aids requires the cooperation of the hearing aid manufacturer, the audiologist, cellular telephone manufacturers, and the telephone user. Individuals with hearing loss should work with their cellular service provider in finding an amplified telephone that works well with their particular hearing aid. One solution is to use Bluetooth to connect the cellular phone directly to the hearing aid. Bluetooth connectivity provides a direct link to the hearing aid, permitting the hearing aid user to access his or her personal amplification while listening on the cellular telephone.

Smartphone technology can also serve as a sophisticated remote control using Bluetooth connectivity to change volume and manipulate frequencies while using the telephone microphone as a remote microphone. Hearing aid wearers can adjust the device for a particular setting, such as a weekly board meeting. When they return to that location, the geotracker on their smartphone can identify the location and ask the wearer if he or she wants last week's successful settings! This is truly not your mother's hearing aid.

Cellular phones have advanced the use of texting or typing messages rather than calling, so individuals with hearing loss simply type and read messages rather

Direct audio input (DAI) is a way to connect some BTE hearing aids to external sound sources, such as MP3 players, computers, or televisions. DAI reduces the effects of background noise and permits the user to hear the device using the amplification parameters of his or her hearing aid. Hearing aids have special connectors on the bottom for DAI.

than try to hear. Videoconference calls (e.g., Skype), e-mail, and Facebook are also available for all with computer Internet service access. Videoconferencing has proven to be a true boon to individuals who are fluent in American Sign Language, as the users can see full views of the individual signing, permitting better understanding of the message. Gone are the days when the Deaf individual needed to purchase expensive add-on telephone equipment, such as a Telecommunication Device for the Deaf (TDD). Refer to the shaded text for a brief explanation of older systems.

In the not-so-distant past, Deaf individuals used text telephones or Telecommunication Device for the Deaf (TDD) or, the older term for the same device, Teletypewriters (TTY). These devices attached to landline telephones by coupling to the headset of the telephone. Both users needed TDDs so that each could type messages on the device keyboard. The message was transmitted via a modem through the telephone line to the receiver's keyboard to an LED screen or printout. TDDs were a major part of the Telephone Relay Service, which permitted calls from individuals using TDDs to individuals with standard telephones. Now, the caller can text a message to a central relay operator who then calls and speaks to the end user with the message. This service is provided in real time and is funded by a charge on all landline telephone user bills.

Individuals who cannot hear the telephone ringing can use visual alerting devices, such as a lamp that blinks to signal that the telephone ringing. Telephones can also be hooked up to louder ringers or bells, or extra remote ringers can be placed throughout the house to aid in hearing them. Cellular telephones should be set to vibrate and ring simultaneously or through the use of an app; they will vibrate and flash to signal incoming calls.

Television Assistive Technologies. FM, infrared, hardwire, and audio-loop systems can all be modified or specifically built to improve television listening. Individuals either use their own hearing aids through direct audio connections or telecoils or use lightweight headsets with volume controls. Another excellent option for television viewing is closed captioning. As of July 1, 1993, all televisions 13 inches or larger manufactured or sold in the United States needed to have closed-caption ability. Captions have not only benefited individuals with hearing loss but have also been cited as being helpful to individuals learning to read English and by anyone stuck in a noisy airport waiting for departure time (McCall & Craig, 2009).

Alert/Alarm Assistive Technologies. Alerting devices serve the dual purpose of informing individuals of potentially dangerous situations and providing the convenience of being aware of sounds in their environments. The latter includes flashing lights associated with the telephone ringing, doorbell ringing, or microwave buzzing. Individuals can be "gently" awoken by a shaking alarm clock or remember an appointment by a vibrating watch or telephone alarm. Multipurpose devices can flash or vibrate for doorbells, smoke alarms, carbon monoxide detectors, baby cries, or kitchen timers. Again, a variety of cellular phone apps exist that will sense sounds in the environment and create specific alerts for that sound. For example, the baby crying would cause the screen to flash, while the doorbell may make the phone vibrate.

Apps are truly blurring the lines between what is a hearing aid, a hearing assistive technology, and a cellular phone. Besides using the cell phone microphone as a remote microphone for the hearing aid or having the phone flash when the dog barks, apps permit real-time voice-to-text dictation and provide subtitles for video viewing. Certain apps can permit the user to perform a miniature self-hearing test and then use that information to change the volume of the phone to match the "self-audiogram."

Perhaps one of the most enjoyable alerting devices is the "hearing dog." Hearing dogs, or dogs for the deaf, are trained to bark or come get the individual if the telephone or doorbell rings or to lead an individual outside and away from a sound, such as a fire alarm. Hearing dogs can also be trained to respond to noises in the environment, such as cars honking or the beeping sounds of equipment backing up. The Americans with Disabilities Act (ADA, 1990) ensures that individuals with hearing dogs have access to all public spaces.

The Role of the Audiologist in Assistive Listening/Hearing Assistive Technology Systems

Audiologists serve as the logical service provider for many HATS, as the systems require compatibility with personal hearing aids and/or specific programming for the type and degree of hearing loss. Audiologists have the necessary training in determining what devices will work well in a given listening situation because they are aware of the benefits and constraints of the systems. In keeping with the current mind-set of providing universal information access to all individuals, HATS permit greater autonomy for individuals who are deaf or hard of hearing, and audiologists need to advocate for the installation and use of such systems in public environments. Audiologists should also serve as the primary source of information on personal HATS, helping the client, family, and caregivers understand how to appropriately use and care for the device. The aging of the population will only serve to increase the market for assistive technology, providing an obvious financial incentive for audiologists, but, more important, HATS are an integral part of hearing health care. Audiologists who are well versed in assistive technologies can use HATS to help alleviate the ongoing stress of trying to communicate for individuals with hearing loss and their families.

Verifying and Validating the Fitting of HATS

The decision to fit a HATS should be made based on client need and listening situation. Audiologists can use the client case history or responses on specific background noise or listening situation questions on self-assessment tools, such as the Abbreviated Profile of Hearing Aid Benefit (APHAB; Cox & Alexander, 1995) or the Hearing Performance Inventory—Revised (HPI-R; Lamb, Owens, & Schuber, 1983). For example, a client who reports difficulty when listening to television may benefit from a television amplifier/streamer connection to his or her hearing aid, while another may complain of background noise issues and could use a remote microphone. The client should also be questioned about his or her interest and motivation in using a HATS and demonstrate an ability to use the device or have a communication partner who can aid him or her in its use.

Validation or real-world worthiness of the HATS can be measured through client report of hours or time of use or through improvement on a self-report validation scale. One more objective validation measure would be to have successful use of the HATS as a goal on an outcome measure, such as the Client Oriented Scale of Improvement (COSI; Dillon et al., 1997). The Veterans Administration has an excellent comprehensive protocol for selection, verification, and validation of FM systems and HATS/ALDS (see recommended readings) that could serve as a model for audiologists interested in developing a HATS/ALDS program for their clinic.

THE BOTTOM LINE: COST MANAGEMENT AND PAYMENT FOR HEARING AIDS AND HATS

Individuals and families note that one of the primary barriers to purchasing hearing aids is cost (Abrams & Kihm, 2015). Price per unit varies from around $1000 per instrument up to $4000 per aid, depending on the sophistication of the device (number of automatic programs, noise-canceling algorithms, Bluetooth capability, etc.) and geographic location of the clinic (rental expense, employee salaries, etc.).

The Americans with Disabilities Act (1990) was signed into law by President George H. W. Bush. The law is modeled after civil rights legislation and prohibits discrimination based on disability defined as a physical or mental impairment that substantially limits a major life activity. The law was expanded in 2008 to include more protections for disabled workers (ADA Amendments Act, 2008), including those with hearing loss.

Currently, hearing aids are usually sold as "bundled" deals that include the instrument, earmold, fitting expense, warranty, and a given number of office visits or other perks, such as batteries. Although this means little out-of-pocket expense while the instrument is covered, the initial price is much higher than simply buying the hearing aid and paying for the warranty or office visit as needed. To bundle or not to bundle, however, remains a question to be played out as audiologists determine what works best for business profitability.

Other factors are also rapidly impacting and changing the hearing aid market. Hearing aids are being covered by more health insurance policies, with individual policyholders being given specific funding amounts every few years to put toward hearing aids. Other plans have audiologists on contract as preferred providers or send the hearing aid to the individual prefit, with an audiologist in the region available for any issues. The latter model has, however, been called into question by various state licensure boards as being unethical or going against state hearing aid sales regulations. In some states, hearing aids can be purchased online, but the old maxim "let the buyer beware" certainly applies. Hearing aids are sophisticated medical devices that can, when misfit, cause harm. They are not your usual Amazon or Craigslist fare. As an alternative, all audiologists should have a go-to list of local, state, and national foundations, charities, and hearing aid companies that are willing to pay for or work with the client in providing access to hearing health care.

CONCLUDING REMARKS

Hearing aids and hearing assistive technology are great rehabilitative tools for persons with hearing loss, but they will not restore hearing to normal. Modern technology has greatly enhanced the benefits our patients can receive from amplification. Audiologists need to remain abreast of new advances in both technology and fitting procedures to provide their patients with the best care. Dispensing of hearing aids and other amplification devices can be some of the most rewarding work in the field of audiology. Providing amplification can truly change the quality of life of persons with hearing loss, allowing them to be part of their family, in society and, in the case of children, providing them with the needed auditory information for both speech and language development and educational advancement.

Summary Points

- The basic components of a hearing aid are the microphone, amplifier, and speaker (receiver). Using algorithms designed to improve speech perception, modern digital instruments are programmed to individualize the fitting.

- Hearing aids come in a variety of styles, including BTE, ITE, ITC, and CIC models.

- Earmolds and all ITE hearing aid shells are often molded to fit the client's ear and couple the hearing aid to the ear. The audiologist can use the earmold's style, tubing, venting, and damping to change the sound going into the ear.

- Hearing aids are appropriate for individuals with hearing loss that cannot be medically or surgically remediated. The fitting process must include a full hearing evaluation and an evaluation of the client's communication difficulties and motivation.

- Most individuals with hearing loss benefit from wearing two hearing aids: a binaural fitting. A hearing aid in both ears improves listening in background noise and helps in sound localization.

- Hearing aid fitting protocols must include selection of the device, quality control, orientation/fitting, and validation with outcome measures. All aspects of the protocol are vital to a successful hearing aid fitting.

- Individuals with unilateral hearing loss can benefit from CROS hearing aids or implantable bone-anchored hearing aids.

- Successful pediatric fittings require a team approach with members including the audiologist, speech pathologist, teachers of the deaf and hard of hearing, and the parents. The audiologist must ensure that the wearer or, in the case of the pediatric fitting, the caregivers know how to remove and work the controls, troubleshoot the instrument, do a listening check, and care for and clean the instruments.

- HATS/ALDs are designed for specific listening situations, such as television, telephone, or auditorium listening. ALDs can be helpful for people with hearing loss and also helpful to all of us when in difficult listening environments, such as watching television in the airport by using the captions.

Supplementary Learning Activities

See www.isu/edu/audiology/rehab to carry out these activities. We encourage you to use these to supplement your learning. Your instructor may give specific assignments that involve a particular activity.

1. Hearing Aid Experience: This activity provides the student with an experience with a hearing aid under two options. Option 1 involves wearing a hearing aid under controlled conditions. Using the information related to this chapter found on the book's website, the student is directed on the correct way to place an instructor-supplied BTE hearing aid (programmed for minimal gain/output) in his or her ear. After using the hearing aid in three or four different listening situations (watching television, taking a walk, socializing, attending class, etc.), the student might write a one- to two-page paper describing his or her experiences. For option 2, the student wears a nonfunctioning BTE hearing aid in three or four situations, noting the reactions he or she observes (from others as well as his or her own reactions as a hearing aid user). Again, students may be asked by the instructor to write a brief summary of the experience.

2. Gathering Information about Hearing Aids/HATS: The student accesses one website for a major hearing aid manufacturer and gathers information regarding the contents of that site (hearing aid models, features of each, etc.) and may be assigned to write a brief one- to two-page summary. The student could do the same thing for a major manufacturer/distributor of HATS.

3. To help in applying new information about hearing aids to the real world, the students could make arrangements with the audiology clinic at their university to observe a clinical activity involving hearing aids (hearing aid selection, hearing aid fitting/verification, hearing aid orientation, etc.). Note the process used and the outcome.

4. Students could conduct and film interviews with individuals with hearing loss regarding their path in choosing HATS, hearing aids, and/or surgical options. Questions could include the pros and cons of different device choices and how users learn about options in technology.

5. The class could develop a list of local venues who provide HATS and provide copies of the list to local audiologists.

6. "A Day in the Life": In this activity, students work in groups to design a "smart" technology day for an individual with hearing loss.

Recommended Reading

American Speech-Language-Hearing Association. (n.d.). *Hearing assistive technology*. Retrieved from http://www.asha.org, 2016.

Dillon, H. (2012). *Hearing Aids* (2nd ed.). New York: Thieme.

Gelfand, S. (2009). *Essentials of audiology*. New York: Thieme.

Kompis, M., Caversaccio, M., Arnold, W., & Randolph, G. (2011). *Implantable bone conduction hearing aids*. Basel: S. Karger.

Johnson, C. E. (2012). *Introduction to auditory rehabilitation: A contemporary approach*. Boston: Allyn & Bacon.

Johnson, C. E., & Danhauer, J. L. (2002). *Handbook of outcome measurement in audiology*. Independence, KY: Thomson Delmar Learning.

Katz, J., Chasin, M., English, K., Hood, L. J., & Tillery, K. L. (2014). *The handbook of clinical audiology* (7th ed.). New York: Wolters Kluwer.

Madell, J., & Flexer, C. (2008). Hearing aids for infants and children. In *Pediatric audiology: diagnosis, technology, and management* (pp. 168–170). New York: Thieme.

Madell, J., & Flexer, C. (2011). *Pediatric audiology casebook*. New York: Thieme.

Newton, V. (2009). Managing the listening environment: Classroom acoustics and assistive listening devices. In *Paediatric audiological medicine* (pp. 312–387). Chichester: Wiley.

Roeser, R. (2013). *Audiology desk reference: A guide to the practice of audiology*. New York: Thieme.

Valente, M., Hosford-Dunn, H., & Roeser, R. (2008). Hearing aid selection and fitting in adults. In *Audiology: Treatment* (pp. 119–158). New York: Thieme.

Recommended Websites

American Academy of Audiology:
http://www.audiology.org

American Speech-Language-Hearing Association:
http://www.asha.org

Cochlear BAHA
http://www.cochlear.com

Envoy Medical, Esteem Middle Ear Implant:
http://www.esteemhearing.com

Harc Mercantile:
http://www.harcmercantile.com

Harris Communications:
http://www.harriscomm.com

Hearing Aid Research Laboratory:
http://www.harlmemphis.org

Hearing Loss Association of America:
http://www.hearingloss.org

Idaho State University Communication Sciences and Disorders:
http://www.isu.edu/csd

National Acoustics Laboratory (Australia):
http://www.nal.gov.au

The Oticon Ponto:
http://www.oticonmedical.com

Otologics:
http://www.otologics.com

The Oticon Ponto:
http://www.oticonmedical.com/ponto/us/medical

The Phonak Lyric:
http://www.phonak.com

TV Ears:
http://www.tvears.com

Williams Sound:
http://www.williamssound.com

References

Abrams HB, Kihm J. (2015). An introduction to MarkeTrak IX: A new baseline for the hearing aid market. *Hearing Review*, 22(6), 16–21. http://www.hearingreview.com/article/introduction-marketrak-ix-new-baseline-hearing-aid-market

American National Standards Institute. (2009). *Specification of hearing aid characteristics* (ANSI S3.22-2009). New York: Author.

Americans with Disabilities Act. (1990). Public Law 101-336, 42 USC Sec. 12101. Equal opportunity for the disabled. Washington, DC: U.S. Government Printing Office.

ADA Amendments Act. (2008). Public Law 110-325, 122 Stat. 3553. Washington, DC: U.S. Government Printing Office.

Anderson, K. (2002). *Early listening function: Discovery tool for parents and caregivers of infants and toddlers*. Retrieved from http://www.phonak.com, 2016.

Bauman, N. (2012). *The Hearing Aid Museum website*. Retrieved from http://hearingaidmuseum.com, 2016.

Byrne, D., Dillon, H., Ching, T., Katsch, R., & Keidser, G. (2001). NALNL1 procedure for fitting nonlinear hearing aids: Characteristics and comparisons with other procedures. *Journal of the American Academy of Audiology*, 12, 37–51.

Ching, T., O'Brien, A., Dillon, H., Chalupper, J., Hartley, L., Hartley, D., et al. (2009). Directional effects on infants and young children in real life: Implications for amplification. *Journal of Speech, Language, and Hearing Research*, 52, 1241–1254.

Christensen, L., Smith-Olinde, L., Kimberlain, J., Richter, G., & Dornhoffer, J. (2010). Comparison of traditional bone-conduction hearing aids with the Baha® system. *Journal of the American Academy of Audiology*, 21, 267–273.

Cox, R. M. (2005). Evidence-based practice in provision of amplification. *Journal of the American Academy of Audiology*, 16(7), 419–435.

Cox, R. M., & Alexander, G. C. (1995) The Abbreviated Profile of Hearing Aid Benefit (APHAB). *Ear and Hearing*, 16, 176–186.

Cox, R. M., & Alexander, G. C. (2001). *International Outcomes Inventory for Hearing Aids*. Paper presented at the annual meeting of the American Auditory Society, Scottsdale, AZ.

Cox, R. M., Alexander, G. C., Taylor, I. M., & Gray, G. A. (1997). The Contour Test of Loudness Perception. *Ear and Hearing*, 18, 388–400.

Cox, R., & Gilmore, C. (1986). Damping the hearing aid frequency response: Effects on speech clarity and preferred listening level. *Journal of Speech and Hearing Research*, 29, 357–365.

Cox R. M., Hyde, M., Gatehouse, S., Noble, W., Dillion, H., Bentler, R.,et al. (2000). Optimal outcome measures, research priorities and international cooperation. *Ear and Hearing*, 21, 106S–115S.

Dillon, H., James, A., & Ginis, J. (1997). Client Oriented Scale of Improvement (COSI) and its relationship to several other measures of benefit and satisfaction provided by hearing aids. *Journal of the American Academy of Audiology*, 8(1), 27–43.

Gatehouse, S. (1999). Glasgow Hearing Aid Benefit Profile: Derivation and validation of a client-centered outcome measure for hearing-aid services. *Journal of the American Academy of Audiology*, 10, 80–103.

Hirsch, I., Davis, H., Silverman, S. R., Reynolds, E. G., Eldert, E., & Benson, R. W. (1952). Development of materials for speech audiometry. *Journal of Speech and Hearing Disorders, 17,* 321–337.

Hodes, M., Schow, R., & Brockett, J. (2009). New support for hearing aid outcome measures: The computerized SAC and SOAC. *Hearing Review, 16*(12), 26–36.

Kahue, C. N., M. L. Carlson, Daugherty, J., Haynes, D., & Glancock, M.. (2014). Middle ear implants for rehabilitation of sensorineural hearing loss: A systematic review of FDA approved devices. *Otology and Neurotology, 35*(7), 1228–1237.

Kemker, B., Goshorn, E., & Kaplan, H. (2015). Analysis of hearing instrument use, satisfaction, and operation in independent male veterans. *Asia Pacific Speech, Language and Hearing, 15*(1), 19–28.

Killion, M., & Mueller, H. G. (2010). Twenty years later: A new count-the-dot method. *Hearing Journal, 10,* 12–14, 16–17.

Killion, M. C., Niquette, P. A., Gudmundsen, G. I., Revit, L. J., & Banerjee, S. (2004). Development of a quick speech-in-noise test for measuring signal-to-noise ratio loss in normal-hearing and hearing-impaired listeners. *Journal of the Acoustical Society of America, 116*(4), 2395–2405.

Kricos, P. (2010, September/October). Looping America: One way to improve accessibility for people with hearing loss. *Audiology Today,* 38–43.

Kuk, F., & Baekgaard, L. (2008). Hearing aid selection and BTEs: Choosing among various "open ear" and "receiver in canal" options. *Hearing Review, 15*(3), 22–36.

McCall, W. G., & Craig, C. (2009). Same-Language-Subtitling (SLS): Using subtitled music video for reading growth. In G. Siemens & C. Fulford (Eds.), *Proceedings of World Conference on Educational Multimedia, Hypermedia and Telecommunications 2009* (pp. 3983–3992). Chesapeake, VA: Association for the Advancement of Computing in Education. Retrieved from http://www.editlib.org/p/32055, 2016.

Mueller, G., & Killion, M. (1990). An easy method for calculation of the Articulation Index. *Hearing Journal, 45*(9), 14–17.

Nabelek, A. K., Tucker, F. M., & Letowski, T. R. (1991). Toleration of background noises: Relationship with patterns of hearing aid use by elderly persons. *Journal of Speech and Hearing Research, 34,* 679–685.

Neuman, A. (1993). *Hearing aids: Recent developments.* Baltimore: York Press.

Nilsson, M., Soli, S. D., & Sullivan, J. A. (1994). Development of the Hearing in Noise Test for the measurement of speech reception thresholds in quiet and in noise. *Journal of the Acoustical Society of America, 95*(2), 1085–1099.

Phonak Hearing Instruments. (2016). *Lyric hearing.* Retrieved March 15, 2016 from https://www.phonak.com/en_us/hearing-aids/lyric-invisible-hearing-aids.html

Pollack, M. (1988). *History and development of hearing aids: Amplification for the hearing impaired* (3rd ed.). Orlando, FL: Grune & Stratton.

Robbins, A., Renshaw, J., & Berry, S. (2001). Evaluating meaningful auditory integration in profoundly hearing-impaired children. *American Journal of Otology, 12*(3), 144–150.

Schow, R. L. (2001). A standardized AR battery for dispensers. *Hearing Journal, 54*(8), 10–20.

Schow, R. L., & Nerbonne, M. (1982). Communication screening profile: Use with elderly clients. *Ear and Hearing, 3*(3), 133–147.

Scollie, S., Ching, T. Y. C., Seewald, R., Dillon, H., Britton, L., Steinberg, J., et al. (2010). Children's speech perception and loudness ratings when fitted with hearing aids using the DSL v4.1 and the NAL-NL1 prescriptions. *International Journal of Audiology, 49,* S26–S34.

Seewald, R. C., Moodie, S. T., & Scollie, S. D. (2005). The DSL method for pediatric hearing instrument fitting: Historical perspective and current issues. *Trends in Amplification, 9*(4), 145–157.

Staab, W. (2015). April 28, 2015 hearinghealthmatters.org, retrieved 2016.

Stephens, S., & Goodwin, J. (1984). Non-electric aids to hearing a short history. *International Journal of Audiology, 23*(2), 215–240.

Sweetow, R. & Sabes, J. (2006). The need for and development of an adaptive Listening and Communication Enhancement (LACE®) program. *Journal of the American Academy of Audiology, 17,* 538–558.

Tillman, T. W., & Carhart, R. (1966). *An expanded test for speech discrimination utilizing CNC monosyllabic words.* Northwestern University Auditory Test No. 6 (U.S. Air

Force School of Aviation Medicine Report SAM-TR-66-55). Brooks Air Force Base, TX: USAF School of Aerospace Medicine.

Valente, M. (2002). *Hearing aids: Standards, options, and limitations* (2nd ed.). New York: Thieme.

Valente, M., Abrams, H., Benson, D., Chisolm, T., Citron, D., Hampton, D., et al. (2008). Guidelines for the audiologic management of adult hearing impairment. *Audiology Today, 18*(5), 32–36.

Ventry, I. M., & Weinstein, B. E. (1982). The Hearing Handicap Inventory for the Elderly: A new tool. *Ear and Hearing, 3*, 128–134.

Wilson, R. H. (2003). Development of a speech in multitalker babble paradigm to assess word-recognition performance. *Journal of the American Academy of Audiology, 14*, 453–470.

Zimmerman-Phillips, S., Osberger, M., & Robbins, A. (1997). *Assessment of auditory skills in children two years of age or younger.* Paper presented at the Fifth International Cochlear Implant Conference, New York.

Cochlear Implants

Alice E. Holmes

CONTENTS

Visit the companion website when you see this icon to learn more about the topic nearby in the text.

Learning Outcomes

After reading this chapter, you will be able to

- List the major components of a typical cochlear implant system
- Identify the three major companies currently marketing cochlear implants in the United States with Food and Drug Administration approval
- List seven potential members of a cochlear implant team
- Describe the candidacy requirements for a cochlear implant currently being utilized for an adult and for a child
- Explain what *hook-up* and *MAP* refer to regarding a cochlear implant
- Describe the main distinction in how a "hybrid" cochlear implant functions when compared to a conventional cochlear implant

INTRODUCTION

Breakthroughs in audiology now allow us to assist persons in ways never thought of 40 years ago. Specializations within audiologic rehabilitation have developed for helping those with severe to profound hearing loss, and many now have the potential to receive sound information through the use of cochlear implants and other specialized instruments. Not all audiologists deal with these issues commonly in their practices, but they need to know when to refer their patients to these specialized audiology clinics. This chapter provides an overview of these specialized options in audiologic rehabilitation.

Most persons who are diagnosed with a sensorineural hearing loss are fitted with hearing aids and can receive varying amounts of benefit from these devices. Unfortunately, for some individuals with severe to profound hearing loss, these traditional amplification devices may offer only limited or no help, even with extensive experience and audiologic rehabilitation. Even the most powerful amplifiers are unable to provide meaningful information for environmental sound awareness or speech perception for persons with little or no residual hearing. Cochlear implant technology has offered many of these individuals an alternative means to receive some important information from their limited auditory systems.

A cochlear implant is a device that electrically stimulates the auditory nerve of patients with severe to profound hearing loss to provide them with sound and speech information. It is not an amplifier that increases the level of the acoustic signal but rather a surgically implanted device that bypasses the peripheral auditory system to directly simulate the auditory nerve. The cochlear implant does not restore normal hearing. Cochlear implant recipients vary in the amount of benefit that they receive from the device. Some individuals are

Cochlear implant: A device that electrically stimulates the auditory nerve of patients with severe to profound hearing loss to provide them with sound and speech information.

Open-set speech perception tests: Listener has an unlimited number of response possibilities.

Closed-set speech perception tests: Listener is given a choice of multiple responses.

provided with auditory awareness, detection of environmental sounds, and improvement in their speechreading abilities, while other patients are able to achieve open-set speech perception without visual cues. Many individuals are able to conduct conversations over the telephone.

How Does a Cochlear Implant Work?

Several cochlear implant systems are available worldwide. Each has its own unique characteristics, advantages, and disadvantages, but all operate using the same basic principles. All cochlear implant systems commonly in use consist of an externally worn headset connected to an ear-level or body-worn speech processor with a battery source and a surgically implanted internal receiver stimulator attached to the electrode array that is placed in the cochlea.

Figure 3.1 shows one of the commercially available cochlear implant systems with an external ear-level speech processor and an internal receiver stimulator attached to an electrode array. The internal receiver stimulator is surgically implanted in the mastoid bone behind the pinna, and the electrode array is threaded through the middle ear space into the cochlea. The ear-level processor shown is a behind-the-ear device consisting of a microphone, a speech processor, and a battery. It is connected via wire to a transmitter coil or antenna with a magnet that adheres to the head over the skin where the receiver stimulator is placed. The microphone picks up the sound wave, converts it into an electrical signal, and sends it to the speech processor. The speech processor codes the information using a device-specific strategy and sends it to the external transmitter coil. The coil sends the information through the skin via FM radio waves to an internal receiver stimulator, which in turn sends the information to the implanted electrodes that stimulate the available auditory nerve fibers. The auditory nerve then sends the information to the brain so that the person can perceive sound stimulation. This all occurs in a matter of microseconds.

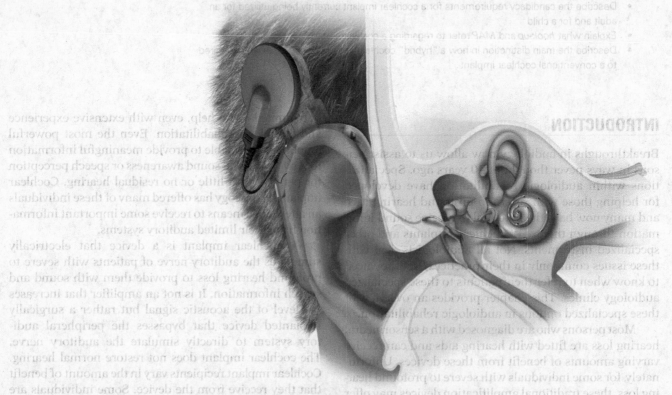

FIGURE 3.1 **Components of a cochlear implant system.**

Source: Image Courtesy of Cochlear Americas, © 2011.

History of Cochlear Implants

In 1972, the first wearable cochlear implant was implanted in an adult at the House Ear Institute. The House/3M device consisted of a single electrode implanted in the basal end of the cochlea with a ground electrode placed in the Eustachian tube. This device was capable of providing the patient with information on the presence or absence of sound, durational cues, and intensity cues. Even with this limited information, many individuals had improved speechreading abilities and were able to learn to identify many environmental sounds with training. Over 1000 persons received this commercially available device. In 1980, the device became available for use in children over the age of 2 years (Wilson, 2000).

Multielectrode devices came into wide use in the 1980s. With these systems, limited frequency cues became available to the patients, and many patients were achieving some open-set speech understanding without the use of visual cues. In 1985, the U.S. Food and Drug Administration (FDA) approved the use of the Nucleus 22-Channel Cochlear Implant System for adults with *postlingual* profound deafness. In 1990, the FDA also approved the use of the device in children over the age of 2 years.

Continued development of cochlear implant systems and the speech-processing strategies over the past two decades have resulted in marked improvements. The 1995 National Institute of Health Consensus Statement on Cochlear Implants reported that the majority of adults with recent processors achieve over 80 percent correct on high-context open-set sentence materials in an auditory-only condition. Most of these individuals became deaf as adults. Cosmetic improvements have included a reduction in the size of the body-worn speech processors and the development of totally ear-level devices.

Postlingual hearing loss occurs after a person has developed speech and language abilities normally (they generally become deaf as adults).

Persons with perilingual hearing loss are those whose hearing loss developed during speech and language development.

Prelingual hearing loss is defined as hearing loss occurring prior to or very early in speech and language development (e.g., born deaf).

Current Systems

Currently, the FDA has granted approval to three companies for cochlear implant systems for general use with both children and adults in the United States. In 2012, worldwide, over 324,200 cochlear implants had been registered from these companies, according to the National Institutes of Health (https://www.nidcd.nih.gov/health/cochlear-implants), and over 50,000 devices have been implanted each year since 2012 (http://www.medel.com/us/cochlear-implants). Many of these users have a cochlear implant in each ear. The products from each of the companies have some unique features, but the patient performance across companies is similar (Firszt et al., 2004). The choice of which device is appropriate for which patient is generally based on the options available.

Cochlear Limited is headquartered in Sydney, Australia, and was the first company to receive FDA approval for multichannel devices in 1985. Its current model is the Nucleus® 6 System (Figure 3.2), which includes the titanium cochlear implant, an ear-level processor, and a remote control. The System has six programs, which suit different hearing environments and can automatically change to use the best program.

All current cochlear implant systems offer remote control options for the recipients. These remote controls give the cochlear implant users the ability to easily change programs, volume controls, and so on.

The HiResolution Advantage System from Advanced Bionics (Figure 3.3) was developed and is manufactured in the United States. This system has the option of either an ear-level processor or a body-worn processor. It has the fastest processing speed in the industry and multiple wearing options. In addition, it has the only processer that can be used in water sports and bathing without enclosing it in a case (Figure 3.4).

The third device approved for use in the United States was developed and is manufactured by MED-EL Corporation in Austria. The SYNCHRONY Cochlear Implant System is MED-EL's technology (Figure 3.5), which includes a titanium implant and a choice of either an ear-level BTE processor (SONNET) or a single-unit speech processor (RONDO). The RONDO headset encases the microphone, speech processor, transmitting coil, and battery pack in a single unit that is worn on the mastoid over the internal receiver/stimulator. The internal implant allows for

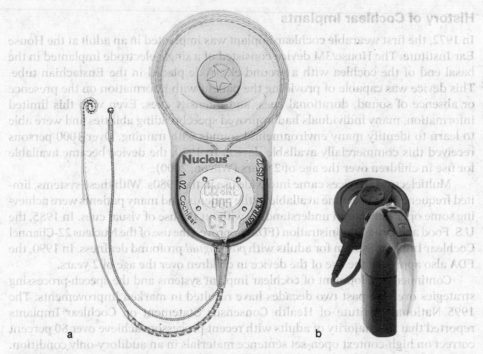

FIGURE 3.2 Nucleus 6 Cochlear implant system: (a) internal titanium cochlear implant, (b) external speech processor and coil.
Source: Images courtesy of Cochlear Americas, © 2017.

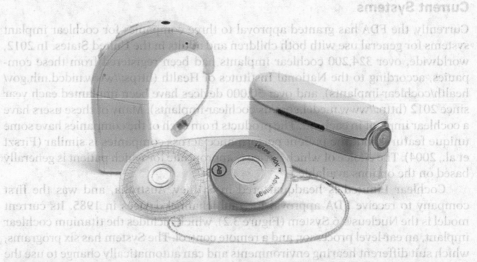

FIGURE 3.3 Advanced Bionics HiResolution System: Naída CI Q70 Ear Level processors, HiRes internal cochlear implant, and a Neptune Swimmable Processor.
Source: Courtesy of Advanced Bionics, LLC.

low- or high-resolution magnetic resonance imaging (MRI) without removal of the internal magnet. The magnet also can be removed if necessary, such as when a clear MRI image of the area near the implant is needed. The other companies require surgical removal of the internal magnet prior to any MRI. For persons who know they may need multiple MRIs, the SYNCHRONY is often the implant of choice.

Two other companies are manufacturing and fitting cochlear implants worldwide that do not currently have FDA approval in the United States. The Neuro System from Oticon Corporation consists of the Neuro Zti implant and an ear-level processor. Nurotron Biotechnology Co. Ltd is a new company that manufactures

The FDA classifies cochlear implants as Class III devices. Manufacturers must submit applications and provide information on the safety and efficacy of the devices, including extensive clinical data. Each new processor, implant, and software package must receive FDA approval for the devices to be implanted, programmed, and serviced in the United States.

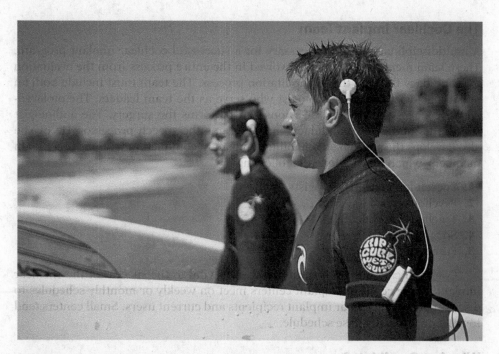

FIGURE 3.4   Two cochlear implant recipients using the Neptune Swimmable Processor.
Source: Courtesy of Advanced Bionics, LLC.

cochlear implants in China. This system has both ear-level and body-worn speech processors that couple to their internal implants.

Companies use their own proprietary coding strategies in their speech processors. The coding strategies are designed to transform the important characteristics of speech or sound input into the electrical pulses that stimulate the auditory nerve. These characteristics include pitch (frequency), loudness (intensity), and phase (timing) cues.

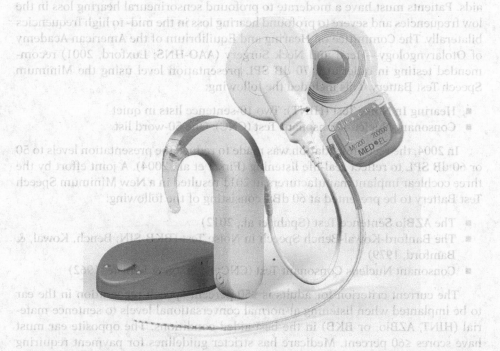

FIGURE 3.5   MED-EL SYNCHRONY cochlear implant system: internal cochlear implant, the SONNET BTE speech processor, and the RONDO single-unit speech processor.
Source: Images courtesy of MED-EL Corporation.

The Cochlear Implant Team

A multidisciplinary team is necessary for a successful cochlear implant program. These team members should be involved in the entire process from the evaluation for candidacy through the re/habilitation process. The team must include both an otolaryngologist and an audiologist who serve as the team leaders. The otolaryngologist makes the medical decisions and performs the surgery. The audiologist determines audiologic candidacy and programs the speech processor. He or she also develops the audiologic rehabilitation plan in conjunction with the other team members, which may include the following:

1. Speech-language pathologists
2. Psychologists
3. Teachers of the deaf
4. Social workers
5. Parents

Communication among team members is vital to the success of the cochlear implant. Large cochlear implant centers meet on weekly or monthly schedules to discuss potential cochlear implant recipients and current users. Small centers tend to meet on a case-by-case schedule.

Who Is a Candidate?

Not everyone is a candidate for a cochlear implant. Candidacy evaluations generally consist of a number of evaluations with several team members. With the improved outcomes, the criteria for implantation have vastly expanded since the 1980s when only adults with profound postlingual hearing loss were eligible. Currently, the FDA has approved the use of cochlear implants in persons over the age of 12 months.

The FDA approves each implant with varying audiologic guidelines based on the clinical data provided to them by the manufacturer. The current most lenient audiologic guidelines (see Table 3.1) are based on the performance of cochlear implant recipients as opposed to those with similar hearing losses wearing hearing aids. Patients must have a moderate to profound sensorineural hearing loss in the low frequencies and severe to profound hearing loss in the mid- to high frequencies bilaterally. The Committee on Hearing and Equilibrium of the American Academy of Otolaryngology—Head and Neck Surgery (AAO-HNS; Luxford, 2001) recommended testing in quiet at a 70 dB SPL presentation level using the Minimum Speech Test Battery. This included the following:

- Hearing In Noise Test (HINT): Two 10-sentence lists in quiet
- Consonant-Nucleus-Consonant Test (CNC): One 50-word list

In 2004, the recommendation was made to reduce the presentation levels to 50 or 60 dB SPL to reflect real-life listening (Firszt et al., 2004). A joint effort by the three cochlear implant manufacturers in 2011 resulted in a New Minimum Speech Test Battery to be presented at 60 dBA consisting of the following:

- The AZBio Sentence Test (Spahr et al., 2012)
- The Banford-Kowal-Bench Speech in Noise Test (BKB-SIN; Bench, Kowal, & Bamford, 1979)
- Consonant Nucleus Consonant Test (CNC; Peterson & Lehiste, 1962)

The current criterion for adults is ≤50 percent speech recognition in the ear to be implanted when listening at normal conversational levels to sentence material (HINT, AZBio, or BKB) in the best-aided conditions. The opposite ear must have scores ≤60 percent. Medicare has stricter guidelines for payment requiring speech recognition scores of 40 percent or less. Currently, there are clinical trials on both adults and elders using more lenient criteria (Gifford, Dorman, Shallop, & Sydlowski, 2010). These criteria with technology are changing rapidly, and it is

TABLE 3.1 Candidacy Guidelines

	Age Group		
	Adults (≥18 Years of Age)	Young Children (12–24 Months)	Older Children (2–18 Years)
Hearing loss	Moderate to profound in the low frequencies; severe to profound in the mid- to high frequencies (≥70 dB HL) bilaterally	Profound (≥90 dB HL) bilaterally	Severe to profound in the low frequencies (≥70 dB HL); profound in the mid- to high frequencies (≥90 dB HL) bilaterally
Aided speech recognition	≤50 percent aided speech recognition on recorded sentence material in the ear to be implanted ≤60 percent aided speech recognition on recorded sentence material in the unimplanted ear	Lack of development in simple auditory skills over a three- to six-month period	≤30 percent best-aided word score at 70 dB HL
Communication/education	Desire to be a part of the hearing world	Therapy program that emphasizes the development of auditory skills	Educational/therapy program that emphasizes the development of auditory skills
Medical	No medical contraindications	No medical contraindications	No medical contraindications
Other	Highly motivated parents Patient has appropriate expectations	Highly motivated patient Parents have appropriate expectations	Highly motivated parents and child Parents and child have appropriate expectations

important for professionals to remain current. As systems and performance with the devices improve, the criteria are expanded.

For children, the FDA-approved audiologic criteria include a bilateral profound hearing loss (≥90 dB HL) for 12- to 24-month-olds and severe to profound sensorineural hearing loss (≥70 dB HL) in 24-month-olds to 18-year-olds with limited benefit from traditional amplification. For a young child, this is often difficult to determine and is defined as little to no progress in auditory development with appropriate amplification and audiologic habilitation. In older children, the criterion is ≤30 percent word recognition at normal conversational levels in the best-aided condition.

Formal evaluations should include standard audiometric unaided test batteries, otoacoustic emissions, aided speech perception testing, and aided speechreading evaluations. Speech and language evaluations should be completed on all children and all adults with prelingual and perilingual hearing loss. Otologic-medical evaluations are done by the physician. *MRIs* or *CT scans* are necessary to determine if the device can be implanted.

In addition to the audiometric guidelines for sensorineural hearing loss listed above, several other criteria are required prior to a person's receiving a cochlear implant. There should be no medical contraindications, such as the absence of the VIII nerve. The person must be free of active middle ear infections and be able to undergo surgery and anesthesia.

Patients and their families also should be counseled on the costs of cochlear implantation, and insurance reimbursement information needs to be provided. The cost of the cochlear implant system, surgery, and rehabilitative program often

MRI: Magnetic resonance imaging provides information on the soft tissue of the ear.

CT scan: Computerized tomography scans of the temporal bone provide information on the bony anatomy of the cochlea.

ranges from $70,000 to $90,000. Most major insurance carriers (e.g., Blue Cross/ Blue Shield), Medicare, and, in some states, Medicaid cover the procedure. Vocational rehabilitation services in some states also will pay for the cochlear implant. Several studies on the cost utility of the procedures have shown the cochlear implant to be a cost-effective procedure that often results in less expensive educational training for the recipient and more employability.

Candidacy for Adults. Adults must have had at least a three- to six-month trial period with appropriate amplification and show limited benefit from the hearing aids as defined by 50 percent or less auditory-only speech recognition performance with open-set sentences. Individuals must have a strong support system and be motivated to undergo the rehabilitative process of speech processor programming and audiologic rehabilitation. They must have realistic expectations. Honest counseling about the range of benefits that people receive is necessary. The limitations of the device need to be covered. Potential candidates need to be told that not everyone is able to use the telephone even after training. Some individuals may receive only enhancement of their speechreading abilities and awareness of environmental sounds. It is helpful to have them contact other patients who have the cochlear implant. Caution should be taken not to have them talk only to the highest-functioning users, as this often leads to unrealistic expectations. The team leaders may make the appropriate referrals for further evaluations to other team members, such as the psychologist, if it is suspected that there may be problems with the patient's or family members' expectations.

Individuals must also want to be part of the hearing world. Adults with prelingual hearing loss (e.g., born deaf) have poorer prognoses for success with a cochlear implant. Although speechreading abilities may be improved in these individuals, very few have achieved any open-set speech perception without visual cues. This is particularly true in those individuals who lack oral communication skills. Referrals for psychological and speech-language pathology consultations are often necessary in this population.

Candidacy for Children. Candidacy for children is sometimes very difficult to determine and should be done by the entire team of professionals mentioned above. Children under the age of 24 months should have at least a three-month trial period with appropriate and consistent binaural hearing aid use, and older children should have at least a six-month trial period. They must be receiving auditory training during that period (see Chapter 4). Hearing loss from some etiologies, such as

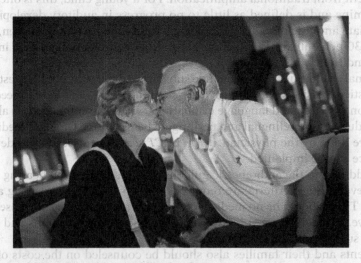

FIGURE 3.6 Older adult with a cochlear implant.
Source: Image courtesy of Cochlear Americas, ©2017.

meningitis, can cause ossification of the cochlea soon after onset. In these cases, the hearing trial may be decreased to one or two months. Limited benefit from amplification in young children is defined as lack of development in simple auditory skills over a three- to six-month period. In older children, when speech perception tests can be completed, limited benefit is defined as scores of 30 percent or less with open-set material.

Case 3.1. SK

SK was an 89-year-old who had a bilateral profound hearing loss for approximately two years. He relied on his wife for all communications. He was implanted in our facility and received good benefit from his cochlear implant as measured by a 92 percent score on the HINT in quiet. At the time of his initial evaluation, his wife had been diagnosed with Alzheimer's disease. About one year after he received his implant, his wife's condition had declined enough that their roles were reversed, and he became her caregiver. Due in part to the benefits derived from the implant, both were able to remain in their home together, and neither had to be institutionalized. There is no upper age limit for cochlear implantation. As long as the person meets all other criteria, he or she is a candidate. The issue is quality of life, not longevity.

The earliest recommended age by the FDA for the implantation is 12 months. The prognosis for development of speech and language is better with early intervention and implantation (Niparko et al., 2010; Robbins et al., 2004). In some cases of definitive diagnosis of profound hearing loss, the surgery can be done earlier (Colletti et al., 2005). The key issue is appropriate diagnosis. It is very difficult to accurately predict an audiogram and amplification potential benefit from objective measures, such as auditory brain stem response (ABR) and auditory steady-state response (ASSR) testing, or from behavioral testing. Implanting a very young child should be considered only after a comprehensive audiologic evaluation by a skilled pediatric audiologist. Although the FDA recommends implanting children only after the age of 12 months, several clinical studies have demonstrated the benefits and safety of implanting infants with profound hearing loss under the age of 1 with cochlear implants, using teams of experienced surgeons, pediatric anesthesiologists, pediatric audiologists, and speech-language pathologists (Cosetti & Roland, 2010).

Motivation and expectations of the family must be assessed, and they must be counseled to have appropriate expectations. Both the psychologist and the social worker on the team are helpful in assessing the family situation and assisting with compliance after the child receives the implant. Many families hope that the cochlear implant will correct the child's hearing. They must be told that the implant is not a cure and will not give the child normal hearing. As with adult recipients, these children's parents should be given the opportunity to talk with other families who have gone through the process with their child. They need to understand that intensive therapy will be a very important part of the child's audiologic and

---

Case 3.2. KP

KP was identified with a profound sensorineural hearing loss through the universal newborn screening program at the hospital where she was born. She was fit with power behind-the-ear hearing aids at age 6 weeks, and she and her parents attended an auditory verbal therapy program starting at 3 months of age. She was a consistent hearing aid user, but it was determined that she was receiving little benefit from traditional amplification. At age 13 months, she received a cochlear implant in her right ear and continued to wear a hearing aid in her left ear. Her parents continued with auditory verbal therapy, and by age 5 years, KP was able to enroll and succeed in a regular kindergarten classroom. At age 6 years, she was implanted in her left ear and is now a bilateral implant user. She is currently in middle school in regular classrooms with normal speech and language abilities.)

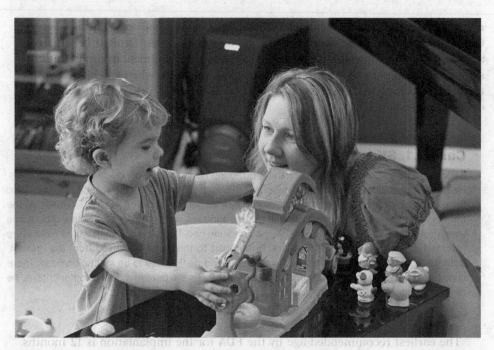

FIGURE 3.7 **Parent interacting in a language-rich environment with her toddler who has a cochlear implant.**
Source: Image courtesy of Cochlear Americas, © 2017.

communication development. It is important to have all members of the team, including the teacher of the deaf and the speech-language pathologist, active in the process. They can provide much of the support needed in training the child and family members.

The communication mode that the child uses does not determine candidacy, but the child's educational program must emphasize the development of auditory skills. Children trained in an auditory-verbal or auditory-visual mode of communication do progress more rapidly with their implants. Children placed in total communication programs do receive benefit from the implant if audition and speech are also encouraged along with signing (Meyer, Svirsky, Kirk, & Miyamoto, 1998).

Teenagers pose an additional challenge when determining candidacy. Sometimes, well-meaning relatives and friends who want the child to be part of the hearing world make inappropriate referrals. If the teen has some oral speech and language skills and wants the implant for him- or herself, then he or she may be a candidate. However, many of the teenagers themselves have no desire or motivation to get a cochlear implant. In addition, the plasticity of the auditory system appears to decline rapidly after about 6 years of age. Therefore, congenitally deafened teens have poorer prognoses for success with an implant, much like that of prelingual adults. They also may have made the choice to enter the Deaf community and have no interest in hearing.

The Nottingham Children's Implant Profile (NChIP; Nikolopoulos, Archbold, & Gregory, 2005) is a good tool for summarizing the evaluation process for children. Ten items are scored by the implant team as "no concern (0), mild to moderate concern (1), or great concern (2)." Items cover the children's demographic details (chronological age and duration of deafness), medical and radiological conditions, the outcomes of audiologic assessments, language and speech abilities, multiple handicaps or disabilities, family structure and support, educational environment, the availability of support services, expectations of the family and deaf child, cognitive abilities, and learning style. Patients with a high NChIP score are not deemed appropriate candidates for a cochlear implant.

Deaf Culture and Cochlear Implants

The Deaf community defines Deafness with a capital "D" as a culture rather than a disability. It is characterized by having its own language, American Sign Language (ASL). Some individuals within the Deaf community have expressed strong opinions against the use of cochlear implants, especially in children. They resent anyone who is trying to "fix a Deaf child." They have likened cochlear implants to foot binding in ancient China by trying to shape the child into actively using hearing. Many of their feelings stem from years of professionals forcing oral programming for all children with hearing loss and their own frustrations with traditional hearing aids.

Over the past 15 years, the National Association of the Deaf (NAD) has softened its criticisms of cochlear implants. In 1990, the organization came out in strong opposition to the FDA approval of cochlear implants in children, stating that the research being conducted on children had no regard for the child's quality of life as a deaf adult. In its 2000 Position Statement on Cochlear Implants, the NAD recognized the technology of cochlear implants as a tool for use with some forms of communication. It asserted that the parents have the right to choose the cochlear implant but emphasized that parents must be given all the options, including the option of sign language and the choice to be part of the Deaf world instead of the hearing world. They continue to assert that young prelingually deafened children do not have the auditory foundation to learn spoken language easily, and therefore cochlear implants in these children may have less-than-favorable results. This is in direct conflict with data by Miyamoto, Osberger, Robbins, Myres, and Kessler (1993) and Waltzman and Cohen (1998) that demonstrated that children implanted at a young age received significant speech perception benefits.

Implant teams must make parents aware of the Deaf culture issues. The parents do need to make informed decisions with knowledge of all options. Implant teams should be cognizant of the Deaf culture issues and be prepared to address them when counseling parents. It is also important to provide information to Deaf clubs on the current status of cochlear implants and the possible benefits and limitations of the devices.

Treatment Plans for Cochlear Implant Recipients

Once the evaluation and patient counseling have been completed and the decision has been made to proceed with the cochlear implant, the implant team may suggest that the patient go through some pretraining. With adults and older children, the pretraining may include speechreading therapy and training in the use of communication strategies for communication breakdowns (Chapters 4, 5, and 10). For children, the pretraining may include conditioning for play audiometry using tactile or visual stimulation, which then will allow for more accurate assessment of hearing sensitivity with and without the implant.

Surgery.   The cochlear implant surgery is completed under general anesthesia. Typically, the surgeon makes an incision behind the ear and drills a small area in the mastoid bone for the placement of the receiver stimulator and the insertion of the electrode array. The electrode array is then threaded through the mastoid and the middle ear cavity and then inserted in the scala tympani of the cochlea through the round window, or the *cochleostomy* technique is used. Insertion depths can range up to 30 mm depending on the implant system being used. Sutures are then made to secure the implant in place. The operation normally ranges from one to three hours and usually is done on an outpatient basis.

After surgical placement of the internal receiver/stimulator and the electrode array, the patient must wait approximately two to three weeks before the external headset and speech processor can be fitted. This waiting period allows for healing of the incision area prior to placing the magnet on the sensitive surface where the external transmitter is placed.

Cochleostomy technique is when the surgeon drills a small hole in the promontory of the cochlea to insert the electrode array into the scala tympani, as opposed to a round window approach where the electrode array is threaded through the round window.

Hook-Up.   The initial fitting and programming of the cochlear implant, commonly called the hook-up, usually takes one and a half to two hours. During the hook-up, or fitting of the headset and speech processor, the audiologist must program the speech processor using a specific manufacturer-designed diagnostic programming

MAP: Cochlear implant program that encodes the acoustic signal and translates it into electrical stimulation levels based on the measured levels.

system interfaced with a personal computer. This system consists of a manufacture-specific interface between the personal computer and the speech processor.

All the current generation implants have the capability of testing the integrity of the internal device by using a technique called telemetry (Abbas & Brown, 2000; Mens, 2007). Electrode voltages and impedances can be measured when current is supplied through the system. In this manner, the audiologist can check the internal device prior to programming the system. If any of the electrodes are found to be out of compliance with standard values, they will not be programmed for use. In some implant centers, telemetry is also completed by the audiologist in the operating room at the time of surgery to ensure proper device functioning before surgical closure.

In order to create the program, or *MAP*, for the speech processor, the audiologist must determine the electrical dynamic range for each electrode used (Figure 3.5). The programming system delivers an electrical current through the cochlear implant system to each electrode in order to obtain the electrical maximal or most comfortable level of current that is comfortably loud (C- or M-level) measures. Each manufacturer uses a measure for maximum comfort level (C) or most comfortable loudness level (M) in programming the cochlear implants to assure that the current level is always within a comfortable loudness level for the user. In addition, the T-level, or minimum stimulation level, is the softest electrical current that produces an auditory sensation by the patient 100 percent of the time and is used by some of the implant systems in programming. The speech processor is then programmed or "mapped" using one of the several encoding strategies so that the electrical current delivered to the implant will be within this measured dynamic range between T- and C- or M-levels or the estimated dynamic ranges when T-levels are not obtained. Obviously, T- and C- or M-levels are much easier to obtain on adults and older children with postlingual hearing loss. Techniques for testing the T-levels in young children are similar to testing pure tone hearing thresholds, ranging from observational testing to conditioned play audiometry. Using a team approach with two audiologists is very helpful when programming or mapping the cochlear implants of young children. Obtaining the C- or M-level in children is a challenging task, with the audiologist often relying totally on behavioral observation.

Neural response telemetry (NRT; Cochlear Corp.), neural response imaging (NRI; Advanced Bionics), and auditory response telemetry (ART; MED-EL) are objective techniques that can be used to estimate the dynamic ranges in young children or difficult-to-test patients. NRT, NRI, and ART offer a means of testing the electrically evoked compound action potential (ECAP) of the nerve using two of the electrodes in the array as recording electrodes and two as stimulating electrodes. No additional equipment is necessary. From these measures, T- and C- or M-levels can be estimated (Abbas & Brown, 2000; Mens, 2007). With children, audiologists will often evaluate only a limited number of electrodes spaced throughout the electrode array during the initial hook-up and either estimate the levels for the other electrodes or include only the tested electrodes in the initial program. These ECAP measures are often taken in the operating room to give the audiologist starting points for programming on the day of the hook-up. Even though these measures do not directly relate to behaviorally measured levels, they can help tremendously in training behavioral methods for testing.

Neural response telemetry (NRT)/neural response imaging (NRI)/auditory response telemetry (ART): Allows the implant system to function as a miniature evoked potential system by sampling and recording action potentials generated by electrical stimulation without additional equipment.

After levels are established and the MAP is created, the microphone is then activated so that the patient is able to hear speech and sounds in the environment. The initial reaction to speech varies among patients. Most adults describe speech as sounding mechanical and cartoonlike. Children often react with tears. This is understandable, considering that they may have no concept of what sound and hearing are and may find the stimulation frightening. Often, they are hearing their own voice, including their crying, for the first time. As they are calmed down, they often realize that when they stopped crying, the stimulation stopped. This can be the first step to auditory awareness.

All current generation systems have multiple memories that allow the audiologist to save more than one MAP in the speech processors. This is very helpful to the

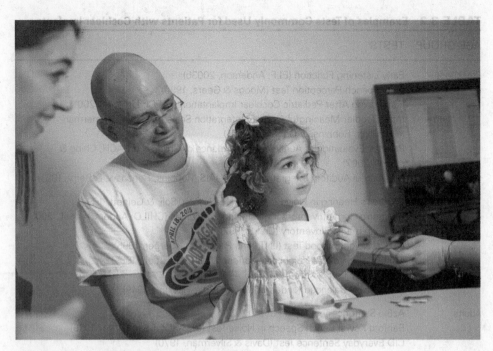

FIGURE 3.8   Programming a child patient.
Source: UF Health photography/Mindy Miller.

audiologist since, due to *acclimatization to sound*, the initial measured levels are often not the final values. Higher current values can be used to make alternative MAPs, which can be saved into the processor's multiple memories so that patients have the option of increasing the power between clinic visits. After their MAP has stabilized, different programs can be designed for various listening situations, such as everyday listening, listening in noisy settings, or music.

The patient and family should also be instructed on the daily care and maintenance of the system. They must know how to place the processor and coil on the head, change batteries, manipulate the controls, and troubleshoot the unit. Parents need to be shown how to check the system prior to putting it on the child. Spare cords or cables should be supplied. Suggestions on wearing the units using clips, belts, or harnesses should be given. Accessories should be explained and demonstrated. Warnings on the dangers of *electrostatic discharge* (ESD) should be given, as well as any other safety factors. Static electricity can corrupt stored programs or, in rare cases, cause damage to the internal unit when the external device is being worn. Parents are told to remove the device when their child plays on plastic slides or on other static-generating materials. Warranty and loss and damage insurance information should be covered.

The patients or the parents of young users are asked to keep a diary or log of their listening experiences. They are asked to record both positive and negative experiences. Significant others are also asked to keep a record of their observations when they are with the implant user. This helps in reprogramming the units on subsequent visits and also in developing the most appropriate treatment plans.

Follow-Up Programming and Therapy.   The second programming session is usually performed within one week of the initial hook-up. Review of the patient diary and experiences with the implant are helpful in determining if the programs provided sufficient power for sound awareness and detection or if any sounds were uncomfortably loud, indicating that the C- or M-levels were set too high. During this visit, the measured values are reevaluated, and new MAPs are placed in the processor.

Acclimatization to sound: Adaptation to sound stimulation that changes the measured T- and C- or M-levels, allowing the individual to tolerate higher levels.

Electrostatic discharge (ESD): Occurs when static electricity (accumulation of electrical charge) transfers between two objects charged to different levels.

TABLE 3.2   Examples of Tests Commonly Used for Patients with Cochlear Implants

AGE-GROUP	TESTS
Preschool	Early Listening Function (ELF; Anderson, 2003b) Early Speech Perception Test (Moogs & Geers, 1990) Functioning After Pediatric Cochlear Implantation (FAPCI; Lin et al., 2001) Infant Toddler Meaningful Auditory Integration Scale (IT-MAIS; Zimmerman-Phillips, Robbins, & Osberger, 2001) Parents' Evaluation of Aural/Oral Performance of Children (PEACH; Ching & Hill, 2007) Meaningful Auditory Integration Scale (MAIS; Robbins, Renshaw, & Berry, 1991)
School age	Children's Hearing in Noise Test (C-HINT; Nilsson, Soli, & Gelnett, 1996) Children's Home Inventory for Listening Difficulties (CHILD; Anderson et al., 2003a) Craig Lip-reading Inventory (Craig, 1992) Lexical Neighborhood Test (LNT; Kirk, Pisoni, & Osberger, 1995) Multisyllabic Lexical Neighborhood Test (MLNT; Kirk et al., 1995) NU-Chips (Elliott & Katz, 1980) Phonetically Balanced Kindergarten Test (PBK; Haskins, 1949)
Adults	AzBio Sentence Test (Spahr et al., 2012) Banford Kowal Bench Speech in Noise Test (BKB-SIN; Bench et al., 1979) CID Everyday Sentence Test (Davis & Silverman, 1970) Consonant Nucleus Consonant Test (CNC; Peterson & Lehiste, 1962) CUNY Sentence Test (Boothroyd, Hanin, & Hnath, 1985) Hearing in Noise Test (HINT; Nilsson, Soli, & Sullivan, 1994) Minimal Auditory Test Battery (MAC; Owens, Kessler, Tellen, & Shubert, 1981) NU-6 Monosyllabic Word Test (Tillman & Carhart, 1966)

Speech tracking: A therapeutic procedure in which subjects are presented with prose and asked to repeat verbatim what they hear (De Filippo & Scott, 1978). See Chapter 4 and Supplementary Learning Activity 4.

During this session, an initial screening of the patient's abilities should be completed. Table 3.2 contains examples of tests commonly used for patients with cochlear implants. Children should be tested using various auditory training screening materials that are age appropriate. These results will help guide the treatment plan. Auditory training programs developed for aided children with hearing loss can be used with cochlear implant users as well. Excellent reviews of screening devices and suggestions for treatment plans can be found in Estabrooks (1998) and Nevins and Chute (1996).

For adults, several programmed therapy plans have been developed for implant users. These include screening tests to help the clinician in determining the starting point in the plans (Cochlear Corporation, 1998; Wayner & Abrahamson, 1998). Auditory training methods such as *speech tracking* are extremely helpful in both treatment and monitoring progress with the device. Various therapy materials are available to the clinician through each of the implant manufacturers (see "Recommended Websites" at the end of this chapter). Software programs, such as Angel Sound (http://angelsound.tigerspeech.com), are available for both children and adults and can be used both in the clinic and at home. Each of the implant companies offers a variety of audiologic rehabilitation programs and activities for cochlear implant users to use at home.

The amount and length of therapy with the cochlear implant depend on the patient, but all cochlear implant patients, regardless of age, will benefit from an audiologic therapy plan based on their needs. In many cases, the implant user will receive device programming and monitoring at the cochlear implant center and other audiologic re/habilitation and speech-language therapy through schools or local audiologists and therapists. A coordinated effort on the part of all professionals and parents is very important in developing and implementing the treatment plans. Face-to-face meetings, teleconferencing, written reports, and e-mail are all means of maintaining contact with all parties involved. Parent-maintained notebooks that all professionals may use are also excellent. By having the parent in charge of a notebook that has records and communications to be shared by professionals, the parent can be empowered to be part of the process. Teachers and therapists who are not familiar with implants need to be provided with literature on cochlear implants and given instructions on how to check and troubleshoot the devices. They need to understand that the cochlear implant is designed to give the child more auditory information. They can still use similar teaching techniques with these children as they used prior to the implant, but they need to raise their expectations concerning what the child can accomplish using audition. The habilitation programming discussions in Chapter 9 can easily be adapted for cochlear implant users. In working with a young child who is learning to listen through a cochlear implant, the focus should be on listening. The child's world needs to have rich, repetitive spoken language. Information needs to be given auditorially first, and then visual cues can be incorporated. Parents need to be involved because they are the true teachers and therapists for their children.

Programming follow-ups for adult patients with postlingual hearing loss usually consist of approximately six visits in the first two months of use, then at three months, six months, and annually thereafter. For young children, the programming schedule suggested is weekly visits for two months, then at six months, nine months, and every six months thereafter. These schedules can be modified to include more or fewer visits depending on the person's adaptation to the implant, auditory responsiveness, and ease of programming.

Variables Affecting Performance

As stated previously, patient performance varies greatly among cochlear implant users. Many users are able to achieve open-set speech recognition even in the presence of background noise, whereas some patients receive only improvement in their speechreading abilities and awareness of environmental sounds. Numerous studies have demonstrated that the overall quality of life improves significantly in both children and adults after they receive cochlear implants (Gaylor et al., 2013). Children who receive cochlear implants along with appropriate therapy have improved speech perception, speech and language development, and reading as compared to children with similar hearing losses who are not implanted. Many children who are implanted at a young age achieve performance similar to normal-hearing peers in both language and reading abilities (Dunn et al., 2014; Niparko et al., 2010; Wang et al., 2008).

Age of onset, length of deafness, age of implantation, length of implant use, etiology of the hearing loss, *nerve survival*, mode of communication, cochlear implant technology, surgical issues, audiologic re/habilitation methods, and motivation are examples of variables that affect success with the implant. Some of these are known factors, such as age of onset and length of deafness. Studies have shown that the shorter the length of severe to profound hearing loss and the better the pre-implant discrimination score, the better the prognosis for benefit from the cochlear implant (Rubenstein, Parkenson, Tyler, & Gantz, 1999; Zwolan et al., 2014). Others are unknown quantities, such as the amount of *nerve survival*, both prior to and following surgical insertion of the electrode array. Patients, parents, and significant others need to be made aware of the many variables that can affect performance.

Nerve survival: The VIII nerve fibers that are available for stimulation.

Bilateral Hearing with Cochlear Implants

Recent studies have shown that some of the benefits of binaural hearing, such as localization and improved hearing in noise, can be accomplished using *bimodal* hearing when the patient wears a hearing aid in the ear opposite the cochlear implant (Ching, Incerti, & Hill, 2004; Ching, Psarros, Hill, Dillon, & Incerti, 2001; Crew, Galvin, Landsberger, & Fu, 2015; Illg et al., 2014; Kong et al., 2012; Seeber, Baumann, & Fastl, 2004; Sheffield & Gifford, 2014). Research has indicated that the hearing aid, even in cases with profound hearing loss, can provide the patients

A bimodal fitting is when there is a hearing aid in one ear and a cochlear implant in the other ear.

with prosody information that cannot be provided by current generation implants. Prosody or suprasegmental information includes rhythm, stress, and intonation that can help in understanding in noise, music appreciation, and hearing emotion in speech. Even patients with a corner audiogram can receive some benefit from a hearing aid in the opposite ear to supplement what they are receiving from the cochlear implant. Therefore, a hearing aid trial in the opposite ear is recommended for all patients receiving unilateral cochlear implants. Hearing aid fitting practices for bimodal users vary greatly (Siburt & Holmes, 2015). Best fitting practices for bimodal cochlear implant users have yet to be developed.

Bilateral cochlear implants involve having an implant in both ears.

   Bilateral cochlear implantation is becoming more common worldwide and has also shown significant improvement in localization and hearing in noise in adults (Neuman, Haravon, Sislioan, & Waltzman, 2007; Ramsden et al., 2005; Sheffield & Gifford, 2014; van Hoesel, 2004; van Schoonhovan et al., 2013). The binaural benefits in children have also demonstrated improved localization abilities (Grieco-Calub & Litovsky, 2010) and improved speech understanding in noise (Sparreboom et al., 2010). The possible benefits of bilateral cochlear implantation must be weighed against the possible disadvantages. The cost of bilateral implantation will be $60,000 to $80,000 greater than with a unilateral cochlear implant. Summerfield, Lovett, Bellenger, and Batten (2010) studied the cost-effectiveness of bilateral cochlear implantation in the pediatric population and found mixed results in that there was an improvement in quality of life with the second implant, but its cost-effectiveness was questionable. Monetary costs are not the only consideration. Surgical risks are also increased. In addition, one must consider the possibility that some future device may be developed that could be used only in an ear that had never had an implant. With the rapid changes in technology, if the child only has the implant in one ear, the other ear would be available so that the new procedure could be performed. When reviewing the options for a young child whose expected life span is 70 to 75 years, the importance of keeping one ear open for future options needs to be considered.

   The decision between bimodal stimulation or bilateral implantation must be made on an individual basis. Cullington and Zeng (2011) studied matched groups of bimodal and bilateral cochlear implant adult users and found similar results for each group in speech recognition in noise, music perception, identifying tone of voice, and discriminating different talkers. Gifford et al. (2015) found that even in patients with high performance unilaterally, the second implant afforded them improvements in difficult noise situations. In children, Litovsky et al. (2006) found that children with bilateral implants could localize better than unilateral users, but some of the bimodal children could perform localization tasks at the same level that the average bilateral user functioned. More research is needed to determine the best way to afford bilateral listening to the cochlear implant user. Currently, many clinics recommend unilateral cochlear implant surgery with the use of a hearing aid in the opposite ear. If, after a trial period, the patient does not receive any benefit from the bimodal condition compared to the cochlear implant–alone condition, a second implant should be considered. Some clinics are recommending simultaneous bilateral implantation (both ears during the same surgery) for infants and young children with bilateral profound hearing loss so that the child has the best possible hearing for the development of speech and language. Others are recommending a trial with bimodal stimulation to allow the child the ability to hear prosody information from the hearing aid during the early development of speech and language before receiving a second cochlear implant (Nittrourer & Chapman, 2009). Bilateral implantation would then be considered if testing shows no benefit from the hearing aid in the opposite ear.

Auditory Brainstem Implant

An auditory brainstem implant (ABI) has been developed for individuals with *neurofibromatosis* (NF2) who are deafened from bilateral VIII nerve tumors. The implant is placed on the cochlear nucleus of the brain stem during the surgery to remove

Case 3.3. May

May was identified through newborn screening in the hospital two days after birth. She was fitted with hearing aids bilaterally at 8 weeks of age, and her parents started with her in a total communication therapy program that emphasized auditory training. At 13 months she was showing little to no progress in her speech/auditory development, and she was evaluated for a cochlear implant. At 15 months she was implanted. She continued using total communication, but speech and audition were emphasized in her therapy at home and by her family. May is now 9 years old and is in a regular classroom performing well educationally. She rarely uses sign language unless with her Deaf friends. Her speech and language development is at the level of her normal-hearing peers. She is active in Girl Scouts and sports at her school. The cochlear implant has given her a chance to function as a well-adjusted happy young lady in the hearing world.

the tumor. To date, over 600 patients have received the ABI, and in early November 2000, the Nucleus 24 ABI was approved by the FDA for use in cases of neurofibromatosis for patients over the age of 12 years (Cochlear Corporation, 2000). Results with this implant are similar to early generation multi-electrode implants and show promise to those who have not been able to benefit from cochlear implants because they lack functioning VIII nerves. MedEl Corporation also has an ABI that is not yet FDA approved but is being implanted in other parts of the world. Researchers have ongoing clinical trials for individuals who cannot benefit from a cochlear implant and do not have NF2 (Yamazaki, 2014).

> Neurofibromatosis is a genetic disorder that causes tumors to develop anywhere in the nervous system. The tumors are common on the auditory nerve and the other cranial nerves, causing hearing loss, cardiovascular issues, vision loss, and other problems.

Electroacoustic Stimulation

Electroacoustic stimulation is a new research and clinical branch in cochlear implants (Adunka, Pillsbury, Adunka, & Buchman, 2010; Gantz et al., 2009). Many individuals have usable hearing in the low- to mid-frequency range but have no hearing in higher frequencies. These people with "dead regions" of the cochlea receive little to no high-frequency information from hearing aids. With electroacoustic stimulation, the cochlear implant electrode array is placed only in the basal to mid-portions of the cochlea and programmed for high-frequency sounds. At the same time, the low to mid-frequencies are amplified using standard hearing aid technology. This cochlear implant/hearing aid combination could help many individuals who currently do not qualify for cochlear implants but are dissatisfied with their hearing aids because the higher pitches cannot be amplified.

The term *hybrid cochlear implant* refers to the Cochlear Corporation's system, whereas MED-EL simply refers to it as electroacoustic stimulation. In March 2014, the FDA approved the use of the Hybrid L24 Cochlear Implant for adults over the age of 18 years. For these electroacoustic systems, both the hearing aid and the speech processor are encased in the behind-the-ear device. The electrical stimulation for high-frequency signals goes through the cochlear implant system the same as with a standard cochlear implant, whereas the acoustic signal is processed through the digital hearing aid portion and sent through the earmold the same as a standard air conduction hearing aid (Figure 3.9). According to the FDA, to qualify for an electroacoustic device, a person must be over the age of 18 years and have low-frequency hearing thresholds in the normal to moderate range through 500 Hz and a severe to profound sensorineural hearing loss averaging 70 dB or poorer for 2000, 3000, and 4000 Hz. Speech recognition testing using monosyllabic consonant-nucleus-consonant (CNC) words must be ≤60 percent in the ear to be implanted and ≤80 percent in the other ear. MED-EL and Advanced Bionics have active clinical trials investigating the benefits of electroacoustic stimulation.

Irving et al. (2014) outlined two areas of research needed to improve electroacoustic stimulation performance. First, we need to better understand how electroacoustic stimulation is processed at the level of the brain, and, second, we need

FIGURE 3.9 Nucleus 6 Hybrid System.
Source: Image courtesy of Cochlear Americas,
© 2017.

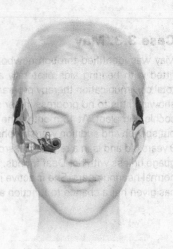

to continue to refine practices to reduce or prevent further hearing loss in these patients. Ongoing research is being done on how to program both the acoustic and the electrical signals to best serve the patients. Patients have significantly better speech recognition in both quiet and noise with electroacoustic stimulation, but in a carefully controlled multicenter study (Gantz et al., 2009) with 87 patients, eight patients lost all of their residual acoustic hearing, and 17 had significant loss of their residual acoustic hearing due to the surgery. Jurawitz et al. (2014) reported a 91 percent preservation rate at the initial activation of the cochlear implant for 87 patients and a 75 percent preservation rate in the one to five years postactivation. Improved surgical techniques designed to preserve acoustic hearing are being developed (Prentiss, Sykes, & Staecker, 2010) so that this technology can be made available to patients in clinical settings. Surgeries designed to preserve residual hearing are often termed *soft surgeries*. Newer implant designs and surgical techniques along with drug therapies are being developed and studied to improve hearing preservation in all implant systems (Santa Maria et al., 2014).

Advances in cochlear implants are occurring rapidly in design, programming techniques, coding strategies, and determining candidacy. Both internal and external devices are becoming smaller. The introduction of behind-the-ear speech processors has provided cosmetic advantages that are particularly attractive to adolescent and young adult users. With improvements in hearing preservation, electroacoustic stimulation will offer another alternative to persons with poor high-frequency hearing.

Summary Points

- The scope of audiologic rehabilitation has increased dramatically in the past two decades. Clinicians must keep current on new technologies and techniques to aid their patients in all types of disorders that involve the auditory system.

- Cochlear implants offer an alternative for sound stimulation to individuals who receive limited benefits from traditional amplification.

- Careful evaluation by a team of professionals is needed to determine candidacy for cochlear implantation and to develop the appropriate treatment plans for these individuals.

- Audiologic rehabilitation is an integral part of the cochlear implant process, including speech processor programming and training. With training, the cochlear implant can improve the quality of life for persons with severe to profound hearing loss.

Supplementary Learning Activities

See www.isu.edu/csed/audiology/rehab to carry out these activities. We encourage you to use these to supplement your learning. Your instructor may give specific assignments that involve a particular activity.

1. Interview a cochlear implant recipient or the parents of a cochlear implant recipient. Gather information about the recipient's background, hearing loss, speech/language development, educational history, previous hearing aid use, type of implant, when he or she was first implanted, the recipient's experiences with the implant, and any other pertinent factors.

2. View the movies *Sound and Fury* (2000) and *Sound and Fury: 6 Years Later* (2006), both directed by Josh Aronson. Also watch the TED talk *The Heather World: Heather Artinian at TEDxGeorgetown* and write a summary on how the opinions of cochlear implants have changed in the Deaf community.

3. Examine a website for a cochlear implant manufacturer. Look over the information about the device that a particular manufacturer produces and markets, along with associated information concerning candidacy, cost, or other parameters. Write a brief summary of what you found, along with your impressions.

4. Attend a local Hearing Loss Association meeting in your area and listen to adults who are hearing aid and/or cochlear implant users. Write a brief discussion paper on the benefits of each from the user's perspective.

Recommended Reading

Chorost, M. (2005). *How becoming part computer made me more human.* New York: Houghton Mifflin.

Chorost, M. (2006). *Rebuilt: My journey back to the hearing world.* New York: Houghton Mifflin.

Chute, P. M., & Nevins, M. E. (2006). *School professionals working with children with cochlear implants.* San Diego, CA: Plural.

Cooper, H. R., & Craddock, L. C. (2006). *Cochlear implants: A practical guide.* West Sussex: Whurr Publishers.

Farley, C. (2002). *Bridge to sound with a "bionic" ear.* Wayzata, MN: Periscope Press.

Gifford, R. H. (2014). *Cochlear Implant Patient Assessment.* San Diego, CA: Plural Publishing.

Moller, A. R. (2006). *Cochlear and brainstem implants.* Basel: Karger.

Niparko, J. K. (2000). *Cochlear implants: Principles and practices.* Philadelphia: Lippincott Williams & Wilkins.

Wayner, D., & Abrahamson, J. (1998). *Learning to hear again with a cochlear implant: An audiologic rehabilitation curriculum guide.* Austin, TX: Hear Again.

Wolfe, J., & Schafer, F. (2014). *Programming cochlear implants* (2nd ed.). San Diego, CA: Plural.

Recommended Websites

Nucleus Cochlear Implant Systems:
http://www.cochlear.com

Advanced Bionics Cochlear Implant Systems:
http://www.cochlearimplant.com

MED-EL Cochlear Implant Systems:
http://www.medel.com

National Association of the Deaf (NAD):
http://www.nad.org

Cochlear Implants in Adults and Children, National Institutes of Health, Consensus Development Conference Statement, May 15–17, 1995:
http://consensus:nih.gov

AAA Position Statement on Cochlear Implants in Children:
http://www.audiology.org

References

Abbas, P. J., & Brown, C. J., and Etler, C.P. (2000). Electrophysiology and device telemetry. In S. B. Waltzman & N. L. Cohen (Eds.), *Cochlear implants*. New York: Thieme.

Adunka, O. F., Pillsbury, H. C., Adunka, M. C., & Buchman, C. A. (2010). Is electric acoustic stimulation better than conventional cochlear implantation for speech perception in quiet? *Otology and Neurotology*, *31*(7), 1049–1054.

Anderson, K. L. (2003a). CHILD—Children's Home Inventory for Listening Difficulties. Retrieved 2016 from http://www.phonak.com/diagnostic.

Anderson, K. L. (2003b). ELF—Early Listening Function. Retrieved 2016 from http://www.phonak.com/diagnostic.

Bench, J., Kowal, A., & Bamford, J. (1979). The BKB (Bamford-Kowal-Bench) sentence lists for partially-hearing children. *British Journal of Audiology*, *13*, 108–112.

Boothroyd, A., Hanin, L., & Hnath, T. (1985). *A sentence test of speech perception: Reliability, set equivalence and short term learning: Internal report RCI 10*. New York: Speech and Hearing Sciences Research Center, City University of New York.

Ching, T. Y., & Hill, M. (2007). Parents' evaluation of aural/oral performance of children (PEACH) scale: Normative data. *Journal of the American Academy of Audiology*, *18*(3), 220–235.

Ching, T. Y. C., Incerti, P., & Hill, M. (2004). Binaural benefits for adults who use hearing aids and cochlear implants in opposite ears. *Ear and Hearing*, *25*, 9–21.

Ching, T. Y. C., Psarros, C., Hill, M., Dillon, H., & Incerti, P. (2001). Should children who use cochlear implants wear hearing aids in the opposite ear? *Ear and Hearing*, *22*, 365–380.

Craig, W. N. (1992). *Craig Lip-Reading Inventory: Word Recognition*. Englewood, CO: Resource Point.

Cochlear Corporation. (1998). *Rehabilitation manual*. Englewood, CO: Author.

Cochlear Corporation. (2000). *Nucleus24ABI: The multichannel auditory brainstem implant*. Englewood, CO: Author.

Colletti, V., Carner, M., Miorelli, V., Guida, M., Colletti, I., & Fiorino, F. G. (2005). Cochlear implantation at under 12 months: Report on 10 patients. *Laryngoscope*, *115*(3), 445–449.

Cosetti, M., & Roland, J. T., Jr. (2010). Cochlear implantation in the very young child: Issues unique to the under-1 population. *Trends in Amplification*, *14*(1), 46–57.

Crew, J. D., Galvin, J. J., III, Landsberger, D. M., & Fu, Q. (2015). Contribution of electric and acoustic hearing to bimodal speech and music perception. *PLOS ONE*, *10*(3), 1–18.

Cullington, H, E., & Zeng, F. G. (2011). Comparison of bimodal and bilateral cochlear implant users on speech recognition with competing talker, music perception, affective prosody discrimination, and talker identification. *Ear and Hearing*, *32*(1), 16–32.

Davis, H., & Silverman, R. (1970). *Hearing and deafness*. New York: Holt, Rinehart and Winston.

DeFilippo, C. L., & Scott, B. L. (1978). A method for training and evaluating the reception of ongoing speech. *Journal of the Acoustical Society of America*, *63*, 1186–1192.

Dunn, C. C., Walker, E. A., Oleson, J., Kenworthy, M., Van Voorst, T., Tombin, B., et al. (2014). Longitudinal speech perception and language performance in pediatric cochlear implant users: The effect of age at implantation. *Ear and Hearing*, *35*(2), 148–160.

Elliot, L. L., & Katz, D. (1980). *Development of a new children's test of speech discrimination* (Technical manual). St. Louis, MO: Auditec.

Estabrooks, W. (1998). *Cochlear implants for kids*. Washington, DC: Alexander Graham Bell Association for the Deaf.

Firszt, J. B., Holden, L. K., Skinner, M. W., Tobey, E. A., Peterson, A., Gaggl, W., et al. (2004). Recognition of speech presented at soft to loud levels by adult cochlear implant recipients of three cochlear implant systems. *Ear and Hearing*, *25*(4), 375–387.

Gantz, B. J., Hansen, M. R., Turner, C. W., Oleson, J. J., Reiss, L. A., & Parkinson, A. J. (2009). Hybrid 10 clinical trial: Preliminary results. *Audiology and Neurotology*, *14*(Suppl. 1), 32–38.

Gaylor, J. M., Raman, G., Chung, M., Lee, J., Rao, M., and Lau, J. (2013). Cochlear implantation in adults: A systematic review and meta-analysis. *JAMA Otolaryngology—Head and Neck Surgery*, *139*(3), 265–272.

Gifford, R. H., Driscoll, C. L. W., Davis, T., & Gifford, R. (2015). A within-subject comparison of bimodal hearing, bilateral cochlear implantation, and bilateral cochlear implantation with bilateral hearing preservation: High-performing patients. *Otology and Neurotology*, *36*(8), 1331–1337.

Gifford, R. H., Dorman, M. F., Shallop, J. K., & Sydlowski, S. A. (2010). Evidence for the expansion of adult cochlear implant candidacy. *Ear and Hearing*, *31*(2), 186–194.

Grieco-Calub, T. M., & Litovsky, R. Y. (2010). Sound localization skills in children who use bilateral cochlear implants and in children with normal acoustic hearing. *Ear and Hearing*, *31*(5), 645–656.

Haskins, H. A. (1949). *A phonetically balanced test of speech discrimination for children*. Master's thesis, Northwestern University, Evanston, IL.

Illg, A., Bojanowicz, M., Lesinski- Schiedat, A., Lenarz, T., & Buchner, A. (2014). Evaluation of the bimodal benefit in a large cohort of cochlear implant subjects using a contralateral hearing aid. *Otology and Neurotology*, *35*(9), e240–e244.

Irving, S., Gillespie, L., Richardson, R., Rowe, D., Fallon, J., & Wise, A. (2014). *Electroacoustic stimulation: Now and into the future*. New York, NY, BioMed Research International.

Jurawitz, M. C., Buchner, A., Harpel, M., Schussler, M., & Majdoni, O. (2014). Hearing preservation outcomes with different cochlear implant electrodes: Nucleus Hybrid-L24 and Nucleus Freedom CI422. *Audiology and Neurotology*, *19*, 293–309.

Kirk, K. I., Pisoni, D. B., & Osberger, M. J. (1995). Lexical effects on spoken word recognition by pediatric cochlear implant users. *Ear and Hearing*, *16*, 470–481.

Kong Y., Muloingi, A., & Marozeau, J. (2012). Timbre and speech perception in bimodal and bilateral cochlear-implant listeners. *Ear and Hearing*, *33*(5), 645–659.

Lin, F. R., Ceh, K., Bervinchak, D., Riley, A., Miech, R., & Niparko, J. (2007). Development of a communicative performance scale for pediatric cochlear implantation. *Ear and Hearing*, *28*(5), 703–712.

Litovsky, R. Y., Johnstone, P. M., Godar, S., Agrawal, S., Parkinson, A., Peters, R., et al. (2006). Bilateral cochlear implants in children: Localization acuity measured with minimum audible angle. *Ear and Hearing*, *27*(1), 43–59.

Luxford, W. M. (2001). Minimum speech test battery for postlingually deafened adult cochlear implant patients. *Archives of Otolaryngology—Head and Neck Surgery*, *124*(2), 125–126.

Mens, L. H. (2007). Advances in cochlear implant telemetry: Evoked neural responses, electrical field imaging, and technical integrity. *Trends in Amplification*, *11*(3), 143–159.

Meyer, T., Svirsky, M., Kirk, K., & Miyamoto, R. (1998). Improvements in speech perception by children with profound prelingual hearing loss: Effects of device, communication mode, and chronological age. *Journal of Speech Hearing Research*, *41*, 846–858.

Miyamoto, R., Osberger, M., Robbins, A., Myres, W., & Kessler, K. (1993). Prelingually deafened children's performance with the Nucleus multichannel cochlear implant. *American Journal of Otology*, *14*, 437–445.

Moogs, J. S., & Geers, A. E. (1990). *Early Speech Perception Test for Profoundly Hearing-Impaired Children*. St. Louis, MO: Central Institute for the Deaf.

National Association of the Deaf. (2001, January). *NAD position statement on cochlear implants.* NAD Broadcaster. Silver Springs, MD.

National Institutes of Health. (1995, May 15–17). *Cochlear implants in adults and children.* National Institutes of Health, Consensus Development Conference Statement. Washington, DC: Author.

Neuman, A. C., Haravon, A., Sislioan, N., & Waltzman, S. B. (2007). Sound-direction identification with bilateral cochlear implants. *Ear and Hearing, 28*(1), 73–82.

Nevins, M. E., & Chute, P. M. (1996). *Children with cochlear implants in educational settings.* San Diego, CA: Singular Publishing Group.

Nikolopoulos, T. P., Archbold, S. M., & Gregory, S. (2005). Young deaf children with hearing aids or cochlear implants: Early assessment package for monitoring progress. *International Journal of Pediatric Otorhinolaryngology, 69*(2), 175–186.

Nilsson, M. J., Soli, S. D., & Gelnett, D. J. (1996). *Development of the Hearing in Noise Test for Children (HINT-C).* Los Angeles: House Ear Institute.

Nilsson, M. J., Soli, S. D., & Sullivan, J. A. (1994). Development of the Hearing in Noise Test for the measurement of speech reception in quiet and in noise. *Journal of the Acoustical Society of America, 95*, 1085–1099.

Niparko, J. K., Tobey, E. A., Thal, D. J., Eisenberg, L., Wang, N., & Quittner, A. (2010). Spoken language development in children following cochlear implantation. *Journal of the American Medical Association, 303*(15), 1498–1506.

Nittrourer, S., & Chapman, C. (2009). The effects of bilateral electric and bimodal electric-acoustic stimulation on language development. *Trends in Amplification, 13*(3), 190–205.

Owens, E., Kessler, D. K., Tellen, C. C., & Shubert, E. D. (1981). Minimal Auditory Test Battery (MAC) battery. *Hearing Aid Journal, 9*, 32.

Peterson, G., & Lehiste, I. (1962). Revised CNC lists for auditory tests. *Journal of Speech and Hearing Disorders, 27*, 62–70.

Prentiss, S., Sykes, K., & Staecker, H. (2010). Partial deafness cochlear implantation at the University of Kansas: Techniques and outcomes. *Journal of the American Academy of Audiology, 21*(3), 197–203.

Ramsden, R., Greenham, P., O'Driscoll, M., Mawman, D., Proops, D., Craddock, L., et al. (2005). Evaluation of bilaterally implanted adult subjects with the Nucleus 24 implant system. *Otology and Neurotology, 26*(5), 988–998.

Robbins, A., Koch, D., Osberger, M. Zimmerman-Phillips, S., & Kishon-Rabin, L. (2004). Effect of age at cochlear implantation on auditory skill development in infants and toddlers. *Archives of Otolaryngology—Head and Neck Surgery, 130*, 570–574.

Robbins, A. M., Renshaw, J. J., & Berry, S. W. (1991). Evaluating meaningful auditory integration in profoundly hearing-impaired children. *American Journal of Otolaryngology, 12*(Suppl.), 144–150.

Rubinstein, J. T., Parkenson, W. S., Tyler, R. S., & Gantz, B. J. (1999). Residual speech recognition and cochlear implant performance: Effects of implantation criteria. *American Journal of Otology, 20*, 445–452.

Santa Maria, P. L., Gluth, M. B., Yuan, Y., Atlas, M., & Blevins, N.. (2014). Hearing preservation surgery for cochlear implantation: A meta-analysis. *Otology and Neurotology, 35*, e256–e269.

Seeber, B. U., Baumann, U., & Fastl, H. (2004). Localization ability with bimodal hearing aids and bilateral cochlear implants. *Journal of Acoustical Society of America, 116*(3), 1698–709.

Sheffield, S. W., & Gifford, R. H. (2014). The benefits of bimodal hearing: Effect of frequency region and acoustic bandwidth. *Audiology and Neurotology, 19*(3), 151–163.

Siburt, H., & Holmes, A. E. (2015). Bimodal programming: A survey of current clinical practice. *American Journal of Audiology, 24*(2), 243–249.

Spahr, A. J., Dorman, M. F., Litvak, L. M., Van Wie, S., Gifford, R. H., Loizou, P. C., et al. (2012). Development and validation of the AzBio sentence lists. *Ear and Hearing, 33*, 112–117.

Sparreboom, M., van Schoonhoven, J., van Zanten, B. G., Scholten, R. (2010). The effectiveness of bilateral cochlear implants for severe-to-profound deafness in children: A systematic review. *Otology and Neurotology, 31*(7), 1062–1071.

Summerfield, A. Q., Lovett, R. E., Bellenger, H., & Batten, G. (2010). Estimates of the cost-effectiveness of pediatric bilateral cochlear implantation. *Ear and Hearing*, *31*(5), 611–624.

Tillman, T. W., & Carhart, R. (1966). An expanded test for speech discrimination utilizing CNC monosyllabic words. Northwestern University Test No. 6. Brooks Air Force Base, TX: USAF School of Aerospace Medicine Technical Report.

van Hoesel, R. J. (2004). Exploring the benefits of bilateral cochlear implants. *Audiologic Neurootology*, *9*(4), 234–246.

van Schoonhoven, J., Sparreboom, M., van Zanten, B., Schatten, R. Mylanus, E., Dreschler, W., et al. (2013). The effectiveness of bilateral cochlear implants for severe-to-profound deafness in adults: A systematic review. *Otology and Neurotology*, *34*(2), 190–198.

Waltzman, S. B., & Cohen, N. L. (1998). Cochlear implantation in children younger than 2 years old. *American Journal of Otology*, *19*, 1083–1087.

Wang, N. Y., Eisenber, L., Johnson, K., Fink, N., Tobey, E., Alexandra, L., et al. (2008). Tracking development of speech recognition: Longitudinal data from hierarchical assessments in the Childhood Development After Cochlear Implantation Study. *Otology and Neurotology*, *29*(2), 240–245.

Wayner, D. S., & Abrahamson, J. E. (1998). *Learning to hear again with a cochlear implant: An audiologic rehabilitation curriculum guide.* Austin, TX: Hear Again.

Wilson, B. S. (2000). Cochlear implant technology. In J. K. Niparko (Ed.), *Cochlear implants: Principles and practices.* Philadelphia: Lippincott Williams & Wilkins.

Yamazaki, H. (2014). Auditory brainstem implant. In *Regenerative medicine for the inner ear* (pp. 165–177). Tokyo: Springer.

Zimmerman-Phillips, S., Robbins, A. M., & Osberger, M. J. (2001). *Infant-Toddler Meaningful Integration Scale.* Sylmar, CA: Advanced Bionics Corp.

Zwolan, T. A., Henion, K., et al. (2014). The role of age on cochlear implant performance, use, and health utility: A multicenter clinical trial. *Otology and Neurotology*, *35*(9), 1560–1568

4

Auditory Stimuli in Communication

Michael A. Nerbonne, Ronald L. Schow, Kristina M. Blaiser

CONTENTS

Visit the companion website when you see this icon to learn more about the topic nearby in the text.

Learning Outcomes

After reading this chapter, you will be able to

- List and describe the main physical parameters associated with the acoustics of speech
- Explain the differences between auditory detection, discrimination, identification, and comprehension
- Describe how redundancy and noise can influence speech perception
- Define linguistic constraint and describe two examples
- Describe in specific terms how intensity and frequency features of hearing loss impact the perception of speech
- Differentiate between analytic and synthetic approaches to auditory training
- List and explain four anticipatory and repair strategies used in communication
- Compare passive, aggressive, and assertive listeners

INTRODUCTION

The importance that communication plays in our lives cannot be overstated. Communication can take a variety of forms and involves one or more of our sensory modalities. The form of communication most often used to express oneself, oral communication, involves utilization of speech. This creates an extraordinary dependence on the sense of hearing in order to receive and perceive accurately the complex network of auditory stimuli that make up speech. The sense of hearing, therefore, is crucial to the process of oral (verbal) communication.

Hearing loss has significant impacts on communication for both pediatric and adult populations. In older children and adults, who have already developed language and oral communication abilities, hearing loss can impact social interactions and access to educational or vocational information and lead to challenges in the individual's ability to communicate. In infants and young children, who are still in the process of learning language, a hearing loss can impact the ability to fully access speech and language and can lead to deficits across communication domains, particularly when the family uses spoken language. Based on the critical role of audition in communication, audiologic rehabilitation represents an extremely important process whereby an individual's diminished ability to communicate as the result of a hearing loss can, it is hoped, be sharpened and improved. Auditory training is an integral part of the aural rehabilitation process. This involves helping the child or adult with a hearing loss to maximize the use of residual hearing or what is heard through their hearing technology (such as cochlear implants).

This chapter provides information regarding auditory training with patients with hearing loss, including objectives and applications, assessment of auditory skills prior to therapy, and exposure to some of the past and present approaches to providing auditory training. Because of the conviction that the professional providing auditory training must be familiar with the basic aspects of oral communication, information is also provided about the oral communication process. This includes the introduction of a communication model, information regarding auditory perception and the acoustics of speech, and a discussion of the possible effects of hearing loss on speech perception.

A COMMUNICATION MODEL

Basic oral communication involves a *speaker*, a *message*, *feedback*, a *listener*, and the *environment* where the communication takes place.

Although a portion of the communication that normally takes place between individuals is nonverbal, we remain heavily dependent on our ability to receive and interpret auditory stimuli presented during oral communication. Successful oral communication involves a number of key components that deserve elaboration so that the reader may gain an appreciation of the basic process. All oral communication must originate with a *source* or *speaker* who has both a purpose for engaging in communication and the ability to properly encode and articulate the thought to be conveyed. The actual thought to be expressed is termed the *message*. The message is made up of auditory stimuli organized in meaningful linguistic units. Visual and tactile cues are also provided by the speaker in conjunction with the production of the auditory message. Another critical component of the process is the auditory *feedback* provided to the speaker while producing speech, which then provides an opportunity for any needed adjustments or corrections to occur. The communication situation in which the message is conveyed is referred to as the *environment*. Factors associated with the environment, such as the presence of competing background noise, can drastically alter the amount and quality of the communication that takes place. The final major component of the communication process is the *receiver* or *listener*, who is charged with the responsibility of receiving and properly decoding and interpreting the speaker's intended thought. The listener also provides additional feedback to the speaker about how the message is being received.

These basic components of the oral communication process and their sequence are found in Figure 4.1. All the major components are equally important in accomplishing the desired end: communication. Disruption or elimination of any one

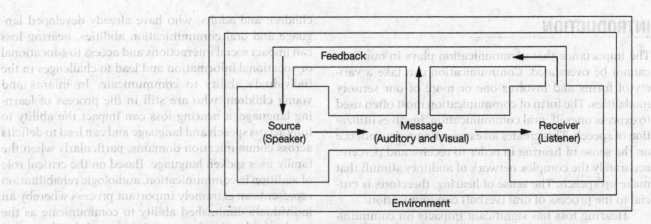

FIGURE 4.1 A simple model of the oral, or verbal, communication process.

part may result in partial or complete failure of the communication process. Proper application of this communication model is of concern to us throughout the chapter and the entire book.

AUDITORY PERCEPTION

Our ability to communicate verbally with others depends to a great extent on the quality of our auditory perception of the various segmental (individual speech sounds) and suprasegmental (rate, rhythm, intonation) elements that make up speech. The following sections focus on the basic aspects of auditory perception: the intensity, frequency, and duration components of speech and transitional cues. The impact of hearing loss on speech perception is also discussed.

Development of Auditory Skills

It is both important and amazing to realize that the unborn infant possesses a functional auditory system that allows the child to begin perceiving auditory stimuli several weeks prior to birth. This is followed by further development and refinement in the neonate's auditory-processing skills in the days and weeks immediately following birth. As a result, the newborn infant not only is capable of detecting auditory stimuli but also can make gross discriminations between various auditory signals on the basis of frequency and intensity parameters. This process of selective listening is extended to speech stimuli within a few weeks following birth. The rather rapid emergence of auditory skills, as described by Northern and Downs (2014), is crucial for the development of speech-processing abilities as well as the emergence of speech and language in the infant. Without the benefit of a normal-functioning auditory system and extensive exposure to auditory stimuli, however, the development of auditory and speech-language skills may be seriously affected.

> The normal development of speech and language is heavily dependent on the infant's acquisition of auditory skills.

Basic Perception Abilities

Although the human auditory system has sophisticated perceptual capabilities, it is limited, to some extent, in terms of the signals it can process. Optimally, the normal human ear is capable of perceiving auditory signals comprising frequencies ranging from about 20 to 20,000 Hz. Stimuli made up entirely of frequencies below and above these limits cannot be detected. Intensity limits, as shown in Figure 4.2, vary as a function of the frequency of the auditory stimulus. The maximum range of intensity we are capable of processing occurs at 3000 to 4000 Hz and varies from about 0 dB SPL to approximately 130 to 140 dB SPL. Signals with intensity of less than 0 dB SPL are generally not perceived; in contrast, signals in excess of 130 to 140 dB SPL produce the sensations of feeling and pain rather than hearing.

> *Detection* simply involves knowing that a sound is present, whereas *discrimination* is the ability to distinguish when two separate sounds are different.

In addition to the detection of acoustic signals, the human ear is also able to discriminate different stimuli on the basis of only minor differences in their acoustical properties. Our ability to discriminate changes in the frequency, intensity, or duration of a signal is influenced by the magnitude of each of the other factors. Stevens and Davis (1938) estimated that the normal ear is capable of perceiving approximately 340,000 distinguishable tones within the audible range of hearing. This total number was based only on frequency and intensity variations of the stimuli, but it suggests that our auditory system possesses amazing discrimination powers.

Acoustics of Speech

Knowledge about the acoustical properties of speech is important for understanding how speech is perceived. Therefore, basic information relevant to this process is covered in the following sections.

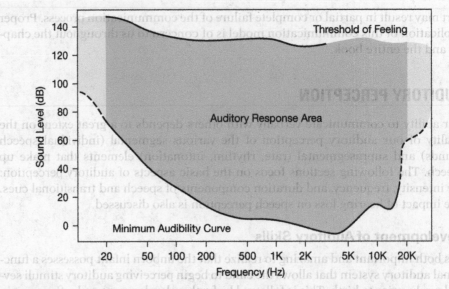

FIGURE 4.2   The auditory response area for persons with normal hearing.

Source: Based on Durrant, J. D., & Lovrinic, J. H. (1995). *Bases of hearing science* (3rd ed.). Baltimore: Williams & Wilkins.

Intensity Parameters of Speech.   The normal human ear is capable of processing signals within an intensity range approaching 130 dB; however, the range of intensity normally found in speech is relatively small. The average intensity of speech, when measured at a distance of approximately 1 meter from the speaker, approximates 65 dB SPL. This corresponds to a value of about 45 dB HL when expressed audiometrically. The average shout will approach 85 dB SPL (65 dB HL), and faint speech occurs at about 45 dB SPL (25 dB HL). Thus, a potential range of about 40 dB exists between the average intensities found, with the softest and loudest speech that we are exposed to in common communication situations. Factors such as distance between the speaker and listener can influence the actual intensity levels for a given communication situation.

Considerable variability exists in the acoustical energy normally associated with individual speech sounds. Table 4.1 lists the relative phonetic powers of the phonemes, as reported by Fletcher (1953). As illustrated, the most powerful

Vowels are produced with greater intensity than consonants, and males tend to speak louder than females.

TABLE 4.1   Relative Phonetic Power of Speech Sounds as Produced by an Average Speaker

ɔ	680	l	100	t	15
ɑ	600	ʃ	80	g	15
ʌ	510	ŋ	73	k	13
Æ	490	m	52	v	12
ʊ	460	tʃ	42	ð	11
ɛ	350	n	36	b	7
U	310	dʒ	23	d	7
L	260	ʒ	20	p	6
I	220	z	16	f	5
R	210	s	16	θ	1

Source: Based on Fletcher (1953).

phoneme, /ɔ/, possesses an average of about 680 times as much energy as the weakest phoneme, /θ/, representing an average overall difference in intensity between the two speech sounds of approximately 28 dB. Since a considerable amount of variability also exists in the intensity of individual voices, Fletcher estimated that, collectively, different speakers may produce variations in the intensity of these two phonemes as great as 56 dB. The relative power of vowels, according to Fletcher, is significantly greater than that of consonants, with the weakest vowel, /i/, having more energy than the most powerful consonant. Further, typical male speakers produce speech with an overall intensity that is about 3 dB greater than that of female speakers.

Frequency Parameters of Speech.   The overall spectrum of speech, as seen in Figure 4.3, is composed of acoustical energy from approximately 50 to 10,000 Hz (Denes & Pinson, 1993). Closer examination of this figure also reveals that the greatest amount of energy found in speech generally is associated with frequencies below 1000 Hz. Above this frequency region, the energy of speech decreases at about a 9 dB/octave rate. The concentration of energy in the lower frequencies can be attributed largely to the fundamental frequency of the adult human voice (males, 130 Hz; females, 260 Hz) and the high intensity and spectral characteristics associated with the production of vowels. As shown in Figure 4.3, the greatest energy for male speech is around 500 Hz. This is due to resonance in the vocal tract rather than just fundamental frequency. It should be noted that the fundamental frequency of children is substantially higher than that of adults, around 400 Hz (Hegde, 2010). As a result, the major energy concentration for this age-group occurs higher on the frequency scale than for adults.

A key aspect of speech production and perception is the information associated with the segmental elements of speech. The segmental components consist of the numerous features associated with the individual vowel and consonant phonemes of the language. The vowels in English are composed mainly of low- and mid-frequency energy and, as indicated earlier, contribute most of the acoustic power in speech. Specifically, the frequency spectrum of each vowel contains at least two or three areas of energy concentration that result from the resonances that occur in the vocal tract during phonation. These points of peak amplitude are referred to as *formants*, and

Formant refers to a band of frequencies that are resonated, or boosted in energy, by the vocal tract.

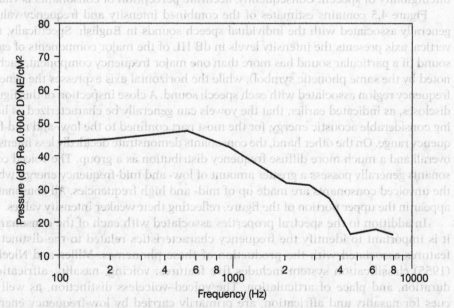

FIGURE 4.3   Long-interval acoustic spectrum of male voices. Measurement made with microphone 18 inches from speaker's lips.

Source: Based on Miller (1951).

This formant frequency graph and a complete learning module on speech acoustics can be found on the text website.

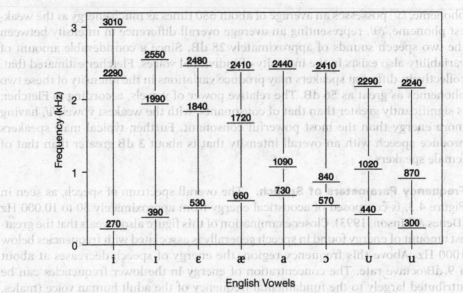

FIGURE 4.4 Mean values of formant frequencies of vowels of American English for adult males.

Source: Based on Peterson & Barney (1952).

Consonant perception plays a major role in comprehending speech.

their location and pattern on the frequency continuum are unique for each vowel. Figure 4.4 illustrates the approximate location of the major formants associated with the vowels, as spoken by adult males. Formants provide important acoustic cues for the identification of vowels. However, it is important to note that even though each of the vowels has several formants, we need to hear only the first two or three to be able to perceive accurately the vowel spoken (Peterson & Barney, 1952).

The consonants in English display a broader high-frequency spectral composition than do vowels. This is particularly true for those consonants for which voicing is not utilized and whose production involves substantial constriction of the articulators. Although they contain relatively little overall energy, or intensity, when compared with vowels, consonants are extremely important in determining the intelligibility of speech. Consequently, accurate perception of consonants is vital.

Figure 4.5 contains estimates of the combined intensity and frequency values generally associated with the individual speech sounds in English. Specifically, the vertical axis presents the intensity levels in dB HL of the major components of each sound (if a particular sound has more than one major frequency component, each is noted by the same phonetic symbol), while the horizontal axis expresses the general frequency region associated with each speech sound. A close inspection of this figure discloses, as indicated earlier, that the vowels can generally be characterized as having considerable acoustic energy, for the most part confined to the low- and mid-frequency range. On the other hand, the consonants demonstrate decidedly less intensity overall and a much more diffuse frequency distribution as a group. The voiced consonants generally possess a greater amount of low- and mid-frequency energy, while the unvoiced consonants are made up of mid- and high frequencies. All consonants appear in the upper portion of the figure, reflecting their weaker intensity values.

Voicing, nasality, duration, and place of articulation are key distinctive features found in speech.

In addition to the spectral properties associated with each of the consonants, it is important to identify the frequency characteristics related to the distinctive features associated with the production of these phonemes. Miller and Nicely's (1955) classification system includes five features: voicing, nasality, affrication, duration, and place of articulation. The voiced–voiceless distinction, as well as cues for nasality and affrication, are primarily carried by low-frequency energy. Information about place of articulation, on the other hand, is contained in the higher frequencies. Table 4.2 categorizes each consonant phoneme by its place and manner of articulation and voicing features.

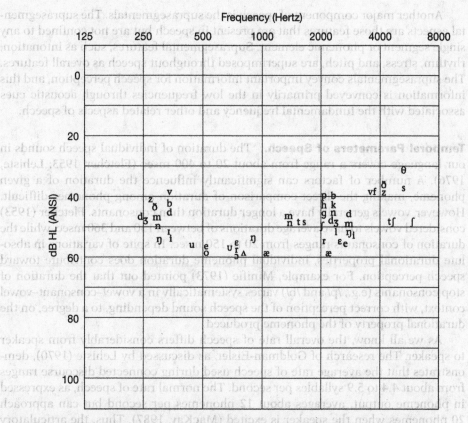

Frequency (Hertz)

FIGURE 4.5 Intensity and frequency distribution of speech sounds in the English language. The values given should be considered only approximations and are based on data reported by Fletcher (1953) and Ling and Ling (1978). Sounds with more than one major component appear in more than one location in the figure.

TABLE 4.2 Categorizing Consonants on the Basis of Manner and Place of Articulation and Voicing

Manner of Articulation	Place of Articulation						
	Bilabial	Labiodental	Linguadental	Alveolar	Palatal	Velar	Glottal
Plosives or Stops	p			t		k	
	b			d		g	
Fricatives		f	θ	s	ʃ		h
		v	ð	z	ʒ		
Affricates					tʃ		
					dʒ		
Nasal	m			n		ŋ	
Liquid				l, r			
Glide	w				j		

Note: Voiceless consonants are listed first, with voiced consonants underneath.

The segmental components of speech are the features associated with the individual speech sounds. The suprasegmental components (rhythm and prosody, pitch, rate) are overall features of speech that are superimposed on phonemes and words.

Another major component of speech is the suprasegmentals. The suprasegmental aspects are those features that are present in speech but are not confined to any single segment or phonemic element. Suprasegmental features, such as intonation, rhythm, stress, and pitch, are superimposed throughout speech as overall features. The suprasegmentals convey important information for speech perception, and this information is conveyed primarily in the low frequencies through acoustic cues associated with the fundamental frequency and other related aspects of speech.

The duration of vowels generally is longer than for consonants.

Temporal Parameters of Speech. The duration of individual speech sounds in our language covers a range from about 20 to 400 msec (Fletcher, 1953; Lehiste, 1976). A number of factors can significantly influence the duration of a given phoneme, making the direct comparison of duration among phonemes difficult. However, vowels generally have a longer duration than consonants. Fletcher (1953) considered vowels to have average durations of between 130 and 360 msec, while the duration of consonants ranges from 20 to 150 msec. In spite of variations in absolute durational properties, individual phoneme duration does contribute toward speech perception. For example, Minifie (1973) pointed out that the duration of stop consonants (e.g., /p/ and /b/) varies systematically in a vowel–consonant–vowel context, with correct perception of the speech sound depending, to a degree, on the durational property of the phoneme produced.

As we all know, the overall rate of speech differs considerably from speaker to speaker. The research of Goldman-Eisler, as discussed by Lehiste (1970), demonstrates that the average rate of speech used during connected discourse ranges from about 4.4 to 5.9 syllables per second. The normal rate of speech, as expressed in phoneme output, averages about 12 phonemes per second but can approach 20 phonemes when the speaker is excited (MacKay, 1987). Thus, the articulatory process is swift and capable of producing a flood of speech sounds and words that must be processed as effectively, or listener, as they were produced by the speaker. Both of these are challenging tasks!

Transitional cues result from the influences of coarticulation of individual speech sounds when combined into words, phrases, and so on.

Transitional Cues. The intensity, frequency, and durational properties of a given phoneme spoken in isolation are altered significantly when the phoneme is produced with other phonemes in conversational speech. In conversational speech, the dynamic movements of the articulators in the production of adjacent phonemes produce acoustical by-products, termed *transitional cues*. These cues make up a large portion of the total speech signal and are very important in the perception of speech since they contain valuable information related to individual phoneme perception, especially for diphthongs and consonants.

For example, the second and third formants of vowels often contain transitions in frequency produced by the flowing movement of the articulators that signal the presence of particular consonants that immediately follow. These formant transitions occur as the vocal resonances shift during articulation of vowels and consonants, which are combined in speech. Likewise, the durational aspects of vowels in connected speech can be altered to convey information regarding the phoneme to follow. For example, a voiced consonant in the final position is often accompanied by increased duration of the vowel immediately before it. The prolonged vowel duration contributes to our perception of voicing in the consonant that follows. This is an example of why formant transitional cues are a vital part of the speech signal and are quite important for speech perception.

Speech Perception and Comprehension

Our discussion has emphasized the segmental and suprasegmental aspects that constitute speech. The organization and production of these crucial elements into a meaningful oral message by the speaker and the accurate reception of this dynamic signal by the listener represent a highly complex, sophisticated process. However, mere reception of the segmented and suprasegmental elements of speech by a listener does not ensure proper perception of the message. Perception of speech implies understanding and comprehension, and the reception of speech by the auditory mechanism is only a first step in its perception.

In its most basic form, the perception of speech may be thought of as involving a number of important components. Among these are the following:

Detection. This basic aspect of auditory perception simply involves being aware of sound. The primary question asked related to detection is, "Do you hear the sound, yes or no?" Our ability to detect speech is influenced by our hearing acuity and the intensity level of the speech signal.

Discrimination. Speech discrimination refers to the ability to distinguish among the individual speech stimuli (phonemes, syllables, etc.) of our language. The question asked related to discrimination is, "Do the two sounds sound the same or different?"

Identification. The ability to identify or label what one has heard by pointing to or naming. The identification-related question is, "What is that sound?"

Attention. A fundamental ingredient in the perception of speech relates to attending to or focusing on the speaker and the message being conveyed. The degree and quality of the listener's attention will influence how well speech is perceived.

Memory. A key component in speech perception is the ability to retain or store verbal information for relatively brief periods or, in some instances, extended lengths of time. Memory is also fundamental to other components of speech perception and enables us to combine individual speech units for the purpose of deriving meaning from an entire verbal message rather than from each individual unit of the message.

Closure. The perceived speech elements must be brought together into a meaningful whole. This process, termed *closure,* helps a person to recognize speech even when some cues are absent, as with hearing loss.

Comprehension. Full perception and understanding of the meaning of an auditory message. In comprehension the question asked is, "What does that mean?"

Our task in audiologic rehabilitation is to consider what is currently known concerning speech perception as we address the needs of individuals with hearing problems.

Speech Perception and Hearing Loss

Our success in processing speech is closely related to a number of important factors, and some of these are discussed in the next section.

Physical Properties.   Information concerning the physical properties of speech is most relevant when considering the relationship between the perception of speech and hearing loss because the degree of our success in processing speech appears closely related to our ability to receive the coded acoustical information that makes up the signal.

The normal ear is well equipped to receive and process speech in most situations. Since most speech is normally presented at average intensity levels of around 45 dB HL, it is well within the sensitivity range of the normal human ear. Also, although we are capable of hearing auditory signals ranging in frequency from about 20 to 20,000 Hz, only a portion of the entire range is required for the reception of speech since speech contains energy from roughly 50 to 10,000 Hz. Consequently, in most listening conditions, those with normal hearing will experience little, if any, difficulty in adequately hearing the speech sounds found in oral communication.

Consonant perception tends to be disrupted more by hearing loss than is vowel perception.

The same does not hold true for persons with hearing loss. No longer are the intensity and frequency ranges of the ear with hearing loss always sufficient to provide total perception of the speech signal. One or both of these stimulus parameters may be limited such that it becomes difficult to hear specific speech sounds adequately for identification purposes. For example, a person with 50-dB thresholds from 2000 to 8000 Hz would have considerable difficulty perceiving the phonemes with spectral compositions that involve primarily those higher frequencies. The information in Figure 4.5 regarding the relative frequency and intensity characteristics of individual speech sounds as spoken at a typical conversation level helps in understanding why this occurs.

While factors such as type of hearing loss and test materials used can influence the outcome of investigations concerning hearing loss and the perception of phonemes, some general patterns of speech perception difficulties have been observed for persons with hearing loss. For example, most listeners with hearing loss experience only minimal difficulty in vowel perception (Owens, Benedict, & Schubert, 1971). Specifically, in the research by Owens et al. (1971), the vowel phonemes /ɛ/ and /o/ were found to have the highest probability of error. Only when the degree of the hearing loss is severe to profound does the perception of vowels become significantly altered (Erber, 1979). Consonant perception, however, presents a far more difficult listening task for those with hearing loss. Owens (1978) found phonemes such as /s/, /p/, /k/, /d/, and /θ/ to be among the most frequently missed by adults with sensorineural hearing loss. He also found misperceptions to be more frequent for phonemes in the final position of words than in the initial position. The most common errors in consonant phoneme perception occur with the place of articulation feature, followed by manner of articulation. Errors in the perception of nasality and voice among consonants are generally far less frequent.

Owens and his colleagues conducted a series of investigations regarding the perception of consonants. In one such study, Owens, Benedict, and Schubert (1972) examined the relationship between the configuration of the audiogram and the specific consonant perceptual errors made by a group of individuals with hearing loss. The /s/, /ʃ/, /tʃ/, and /dʒ/ and the /t/ and /θ/ in the initial position only were found to be difficult for listeners with sloping configurations on the audiogram. The authors noted that these phonemes became increasingly difficult to hear accurately as the steepness of the sloping high-frequency hearing loss increased. Correct recognition of /s/ and the initial /t/ and /θ/ were found to be closely related to hearing sensitivity above 2000 Hz, while perception of /ʃ/, /tʃ/, and /dʒ/ was very dependent on sensitivity between 1000 and 2000 Hz. These findings point out the crucial role that hearing in this frequency region plays in the perception of several consonant phonemes. A similar study by Sher and Owens (1974) with listeners having high-frequency loss confirmed that individuals with normal hearing to 2000 Hz and a sharp-sloping sensitivity loss for frequencies above that experience difficulty in adequately hearing a number of consonant phonemes. These authors pointed out that information concerning specific phoneme errors is useful in establishing audiologic rehabilitation strategies for persons with hearing losses of this type. More recent work by Stelmachowicz, Pittman, Hoover, and Lewis (2001) has demonstrated similar findings, suggesting that, even with well-fit hearing technology, high-frequency phoneme perception may be difficult to achieve for individuals with hearing loss.

As can be seen, the actual overall degree of difficulty in speech perception imposed on an individual is closely related to the intensity and frequency features of speech and the intensity and frequency features of the hearing loss found on the conventional audiogram. However, difficulty with speech perception can also be influenced by other related variables that are discussed elsewhere in this chapter and throughout the text. Therefore, while the audiogram usually is our most useful single predictor of a person's speech perception abilities, other factors to be discussed in the next section must be considered as well.

Redundancy and Noise. The perception of speech is a highly complex process that involves more than the acoustics of speech or the hearing abilities of the listener, even though these are important variables to be sure. Ultimately, for oral communication to be successful, sufficient information must be present in the message of interest for it to be perceived. The amount of information available for a given communication situation is closely associated with the concepts of redundancy and noise.

Conversational speech generally can be described as being highly redundant. That is, it contains information from a variety of sources that is available for a listener to use in comprehending a message, even though portions of the communication may not have been heard. The degree of redundancy in oral communication varies from one expression to the next, so the extent to which a listener can predict what was said will also vary. Basically, the more redundant a message, the more readily it can be perceived by the listener, especially in difficult listening situations. A number of factors present in a given communication situation can influence the amount of redundancy present, and Table 4.3 provides a list of some of these.

Among the many factors associated with the redundancy, or predictability, found in conversational speech for the listener to use for perception are syntactic, semantic, and situational constraints (see Table 4.4). Syntactic, or structural, constraints relate to the predictable manner in which linguistic units are chained together according to the rules associated with acceptable English. The selection and use of phonemes and words in an utterance are strongly influenced by these rules, making it easier for the listener to predict what is to follow after having heard only the initial portion of the sentence. Such syntactic clues can be used in conjunction with another factor related to redundancy, namely, semantic constraints, which allow the listener to predict the type of vocabulary and expressions to be used based on the general semantic content of the expression. When the topic of conversation is food, for example, the listener can expect to hear a rather restricted range of vocabulary peculiar to that particular topic. Use of this small range of words will increase the redundancy of the message, making it easier to predict what is said. Situational constraints also create redundancy. Our conversational partner, the location of the conversation, the time of day it takes place, and other similar factors all influence what we say and how we say it, which also can make conversational speech more predictable. All these types of constraints, along with other factors listed in Table 4.3, collectively produce the redundancy that makes the perception of speech easier for us all.

The redundancy of speech relates to its predictability; the greater the redundancy, the better the odds will be that a listener can guess what was said, even when he or she did not hear the entire message.

The more redundant a message, the more readily it can be perceived by the listener, especially in difficult listening situations.

TABLE 4.3   A Partial List of Factors That Can Influence the Amount of Redundancy in Speech

Within the speaker	Compliance with the rules of the language
	Use of appropriate articulation, intonation, stress
	Size and appropriateness of the vocabulary used to convey the message
Within the message	Number of syllables, words, etc.
	Amount of context
	Frequency composition of the speech signal
	Intensity of the speech signal
Within the communication environment	Amount of acoustic noise
	Degree of reverberation
	Number of situational cues present that are related to the message
Within the listener	Familiarity with the rules of the language
	Familiarity with the vocabulary of the message
	Knowledge of the topic of conversation
	Hearing abilities

Source: Adapted from Sanders (1971).

TABLE 4.4 **Examples of Linguistic Constraints Available to Enhance Speech Perception**

Syntactic constraints: Refer to the fact that every language is governed by a set of grammatical rules that specifies the relationship between words used to communicate. For example, adjectives may be used to qualify nouns (as in "the *blue* shoes"); adjectives are not used to qualify verbs (as in "he *blue* ran").

Semantic constraints: Refer to the fact that the words used in a sentence are usually related to each other in a meaningful way. For example, although the sentence "Put the salt on the cloud" is syntactically correct, semantically it is highly improbable.

Situational constraints: Refer to the fact that language usually takes place within a physical and social context. Generally, the use of language bears some relationship with the context in which it is used. For example, in a stadium, during a football game, it is more likely that the topic of discussion will center around sports-related activities than around religious beliefs and values.

Source: Adapted from Gagne and Jennings (2000).

Noise can be considered to refer to a variety of variables that can be counterproductive to communication, not only competing auditory noise.

Noise in oral communication refers to a host of factors that can actually reduce the amount of information present for the listener to use. In this context, "noise" refers to a variety of variables that can be counterproductive to communication, not only competing auditory noise. Table 4.5 provides a partial list of the potential sources of noise associated with oral communication with which the listener must contend. Each of these factors may reduce the amount of information in a spoken message, thus reducing the amount of redundancy, or predictability, that is available for the listener to use in perceiving speech.

Noise impacts both the quantity (how much someone hears) and the quality (the fidelity of the acoustic signal) of what someone hears. This can impact children even more than adults. For example, children may not have the linguistic knowledge to "fill in the gaps" of a sentence that is presented in a noisy environment. They also may miss the meanings of words or the production of phonemes that are less acoustically important. Even with the most advanced hearing technology, clinicians, family members, and audiologists can work together to promote listening environments that are conducive to spoken language learning.

Thus, the degree of information available for the listener to use in perceiving a message is influenced in a positive or negative manner by a number of related variables that are part of oral communication. For the listener, particularly one with hearing loss, the importance of each of these variables to the process of speech perception cannot be overstated. In addition, as previously stated, children with prelinguistic hearing loss, or hearing loss that exists prior to language development, need more help decoding the language than an older child or adult who has a hearing loss after language has already been established.

TABLE 4.5 **Some Potential Sources of Noise in Oral Communication**

Within the speaker	Poor syntax
	Abnormal articulation
	Improper stress or inflection
Within the communication environment	Abnormal lighting
	Competing or distracting visual stimuli
	Competing or distracting auditory stimuli
	Reverberation
Within the listener	Lack of familiarity with the rules of the language
	Inability to identify the topic of the message
	Poor listening skills

Source: Adapted from Sanders (1971).

THE AUDITORY TRAINING PROCESS

Traditionally, auditory training has been considered a major component of the audiologic rehabilitation process. Thus, its potential in assisting those with hearing loss has been expressed in major textbooks within the field of audiology both in the past (Davis & Hardick, 1981; Oyer, 1966) and more recently (Montano & Spitzer, 2013; Cole & Flexer, 2015; Tye-Murray, 2015).

The intent of the next major section of this chapter is to familiarize the reader with both the traditional and the current forms of auditory training and how they fit into the entire audiologic rehabilitation process.

Definition and Application of Auditory Training

Numerous attempts have been made to define auditory training in the past. Although similar in some respects, these definitions vary considerably according to the orientation of the definer and special considerations associated with hearing loss, such as its degree and time of onset.

Probably the most commonly referred to definition of auditory training is attributed to Carhart (1960), who considered auditory training a process of teaching the child or adult with hearing loss to take full advantage of available auditory clues. As a result, Carhart recommended an emphasis in therapy on developing an awareness of sound, gross discrimination of nonverbal stimuli, and gross and fine discrimination of speech.

Later, in discussing the use of auditory training with children, Erber (1982) described it as "the creation of special communication conditions in which teachers and audiologists help hearing-impaired children acquire many of the auditory perception abilities that normally hearing children acquire naturally without their intervention" (p. 1). Erber stated further, "Our intent is to help the hearing-impaired child apply his or her impaired auditory sense to the fullest capacity in language communication, regardless of the degree of damage to the auditory system. Usually progress is achieved through careful application of amplification devices and through special teaching techniques" (p. 29).

When considering auditory training for adults, two general objectives are usually relevant: (1) learning to maximize the use of auditory and other related cues available for the perception of speech and (2) adjustment and orientation to facilitate the optimum use of hearing aids and cochlear implants.

Inherent in the various views of auditory training, as well as those of other professionals in audiologic rehabilitation, is the notion that persons with hearing loss can be trained to maximize the use of whatever amount of hearing they possess. Today, this is particularly true because of the advances in hearing technology, such as digital hearing aids and cochlear implants. The ultimate aim of auditory training is to achieve maximum communication potential through developing the auditory sensory channel, often with the use of appropriately fit hearing technology, to its fullest. In a sense, auditory training is often designed to improve one's listening skills, which will result in improved speech perception. Although the primary goal of auditory training is usually to maximize receptive communication abilities, it is important to point out that achieving this basic goal can result in other important accomplishments as well, including acquisition of more proficient speech and language skills, educational and vocational advancement, and successful psychosocial adjustment. As indicated earlier, if the communication skills of persons with hearing loss can be improved, other areas of concern, such as educational progress, will be facilitated as well.

Early Efforts in Auditory Training

The earliest efforts in auditory training date back at least to the nineteenth century. Individuals in Europe used auditory training with those having hearing loss throughout

The hearing abilities that a person with hearing loss has left are often referred to as residual hearing.

the 1800s, with some success noted. Impressed with their accomplishments,ts, Goldstein (1939) introduced a similar approach to auditory training in the United States in the late 1890s and early 1900s. Known as the Acoustic Method, this approach centered around systematic stimulation with individual speech sounds, syllables, words, and sentences to improve speech perception and to aid deaf persons in their own speech production. The Acoustic Method was utilized in a number of facilities throughout the country, including the Central Institute for the Deaf in St. Louis, Missouri, which Goldstein founded. Goldstein exerted a significant influence on the thinking of many professionals over the years regarding the potential of auditory training with persons with hearing loss.

Until World War II, the primary focus of auditory training was its use with severely/profoundly deaf children in an effort to facilitate speech and language acquisition and increase their educational potential. However, the activities that occurred at Veterans Administration audiology centers during World War II served to demonstrate on a large scale that adults with mild to severe hearing losses could profit from auditory training as well. Led by Raymond Carhart, personnel in these centers developed and applied auditory training exercises with large numbers of adults, most with noise-induced hearing loss. Carhart (1960) later authored a book chapter that influenced the thinking of audiologists regarding auditory training with children and adults for years to come.

Raymond Carhart made many contributions to the profession of audiology and is considered by many to be the Father of Audiology.

Carhart.   Carhart's approach to auditory training for prelingually deafened children was based on his belief that since listening skills are normally learned early in life, the child possessing a significant hearing loss at birth or soon after will not move through the normal developmental stages important in acquiring these skills. Likewise, when a hearing loss occurs in later childhood or in adulthood, some of the person's auditory skills may become deficient even though they were intact prior to the onset of the hearing loss. In each instance, Carhart believed that auditory training was warranted.

Childhood Procedures.   Carhart outlined four major steps or objectives involved in auditory training for children with prelingual deafness:

1. Development of awareness of sound
2. Development of gross discriminations
3. Development of broad discriminations among simple speech patterns
4. Development of finer discriminations for speech

Development of an awareness of auditory stimuli and the significance of sound involves having the child acknowledge the presence and absence of sound and the importance of sound in his or her world. The development of gross discrimination initially involves demonstrating with various noisemakers that sounds differ. Once the child can successfully discriminate grossly different sounds, he or she is exposed to finer types of discrimination tasks that include variation in the frequency, intensity, and durational properties of sound. When the child is able to recognize the presence of sound and can perceive gross differences with nonverbal stimuli, Carhart's approach calls for the introduction of activities directed toward learning gross discrimination for speech signals. The final phase consists of training the child to make fine discriminations of speech stimuli in connected discourse and integrating an increased vocabulary to enable him or her to follow connected speech in a more rapid and accurate fashion. Carhart also felt that the use of vision by the child should be encouraged in most auditory training activities.

Adult Procedures.   Because adults who acquire a hearing loss later in life retain a portion of their original auditory skills, Carhart recommended that auditory training with adults focus on reeducating a skill diminished as a consequence of the hearing loss. Initially, Carhart felt that it was important to establish "an attitude of critical listening" in the individual. This involves being attentive to the subtle differences among sounds and can involve a considerable amount of analytic drill work on the perception of phonemes that are difficult for the adult with hearing loss to perceive. Lists of matched syllables and words that contain the troublesome phonemes, such as *she-fee*, *so-tho*, *met-let*, or *mash-math*, are read to the individual, who repeats them back. Such training should also include phrases and sentences, with the goal of developing as rapid and precise a recognition of the phonetic elements as is possible within the limitations imposed by the person's hearing loss. Speechreading combined with a person's hearing was also encouraged by Carhart during a portion of the auditory training sessions.

Because we often communicate under less-than-ideal listening circumstances, Carhart advocated that auditory training sessions for adults be conducted in three commonly encountered situations: (1) relatively intense background noise, (2) the presence of a competing speech signal, and (3) listening on the telephone. This emphasis on practice in speech perception under listening conditions with decreasing amounts of redundancy has been emphasized more recently, as noted by Sweetow and Henderson-Sabes (2009).

According to Carhart, the use of hearing aids (and cochlear implants) is vital in auditory training, and he recommended that they be utilized as early as possible in the auditory training program. These recommendations were consistent with Carhart's belief that systematic exposure to sound during auditory training was an ideal means of allowing a person to adequately adjust to hearing aids and assist in using them as optimally as possible.

Analytic auditory training employs a "bottoms-up" approach that focuses mainly on enhancing perception of small segments of speech (phonemes, syllables, words).

CURRENT APPROACHES TO AUDITORY TRAINING

The basic intent of more recent methods of auditory training remains the same, that is, to maximize communication potential by developing to its fullest the auditory channel of the person with hearing loss. This next section discusses how this form of audiologic rehabilitation currently is being applied with those experiencing hearing loss.

Candidacy for Auditory Training

In recent times, auditory training therapy is used routinely with children who use hearing technology such as hearing aids and/or cochlear implants. Auditory training can be beneficial for young children with cochlear implants and/or hearing aids to help the child understand and make use of sound as part of spoken language development and communication. Because children are identified at earlier ages, auditory training has evolved to helping to integrate listening skills into daily communication and early language learning.

Adults with newly fit hearing aids or cochlear implants also can benefit from auditory training. There is strong evidence that a structured program of listening training enhances the benefits derived from a cochlear implant. Although extensive auditory training typically has not been utilized routinely in the past with hard of hearing adults, certain factors, such as exceptionally poor speech perception and/ or a severe to profound degree of loss, resulted in its application on a selective basis. However, in recent times, its use with hard of hearing adults on a more routine basis has been advocated by many in conjunction with facilitating the effective use of hearing aids.

Assessment of Auditory Skills

An integral part of a comprehensive auditory training program is the assessment of individual auditory skills. Before, during, and at the conclusion of auditory training, the clinician should attempt to evaluate the auditory abilities of the person with hearing loss. Information of this nature is important for several reasons, including the following:

1. Determining whether auditory training appears warranted
2. Providing a basis for comparison with posttherapy performance to assess how much improvement in auditory performance, particularly speech perception, has occurred
3. Identifying specific areas of auditory perception to concentrate on in future auditory training

The nature of the auditory testing that takes place will vary considerably, depending on a number of variables, such as the age of the client, his or her language skills, and the type and degree of the hearing loss. The clinician must exercise care in selecting appropriate test materials for the individual patient, particularly with regard to the language levels required for a given test. Actually, when testing speech perception performance via hearing or vision, a number of variables need to be kept in mind that can influence the degree of difficulty of the perceptual task. These include the following:

- The nature of the perceptual task (detection, discrimination, identification, comprehension)
- The use of either an open-set or a closed-set (e.g., multiple-choice) response format
- The degree of context present (e.g., monosyllables presented in isolation or sentences)
- The level of sophistication and the age level of the vocabulary used in the test (instructions and test items)
- The signal-to-noise ratio present (figure–ground)

Manipulation of any one of these variables can make the test either easier or harder for an individual, and the clinician should be mindful of all this when selecting and administering tests. A variety of tests, both formal and informal, should be available for assessment purposes so that the particular needs of each individual can be met adequately.

Evaluating Children. Both the amount and the difficulty of testing appropriate for young children are limited by their physical and cognitive development. Therefore, informal testing and observation are relied on heavily with this age-group. For the infant, the initial goal of assessment for auditory training purposes may not center on speech perception. Rather, an effort may be made to better understand how well the hearing technology is fit for the child's particular hearing loss, to identify the extent to which auditory skills have emerged (e.g., gross discrimination and localization of a variety of stimuli), and to make programming changes as needed. Once this information is known, a specific program for developing auditory skills, such as that described in Chapter 9, can be implemented in conjunction with therapy related to development of speech and language. It is important that audiologists, parents/caregivers, and early interventionists collaborate to ensure that the child's hearing technology is well fit and providing the child with the acoustic access needed to develop spoken communication. Parent-completed questionnaires, such as the LittlEARS (Tsiakpini et al., 2004), the Parent's Evaluation of Aural/Oral Performance of Children (PEACH; Ching & Hill, 2005), and the Infant-Toddler Meaningful Auditory Integration Scale (ITMAIS; Zimmerman-Phillips, Osberger, & Robbins, 1997), help provide audiologists with a framework of understanding how the hearing technology is working and whether any programming changes are needed.

For older children, more formal, in-depth assessment of overall speech perception abilities generally is possible. Specifically, materials have been developed that require the child to respond in a prescribed manner to individual words or phonemes presented at a comfortable listening level. Some of the commonly used

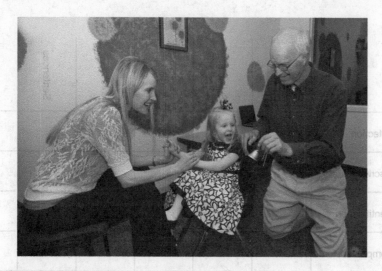

Informal assessment of auditory awareness/localization skills

formal tests of this type that have been designed for assessing speech perception in children with hearing loss include the following:

1. Word Intelligibility by Picture Identification (WIPI; Ross & Lerman, 1970). The authors of the WIPI modified an existing test for children (Myatt & Landes, 1963) to include only vocabulary appropriate for children with hearing loss. The WIPI includes four lists, each of which contains 25 monosyllabic words. The child provides a picture-pointing response in a closed-set format. According to the authors, the test is suitable for use with children with hearing loss and limited receptive and expressive language abilities.

2. Northwestern University Children's Perception of Speech (NU-CHIPS; Katz & Elliott, 1978). This test consists of 50 monosyllabic nouns that have been scrambled to form four individual lists. Like the WIPI, the NU-CHIPS uses a response format that requires that the child point to the one picture from several options that best represents the test items. Because of the basic vocabulary included and the nonverbal response format, use of the NU-CHIPS with many children with hearing loss appears appropriate.

3. Six Sound Test (Ling, 1976, 1989). Six isolated phonemes (/m/, /a/, /u/, /i/, /s/, and /ʃ/) are spoken to the child at a normal conversational level. Those with usable residual hearing up to 1000 Hz should be able to detect the vowels. Children with some residual hearing up to 2000 Hz should detect /ʃ/, and those with residual hearing up to 4000 Hz (not worse than 90 dB HL at 4000 Hz) should detect /s/.

Additional test batteries are designed to assess varied aspects of auditory skill development in children. Examples include the following:

1. Early Speech Perception Test (ESP; Moog & Geers, 1990). ESP consists of a series of subtests that assess pattern and word perception using a closed-set format. The results allow children to be placed into four speech perception categories: (1) no pattern perception, (2) pattern perception, (3) some word identification, and (4) consistent word identification. A Low Verbal version also has been developed for use with children having restricted vocabulary.

2. Glendonald Auditory Screen Procedure (GASP), developed at the Glendonald Auditory School for the Deaf in Australia (Erber, 1982). GASP is based on a model of auditory perception described in the next section of this chapter (see Figure 4.6). The basic test battery associated with GASP consists of three subtests of speech perception: (1) phoneme detection, (2) word identification, and (3) sentence comprehension. The GASP phoneme detection subtest is similar in format to the Six Sound Test developed by Ling (1976, 1989). According to

Tests use either a closed-set or an open-set format. A closed-set format for a test of speech perception involves presenting a test item (e.g., a word) and having the listener choose the correct response from a limited set of options (multiple choice). In an open-set format, the listener can respond with any word he or she feels is correct.

Speech Stimulus

	Speech Elements	Syllables	Words	Phrases	Sentences	Connected Discourse
Detection	1					
Discrimination						
Identification			2			
Comprehension					3	

Response Task

FIGURE 4.6 An auditory stimulus–response matrix showing the three GASP subtests: Phoneme Detection (1), Word Identification (2), and Sentence (Question) Comprehension (3).

Source: Erber, N. (1982). *Auditory training.* Washington, DC: Alexander Graham Bell Association for the Deaf. Reprinted by permission.

Figure–ground refers to the ability to perceive a target signal that is presented simultaneously with other competing signals.

Word recognition testing typically involves presenting a 25- or 50-word list of monosyllabic words at a comfortable intensity level for the listener. A percent correct score is calculated.

Erber, the results from GASP can aid in planning auditory training because the child's performance on the subtests is predictive of other, related auditory tasks.

3. Developmental Approach to Successful Listening Test (DASL II; Stout & Windle, 1994). This comprehensive test of auditory skills evaluates numerous aspects of sound awareness, phonetic listening, and auditory comprehension. Children from 3 years of age can be evaluated with the DASL Test, and some normative information is available for children with varying degrees of hearing loss.

All these tests attempt to take into account potential limitations of a child's receptive vocabulary level and ability to respond orally. However, the variability observed in the receptive and expressive communication skills of these children makes it unwise to draw any firm generalization about the specific age range of children for whom any of these tests are suited. Vocabulary development and expressive language skills, rather than chronological age, is a key consideration in selecting the appropriate test to use.

Evaluating Adults. A number of formal tests of speech perception also are available for use with adults. Any of the traditional monosyllabic word lists, such as the Northwestern University Auditory Test No. 6 (Tillman & Carhart, 1966), may be employed to evaluate overall word-recognition abilities.

Other tests allow for more in-depth assessment of the perception of consonants, which can be especially difficult for persons with hearing loss to perceive accurately. For example, Owens and Schubert (1977) produced a 100-item, multiple-choice consonant perception test called the California Consonant Test (CCT). Thirty-six of the test items assess consonant perception in the initial word position, while 64 items test perception in the final position. Each of the 100 items is presented to the listener in a closed-set, multiple-choice format, as shown in Figure 4.7. Research by Schwartz and Surr (1979) demonstrated that, compared to the Northwestern University Auditory Test No. 6, the CCT is more sensitive to the speech recognition difficulties experienced by individuals with high-frequency hearing loss. Consequently, the CCT is frequently relied on in assessing the speech recognition abilities of adult patients.

Tests that employ sentence-type stimuli also can be informative. Kalikow, Stevens, and Elliott (1977) developed a test called Speech Perception in Noise (SPIN).

ROBE	_____	MAP	_____	BAIL	_____
RODE	_____	MATCH	_____	JAIL	_____
ROSE	_____	MATH	_____	DALE	_____
ROVE	_____	MAT	_____	GALE	_____

LASS	_____	DIES	_____	LEAF	_____
LAUGH	_____	DIED	_____	LEASE	_____
LATCH	_____	DIVE	_____	LEACH	_____
LASH	_____	DINE	_____	LEASH	_____

FIN	_____	PEAK	_____	RAISE	_____
PIN	_____	PEACH	_____	RAID	_____
KIN	_____	PEAT	_____	RAGE	_____
TIN	_____	PEEP	_____	RAVE	_____

FIGURE 4.7   Examples of multiple-choice test items for the California Consonant Test.
Source: Based on Owens & Schubert (1977).

This test is unique in that it attempts to assess a listener's utilization of both linguistic and situational cues in the perception of speech. Sentence material is presented against a background of speech babble, with the listener's task being to identify the final word in the sentence. Ten 50-item forms of SPIN have been generated, each version containing sentences with either high or low predictability relative to the final word in each sentence. Examples of each are shown in Table 4.6. Bilger, Rzcezkowski, Nuetzel, and Rabinowitz (1979) have revised the forms to make them more equivalent to each other. The SPIN test can provide important information concerning how effectively a given listener makes use of contextual information in the perception of speech, in addition to providing insight regarding how the listener perceives the acoustical properties of speech.

The Central Institute for the Deaf (CID) Everyday Speech Sentences (Davis & Silverman, 1978) has been used extensively for several decades to evaluate a listener's ability to perceive connected discourse. They consist of 10 sets of 10 sentences, as shown in Table 4.7. The sentences vary in length and form and possess several characteristics associated with typical conversation.

Results of these tests, as well as others, should provide the clinician with specific information concerning a client's consonant perception in a word and/or sentence context as well as the ability to comprehend speech in sentence form.

Additional information about speech perception can be gained by introducing competing noise to the test situation and varying the degree of redundancy in the test material. Commonly used tests of this type include the Hearing in Noise Test (HINT; Nilsson, Soli, & Sullivan, 1994) and Quick Speech in Noise (QuickSIN; Etymotic Research, 2001). Also, addition of visual cues via speechreading during test administration in a bisensory perceptual condition can provide useful information regarding a person's overall integrative skills (see Chapters 5 and 10).

Speech babble is a recording of several people talking at once.

TABLE 4.6   Examples of Low- and High-Predictability Sentences from the SPIN Test

Sentence	Level of Predictability
The honey bees swarmed round the *hive*.	High
The girl knows about the *swamp*.	Low
The cushion was filled with *foam*.	High
He had considered the *robe*.	Low

Source: Based on Kalikow et al. (1977).

TABLE 4.7   Examples of a 10-Sentence Set of CID Everyday Speech Sentences

1. *It's time* to *go*.
2. *If* you *don't want these old magazines, throw them out*.
3. *Do* you *want to wash up*?
4. It's a *real dark night so watch your driving*.
5. *I'll carry* the *package* for *you*.
6. Did *you forget* to *shut off* the *water*?
7. *Fishing* in a *mountain stream* is my *idea* of a *good time*.
8. *Fathers spend* more *time* with their *children than* they *used to*.
9. *Be careful not to break your glasses*!
10. *I'm sorry*.

Source: Based on Davis & Silverman (1978).

Signal-to-noise ratio refers to comparing the intensity of the signal you wish to hear with all the other auditory signals present in that listening situation.

Owens, Kessler, Telleen, and Schubert (1985) developed a comprehensive set of tests, the Minimal Auditory Capabilities (MAC) Battery, for assessing auditory and visual skills of patients with severe to profound hearing loss. The level of difficulty of the MAC is suitable for individuals for whom conventional speech perception tests may be too challenging, such as with persons having profound hearing loss. Included in the MAC battery are 14 subtests that evaluate both basic and more complex auditory perception abilities involving a variety of listening tasks with speech. One of the subtests also assesses speechreading skills. The battery is presently being used in the evaluation of cases considered for a cochlear implant. Other assessment tools used for this purpose include the Iowa Vowel and Consonant Confusion Tests (Tyler, Preece, & Tye-Murray, 1986), the Banford-Kowal-Bench (BKB) sentences (Bench, Kowal, & Bamford, 1979), and the HINT.

Methods of Auditory Training

The more current approaches to auditory training vary considerably. According to Blamey and Alcantara (1994), it is possible to categorize them into one of four general categories, based on the fundamental strategy stressed in therapy:

1. *Analytic:* Attempts to break speech into smaller components (phoneme, syllable) and incorporate these separately into auditory training exercises. Examples include exercises that emphasize same–different discrimination of vowel or consonant phonemes in syllables (e.g., /bi-ba/), or words (e.g., /kɪp-kɪt/) or that require the listener to identify a word within a closed-set response format (e.g., run–money–bat).

2. *Synthetic:* Emphasizes a more global approach to speech perception, stressing the use of clues derived from the syntax and context of a spoken message to derive understanding. Training synthetically involves the use of meaningful stimuli (words, phrases, sentences). This might involve practicing sentence perception based on prior information about context (e.g., having lunch, a classroom discussion on government) or having the clinician name a topic and present related words or phrases that the individual must repeat back.

3. *Pragmatic:* Involves training the listener to control communication variables, such as the level of speech, the *signal-to-noise ratio*, and the context or complexity of the message, in order to obtain the necessary information via audition for understanding to occur. For example, the person with hearing loss practices how to effectively use conversation repair strategies, such as asking questions or requesting that a statement be repeated or clarified, to comprehend a paragraph read by the clinician. A similar activity centers around the use of QUEST?AR (Erber, 1996). Here, the patient is given a series of questions related to a specified topic, such as those listed in Table 4.8. The patient asks the clinician each question. The clinician answers each question, and the patient then must correctly repeat the answer given before moving on to

TABLE 4.8   Topics and Questions from QUEST?AR[a]

Where did you go?	museum, restaurant, post office, shopping, camping, doctor, zoo, beach, airport, swimming, mountains, picnic, music lesson, Mars, supermarket, and so forth

Questions:

1. Why did you go there?
2. When did you go?
3. How many people went with you?
4. Who were they? (names)
5. What did you take with you?
6. Where is (the place where you went)?
7. How did you get there?
8. What did you see on the way?
9. What time did you get there?
10. What did you do first?
11. What did you see?
12. How many? What colour? etc.
13. What happened at (the place where you went)?
14. What else did you do?
15. What were other people doing at (the place where you went)?
16. What was the most interesting thing that you saw?
17. What was the most interesting thing that you did?
18. What did you buy?
19. What kind? What flavour? What colour? etc.
20. How much did it cost?
21. Did anything unusual happen? What?
22. How long did you stay?
23. What did you do just before you came home?
24. When did you leave?
25. How did you get home?
26. What happened on the way home?
27. What time did you get home?
28. How did you feel then?
29. When are you going back?
30. Do you think that I should go sometime? Why?

[a]QUESTions for Aural Rehabilitation.
Source: Based on Erber (1996).

the next question. This conversation-like therapy strategy can be done in an auditory-only or auditory-visual perceptual mode.

4. *Eclectic:* Includes training that combines most or all of the strategies previously described.

While all the auditory training programs to be described have analytic, synthetic, or pragmatic tendencies, most would best be described as eclectic since more than one general strategy for the training of listening skills typically is used with a given child or adult.

Erber. Erber (1982) has described a flexible and widely used approach to auditory training designed for use primarily with children. This adaptive method is based on a careful analysis of a child's auditory perceptual abilities through the use of the Glendonald Auditory Screening Procedure (GASP) assessment battery (described briefly in the earlier portion of this chapter devoted to assessment). Recall that GASP's approach to evaluating a child's auditory perceptual skills takes into account two major factors: (1) the complexity of the speech stimuli to be perceived (ranging from individual speech elements to connected discourse) and (2) the form of the response required from the child (detection, discrimination, identification, or comprehension). Several levels of stimuli and responses are involved, as shown in Figure 4.6. The GASP test battery initially evaluates only the three stimulus–response combinations indicated in the figure. However, Erber encourages the use of other available test materials to evaluate other stimulus–response combinations from the matrix in Figure 4.6, when appropriate.

Once the child's auditory capabilities are determined, an auditory training program is outlined using the same stimulus–response model as discussed for the GASP assessment when establishing goals and beginning points for therapy. Those stimulus–response combinations found not to be processed well during the GASP assessment phase logically become the same combinations targeted in auditory training activities that follow. Erber's approach is flexible and highly adaptable to children with a wide variety of auditory abilities since the stimulus and response combinations range from the simplest (phoneme detection) to the most complex (sentence comprehension) perceptual tasks.

Erber also described three general styles that the clinician may use during auditory training, depending on the communication setting. These styles differ in specificity, rigidity, and direction and are described in Table 4.9. Adaptive procedures, where the child's responses to speech stimuli are used to determine the next activity, can be employed with any of these styles. In attempting to develop a child's auditory abilities, Erber (1982) stated,

> Auditory training need not follow a developmental plan where, for instance, you practice phoneme detection first and attempt comprehension of connected discourse last. Instead, you might use the "conversational approach" during all daily conversation, and apply the "moderately structured approach" as a follow-up to each class activity. During each activity, you will note consistent errors. Later, you might provide brief periods of specific practice with difficult material. In this way, you can incorporate auditory training into conversation and instruction, rather than treat listening as a skill to be developed independently of communication. (p. 105)

Erber's emphasis on integrating the development of auditory skills into all activities with children with hearing loss is shared by many, including Sanders (1993)

TABLE 4.9 Three General Auditory Training Approaches

Natural conversational approach	1. The teacher eliminates visible cues and speaks to the child in as natural a way as possible, while considering the general situational context and ongoing classroom activity.
	2. The auditory speech perception tasks may be chosen from any cell in the stimulus–response matrix, for example, sentence comprehension.
	3. The teacher adapts to the child's responses by presenting remedial auditory tasks in a systematic manner (modifies stimulus and/or response), derived from any cell in the matrix.
Moderately structured approach	1. The teacher applies a closed-set auditory identification task, but follows this approach activity with some basic speech development procedures and a related comprehension task. Thus, the method retains a degree of flexibility.
	2. The teacher selects the nature and content of words and sentences on the basis of recent class activities.
	3. A few neighboring cells in the stimulus–response matrix are involved (for example, word and sentence identification and sentence comprehension).
Practice on specific tasks	1. The teacher selects the set of acoustic speech stimuli and also the child's range of responses, prepares relevant materials, and plans the development of the task, all according to the child's specific needs for auditory practice.
	2. Attention is directed to a particular listening skill, usually represented by a single cell in the stimulus–response matrix (e.g., phrase discrimination).

Source: Erber, N. (1982). *Auditory training.* Washington, DC: Alexander Graham Bell Association for the Deaf. Reprinted by permission.

and Ling and Ling (1978), who recommend that auditory training "be viewed as a supplement to auditory experience and as an integral part of language and speech training" (p. 113). Thus, therapy directed toward the development of auditory and language skills can and should be done in an integrated, mostly seamless manner.

As mentioned earlier, Erber's levels of perception model (detection, discrimination, identification, and comprehension) are widely used with both children and adults in rehabilitation therapy involving the development and improvement of auditory and visual perceptual skills for speech perception.

DASL II.   Stout and Windle (1994) have developed a sequential, highly structured auditory-training curriculum called the Developmental Approach to Successful Listening II (DASL II). Like Erber's (1982) approach, the DASL II consists of a hierarchy of listening skills that are worked on in relatively brief, individualized sessions.

The DASL II curriculum can be used with persons of any age, but it has been utilized mainly with preschool- and school-age youngsters using either hearing aids or cochlear implants. Three specific areas of auditory skill development are focused on the following:

1. *Sound awareness:* Deals with the development of the basic skills of listening for both environmental and speech sounds. The care/use of hearing aids and cochlear implants is also included.
2. *Phonetic listening:* Includes exposure to fundamental aspects of speech perception, such as the duration, intensity, pitch, and rate of speech. The discrimination and identification of vowels and consonants in isolation and in words are included in this area.
3. *Auditory comprehension:* Emphasizes the understanding of spoken language by the child with hearing loss. Includes a wide range of auditory-processing activities, from basic discrimination of common words to comprehension of complex verbal messages in unstructured situations.

The authors have developed a placement test that enables the clinician to evaluate the child's auditory skills relative to each of these three main areas. Specific subskills are tested, making it possible to determine the particular listening skills that a child has or has not acquired. As with the GASP approach, information from the DASL II placement test enables the clinician to determine the appropriate placement of the child within the auditory skills curriculum. The test's developers provided numerous activity suggestions for the clinician. These address each of the many subskills of the three main areas of listening that make up the DASL II. These are organized from the simplest to the most difficult listening task.

The following example is a list of subskills related to sound awareness that are included in the DASL II. Similar subskill lists and related activities are provided by the developers for all components of the DASL II.

Developing Sound Awareness Subskills

1. Responds to the presence of a loud, low-frequency gross environmental sound. (Example: loud banging on a hard surface)
2. Responds to the presence of a loud speech syllable or word.
3. Responds to the presence of a variety of different gross environmental sounds.
4. Indicates when ongoing environmental sounds stop.
5. Indicates when a sustained speech syllable or word stops.
6. Indicates when teacher or parent turns both hearing aids (or processor) on or off.
7. Discriminates between presence of spoken syllable or word and silence.

8. Discriminates between a variety of familiar environmental sounds in a set of two choices.
9. Discriminates between a variety of familiar environmental sounds in a set of three choices.
10. Discriminates between a variety of environmental sounds in a set of four choices.
11. If the student is amplified binaurally, locates the direction of sound on the same plane.
12. If the student is amplified binaurally, locates the direction of sound on different planes.
13. Identifies common environmental sounds.
14. If the student is amplified binaurally, he or she can detect when one aid is on versus when both aids are on in a structured situation.

Home intervention involves guiding the parents as they carry out important components of an early audiologic rehabilitation program in the home for an infant diagnosed with a hearing loss.

A team approach is encouraged with the DASL II, with the audiologist, speech-language pathologist, classroom teacher, and parents working in a coordinated fashion on relevant subskills. This makes it vital that frequent communication occurs among the team members.

SKI-HI. Watkins (2004) has a comprehensive identification and home intervention treatment curriculum for infants with hearing loss and their families, and it is in wide use nationally (see Chapter 9 for more details). One of the major components of SKI-HI's treatment plan is a developmentally based auditory stimulation–training program. It is utilized in conjunction with language–speech stimulation and consists of four phases and 11 general skills, which are listed in Table 4.10. Although these phases and skills are organized developmentally, infants may not always move sequentially from one phase or skill on the list to the next higher one in

TABLE 4.10   The Four Phases and 11 Skills of the SKI-HI Auditory Program

The approximate time line indicates the estimated amount of time spent by a profoundly deaf infant in each phase. The age of the child on entry into the program and the amount of hearing loss are among the factors that will affect the time needed to progress through the four phases.

Phases	Skills
Phase I (4–7 months)	1. *Attending:* Child is aware of presence of home and/or speech sounds but may not know meanings; stops, listens, etc.
	2. *Early vocalizing:* Child coos, gurgles, repeats syllables, etc.
Phase II (5–16 months)	3. *Recognizing:* Child knows meaning of home and/or speech sounds but may not be able to locate; smiles when hears Daddy home etc.
	4. *Locating:* Child turns to, points to, locates sound sources.
	5. *Vocalizing with inflection:* High/low, loud/soft, and/or, up/down
Phase III (9–14 months)	6. *Hearing at distances and levels:* Child locates sounds far away and/or above and below.
	7. *Producing some vowels and consonants.*
Phase IV (12–18 months)	8. *Environmental discrimination and comprehension:* Child hears differences among and/or understands home sounds.
	9. *Vocal discrimination and comprehension:* Child hears differences (a) among vocal sounds, (b) among words, or (c) among phrases and/or understands them.
	10. *Speech sound discrimination and comprehension:* Child hears differences among and/or understands distinct speech sounds.
	11. *Speech use:* Child imitates and/or uses speech meaningfully.

Source: Adapted from Watkins (2004) and Watkins and Clark (1993).

TABLE 4.11 A Lesson in SKI-HI's Auditory Stimulation and Training Program

Recognition of objects and events from sound source (Phase II, Skill 3, Subskill 6)

Parent objective	Parent will provide repeated meaningful opportunities for his or her child to associate environmental and speech sounds with their source.
Child objective	Child will demonstrate recognition of environmental and speech sounds by realizing their source.
Lesson	Review with the parent the sounds and activities that you have been utilizing for previous work on attending. Continue these activities, ensuring that the child is aware of the source of the sound and that the sounds are relevant to the child.
Materials	Naturally occurring environmental sounds and voice.
Activities	1. Ask everyone who comes to visit to knock several times, pause, and knock again. When someone knocks, take your child to the door and say "listen" etc.
	2. Encourage the child to discover different sounds that toys make by providing him or her playtime with several different-sounding toys.
	3. Stimulate the child to produce sounds by manipulating objects or toys (banging pans, squeezing toy, etc.) and stimulate vocalization by making sounds as you play with the toys.
	4. Imitate the child's actions, such as shaking a rattle, and imitate all vocalizations.
	5. Associate speech with all major movements (e.g., saying "roll" each time you roll the child over and "up" when you pick him or her up).
	6. Stimulate association of particular voices with particular people by having siblings/relatives use voice as they play with the child.

Source: Adapted from Watkins (2004).

a completely predictable manner. SKI-HI provides an extensive description of activities that the clinician and parent or caregiver may utilize in working on subskills related to each of the specific general skills included in each phase of the auditory training program. The structure and completeness of SKI-HI's auditory training component make it user-friendly for parents under the guidance of clinicians. Table 4.11 provides a summary of an example of listening activities that are part of SKI-HI's comprehensive auditory stimulation program.

SPICE. Moog, Biedenstein, and Davidson (1995) developed the Speech Perception Instructional Curriculum and Evaluation (SPICE) to provide a guide for clinicians in evaluating and developing auditory skills in children with severe to profound hearing loss. It contains goals and objectives associated with four levels of speech perception. The first level, *detection*, is intended to establish an awareness and responsiveness to speech. The second and third levels, *suprasegmental* and *vowel and consonant perception*, are worked on in tandem. In the suprasegmental section, children work on differentiating speech based on gross variations in duration, stress, and intonation. In the vowel and consonant section, children begin to make perceptual distinctions among individual word stimuli with similar duration, stress, and intonation features but with different vowels and consonants. With progress, the child is introduced to the fourth level, *connected speech*. Now the emphasis is the perception of words in a more natural environment (phrases and sentences). Activities for SPICE are done with combined auditory–visual presentation as well as auditory-only listening situations. Many of these activities are carried out in short, structured therapy sessions that concentrate on specific listening skills. As the child progresses, the newly acquired skills can be refined further in more natural, informal conversation. Recently, SPICE has been used extensively with children using cochlear implants as an approach to developing listening skills in conjunction with their expanded auditory input.

Connected, or running, speech is natural or conversational speech.

Cochlear Implant Manufacturers. The major cochlear implant manufacturers have made available some excellent supportive programs for developing/improving auditory skills and facilitating the use of cochlear implants for both children and adults. For example, Cochlear Americas has developed a comprehensive series of age-appropriate programs (babies, toddlers, teens, adults) to develop and enhance listening and general skills related to face-to-face and telephone communication as well as listening to music. Information regarding each of these can be accessed at Cochlear Americas' Communication Corner (http://www.cochlear.com). MED-EL has developed a variety of programs to facilitate listening activities for young children, teens, and adults called Sound Scape (http://www.medel.com/us/resources-for-success-soundscape/?titel=SoundScape&). Finally, Advanced Bionics has developed an extensive series of web-based materials called the Listening Room (https://thelisteningroom.com) for parents of recently implanted children as well as members of the cochlear implant team. These materials cover a variety of important topics, including detailed information and activities related to auditory skill development.

Consonant Recognition Training. This approach to auditory training has been used mainly with adults and relies primarily on an analytic approach to facilitate improved speech perception. In addition to its use in auditory training, consonant recognition training frequently incorporates speechreading into a combined auditory–visual training approach. Walden, Erdman, Montgomery, Schwartz, and Prosek, (1981) described consonant recognition training as it was utilized initially at the Walter Reed Army Medical Center. Briefly, a large number of training exercises were developed with each exercise concentrating on a select number of consonants presented in a syllable context. The listener's task is to make same–different judgments between syllable pairs and to identify the nonsense syllables presented individually. The position of the consonants within the syllable is varied between exercises. The person with hearing loss receives immediate feedback regarding the correctness of his or her response. This general procedure allows for intense drill to occur for a select number of consonants during a relatively short therapy session.

Walden and others presented data to support the efficacy of this approach to auditory training. They noted an 11.6 percent average improvement in consonant recognition. More impressively, a 28.2 percent average improvement was found in perception of sentences presented in a combined auditory–visual mode. A follow-up study (Montgomery, Walden, Schwartz, & Prosek, 1984) utilized a similar training protocol for consonant recognition that combined work on speechreading and auditory training. Using sentence material to assess performance, they noted a substantial improvement in speech recognition for adults with hearing loss.

Another investigation (Rubenstein & Boothroyd, 1987) also examined the effectiveness of consonant recognition training as part of a larger study comparing analytic and synthetic therapy approaches to improving speech perception. Rubenstein and Boothroyd found that consonant recognition training did produce modest improvement in speech perception for a group of adults with hearing loss, but the amount of improvement observed was not any greater than was achieved with a synthetic approach to auditory training. However, the results from Kricos and Holmes (1996) did not support the efficacy of consonant recognition training with older adults.

More research needs to be focused on the relative merits of consonant recognition training as it is used in attempting to improve auditory perception. Also needed is further clarification of the basic roles played by auditory and visual speech perception, both individually and when utilized in a combined manner, in the processing of speech by persons with hearing loss (Gagne, 1994; Walden & Grant, 1993). In the meantime, interest in using consonant recognition training continues, and its use has been extended in recent years to include computer-based programming as well (Lansing & Bienvenue, 1994; Tye-Murray, Tyler, Lansing, &

TABLE 4.12 Examples of Anticipatory and Repair Strategies That the Person with Hearing Loss Can Use to Enhance the Extent to Which Hearing Contributes to Speech Perception

Anticipatory Strategies

Minimizing the distance from the speaker

Optimizing the hearing aid volume setting

Reducing the level of competing signals (stereo, TV)

Using situational cues to anticipate topics and words

Repair Strategies

Asking the speaker to repeat all or part of a message

Asking the speaker to rephrase or simplify the message

Asking a follow-up question to either confirm the content of a previous message or to elaborate on it

Bertschy, 1990). Clinicians also can access a wealth of therapy materials useful in this type of analytic approach from Analytika (Plant, 1994).

Communication Training and Therapy.   This common form of audiologic rehabilitation emphasizes the role of communication strategies and pragmatics to facilitate successful communication. The adult with hearing loss is coached regarding those factors in conversational situations that the listener can exercise control of and that can maximize the opportunity to perceive what is spoken. Many of these factors are classified as being either anticipatory or repair strategies for the listener to use. Anticipatory strategies refer to things the listener can do to better prepare for communication or ensure that it will be successful. Some examples of anticipatory strategies that can be helpful are listed in Table 4.12.

Repair strategies involve techniques used to overcome a breakdown in communication that has already occurred. The person with hearing loss (and the speaker as well) can use one or more of these strategies to help with perceiving a given message. Examples of common repair strategies are also given in Table 4.12.

Table 4.13 demonstrates further how repair strategies can be used for specific communication problems. Persons with hearing loss, as well as their communication partners, are encouraged to employ these communication strategies when necessary, which does require some degree of assertiveness and thought on their part as they communicate with others. Successful use of communication strategies also requires that they be used in a diplomatic manner as well (see Conversational Styles box on page 120).

DeFilippo and Scott (1978) developed a technique called *speech tracking*, which can be used in therapy to provide practice in utilizing communication repair strategies in a conversation context. As it is used in therapy centered on improving auditory-speech perception, speech tracking involves having a listener repeat a phrase

TABLE 4.13 Some Communication Problems Commonly Experienced by People with Hearing Loss and Associated (Specific) Requests for Clarification

What Was the Communication Problem?	How You Can Ask for Help
You understood only part of the message.	Repeat the part you understood; ask for the part you didn't understand (e.g., "You flew to *Paris*?")
You couldn't see the speaker's mouth.	"Please put your hand down."
The person was speaking too fast.	"Please speak a little slower."
The person's speech was too soft.	"Please speak a little louder."
The sentence was too long.	"Shorter, please."
The person's speech was not clear.	"Speak a little more clearly, please."
The sentence was too complicated.	"Please say that in a different way."
You don't know what the problem was.	"Please say that again."

Source: Based on Erber (1993).

or sentence presented by a clinician in an auditory-only condition. To assist in perceiving 100 percent of the message, the listener can use various repair strategies, such as requesting that the entire sentence (or portions) be repeated or rephrased until the complete utterance is comprehended. Visual cues may be added for bisensory training as well. Performance in the speech-tracking procedure is monitored by calculating the number of words or sentences correctly repeated by the listener per minute over a set period of time. An example of the tracking method as applied in a therapy session is provided below. (The topic of the sentence is fishing.) (See also Supplementary Learning Activity 4.)

> *Clinician: Dry flies float on the surface.*
> *Listener: Dry ... on the ... ? Please repeat it.*
> *Clinician: Dry flies float on the surface.*
> *Listener: Dry flies ... on the ... ? Please repeat the word after "flies."*
> *Clinician: Float.*
> *Listener: Float?*
> *Clinician: Yes.*
> *Listener: Dry flies float on the water.*
> *Clinician: No. On the surface of the water.*
> *Listener: Oh. Dry flies float on the surface.*
> *Clinician: Yes.*

In recent years, audiologists have frequently included condensed variations of communication training and counseling as an important aspect of audiologic rehabilitation for adults at the time they are fitted with new hearing aids (Beyer & Northern, 2000). Many think that sharing information with the patient about the role of hearing and vision and the use of communication strategies in communicating is a timely and appropriate adjunct to the hearing aid orientation process, and audiologists have begun to do this on a more frequent basis (Kochkin et al., 2010; Schow, Balsara, Smedley, & Whitcomb, 1993). Montgomery (1994) discussed the rationale for providing a brief exposure to auditory rehabilitation at the time the patient who is hard of hearing is fitted with a hearing aid. Montgomery uses the acronym WATCH for his abbreviated program, which includes the following key elements of auditory rehabilitation: W: Watch the talker's mouth (lipreading); A: Ask specific questions (conversation repair strategies); T: Talk about your hearing loss (admission of hearing loss); C: Change the situation (situation control); and H: Health care knowledge (consumer education and awareness). The program, which takes about one hour to share with the new hearing-aid user, is designed to provide important tips for successful communication as well as to "encourage or empower the hearing-impaired patient to take care of his or her communication behavior and take responsibility for its success."

Conversational Styles

It's important to note that persons with hearing loss can react to their hearing problems in either a positive or a negative fashion. This can result in the routine use of one of three general conversational styles for the listener with hearing loss, as summarized below.

Passive: The listener has a tendency to withdraw from conversations and social situations. When unable to hear what is said, this person is prone to bluff or pretend to hear by simply smiling or nodding his or her head. Persons using this approach do very little to facilitate communication.

Aggressive: The listener routinely blames others for communication difficulties (e.g., "Everyone mumbles" or "He does not speak loudly enough"). It is common for listeners using this style to convey a hostile, negative feeling toward their communication partners.

Assertive: The listener takes responsibility for facilitating communication (e.g., turning down the television or stereo during conversation, sitting closer, acknowledging to communication partners that he or she has a hearing loss) and does so in a positive, diplomatic manner.

Three handouts, called HIO BASICS, CLEAR, and SPEECH, developed by Brockett and Schow (2001) and Schow (2001), constitute another approach to providing short-term audiologic rehabilitation. Used *primarily* in conjunction with the fitting/orientation process, these tools involve presenting key aspects of the rehabilitation process. HIO BASICS focuses on presenting information related primarily to the care and effective use of hearing aids. CLEAR provides suggestions for the person with a hearing loss regarding the communication process, while SPEECH gives helpful suggestions for the significant other that are designed to facilitate communication. The latter two handouts are closely tied to Schum's (1989) Clear Speech. More detailed descriptions of all three of these handouts are found in Chapter 10.

Computerized Approaches to Auditory Training.   Computerized approaches to auditory training have emerged in recent times and have shown potential for providing valuable training and information related to enhancing listening skills. For example, CasperSent (Boothroyd, 1987, 2008) is a program involving computer-assisted speech perception testing and training at the sentence level. It consists of 60 sets of sentences involving 12 topics and three sentence types. The sentences can be presented by lipreading only, hearing only, or a combination of the two perceptual modes, and the patient attempts to repeat as much of each sentence as possible. The sentences can be self-administered by the person with hearing loss or by a clinician, and correct/incorrect feedback is provided after each response.

Computer-assisted speech training (CAST; Fu & Galvin, 2008), is another auditory training program developed originally for use with cochlear implant recipients. It includes a variety of training material, including nonspeech signals, such as pure tones and environmental sounds, and speech signals, ranging from phonemes to monosyllabic words and sentences produced by different talkers. The program is adaptive, adjusting the level of difficulty based on patient performance.

Yet another computerized approach to auditory training that has received wide attention and use in recent years is Listening and Communication Enhancement (LACE; Sweetow & Henderson-Sabes, 2004, 2006). LACE is an interactive program designed to improve listening skills. It is intended for use primarily in the patient's home in a self-directed manner. However, an in-office version is now also available. Twenty therapy sessions run 30 minutes apiece each day, five days a week, for approximately four weeks, and focus on perception of degraded speech, developing/refining certain cognitive skills important for listening, and the effective use of communication strategies. Immediate feedback is provided to the patient during the exercises, and progress is monitored electronically. The developers have shown that LACE improved patients' abilities to comprehend speech in noisy environments and increased their confidence in dealing with difficult listening situations. Some difficulties have been noted in motivating patients to complete the entire 20 sessions, and various suggestions have been made for improving compliance. While some information has been obtained that indicates good efficacy for LACE (Song, Skoe, Banai, & Kraus, 2011; Sweetow & Henderson-Sabes, 2006), further information is needed.

Finally, Tyler, Witt, Nunn, and Wang (2010) have developed a home-based listening training system for hearing aid and cochlear implant users that focuses on improving speech perception in the presence of background noise and facilitating localization abilities. Although still in the preliminary stages of development, this approach shows promise as an option for providing auditory training.

In summary, a variety of approaches to auditory training are available for audiologists to employ with their patients. While new hearing aids and cochlear implants often provide the user with a wealth of auditory stimulation, the patient must learn to use this new information effectively in order to receive maximum benefit. This often can be facilitated with auditory training. While more investigation needs to be done related to the efficacy of auditory training, some evidence already exists supporting its effectiveness (Abrams, 2011; Kricos & Holmes, 1996; Sweetow & Palmer, 2005). Given this, audiologists are encouraged to consider providing some form of auditory training more *routinely* as they work with patients with hearing loss.

Summary Points

- Basic oral (verbal) communication involves five key components: the speaker, a message (often with auditory and visual forms), a listener, feedback to the speaker, and the environment in which the communication takes place.

- Both the segmental and the suprasegmental components found in speech contribute to speech perception.

- Hearing loss results in the loss of varying degrees of segmental and suprasegmental information, which leads to problems with speech perception.

- Speech has quite a bit of built-in redundancy, making it possible to figure out what was said even though the listener did not perceive all the acoustical information produced by the speaker.

- Auditory training is intended to facilitate auditory perception in the listener with impaired hearing.

- Long-term auditory training therapy is not done routinely with a majority of cases with hearing loss. However, it can be a key component of audiologic rehabilitation for cochlear implant recipients, those with prelingual onset of hearing loss, and those with severe to profound losses.

- Assessment of auditory skills can provide valuable information regarding candidacy for therapy, can help in identifying areas in need of work in therapy, and can be useful in outcomes assessment.

- Analytic, synthetic, and pragmatic approaches to auditory training currently are employed in a variety of forms for children and adults.

- Passive and aggressive conversational styles are negative, often counterproductive reactions to hearing loss, while the assertive conversational style is a more positive approach that places responsibility on those with hearing loss to assist in facilitating communication.

- Numerous forms of communication strategies are available to assist in making communication more successful.

- A number of models have been developed for providing auditory training on a short-term basis, and these usually are incorporated into the hearing aid fitting process.

Supplementary Learning Activities

See www.isu.edu/csed/audiology/rehab to carry out these activities. We encourage you to use these to supplement your learning. Your instructor may give specific assignments that involve a particular activity.

1. Linguistic Constraints: To demonstrate the concept of linguistic constraint, this activity shows a sentence with four words. Learners begin by guessing what one of the words might be. When a correct word is found, it is displayed. From this, the learner can begin to figure out the other words. The number of tries each word requires is displayed under the word. Common results show many guesses for the first word, fewer for the next, and very few for the last two. A second (and much harder) activity has double the number of words.

2. Cloze Procedure: To demonstrate a listener's ability to "fill in" missing information, two different activities are presented. One activity is a visual-only task displaying a paragraph of information with some words removed. Learners are to figure out the missing information and then check to see if they have the correct words. The second activity is similar, except it brings in the auditory component.

The learner will hear a paragraph with some words removed. He or she can then fill in the missing words and check to see if the information is correct.

3. **Filtered Speech:** This activity allows the listener to hear what speech might sound like when different speech acoustic information has been filtered out. Additional filtered speech simulations can be found on the text website.

4. **Tracking Activity:** Tracking is a way of measuring how many words are recognized over a given time frame. This technique is frequently employed when working with cochlear implant recipients. It requires two people: one to read the material and one (e.g., the cochlear implant recipient) to repeat the material in the exact order of presentation. In the activity, the tracking score is computed in terms of words perceived correctly in order per minute.

Recommended Reading

Erber, N. (1996). *Communication therapy for hearing-impaired adults*. Abbotsford, Australia: Clavis Publishing.

Gagne, J.-P., & Jennings, M. (2000). Audiological rehabilitation intervention services for adults with acquired hearing impairment. In M. Valente, H. Hosford-Dunn, & R. Roeser (Eds.), *Audiology treatment*. New York: Thieme, 563–580.

Kricos, P., & McCarthy, P. (Eds.). (2007). From ear to there: A historical perspective on auditory training. *Seminars in Hearing, 28*(2), 89–98.

Montano, J., & Spitzer, J. (2013). *Adult audiologic rehabilitation*. San Diego, CA: Plural.

Sweetow, R., & Henderson-Sabes, J. (2013). Auditory training. In J. Montano & J. Spitzer (Eds.), *Adult audiologic rehabilitation*. San Diego, CA: Plural, 277–290.

Tye-Murray, N. (2015). *Foundations of aural rehabilitation*. Stamford, CT: Cengage Learning.

Recommended Websites

Listening and Communication Enhancement:
http://www.neurotone.com

Virtual Tour of the Ear:
http://www.augie.edu

Cochlear Implant Manufacturers:
Advanced Bionics
http://www.advancedbionics.com

Cochlear Americas
http://hope.cochlearamericas.com

MED-EL
http://www.medel.com

References

Abrams, H. (2011). *Postfitting rehabilitation: If it works so well, why don't we do it?* http://asha.org

Bench, J., Kowal, A., & Bamford, J. (1979). The BKB (Bamford-Kowal-Bench) sentence lists for partially-hearing children. *British Journal of Audiology, 13*, 108–112.

Beyer, C., & Northern, J. (2000). Audiologic rehabilitation support programs: A network model. *Seminars in Hearing, 21*(3), 257–266.

Bilger, R., Rzcezkowski, C., Nuetzel, J., & Rabinowitz, W. (1979, November). *Evaluation of a test of speech perception in noise (SPIN)*. Paper presented at the annual meeting of the American Speech-Language-Hearing Association, Atlanta, GA.

Blamey, P., & Alcantara, J. (1994). Research in auditory training. In J.-P. Gagne & N. Tye-Murray (Eds.), *Research in audiological rehabilitation* (Monograph). *Journal of the Academy of Rehabilitative Audiology, 27,* 161–192.

Boothroyd, A. (1987). CASPER, computer-assisted speech–perception evaluation and training. In *Proceedings of the 10th Annual Conference of the Rehabilitation Society of North America.* Washington, DC: Association for Advancement of Rehabilitation Technology.

Boothroyd, H. (2008). CasperSent: A program for computer-assisted speech perception testing and training at the sentence level. *Journal of the Academy of Rehabilitative Audiology, 41,* 31–52.

Brockett, J., & Schow, R. (2001). Web site profiles common hearing loss patterns and outcome measures. *Hearing Journal, 54*(8), 20.

Carhart, R. (1960). Auditory training. In H. Davis & R. Silverman (Eds.), *Hearing and deafness* (2nd ed.). New York: Holt, Rinehart and Winston, 346–359.

Ching, T., & Hill, M. (2005). *The Parents' Evaluation of Aural/Oral Performance of Children (PEACH) Diary.* Sydney, Australia: Australian Hearing.

Cole, E., & Flexer, C. (2015). *Children with hearing loss* (3rd ed.). San Diego, CA: Plural.

Davis, H., & Silverman, R. (1978). *Hearing and deafness* (4th ed.) New York: Holt, Rinehart and Winston.

Davis, J., & Hardick, E. (1981). *Rehabilitative audiology for children and adults.* New York: Wiley.

DeFilippo, C., & Scott, B. (1978). A method for training and evaluating the reception of ongoing speech. *Journal of the Acoustical Society of America, 63,* 1186–1192.

Denes, P., & Pinson, E. (1993). *The speech chain* (2nd ed.). New York: Freeman.

Durrant, J., & Lovrinic, J. (1995). *Bases of hearing science* (3rd ed.). Baltimore: Williams & Wilkins.

Erber, N. (1979). Speech perception by profoundly hearing-impaired children. *Journal of Speech and Hearing Disorders, 122,* 255–270.

Erber, N. (1982). *Auditory training.* Washington, DC: Alexander Graham Bell Association for the Deaf.

Erber, N. (1993). *Communication and adult hearing loss.* Abbotsford, Australia: Clavis Publishing.

Erber, N. (1996). *Communication therapy for hearing-impaired adults.* Melbourne, Australia: Clavis Publishing.

Etymotic Research. (2001). *QuickSIN.* Elk Grove Village, IL: Etymotic Research.

Fletcher, H. (1953). *Speech and hearing in communication.* Princeton, NJ: D. Van-Nostrand.

Fu, Q., & Galvin, J. (2008). Maximizing cochlear implant patients' performance with advanced speech training procedures. *Hearing Research, 242,* 198–208.

Gagne, J.-P. (1994). Visual and audiovisual speech perception training: Basic and applied research needs. In J.-P. Gagne & N. Tye-Murray (Eds.), Research in audiological rehabilitation (Monograph). *Journal of the Academy of Rehabilitative Audiology, 27,* 133–160.

Gagne, J.-P., & Jennings, M. (2000). Audiological rehabilitation intervention services for adults with acquired hearing impairment. In M. Valente, H. Hosford-Dunn, & R. Roeser (Eds.), *Audiology treatment.* New York: Thieme.

Goldstein, M. (1939). *The acoustic method of the training of the deaf and hard of hearing child.* St. Louis, MO: Laryngoscope Press.

Hegde, M. (2010). *Introduction to communicative disorders* (4th ed.). Austin, TX: PRO-ED.

Kalikow, D., Stevens, K., & Elliott, L. (1977). Development of a test of speech intelligibility in noise using sentence materials with controlled word predictability. *Journal of the Acoustical Society of America, 61,* 1337–1351.

Katz, D., & Elliott, L. (1978, November). *Development of a new children's speech discrimination test.* Paper presented at the annual meeting of the American Speech-Language-Hearing Association, Chicago, IL.

Kochkin, S., Beck, D., Christensen, L., Compton-Conley, C., Fligor, B., Kricos, P., et al. (2010). Marke Trak VIII: The impact of the hearing healthcare professional on hearing aid use success. *Hearing Review, 17*(4), 12–34.

Kricos, P., & Holmes, A. (1996). Efficacy of audiologic rehabilitation for older adults. *Journal of American Academy of Audiology*, 7(4), 219–229.

Lansing, C., & Bienvenue, L. (1994). Intelligent computer-based systems to document the effectiveness of consonant recognition training. *Volta Review*, 96, 41–49.

Lehiste, I. (1970). *Suprasegmentals*. Cambridge, MA: MIT Press.

Lehiste, I. (1976). Suprasegmental features of speech. In N. J. Lass (Ed.), *Contemporary issues in experimental phonetics* (pp. 225–242). New York: Academic Press.

Ling, D. (1976). *Speech and the hearing-impaired child: Theory and practice*. Washington, DC: Alexander Graham Bell Association for the Deaf.

Ling, D. (1989). *Foundations of spoken language for hearing-impaired children*. Washington, DC: Alexander Graham Bell Association for the Deaf.

Ling, D., & Ling, A. (1978). *Aural rehabilitation*. Washington, DC: Alexander Graham Bell Association for the Deaf.

MacKay, I. (1987). *Phonetics: The science of speech production* (2nd ed.). Austin, TX: PRO-ED.

Miller, G. (1951). *Language and communication*. New York: McGraw-Hill.

Miller, G., & Nicely, P. (1955). Analysis of perceptual confusions among English consonants. *Journal of the Acoustical Society of America*, 27, 338–352.

Minifie, F. (1973). Speech acoustics. In F. Minifie, T. Hixon, & F. Williams (Eds.), *Normal aspects of speech, hearing and language*. Englewood Cliffs, NJ: Prentice Hall, 235–260.

Montano, J., & Spitzer, J. (2013). *Adult audiologic rehabilitation*. San Diego, CA: Plural.

Montgomery, A. (1994). WATCH: A practical approach to brief auditory rehabilitation. *The Hearing Journal*, 47(10), 53–55.

Montgomery, A., Walden, B., Schwartz, D., & Prosek, R. (1984). Training auditory–visual speech recognition in adults with moderate sensorineural hearing loss. *Ear and Hearing*, 5, 30–36.

Moog, J., Biedenstein, J., & Davidson, L. (1995). *The SPICE*. St. Louis, MO: Central Institute for the Deaf.

Moog, J., & Geers, A. (1990). *Early Speech Perception Test*. St. Louis, MO: Central Institute for the Deaf.

Myatt, B., & Landes, B. (1963). Assessing discrimination loss in children. *Archives of Otolaryngology*, 77, 359–362.

Nilsson, M., Soli, S., & Sullivan, J. (1994). Development of the Hearing in Noise Test for the measurement of speech reception thresholds in quiet and noise. *Journal of the Acoustical Society of America*, 87, 1085–1099.

Northern, J., & Downs, M. (2014). *Hearing in children* (6th ed.). San Diego, CA: Plural

Owens, E. (1978). Consonant errors and remediation in sensorineural hearing loss. *Journal of Speech and Hearing Disorders*, 43, 331–347.

Owens, E., Benedict, M., & Schubert, E. (1971). Further investigation of vowel items in multiple-choice discrimination testing. *Journal of Speech and Hearing Research*, 14, 814–847.

Owens, E., Benedict, M., & Schubert, E. (1972). Consonant phoneme errors associated with pure tone configurations and certain types of hearing impairment. *Journal of Speech and Hearing Research*, 15, 308–322.

Owens, E., Kessler, D., Telleen, C., & Schubert, E. (1985). The Minimal Auditory Capabilities (MAC) battery. *Hearing Journal*, 34(9), 32–34.

Owens, E., & Schubert, E. (1977). Development of the California Consonant Test. *Journal of Speech and Hearing Research*, 20, 463–474.

Oyer, H. (1966). *Auditory communication for the hard of hearing*. Englewood Cliffs, NJ: Prentice Hall.

Peterson, G. E., & Barney, H. L. (1952). Control methods used in the study of the vowels. *Journal of the Acoustical Society of America*, 32, 693–703.

Plant, G. (1994). *Analytika*. Somerville, MA: Audiological Engineering Corp.

Ross, M., & Lerman, L. (1970). A picture identification test for hearing impaired children. *Journal of Speech and Hearing Research*, 13, 44–53.

Rubenstein, A., & Boothroyd, A. (1987). Effect of two approaches to auditory training on speech recognition by hearing-impaired adults. *Journal of Speech and Hearing Research*, 30, 153–160.

Sanders, D. (1971). *Aural rehabilitation*. Englewood Cliffs, NJ: Prentice Hall.

Sanders, D. (1993). *Management of hearing handicap* (3rd ed.). Englewood Cliffs, NJ: Prentice Hall.

Schow, R. L. (2001). A standardized AR battery for dispensers. *Hearing Journal*, *54*(2), 10–20.

Schow, R., Balsara, N., Smedley, T., & Whitcomb, C. (1993). Aural rehabilitation by ASHA audiologists: 1980–1990. *American Journal of Audiology*, *2*, 28–37.

Schum, D. (1989). *Clear and conversational speech by untrained talkers: Intelligibility*. Paper presented at the annual meeting of the American Speech-Language-Hearing Association, Seattle, WA.

Schwartz, D., & Surr, R. (1979). Three experiments on the California Consonant Test. *Journal of Speech and Hearing Disorders*, *44*, 61–72.

Sher, A., & Owens, E. (1974). Consonant confusions associated with hearing loss above 2000 Hz. *Journal of Speech and Hearing Research*, *17*, 669–681.

Song, J., Skoe, E., Banai, K., & Kraus, N. (2011). Training to improve speech in noise: Biological mechanisms. *Cerebral Cortex*, *122*, 1890–1898.

Stelmachowicz, P.G., Pittman, A.L., Hoover. B.M., Lewis, D.E. (2001). Effect of stimulus bandwidth on the perception of /s/ in normal- and hearing-impaired children and adults. *Journal of the Acoustical Society of America*, *110*(4), 2183–2190.

Stevens, S., & Davis, H. (1938). *Hearing: Its psychology and physiology*. New York: Wiley.

Stout, G., & Windle, J. (1994). *Developmental Approach to Successful Listening II*. Englewood, CO: Resource Point.

Sweetow, R., & Henderson-Sabes, J. (2004). The case for LACE: Listening and auditory communication enhancement training. *Hearing Journal*, *57*(3), 32–38.

Sweetow, R., Henderson-Sabes, J. (2006). The need for and development of an adaptive Listening and Communication Enhancement (LACE) Program. *Journal of the American Academy of Audiology*, *17*, 538–558.

Sweetow, R., & Henderson-Sabes, J. (2013). Auditory training. In J. Montano & J. Spitzer (Eds.), *Adult audiologic rehabilitation*. San Diego, CA: Plural, 277–290.

Sweetow, R., & Palmer, C. (2005). Efficacy of individual auditory training in adults: A systematic review of the evidence. *Journal of the American Academy of Audiology*, *16*, 494–504.

Tillman, T., & Carhart, R. (1966). *An expanded test for speech discrimination utilizing CNC monosyllabic words*. Northwestern University Auditory Test No. 6 (Technical Report No. SAM-TR55). Brooks Air Force Base, TX: USAF School of Aerospace Medicine.

Tsiakpini, L., Weichbold, V., Kuehn-Inacker, H., Coninx, F., D'Haese, P., & Almadin, S. (2004). *LittlEARS Auditory Questionnaire*. Innsbruck, Austria: MED-EL.

Tye-Murray, N. (2015). *Foundations of aural rehabilitation* (4th ed.). Stamford, CT: Cengage.

Tye-Murray, N., Tyler, R., Lansing, C., & Bertschy, M. (1990). Evaluating the effectiveness of auditory training stimuli using a computerized program. *Volta Review*, *92*, 25–30.

Tyler, R., Preece, J., & Tye-Murray, N. (1986). *The Iowa Phoneme and Sentence Tests*. Iowa City: University of Iowa Hospitals and Clinics.

Tyler, R., Witt, S., Nunn, C., & Wang, W. (2010). Initial development of a spatially separated speech-in-noise and localization training program. *Journal of the American Academy of Audiology*, *21*, 390–403.

Walden, B., Erdman, I., Montgomery, A., Schwartz, D., & Prosek, R. (1981). Some effects of training on speech recognition by hearing-impaired adults. *Journal of Speech and Hearing Research*, *24*, 207–216.

Walden, B., & Grant, K. (1993). Research needs in rehabilitative audiology. In J. Alpiner & P. McCarthy (Eds.), *Rehabilitative audiology: Children and adults*. Baltimore: Williams & Wilkins, 501–528.

Watkins, S. (Ed.). (2004). *SKI-HI curriculum: Family-centered programming for infants and young children with hearing loss*. Logan, UT: Hope, Inc.

Zimmerman-Phillips, S., Osberger, M. F., & Robbins, A. M. (1997). *Infant-Toddler: Meaningful Auditory Integration Scale (IT-MAIS)*. Sylmar, CA: Advanced Bionics Corp.

5

Visual Stimuli in Communication

Nicholas M. Hipskind

CONTENTS

Visit the companion website when you see this icon to learn more about the topic nearby in the text.

Learning Outcomes

After reading this chapter, you will be able to

- List two ways that each of the following components of the speechreading process can influence speechreading performance: speaker, code, environment, and speechreader
- Distinguish between a phoneme and a viseme
- Describe how residual hearing contributes to the success of speechreading
- Explain how the redundancy in speech affects a listener's ability to speechread
- Define clear speech
- Distinguish between analytic and synthetic speechreading
- List four tips for facilitating speechreading
- Describe and distinguish between fingerspelling, sign language, and sign systems
- Explain what an iconic sign is
- Describe the link between cued speech and speechreading

INTRODUCTION

When engaged in conversation, we tend to rely primarily on our hearing to receive and subsequently comprehend the message being conveyed. In addition, given the opportunity, we often look at the speaker in order to obtain further information related to the topic of conversation. The speaker's mouth movements, facial expressions, and hand gestures, as well as various aspects of the physical environment in which the communication takes place, are all potential sources of useful information. Humans learn to use their vision for communication to some extent, especially in

challenging listening situations (e.g., noisy). However, most of us enjoy the benefits of normal hearing and find it unnecessary in most situations to depend on vision to communicate effectively.

The person with hearing loss, on the other hand, is much more dependent on visual cues for communication. The degree to which those with hearing loss need visual information when conversing with someone is proportional to the amount of information that is lost due to the hearing problem. In other words, a person with a severe hearing loss is likely to be more dependent on visual information to communicate than an individual with a mild auditory problem.

Speechreading involves attempting to perceive speech by using visual cues to supplement whatever auditory information is available.

Visual information may be transmitted by means of a manual or an oral communication system. In oral communication, the listener uses visual cues by observing the speaker's mouth, facial expressions, and hand movements to help perceive what is being said. This process is referred to by such terms as lipreading, visual hearing, visual communication, visual listening, or speechreading. Among laypersons, the most popular of these terms is *lipreading*. This term implies that only the lips of the talker provide visual cues. However, because the use of vision for communication involves more than merely watching the speaker's mouth, most professionals prefer the term *speechreading*. Thus, speechreading is used in the remainder of this chapter to refer to visual perception of oral communication.

Manual communication, or *signing*, also relies on a visual system. Manual communication is transmitted via special signs and symbols made with the hands and is received and interpreted visually. This complex form of communication allows for transfer of information via the visual channel when both the sender and the receiver are familiar with the same set of symbols.

This chapter assumes the reader is familiar with phonetics, the written symbols for phonemes.

The intent of this chapter is to discuss the advantages and limitations of vision as part of the audiologic rehabilitation process. Emphasis will be given to the factors that affect speechreading as well as to a discussion of manual communication methods. The reader is reminded that those with hearing loss comprise two populations: the hard of hearing and the deaf. Although frequently classified under the generic term *hearing loss*, these groups have different communication needs and limitations. Therefore, it is unrealistic to expect that a single rehabilitation method can satisfy all their communication needs. Ultimately, it is the clinician's responsibility to select appropriate strategies that will enable the hard of hearing and the deaf to use vision to effectively enhance their communication skills, to achieve educational and vocational success, and to mature emotionally and socially.

FACTORS RELATED TO SPEECHREADING

The variables that affect the speechreading process usually fall in four general areas: the speaker, the signal/code, the environment, and the speechreader. While research has contributed to a better understanding of how speech is processed visually, some of the findings are equivocal and have been found to be difficult to duplicate in the clinical setting. This is not to imply that professionals should ignore available laboratory findings; rather, they must realize the significance of these findings in order to provide individualized patient programming. The following section presents selected experimental evidence regarding factors that have been reported to influence the efficacy of speechreading. Figure 5.1 provides a summary of these factors.

Speaker

Differences among speakers have a greater effect on speechreading than on listening. More than 50 years ago, a positive correlation was shown to exist between speaker–listener familiarity and the information received from speechreading. That is, speechreading performance improves when the speaker is familiar to the receiver (speechreader). Speakers who use appropriate facial expressions and common gestures and who position themselves face-to-face or within a 45-degree angle of the listener also facilitate communication for the speechreader (Berger, 1972a).

A slightly slower to normal speech rate with precise, not exaggerated, articulation is best for speechreading. This is sometimes referred to as clear speech (see Chapter 4).

The rate of normal speech results in the production of as many as 15 phonemes per second. Evidence suggests that the eye may be capable of recording only 8 to 10 discrete movements per second. Thus, at times, a speaker's speaking rate may exceed the listener's visual reception capabilities. Although normal rate of speech may be too fast for optimal visual processing, extremely slowed and exaggerated speech production does not ensure improved comprehension. It has been reported that speakers who use a slightly slower to normal speech rate accompanied by precise, not exaggerated, articulation are the easiest for the speechreader

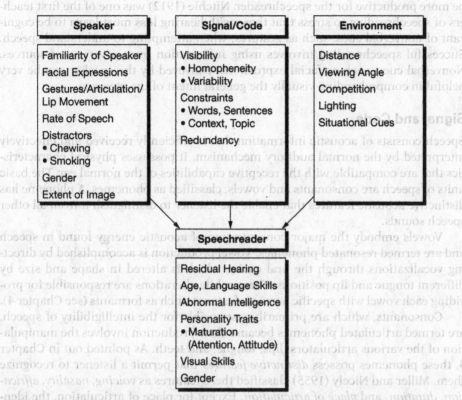

Speaker	Signal/Code	Environment
Familiarity of Speaker	Visibility	Distance
Facial Expressions	• Homopheneity	Viewing Angle
Gestures/Articulation/	• Variability	Competition
Lip Movement	Constraints	Lighting
Rate of Speech	• Words, Sentences	Situational Cues
Distractors	• Context, Topic	
• Chewing	Redundancy	
• Smoking		
Gender		
Extent of Image		

Speechreader

Residual Hearing
Age, Language Skills
Abnormal Intelligence
Personality Traits
• Maturation
  (Attention, Attitude)
Visual Skills
Gender

**FIGURE 5.1   Summary of various factors related to speechreading performance.
Arrows have been drawn from the Speaker, Signal/Code, and Environmental lists to
Speechreader to signify that all these factors influence the speechreader's performance
in addition to those variables that are directly related to the speechreader.**

to understand. Montgomery and Houston (2000) noted that the rapidity of speech
may not be as limiting a factor in determining speechreading success as was once
thought because each phoneme does not have a discrete visual image as speech
is produced. Thus, the speechreader actually may not have to process as many
visual stimuli per second as once thought. In addition, the speaker also should
avoid simultaneous oral activities, such as chewing, smoking, and yawning, when
conversing with a person with hearing loss. Other potentially counterproductive
postures include holding a hand near the mouth while talking and wearing sun-
glasses. While the masking effects of these coincidental activities have not been
documented, they seem likely to complicate an already trying task. With respect
to the gender of speakers, Daly, Bench, and Chappell (1996) demonstrated that
female speakers are easier to speechread than are male speakers. Related to this
finding, little evidence exists concerning the potential influence that gender-related
variables associated with the speaker, such as a moustache or the use of lipstick,
may have on speechreading success.

The speaker may enhance conversational efficiency by complementing
speechreading with appropriate facial expressions and gestures (Sanders, 1993).
From infancy, we learn that the spoken word "no" is accompanied by a stern facial
expression and shaking of the head and/or index finger from side to side. Salu-
tations are made in conjunction with a smile and the extension or wave of the
hand, opening of the arms, and/or puckering of the lips. Similarly, shrugging of
the shoulders has become a universal gesture that augments the verbal phrases
"I don't know" or "I don't care." Consequently, appropriate nonverbal communication is closely associated with the verbal message and is used simultaneously with
speech to provide emphasis and redundancy. This means that situations where the
speechreader can observe both the head and the body of the speaker generally will

be more productive for the speechreader. Nitchie (1912) was one of the first teachers of speechreading to stress that those with hearing loss must learn to be cognizant of nonverbal cues, such as gestures, when attempting to understand speech. Successful speechreading involves using information from a variety of sources. Nonverbal cues, such as facial expressions, conveyed by the speaker can be very helpful in comprehending visually the general intent of the message.

Signal and Code

Speech consists of acoustic information that is efficiently received and effectively interpreted by the normal auditory mechanism. It possesses physical characteristics that are compatible with the receptive capabilities of the normal ear. The basic units of speech are consonants and vowels, classified as phonemes. A phoneme has distinctive acoustic features that enable the listener to distinguish it from all other speech sounds.

Vowels embody the major concentration of acoustic energy found in speech and are termed resonated phonemes. Vowel production is accomplished by directing vocalizations through the oral cavity, which is altered in shape and size by different tongue and lip positions. These subtle alterations are responsible for providing each vowel with specific acoustic features, such as formants (see Chapter 4).

> Distinctive features are unique characteristics of a given phoneme that distinguish one phoneme from another.

Consonants, which are primarily responsible for the intelligibility of speech, are termed articulated phonemes because their production involves the manipulation of the various articulators: lips, tongue, and teeth. As pointed out in Chapter 4, these phonemes possess *distinctive features* that permit a listener to recognize them. Miller and Nicely (1955) classified these features as *voicing, nasality, affrication, duration,* and *place of articulation*. Except for place of articulation, the identifying characteristics of consonants are perceived well on the basis of acoustic information. Although difficult to distinguish acoustically, the place of articulation may be processed to some extent visually due to the visibility of the articulators.

Because many of the 40 or more phonemes used in English demonstrate ambiguous or very limited visible features, an individual who relies solely on vision to understand speech faces much uncertainty. Knowledge of the visual components of speech depends, for the most part, on research using small speech units, that is, consonant–vowel combinations or monosyllabic words (e.g., Jackson, 1988).

> A viseme is a group of phonemes in which each looks alike when spoken.

Visemes.   The number of distinctive visual features of vowels and consonants is reduced to the shape of the mouth for vowels and the place of articulation for consonants. Because the perception of phonemes is primarily an auditory function based on acoustic features, Fisher (1968) coined the term *viseme* to indicate the distinguishable visual characteristics of speech sounds. A viseme, therefore, is a speech sound (phoneme) that has been classified by its place of articulation or by the shape of the mouth. This creates a major limitation for the observer of speech compared to that of the listener. Whereas combinations of auditory distinctive features are unique to each phoneme, several phonemes yield the same viseme, thus limiting the speechreader to the conclusion that one of a group of sounds was uttered.

> Homophenes are words that look alike when spoken, even though they sound different. Homophones are words that sound and look the same but are spelled differently.

Because groups of consonants are produced at the same points of articulation, the phonemes within these groups cannot be differentiated visually without grammatical, phonetic, or lexical information. These visually confusable units of speech are labeled *homophenes*, or different speech sounds that look the same. Similarly, words that look alike are referred to as homophenous words. Look in the mirror and say aloud or have a friend utter the syllables /p/, /b/, and /m/. As you watch and listen simultaneously, the syllables sound so different that you may not notice their visual similarities. However, when these same syllables are formed without voice, you will note that their visual characteristics are indistinguishable. This same type of confusion often occurs among word groups (e.g., *pet*, *bed*, and *men*; *tip*, *limb*, and *dip*; and *cough* and *golf*). However, it has been demonstrated that talkers significantly influence the number of visemes produced (Kricos & Lesner, 1982). That is, some talkers are easier to speechread than are other talkers because they produce more distinctively different viseme groups. It has been estimated that, regardless of the number of viseme categories reported by various authors, in conversational speech nearly 50 percent of the words are indistinguishable visually; that is, they look like other words (Berger, 1972b).

Consonant Visemes. A number of studies have been conducted to determine the number of visemes in spoken English. Jeffers and Barley (1971), Lesner, Sandridge, and Kricos (1987), and many others have determined that there are a limited number of visually distinct patterns that can be made among spoken English consonants. However, these authors do not agree on the number of visemes that can be recognized. Estimates vary from a low of four viseme groups to a high of nine viseme groups.

Table 5.1 lists the homophenous classifications proposed by several authors. Table 5.1 also illustrates the chance for error that a listener has when required to interpret consonant phonemes visually. Except for the *independent visemes* of /r/ and /w/ reported by Binnie, Jackson, and Montgomery (1976) and the /j/ reported by Jeffers and Barley (1971), all consonant viseme clusters contain at least two phonemes. Consequently, on the average, the speechreader has at best a 50 percent chance of correctly identifying a specific isolated phoneme within any group when relying solely on vision.

Vowel Visemes. Although vowels are not considered articulated phonemes, Jeffers and Barley (1971) suggested that vowels can be visually recognized by their movements, that is, by "a recognizable visual motor pattern, usually common to two or more speech sounds" (p. 42). These authors observed seven visually distinct movements when the vowels were produced at a slow rate accompanied with pronounced movement and normal rhythm. When the same phonemes were produced in conversational speech, the number of different movements was reduced to four.

Jeffers and Barley (1971) describe two viewing conditions based on speaker presentation that determine the visually distinct patterns among English phonemes produced in isolation. The first condition is referred to as *ideal*. Under this viewing condition the speaker provides the listener with essentially perfectly articulated

Ideal conditions include optimal distance, viewing angle, speech rate, and an unobstructed, well-lighted view of the speaker without auditory or visual distractions.

TABLE 5.1 **Visemes for English Consonants Determined by Various Researchers**

		Viseme Groups		
Jeffers and Barley (1971)		**Fisher (1968)**		**Binnie et al. (1976)**
Initial[a]		Final[b]		
1. /f, v/	1. /f, v/	1. /f, v/		1. /f, v/
2. /w, r/	2. /p, b, m, d/	2. /p, b/		2. /p, b, m/
3. /p, b, m/	3. /hw, w, r/	3. /ʃ, ʒ, ʤ, ʧ/		3. /w/
4. /θ, ð/	4. /ʃ, t, n, l, s, z/	4. /t, d, n, θ, ð, s,		4. /l, n/
5. /ʃ, ʒ, ʧ, ʤ/	5. /ʤ, j, h/	z, r, l/		5. /ʃ, ʒ/
6. /s, z/	5. /k, g/	5. /k, g, ŋ, m/		6. /r/
7. /j/				7. /θ, ð/
8. /t, d, n, l/				8. /t, d, s, z/
9. /k, g, ŋ/				9. /k, g/

[a]Observed in the initial position.
[b]Observed in the final position.

Note: The order of the visemes is based on the rank ordering of the visual clustering of these phonemes by Binnie et al. (1976).

TABLE 5.2   Visemes for All Speech Sounds Combined in *Ideal* and *Usual* Viewing Conditions

COMBINED CONSONANT AND VOWEL SPEECHREADING MOVEMENTS
IDEAL VIEWING CONDITIONS

Visible	Obscure
1. Lower lip to upper teeth, /f,v/	1. Lips rounded, moderate opening to lips back, narrow opening, /ɔɪ/
2. Lips relaxed, moderate opening to lips puckered, narrow opening, /aʊ/	2. Tongue up or down, /t,d,n,ɪ/
3. Lips puckered, narrow opening, /w,hw,r,u,ʊ,o,oʊ,ɝ/	3. Lips relaxed, moderate opening, /ɛ,æ,ɑ/
4. Lips together, /p,b,m/	4. Lips relaxed, moderate opening to lips back narrow opening, /aɪ/
5. Tongue between teeth, /θ,ð/	5. Tongue back and up, /k,g,ŋ/
6. Lips forward, /ʃ,ʒ,tʃ,dʒ/	
7. Lips back, narrow opening, /i,ɪ,eɪ,e,ʌ,j/	
8. Lips rounded, moderate opening, /ɔ/	
9. Teeth together, /s,z/	

COMBINED CONSONANT AND VOWEL SPEECHREADING MOVEMENTS
USUAL VIEWING CONDITIONS

Visible	Obscure
1. Lower lip to upper teeth, /f, v/	1. Lips forward, /ʃ,ʒ,tʃ,dʒ/
2. Lips puckered, narrow opening, /w,hw,r,u,ʊ,oʊ,ɝ/	2. Lips rounded, moderate opening, /ɔ,ɔɪ/
3. Lips together, /p, b, m/	3. Teeth approximated, /s,z; t,d,n,l;θ,ð; k,g,ŋ;j/
4. Lips relaxed, moderate opening to lips puckered, narrow opening, /aʊ/	4. Lips relaxed, narrow opening, /i,ɪ,eɪ,e,ʌ,ɛ,æ,ɑ,aɪ/
5. Tongue between teeth, /θ,ð/	

The movements are presented in an estimated order of relative visibility with a Visible 1 being most visible and an Obscure 4 or 5 the least visible.

Source: Adapted from Jeffers and Barley (1971).

speech that contains maximal visual cues. The second viewing condition is labeled *usual*. This condition occurs in what can be classified as everyday talking conditions. While the speaker does not intentionally distort his or her speech, he or she articulates in a typical manner that produces fewer visual cues. As can be seen in Table 5.2, these two conditions significantly influence which phonemes are included in which viseme cluster.

In general, it has been demonstrated that there are consistent visual confusions among vowels, frequently with vowels that have similar lip positions and movement (Jackson, Montgomery, & Binnie, 1976; Montgomery & Jackson, 1983). Furthermore, there are vowels that are seldom recognized visually, and, as might be expected, the vowels that are perceived correctly in isolation are not necessarily comprehended visually in conversational speech.

In summary, most of the individual phonemes in our language are not unique visually when spoken, resulting in considerable confusion and misperception for the speechreader. Jeffers and Barley (1971) concluded that under optimal viewing conditions, only about 40 percent of the information regarding consonant sounds provided by audition is available via vision. Furthermore, these authors demonstrated that the speechreader, under ideal viewing conditions, receives only about 33 percent of the information that is contained auditorily in conversational speech (vowels plus consonants). This visual information is reduced to approximately 17 percent (a range of 10 to 25 percent) when the speechreader is viewing conversations under everyday-type listening conditions.

Under ideal conditions, there are 14 total visemes, but under usual conditions, there are nine, as compared to about 40 phonemes (see Table 5.2).

Under ideal conditions, about 33 percent of speech is visible; with usual conditions, 10 to 25 percent is visible.

Visibility

In addition to the fact that a number of speech sounds and words look similar, another related problem for the speechreader is that many speech sounds are not very visible as they are produced. While phonemes such as /p/ or /f/ can be seen quite well, other phonemes, such as /k/ or /t/, are produced in a far less visible manner. In addition, other features, such as *voicing*, are not visible at all. It has been estimated that as many as 60 percent of the English phonemes are not readily visible (Woodward & Barber, 1960).

Visual Intelligibility of Connected Discourse.   Researchers have determined the visemes that viewers can identify at the syllable and word levels, but they are less certain about what is visibly discernible when these speech elements are portions of lengthier utterances. The visual properties of isolated speech units change when placed in sentence form, as does the acoustic waveform itself. Unless there is a visible pause between words, a speechreader presumably perceives an uninterrupted series of articulatory movements of varying degrees of inherent visibility. This sequence is broken only when the speaker pauses, either deliberately or for a breath. As a result, the written message "There is a blue car in our driveway" is spoken /ðɛrɪzeblukarɪnaʊɚdraɪvweɪ/. Connected speech contains numerous articulatory positions and movements that occur in a relatively short period of time. Consequently, the majority of phonemes in conversational speech occur in the medial position. The example just given contains an initial consonant /ð/, a final vowel /eɪ/, with numerous sounds (positions and movements) between these phonemes. Ironically, researchers have not determined the number of visemes that are identifiable when phonemes occur in the medial position.

The nature of grammatical sentence structure imposes constraints on word sequences that are not present when the words are used in isolation. These word arrangement rules change the probabilities of word occurrence. Thus, the receiver's task is altered (theoretically made easier) because of the linguistic information and redundancy provided by connected discourse. Language is structured in a way that provides more information than is absolutely necessary to convey a given meaning or thought. Even if certain fragments of the spoken code are missed, cues or information inherent in the message may assist the receiver in making an accurate prediction of the missing parts. That is, oral language is an orderly process that is governed by the rules of pragmatic, topical, semantic, syntactic, lexical, and phonological constraints that are the sources for linguistic redundancy (Boothroyd, 1988). This redundancy creates the predictability of conversational speech. Table 4.4 in Chapter 4 summarizes several types of linguistic constraints that contribute to this.

Briefly, the pragmatic constraints of language allow for two or more individuals to share thoughts and information orally. Similarly, the topical constraints, which are also referred to as contextual and situational constraints, limit conversation to a specific topic, which, in turn, governs the vocabulary that is appropriate to describe the topic. We use this rule consistently, even though we frequently introduce it in a negative manner. For example, how many times have you said, "Not to change the subject," and then promptly deviated from the original topic of conversation? You are engaging the rule of contextual information, and, regardless of how it is initiated, it provides your receiver with a preparatory set that allows her or him to expect a specific vocabulary concerned with a specific event. The situation or environment determines the manner in which the speaker will describe a certain event. Comedians are masters at using this rule; they alter the language of their "stories" based on the makeup of their audience. Contextual and situational constraints are closely allied and are used interchangeably by some authors. For example, during a televised sporting event, when a coach disputes a decision by a referee, have you noticed how well you perceive what the coach says even though you only have limited auditory and visual cues available? Contextually, you perceive an argument while the situation causes the coach to express himself by using a rather limited and heated vocabulary that enables you to predict the words being used. As illustrated in this instance, the situation in which the conversation occurs provides information that otherwise you may not have been able to obtain by relying solely on the articulatory features of the message for perception.

Redundancy, the result of these constraints, contributes significantly to the information afforded by oral language. Thus, redundancy allows the receiver to predict missed information from the bits of information that have been perceived. To illustrate, "Dogs going" means the same as "The dogs are going away." The latter is grammatically correct and contains redundant information. Plurality is indicated twice (dogs, are), present tense twice (are, going), and the direction twice (going, away). Consequently, it would be possible to miss the words "are" and "away" while still comprehending the message ("dogs going"). If we miss part of a message, linguistic redundancy can enable us to synthesize correctly what we missed. However, as will be mentioned in the discussion of perceptual closure, a minimum amount of information must be perceived before accurate predictions can be made. In the preceding example, the words "dogs" and "away" would have to be processed visually in order for the speechreader to conceptualize the message "The dogs are going away."

Although the constraints of language do not enhance the physical visibility of speech, they help the speechreader follow what has been said. Albright, Hipskind, and Schuckers (1973) demonstrated that speechreaders actually obtain more total information from the redundancy and linguistic rules of spoken language than from phoneme and word visibility. Clouser (1976) concluded that the ratio between the number of consonants and vowels did not determine the visual intelligibility of sentences; rather, he found that short sentences were easier to speechread than longer sentences. In another study related to visual perception of speech, Berger (1972b) determined that familiar and frequently used words were identified visually more often than were words used infrequently. Additional information on redundancy is provided in Tables 4.3 and 4.4 in Chapter 4.

Environment

Circumstances associated with the environments in which the speechreader must communicate can influence the speechreading process considerably. For example, investigators have demonstrated that such factors as distance and viewing angles between the speaker and receiver affect speechreading performance. Erber's (1971) study regarding the influence of distance on the visual perception of speech revealed that speechreading performance was optimal when the speaker was about 5 feet from the speechreader. Although performance decreased beyond 5 feet, it did not drop significantly until the distance exceeded 20 feet. Similarly, there is evidence that simultaneous auditory and visual competition, such as distracters, can have an adverse effect on speechreading under certain conditions (O'Neill & Oyer, 1981). Although the amount of lighting is not an important factor in speechreading, provided a reasonable amount of light is present, Erber (1974) suggested that, for optimal visual reception of speech, illumination should provide a contrast between the background and the speaker's face.

Garstecki (1977) concluded that speechreading performance improved when the spoken message was accompanied by relevant pictorial and auditory cues. This finding was given further support by Garstecki and O'Neill (1980), whose subjects had better speechreading scores when the *CID Everyday Sentences* were presented with appropriate situational cues. In essence, environmental cues provide speechreaders with contextual and situational information, thereby increasing their ability to predict what is being conveyed verbally.

Redundancy determines the predictability of a spoken message. The more redundancy present, the easier speechreading will be.

As noted earlier in the section "Speaker," a 0- to 45-degree viewing angle is best; 90 degrees is not as good. Five to 10 feet from the speaker is a good distance for speechreading.

Speechreader

Reduction of a person's ability to hear (auditory sensitivity, or detection) auditory stimuli is only one of several parameters that contribute to the disabling effects of hearing loss. Other factors, such as auditory perception abilities (discriminating, identifying, comprehending), age of onset of the hearing loss, site(s) of lesions, and the educational and therapeutic management followed, all contribute toward making the hearing loss population extremely heterogeneous. This heterogeneity appears to extend to speechreading because individuals with hearing loss demonstrate considerable variability in their ability to use vision to speechread. Individual differences in speechreading abilities are large. This body of research is summarized by Dodd and Campbell (1987). Some persons possess amazing speechreading abilities, while others are able to perceive very little speech through the visual channel. Ever since speechreading has been included in audiologic rehabilitation, clinicians and researchers have attempted to determine what personal characteristics of the speechreader account for success or failure in speechreading, including variables such as age, gender, intelligence, personality traits, and visual acuity (O'Neill & Oyer, 1981). In general, it is impossible to totally clarify the characteristics associated with success in speechreading. The following is a sampling of the research that has been conducted in this area related to the speechreader.

Age. There appear to be some interactions between a speechreader's age and other attributes that contribute to speechreading ability. Specifically, evidence suggests that speechreading proficiency tends to develop and improve throughout childhood and early adulthood and appears to be closely associated with the emergence of language skills. Even though their speechreading abilities are not fully developed, younger children, even infants, may use speechreading to some extent (Pollack, 1985).

> Young speechreaders show better scores as they get older throughout childhood.

Some older people demonstrate phonemic regression, that is, severe inability to understand speech via hearing, that is not consistent with their audiometric profiles (Gaeth, 1948). This same type of phenomenon may account, in part, for the finding that older individuals do less well in speechreading than their younger counterparts even when visual acuity is controlled. Hefler (1998) suggested that the elderly perform more poorly on experimental speechreading tasks because of the inability to process temporally changing visual information. Finally, it is important to note that decreased visual acuity may also contribute to reduced speechreading skill in the aged.

Gender. This variable has been investigated thoroughly (Dancer, Krain, Thompson, Davis, & Glenn, 1994; Tye-Murray, Murray, & Spehar, 2007). Overall, while adult females tend to achieve slightly higher speechreading scores than do males, the difference generally has been small and nonsignificant.

Intelligence. An abundance of research describes the relationship between speechreading and mental abilities. Generally, no demonstrable positive correlation has been found between understanding speech visually and intelligence, assuming intelligence levels in or above the "low normal" range (Lewis, 1972). However, a study conducted by Smith (1964) with a population of mentally impaired individuals revealed that much-reduced intelligence levels did result in significantly poorer speechreading performance.

> IQ appears to have little effect on speechreading as long as it is not below the normal range.

Personality Traits. As may be expected from the preceding discussion, investigators have not been able to ferret out specific personality traits that differentiate among levels of speechreading proficiency. While motivation is tenuous to assess, most clinicians intuitively concur that highly motivated (competitive) clients tend to speechread more effectively than do unmotivated clients. However, it is apparent that good and poor speechreaders generally cannot be stereotyped based on personality patterns (Giolas, Butterfield, & Weaver, 1974; O'Neill, 1951).

Visual acuity can have a major impact on speechreading success.

Visual Acuity. Hardick, Oyer, and Irion (1970) determined that they could rank successful and unsuccessful speechreaders based on their visual acuity. Lovering (1969) demonstrated that even slight visual acuity problems (20/40 and poorer) had an appreciable, negative effect on speechreading scores. Johnson and Snell (1986) also showed that distance and visual acuity have a significant effect on speechreading.

In support of the argument that good visual acuity is important for successful speechreading performance, Romano and Berlow (1974) concluded that visual acuity must be at least 20/80 before speech can be decoded visually. Recently, a line of research has compared visually evoked responses and speechreading ability. According to the results of this research, a viewer's ability to process speech visually is, in part, a function of the rapidity (latency) with which physical visual stimuli are transduced to neural energy for interpretation at the cortical level (Samar & Sims, 1983, 1984; Shepard, 1982; Summerfield, 1992). While the clinical applicability of this research has not yet been fully realized, visually evoked responses can assist the clinician in understanding a client's ability to process visually oriented information. Potentially, visually evoked responses may provide audiologic rehabilitationists with information regarding a viewer's ability to speechread various types of oral stimuli.

Figure–ground patterning involves an ability to focus on and perceive a target stimulus, or figure, from a background of other stimuli, or ground.

Visual Perception. Based on Gibson's (1969) definition of perception, our eyes receive visual stimuli that are interpreted at a cortical level and provide us with visual information. This information, in turn, enables us to make a selective response to the original stimuli. Thus, when interpreting speech visually, the speechreader first "sees" the movement of the lips, which the cortex classifies as speech. The accuracy of the speechreader's response to these stimuli is partially a function of how well the peripheral-to-central visual process enables him or her to discriminate among the speaker's articulatory movements.

At present, explanations of the way in which the perceptual process develops are theoretical. However, two strategies appear relevant in connection with obtaining information from the environment. The first, figure–ground patterning, is achieved by identifying a target (meaningful) signal that is embedded in similar but ambient stimuli. Observe the following letters:

wabriodraz
opaiblohye
lipreading
iracraxole
mualyocepl

The letters within this rectangle are of the same case and are placed in an order that meets the criterion of structural ordering. That is, all the letter combinations are possible and probable in written English. As noted, however, there is only one string of letters that creates a meaningful word: lipreading (see line 3). Thus, this sequence of printed symbols is the figure, while all the other letters are merely spurious background stimuli. The development of figure–ground patterning skills permits the individual with hearing loss to separate meaningful visual and auditory events from ambient stimuli.

Being able to combine or pull bits of information together in order to figure out what was said is termed *closure*.

As early as 1912, Nitchie claimed that successful speechreaders are intuitive and able to synthesize limited visual input into meaningful wholes. Since then, professionals have concurred that successful speechreaders possess the ability to visually piece together fragmented pictorial and spoken stimuli into meaningful messages. This ability, termed *closure*, is yet another strategy used to obtain information from environmental events. Before this strategy can be used effectively, a person must receive at least minimal stimulation and, more important, must have had prior experience (familiarity) with the whole. Both of the following sentences require that the reader use closure to obtain accurate information:

1. Humpty _____ wall.
2. When you _____ time, you murder _____.

In all probability you had little difficulty supplying the four words, *Dumpty sat on a*, to the first sentence. The second sentence may have been more difficult unless you are familiar with the adage "When you kill time, you murder opportunity." The first sentence provides considerably fewer physical cues than does the second, but experience with and exposure to nursery rhymes permitted you to perceive the whole expression. Effective visual closure skills are essential for those with hearing loss because, due to their disorder and the limited visual cues afforded by speech, they receive fragmented or distorted auditory and visual stimuli. In trying to understand the role of prediction or predictability, it is paramount to realize that we do not merely get some information by perception (processing the stimuli) and some from the context (prediction) and then add the two. If we did, the total information received would be equal to or less than (because of redundancy or correlation) the sum of what we can get from either channel alone. The fact that the total is greater than the sum of both channels (as measured above) implies a facilitating or feedback effect from one to the other. The aural information facilitates visual processing, and the visual information enhances auditory processing.

Hearing. Unfortunately, those with hearing loss generally are not any better at speechreading than are those with normal hearing. Among individuals with hearing loss, however, there is a mild relationship between speechreading proficiency and the degree of hearing loss present. Those persons fortunate to have significant amounts of residual hearing remaining have the potential to speechread more successfully than those with very limited hearing. This occurs because speechreading is enhanced somewhat by the availability of simultaneous auditory cues contained in speech. This is especially apparent in persons beginning to use a cochlear implant, where speechreading performance often improves dramatically relative to what it was previously; because of the additional information provided by the cochlear implant, speechreading becomes somewhat more productive.

It is apparent that numerous factors have an impact on speechreading success. The successful clinician will be familiar with these and take each into account when assisting those with hearing loss in effectively using visual information for communication.

In general, those with hearing loss are not better speechreaders than those with normal hearing.

SPEECHREADING AND HEARING LOSS

Assessing speechreading ability and providing effective speechreading instruction to those with hearing loss are two primary responsibilities of the aural rehabilitationist. The next section outlines some of the ways in which a person's visual communication ability can be evaluated. It also describes several traditional and current approaches to speechreading instruction.

Assessment of Speechreading Ability

Because of the complexities associated with the process, accurate evaluation of speechreading performance is difficult. Professionals have attempted for several decades to develop a means of reliable and valid measurement, but to date no universally acceptable test or battery of tests has emerged for this purpose. Nevertheless, clinicians recognize the importance of assessing speechreading ability to determine if visual communication training is warranted for a particular individual as well as to evaluate the effectiveness of speechreading training. Consequently, a number of formal and informal approaches for measuring speechreading ability are currently in use.

Formal Speechreading Tests. Since the mid-1940s, speechreading tests have been developed, published, and used. These tests, designed specifically to measure

Vision only refers to attempting to perceive speech via visual cues (without voice).

Both speechreading and auditory assessment are influenced by variables that raise or lower scores. These include vocabulary level, context, and response format (see Chapter 4).

the speechreading abilities of adults or children, may consist of syllables, words, sentences, stories, or a combination of these stimuli. Speechreading tests are presented either in a vision-only condition without acoustic cues or in a combined visual-auditory test condition in which the stimuli are both seen and heard by the speechreader. These formal tests sometimes are presented in a prerecorded fashion—videotape, CD, DVD—but often are administered in a live, face-to-face situation where the clinician presents the test stimuli. Although the test contents remain constant, the manner of presentation may vary considerably among clinicians when tests are administered live, which can make interpretation of the results less secure due to the variability created by using different speakers to present the test stimuli (Montgomery, Walden, Schwartz, & Prosek, 1984). Some of these tests are listed in Table 5.3 and in the appendices of this chapter. It should be noted that several tests originally developed to assess auditory speech perception have also been used to evaluate speechreading skills.

Informal Speechreading Tests. Informal tests are developed by the clinician, who selects stimulus materials of his or her choosing. Contents should vary as a function of the client's age and the information sought by the rehabilitationist. Clinicians use a variety of speech forms, including lists of words presented in isolation or in sentences. Sentence items may include statements like "What is your name?" or "Show me a toothbrush." Informal assessment allows the tester to select stimuli that

TABLE 5.3 Formal Speechreading Tests for Adults and Children

Title of Tests	Authors	Content Format
Adults		
How Well Can You Read Lips?	Utley (1946)	Words Sentences Stories
Semi-Diagnostic Test	Hutton, Curry, and Armstrong (1959)	Words
Barley CID Sentences	Barley and Jeffers (1971)	Sentences
CID Everyday Sentence Test	NTID (DVD from Auditec in 2009)	Sentences
Denver Quick Test of Lipreading Ability[a]	Alpiner (1978)	Sentences
Assessment of Adult Speechreading Ability	New York League for the Hard of Hearing (1990)	Sentences Paragraphs
Iowa Phoneme and Sentence Test	Tyler, Preece, and Tye-Murray (1986)	Phonemes and sentences
Children		
Craig Lipreading Inventory[a]	Craig (1964)	Words Sentences
Diagnostic Test of Speechreading	Myklebust and Neyhus (1970)	Questions Commands
Children's Audiovisual Enhancement Test (CAVET)	Tye-Murray and Geers (2002)	Words Phrases Sentences
Multimodal Lexical Sentence Test for Children (MLST-C)	Kirk et al. (2011)	Sentences

[a]See Appendixes 5B and 5C.

are more pertinent for a particular client than items on formal speechreading tests. However, as a result of the loose format and the intent of these tests, the obtained results do not lend themselves well to comparative analysis.

Whether using formal or informal speechreading tests, it is important that the stimuli not be so difficult that they discourage the client or so easy that test scores reflect a ceiling effect (100 percent correct for each viewer). Materials should be selected so that they approximate various types of stimuli encountered by the individual in everyday situations. For children and certain adults (such as those with severe speech or writing problems), the response mode should involve pointing with a multiple-choice format; most adults are capable of responding to (writing or repeating) open-set tests. Because of the various shortcomings of existing speechreading tests, these instruments cannot be expected to provide completely valid measures of speechreading ability but may yield data of some clinical usefulness.

The use of live, face-to-face presentation, although widespread, should be conducted carefully with optimal consideration for distance (5 to 10 feet), lighting (no shadows), and viewing angle (0 to 45 degrees). Even following these precautions, speaker variability will introduce uncertainty into the test situation. Not only will two speakers produce the same speech stimuli somewhat differently, but a single talker, producing the same stimuli twice, also will not do so in precisely the same manner each time. Therefore, it is difficult to compare a person's skills from one testing to another (pre- and post-therapy) or to directly compare the performance of two individuals. Scores obtained through face-to-face test administration, although useful, need to be interpreted carefully.

Assessment of speechreading can involve the presentation of visual stimuli without any associated acoustic cues. Although this yields meaningful information regarding the basic skill of speechreading, additional testing of speechreading ability in a combined auditory–visual fashion is also advocated by many because it more closely resembles ordinary person-to-person communication. Such testing provides a relevant measure of how well a person integrates visual and auditory information, which is how speech perception occurs in most real communication situations.

To estimate how a listener is using vision to supplement audition, present the listener with words and sentences in a vision-only mode, followed by another presentation in a vision-hearing combined (natural) mode. By subtracting the vision-only score from the vision-hearing score, a difference between these two presentation modalities will provide an estimate of the amount of information provided by speechreading for a given individual.

Speechreading abilities can also be assessed informally with auditory-only and auditory–verbal speech tracking. (See Chapter 4 and Supplementary Learning Activity 4.)

Schow (personal communication) noted that when college students with normal hearing are given his filmed version of Utley's (1946) How Well Can You Read Lips? test in a vision-only mode at a 0-degree azimuth, their performance is approximately as follows (see Supplementary Learning Activity 1):

	SENTENCES	WORDS
Mean	35–45%	35–45%
Range	10–70%	25–70%

When given a similar filmed version of the Semi-Diagnostic Test (Hutton et al., 1959), these same students score as follows:

	WORDS	
	0-Degree Azimuth	**90-Degree Azimuth**
Mean	60–65%	50–60%
Range	25–90%	25–75%

The better Semi-Diagnostic scores are probably due to the closed-response set as opposed to the open-response set in the Utley test.

Visual Assessment and Speechreading Evaluation

It is important that assessment of speechreading skills be preceded by a measure of visual acuity. As discussed, there is clear evidence that even mild visual acuity problems can have adverse effects on speechreading performance. It is amazing, therefore, that audiologic rehabilitationists have given only limited attention to measuring basic visual abilities in connection with the assessment and instruction of speechreading with persons having hearing loss. Concern for this is further reinforced by research on visual disorders among those with hearing loss. Evidence indicates that the incidence of ocular anomalies among students with hearing loss is greater than for normal-hearing children of the same age. Campbell, Polomeno, Elder, Murray, and Altosaar (1981) surveyed the literature and found that 38 to 58 percent of persons with hearing loss reportedly have accompanying visual deficiencies. Even more alarming are data from the National Technical Institute for the Deaf (NTID, 1987) showing that, of the total number of students entering the NTID in the past, 65 percent demonstrated defective vision (Johnson, Caccamise, Rothblum, Hamilton, & Howard, 1981). The elderly also present challenges, as their overall visual skills are declining at the same time as their hearing loss emerges. To maximize speech perception, both vision and auditory needs of the individual should be considered. Basic visual skills associated with the detection, recognition, resolution, and localization of visual stimuli are fundamental when assessing a person's visual acuity. Each of these measurements uses static stimuli; that is, the viewer describes specific characteristics of stationary targets that measure a certain aspect of the viewer's visual acuity. Although research on the relationship between visual acuity and speechreading has concentrated on visual *recognition* (commonly referred to as far visual acuity), at least for some clients it may be prudent to determine their ability to *detect*, *resolve*, and *localize* visual test stimuli prior to initiating speechreading therapy.

Hearing Loss and Dependence on Vision

The degree to which persons with hearing loss depend on vision for information is related to the extent of their hearing loss. To paraphrase Ross (1982), there is a world of difference between the deaf, who must communicate mainly through a visual mode (speechreading or manual communication), and the hard of hearing, who communicate primarily through an auditory mode (albeit imperfectly).

Deaf. The deaf, who receive quite limited meaningful auditory cues, must rely more on their vision to keep in contact with their environment. The deaf, by the nature of their disorder, use their vision projectively and are visually oriented. However, as stated throughout this chapter, vision generally is less effective than audition when used to decode spoken language. Therefore, these individuals must learn to decode a foreign language without the benefit of auditory cues. English competency, which is most effectively and efficiently developed via the auditory channel, is essential to communication in our society. By definition, "speechreading is an inherently linguistic activity" (Boothroyd, 1988). The deaf therefore are further disabled in that, before they can gain meaning from speechreading English, they must have developed the linguistic rules of English, which, in turn, are most naturally acquired through aural stimulation. In summary, to benefit from speechreading, the listener–viewers must have a fairly extensive language background. Without this, they are not able to fill in the gaps providing them with information that cannot be obtained through speechreading or hearing (Bevan, 1988). Thus, the deaf face the monumental challenge of having to speechread words that they may never have conceptualized.

Hard of Hearing. Hard of hearing individuals, by definition, possess functional residual hearing, which permits them to receive and ultimately perceive more auditory stimuli within their environment than those who are deaf. This enhanced ability would suggest that they are less dependent on their vision than are the deaf when perceiving speech. Even so, the hard of hearing, who employ their vision to supplement distorted and reduced acoustic stimuli, receive considerably more information from the spoken code than is provided solely by their auditory channel.

Various investigators have assessed the advantages that audition, vision, and a combination of these sensory modalities afford the receiver when decoding spoken stimuli (CHABA, 1991; Massaro, 1987). More recently, the term *audiovisual integration* has been used to describe information obtained from speech that is seen (Tye-Murray, 2009). Few would disagree that using these two senses simultaneously produces better speech reception than using either alone. Likewise, it is clear that vision can provide information to the receiver when decoding speech in the absence of auditory cues. More important, however, even limited auditory input allows the listener to establish a referent from which additional information can be gained visually. Thus, the contributions made by these sensory mechanisms as receptors of speech fall into a hierarchy. That is, when both residual hearing and speechreading are available, the listener with hearing loss tends to do better on a communicative task (see Figure 5.2). For example, if a person achieves a speech recognition score of 50 percent with hearing alone and a speechreading score of 20 percent using similar test material, this individual might achieve a combined auditory–visual score that could approach 80 to 90 percent. In other words, there is more than a simple additive effect from the combination of auditory and visual information. Therefore, the benefits of speechreading need to be strongly emphasized in the auditory rehabilitation provided to those with hearing loss.

Traditional Speechreading Methods

During the early 1900s, four methods of teaching speechreading were popularized in the United States (O'Neill & Oyer, 1981). Three of these methods were nurtured by individuals who had normal hearing until adulthood, at which time they

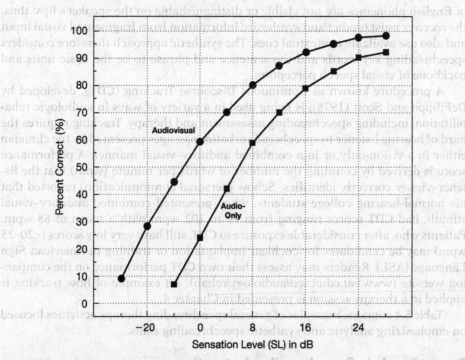

FIGURE 5.2   Mean discrimination scores for normal hearing adults using audiovisual and audio-only speech stimuli (NU-6s).

Source: Based on Binnie (1973).

acquired significant hearing losses. Initially, they sought assistance to overcome the limitations placed on them by their sensory deprivation. Subsequently, they became interested in assisting other hearing-impaired persons in developing speechreading skills, eventually establishing methods that bear their names: the Bruhn (1929) method, the Kinzie method (Kinzie & Kinzie, 1931), and the Nitchie (1912) method. Later, Bunger (1944) wrote a book describing a speechreading method developed by Brauckman in Jena, Germany: the Jena method. Although these original four speechreading methods are seldom used now as they were originally conceived, it is recommended that the interested reader refer to French-St. George and Stoker (1988) for a historical chronicle of speechreading.

Analytic speechreading centers around visually perceiving the details *found in speech.*

Analytic and Synthetic Approaches.   Each of the above original methods for teaching speechreading, as well as the recent approaches used currently, primarily makes use of one of two general approaches (analytic or synthetic) for speechreading instruction. However, for the most part, these incorporate the same general strategies as the analytical and synthetic approaches described in Chapter 4 for auditory training. The analytic approach to speechreading is based on the concept that, before an entire word, sentence, or phrase (the whole) can be identified, it is necessary to perceive visually each of its basic parts. That is, because a word is constructed by placing phonemes in a given sequential order and sentences (thoughts) are constructed by correctly ordering words, it is essential that the viewer initially identify phonemes visually in isolation before attempting to perceive words. Likewise, we must be able to identify individual words before attempting to recognize strings of words (sentences or phrases). Said differently, this approach to speechreading considers the phoneme and syllable to be the key units for visual perception; therefore, these units must be recognized in isolation before comprehension of the whole is probable.

Synthetic speechreading involves grasping the general thought of the speaker through intuitive thinking.

Conversely, the synthetic approach to speechreading emphasizes that the perception of the whole is paramount regardless of which of its parts is perceived visually. Consequently, the speechreader is encouraged to comprehend the general meaning of oral utterances rather than concentrating on accurately identifying each component within the oral message. As noted earlier, a considerable number of English phonemes are not visible or distinguishable on the speaker's lips; thus, the receiver must predict and synthesize information from fragmented visual input and also use available contextual cues. The synthetic approach therefore considers speechreading key words and the sentence and phrase to be the basic units and backbone of visual speech perception.

A procedure known as Continuous Discourse Tracking (CDT), developed by DeFilippo and Scott (1978), is being used in a variety of ways in audiologic rehabilitation, including speechreading assessment and therapy. Tracking requires the hard of hearing listener to speechread verbatim passages presented by the clinician either in a vision-only or in a combined auditory–visual manner. A performance score is derived by counting the number of words per minute (wpm) that the listener–viewer correctly identifies. Schow (personal communication) reported that his normal-hearing college students, when presented combined auditory–visual stimuli, had CDT scores ranging from 76 to 102 wpm with a mean of 88 wpm. Patients who, after considerable exposure to CDT, still have very low scores (<20–25 wpm) may be candidates for cochlear implantation or training in American Sign Language (ASL). Readers may assess their own CDT performance on the companion website (www.isu.edu/csed/audiology/rehab). An example of how tracking is applied in a therapy session is presented in Chapter 4.

Table 5.4 contains examples of general speechreading therapy activities focused on emphasizing analytic and synthetic speechreading skills.

Recent Trends in Speechreading Instruction

The improvements in hearing aids, assistive listening devices, vibrotactile devices, and cochlear implants that have occurred during the past two decades have made it

TABLE 5.4 Examples of Analytical and Synthetic Speechreading Therapy Activities

Analytic Activities

1. Present syllable pairs with initial consonants that are the same or different (e.g., /ba/ and /ba/ or /la/ and /ba/) and ask the speechreader to discriminate if the initial consonant in the syllable pair is the same or different.
2. Present three or four words (e.g., *talk, tool, mop*) and have the speechreader determine which word has /m/ in initial position.
3. Present single words and ask the speechreader to identify each word from a short list of printed words that the speechreader has in front of him or her.

Synthetic Activities

1. Show the speechreader a picture and ask him or her to provide four to six words that logically could be used by someone talking about the picture.
2. Name a topic (e.g., popular television shows) and have the speechreader identify the name of each show that you present.
3. Present a short paragraph and then ask the speechreader to answer three or four questions based on the content of the paragraph.

possible for individuals with hearing loss, especially those with moderate to severe losses, to more effectively use their hearing than in the past in an integrated manner with speechreading. In a sense, this increased potential to greatly improve the communication abilities of those with hearing loss through hearing aids has, in part, led to much less emphasis on long-term, individualized speechreading therapy in rehabilitation programs for most individuals than in the past, particularly those with mild to moderate hearing difficulties. In addition, there is a growing realization that in-depth speechreading therapy mostly produces only modest improvement at best in speechreading performance, and most of this improvement occurs in the very initial portion of therapy. Instead, what currently is done routinely is to remind them of the importance of attending visually while communicating and to encourage them to utilize this potentially helpful information as much as possible as another way, in addition to using hearing aids or cochlear implants, to maximize overall speech perception. Speechreading is still viewed as a useful component of audiological rehabilitation, but in-depth therapy designed to facilitate speechreading skills generally is recommended only on a selective basis for some persons with hearing loss. The next two sections briefly discuss some of the more recent ways in which speechreading has been incorporated into rehabilitation strategies for both children and adults.

Children. There has been a dearth of information available concerning speechreading strategies for this population (Yoshinaga-Itano, 1988). One probable explanation for this is that some therapeutic approaches used with children with hearing loss have focused almost exclusively on maximizing the use of the auditory channel (Pollack, 1964, 1985; Wedenberg, 1951) with little if any attempt made to teach speechreading skills. This auditory-only unisensory philosophy of management is sometimes referred to as the *auditory–verbal approach*. Despite the unisensory orientation of these approaches, children trained in this manner often emerge with effective speechreading skills. Although this approach clearly focuses on processing and using auditory input, speechreading appears to develop synergistically with the acquisition of auditory and language skills (Pollack, 1964).

Other professionals believe that limited speechreading therapy has some relevance to a comprehensive plan for audiologic rehabilitation for children. Yoshinaga-Itano (1988) suggests using what she terms a *holistic approach* when teaching hard of hearing children to speechread. This method differs from the traditional

In the auditory–verbal approach, auditory abilities are developed to the fullest extent possible. Consequently, formal speechreading training is not incorporated into a child's overall program, and speechreading actually is prevented in some therapy activities.

approaches to speechreading in that, rather than using a single technique for all young clients, it focuses on each individual child's motivation, tolerance, and sense of responsibility for communicating. Goals include building the child's knowledge base concerning the speechreading process and having the child develop an appreciation of the benefits that speechreading can provide in perceiving speech. Consequently, the stimuli used are client oriented, and therapy is based on each client's capabilities and needs in real-life situations rather than simply in canned exercises. Therefore, speechreading activities must be interesting and give the child the opportunity to experience frequent success by correctly perceiving what is being presented. Figure 5.3 is an example of an activity that may be appropriate for *some* hard of hearing children. The child is given a worksheet with a picture on it and asked to speechread the key words presented by the clinician or by other children if it is being used in a group session. Beyond providing contextual and situational information, the picture has the potential to stimulate client motivation and interest. As a reward, the clinician may ask the child to color the picture. The clinician is reminded that this is only an example and that the idea and format should be adapted to meet the needs and interests of his or her clients.

Auditory only refers to attempting to perceive speech via hearing (without visual cues).

Some children born with severe to profound hearing losses or who acquire the hearing loss prelingually become potential recipients of limited speechreading therapy if an oral–aural or total communication approach to management is followed. These children are fitted as early as possible with hearing aids binaurally or cochlear implants. As part of an overall management approach, they also are encouraged to use vision and may receive some speechreading therapy, along with extensive auditory training. Both analytic and synthetic training activities are used to develop visual as well as auditory skills. Although a portion of speechreading and auditory skill development is done in *vision-only* or *auditory-only* conditions, many professionals currently advocate using both vision and audition together. Expressions with visual and auditory stimuli presented simultaneously are more natural and provide an opportunity to integrate the auditory and visual cues that are available. More information on the application of speechreading with hearing-impaired children can be obtained in the publications by McCaffrey (1995) and Tye-Murray (1993a, 1993b, 2009).

Adults. As mentioned earlier, speechreading training was frequently provided in the past to adults with hearing loss in an intensive manner over a lengthy period of time, which sometimes extended for weeks and even months. While no longer done routinely, this approach is still used selectively in rare instances, when speech

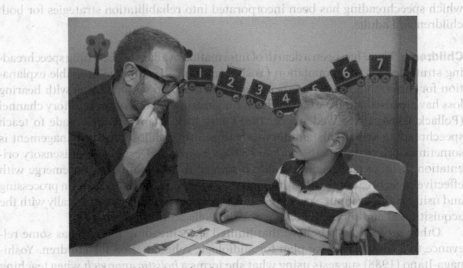

Therapy emphasizing visual cues.

Space Patrol

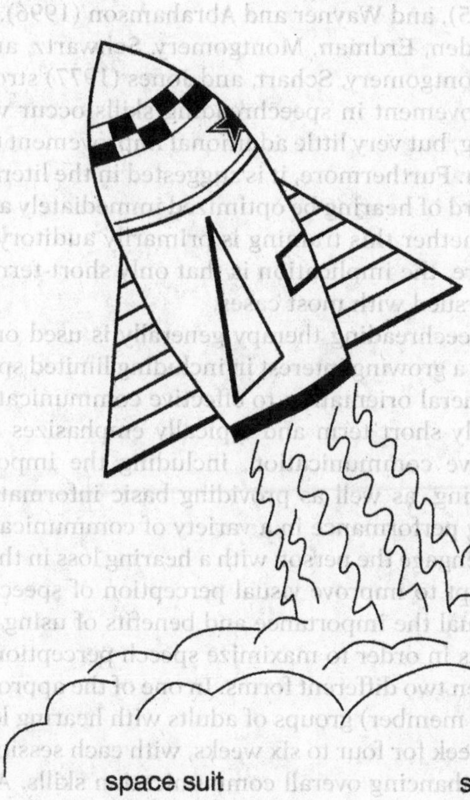

space suit	space helmet
sky	sun
stop	stars

Here is a space ship. Let's take a ride in it. Put on your _____ and your _____ . Step in and sit down. We will see the _____ and the _____ in the _____ . We will not _____ for a long time.

FIGURE 5.3 Example of an exercise used in speechreading therapy with children.

perception is challenging at best, and attempting to maximize the use of visual cues through extensive speechreading therapy is sometimes warranted, even if the benefits derived are limited.

Long-term speechreading therapy typically includes both analytic and synthetic training activities. In addition, clinicians are encouraged to use both visual-only and visual–auditory sensory modalities throughout the therapy program. The level of difficulty for the speechreader can be varied by degrading either the visual or the auditory stimulus. For example, increasing the distance between the speechreader and the clinician will increase the level of difficulty for the speechreading task. Focused speechreading therapy of this nature can be done in either an individualized or a group setting. However, group sessions afford an opportunity for the participants to interact and learn from one another. In some instances, clinicians elect to conduct programs that combine both individual and group sessions for the participants to gain the benefits of each format. Guidance in this application of speechreading, including useful information regarding therapy activities, can be obtained from Feehan, Samuelson, and Seymour (1982), Tye-Murray (2015), and Wayner and Abrahamson (1996). It should be noted that research by Walden, Erdman, Montgomery, Schwartz, and Prosek (1981) and Walden, Prosek, Montgomery, Scharr, and Jones (1977) strongly suggests that demonstrable improvement in speechreading skills occur within the first five or six hours of training, but very little additional improvement (learning) generally is observed thereafter. Furthermore, it is suggested in the literature that sentence recognition by the hard of hearing be optimized immediately after training is started, regardless of whether this training is primarily auditory or visual (Walden et al., 1981). Therefore, the implication is that only short-term involvement should be conducted/pursued with most cases.

Even though long-term speechreading therapy generally is used only in isolated situations, there has been a growing interest in including limited speechreading instruction as part of a general orientation to effective communication skills. This approach is comparatively short term and typically emphasizes a number of key components of effective communication, including the importance of speechreading in communicating, as well as providing basic information about how to enhance speechreading performance in a variety of communicative situations. The intent here is not to engage the person with a hearing loss in therapy and drill-like activities in an attempt to improve visual perception of speech. Rather, it is to highlight to the individual the importance and benefits of using the visual skills that he or she already has in order to maximize speech perception abilities. This strategy has generally taken two different forms. In one of the approaches, clinicians organize small (6 to 12 member) groups of adults with hearing loss. These groups typically meet once a week for four to six weeks, with each session devoted to a general topic related to enhancing overall communication skills. Among the more common topics included are the following:

1. Understanding hearing loss
2. Using assistive listening devices
3. Using communication strategies and speechreading
4. Effective use of hearing aids

The session devoted to speechreading often includes general information about the speechreading process as well as tips for effective speechreading (Table 5.5).

Another approach used is to provide a streamlined and condensed version of the same type of communication-related information and helpful hints. This can be done in one session, often when the individual is fitted with hearing aids. One example of this is the CLEAR program (Schow, 2001) described in Chapter 10. The "L" in CLEAR emphasizes the necessity to "look at" and "lipread" the talker. WATCH (Montgomery, 1994) is another method designed to help reinforce the importance of observing the talker. The "W" in this program is for "Watch the talker's mouth." Both CLEAR and WATCH are designed to illustrate the importance

Speechreading skills appear to improve in the first few hours of training, but afterward, there is very little additional improvement.

Group audiologic rehabilitation sessions often focus on these four main topics.

TABLE 5.5 Tips for Speechreading

Be relatively close to the person(s) with whom you are communicating.

Watch the speaker's mouth, facial expressions, and hand gestures as much as possible.

Be aware of the topic of conversation and contextual cues.

Maximize your hearing (hearing aids and assistive listening devices at optimum volume and minimize background noise).

Let the talker know that you have a hearing loss and request that he or she face you as much as possible.

of seeing as well as listening during conversation. More information on WATCH can be found in Chapter 4.

Since hearing loss is an invisible disorder and since hard of hearing individuals comprehend much of what is said yet misinterpret a significant amount of conversation, the general populace and, frequently, significant others are unaware of the deleterious effects of hearing loss, especially on oral communication. SPEECH (see Chapter 10) is a related program designed to help normal-hearing people communicate effectively with individuals who have a hearing loss.

Speechreading instruction can occur in ways other than the traditional face-to-face approach. For example, individuals can use a variety of self-instructional programs to improve speechreading skills that are available in CD/DVD formats, such as *Conversation Made Easy*, developed by Tye-Murray et al. (2002), and CasperSent, created by Boothroyd (2008). Additional self-help materials include a comprehensive, six-part set of DVDs called *Read My Lips*, developed by Russell (1987); *Seeing and Hearing Speech*, available through Sensimetrics (2002); *I See What You Say* (Kleeman, 1996); and Read My Quips (www.sensesynergy.com). Most of these materials provide instruction and practice with analytic and synthetic speechreading tasks and include practice for speech perception in vision-only, auditory-only, and combined modes as well.

Case 5.1

The importance of using a *preparatory set* with the hard of hearing during oral communication needs to be emphasized because it is frequently underutilized. Tye-Murray (2015) refers to this as providing *topical cues* for the listener. In fact, normal-hearing listeners use this strategy with regularity during conversation. They will say, "Not to change the topic, but..." and proceed to change the topic. However, they have provided the listener with a "preparation" for the new topic, and generally the listener will be able to follow the ensuing conversation. As an example, in a recent audiologic rehabilitation adult support group, a retired professor expressed that he was having great difficulty in most communication situations. He stated that he was not able to gain much information either from audition, via his digital hearing aids, or from his vision. However, when the audiologist said, "Let's talk about what you did yesterday," the patient had little difficulty conversing. When the audiologist injected, "Now let's talk about your favorite hobby—golf," the patient became even more accurate in his exchange of information. His ability to receive and express appropriately and accurately continued when the audiologist alerted him that they were now going to discuss current events. What became evident during this therapy session was that this hard of hearing person was able to use his audition and vision far more effectively to decode conversational speech if he knew the topic(s) to be discussed and the general context. These make overall perception of the message more likely.

Tye-Murray (2009) lists several reasons to use computerized speechreading instruction to supplement the traditional forms of audiologic rehabilitation:

1. A variety of stimuli can be viewed by the patient in a short period of time.
2. The patient's responses are recorded within and between training sessions.
3. The patient may view a number of different talkers during a single session.
4. If the program is interactive, the patient's response determines the ensuing stimulus.
5. The patient determines the pace of the instruction.
6. The instruction occurs at the patient's convenience.

However, it also is clear that the traditional face-to-face format, involving both patient and clinician, will continue to be an important and viable format for audiologic rehabilitation as well.

MANUAL COMMUNICATION

Vision can be used by individuals with hearing loss for communication in another manner besides speechreading. Physical gestures and facial expressions have always been used by humans to express emotions and to share information. The transmission of thoughts in this manner undoubtedly preceded the verbal form of communication. As stated earlier in this chapter, manual communication is comprised of specific gestural codes. That is, a visual message is transmitted by the fingers, hands, arms, and bodily postures using specific signs or fingerspelling. In general, manual communication is used by a high percentage of the Deaf to communicate with other individuals also having manual communication skills. The various forms of manual communication are used in isolation or in combination with speech.

Types of Manual Communication

Numerous forms of manual communications have evolved. The major types, along with spoken English, are briefly described and compared in Table 5.6 (Smith, personal communication, 1984). Smith pointed out that the only two pure languages represented in this group are English and American Sign Language.

Cheremes are the most basic and visually distinct units of sign language.

American Sign Language. American Sign Language, also referred to as ASL or Ameslan, was the first form of manual communication established, independent of existing oral languages, by the Deaf. Consequently, the original sign language was indeed a unique "natural" language. Approximately 500,000 to 2,000,000 persons with either hearing loss or normal hearing use this language today (Lane, Hoffmeister, & Bahan, 1996). This widespread usage is due, in part, to an increasing number of basic introductory courses in sign language now offered at many universities and in communities. However, the emergence of cochlear implants as a common component of spoken language intervention with many Deaf infants may result in a reduction in this number in the future. Interestingly, some individuals learn ASL mainly via their deaf peers and professionals rather than from their parents. The signs associated with ASL possess four identifying physical characteristics: hand configuration, movement, location, and orientation. In fact, Stokoe (1978) claims that there are 19 basic symbols for hand shapes, 12 basic symbols for locations, and 24 basic symbols for movement. Although these parameters, referred to as *cheremes* by Stokoe, Casterline, and Croneberg (1965), are different from spoken lexical items, they may be viewed as analogous to the distinctive features of speech. These features are illustrated in Figure 5.4. The prosodic features of ASL are provided by facial expressions, head tilts, body movement, and eye gazes (Vernon & Andrews, 1990).

Because ASL is a language, it consists of words. However, there is not a corresponding sign to represent each English word, just as there is no unique relationship between the words used in English, French, Portuguese, Chinese, or Japanese. All languages were developed using a common code for the exchange of information. Also, the structure of each language is as unique as is its vocabulary (code). Thus, "Ni qui guo zhong-guo mei-you?" probably looks and sounds peculiar and unintelligible to those of us native to the United States, but the sentence is logical and meaningful to someone in Taiwan. Similarly, ASL is not a form of English but rather a distinct language produced manually that requires just as unique a translation of English as does any foreign language.

Iconic signs closely represent the respective actions or things. They are easily presented and understood, sometimes even by those not fluent in signing.

Some of the over 6,000 signs that are part of ASL can be decoded intuitively. These signs are classified as iconic, meaning that they are imageries of the concepts they represent. The signs in Figure 5.5 will be familiar to most readers, even those who have never been exposed to manual communication, specifically ASL.

TABLE 5.6 Forms of Manual and Spoken Communication

American Sign Language (ASL)	Pidgin Signed English (PSE)	Signed English	Linguistics of Visual English (LOVE)	Signing Exact English (SEE II)	Seeing Essential English (SEE I)	Finger-Spelling	Cued Speech	English
Independent language; visual manual mode; own grammar; own syntax; signs are meaning based; has dialects, regionalisms, slang, puns; wide range of vocabulary covering minute differences in meaning; may borrow from other languages	A combination of elements from ASL and the sign systems, ranging from the more ASL-like (occasionally called Ameslish) to the more English-like (sometimes called CASE—Conceptually Accurate Signed English); usually contains few if any sign markers (see "Signed English") yet makes frequent use of fingerspelled English words; used in conjunction with speech or mouthing words in interpreting and college teaching; signs are meaning based	Signed in accordance with English grammar, but signs are meaning based; specially invented sign markers for important affixes in English; invented by Bornstein; used widely in education	Essentially the same as SEE II, but has a method of writing each sign; used in education; invented by Wampler; usage is diminishing	Signs are word based; special signs for all affixes in English; signed in strict accordance with English; invented by Zawolkow, Pfetzing, and Gustason; widely used in education; very influential	Signs are based on word roots (morphemes) (trans/port/a/tion); an extreme form of word-based signs; invented by Anthony; not popular in United States but still common in Iowa and Colorado schools for the deaf; signs for all affixes	Manual representation of the written language; one hand shape for each letter of alphabet; used to borrow English words in ASL; when used with speech and speechreading, it is called the Rochester Method	Employs eight hand shapes in four positions on the face; used in conjunction with lip movements to enable a deaf person to lipread more easily; based on sound with the syllable as the basic unit; devised by Orin Cornett at Gallaudet College	Independent language; aural–oral mode; own grammar; own syntax; words are meaning based; contains dialects, regionalisms, slang, puns; can be written; wide range of vocabulary covering minute differences in meaning; may borrow from other languages; is verbal but also makes use of nonverbal elements

Artificial pedagogical systems, invented for educational purposes

Nonverbal communication: natural gestures, facial expression, body movements, body language, pantomime

Source: Based on W. H. Smith, personal communication, 1984.

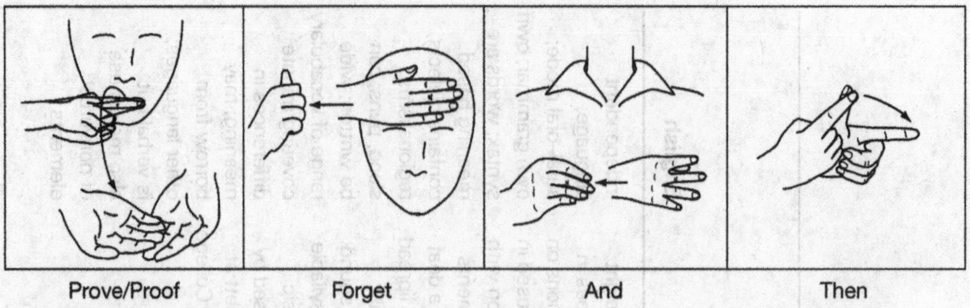

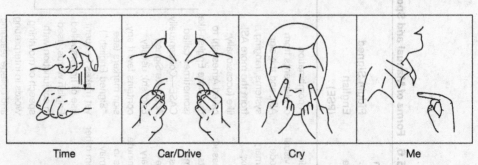

Prove/Proof   Forget   And   Then

FIGURE 5.4 **Four signs used in ASL representing the features of hand shape (DEZ), movement/signation (SIG), tabulation where sign is produced (TAB), and palmar direction of the hands.**
Source: Based on Riekehof (1978).

Signed English Systems. There is evidence that only Deaf adults are truly proficient at using ASL. When many hearing individuals attempt to communicate manually using ASL, they often attempt to use the signs of ASL in a manner that more closely resembles English grammatically. This counterpart to ASL is commonly referred to as Pidgin Sign Language. In other words, Pidgin Sign Language involves combining ASL with English to some extent. If the signer makes English-related modifications, then the result is Pidgin Signed English.

Other attempts have been made to seriously alter ASL so that it closely resembles English, and these are referred to as manually coded English or sign systems. Since sign systems more closely resemble English than ASL, they are often used in an educational setting to minimize the differences that exist between spoken and written English and ASL.

Signed English is a system in which the English words that appear in a message are signed in that same order. To indicate tense, person, plurality, and possession, a sign marker is used as a suffix to the signed word. Seeing Essential English (SEE I) was developed by David Anthony, a deaf individual, as a means of presenting English visually to the deaf as it is presented auditorily to normal-hearing children. Anthony suggested that the word order of the message parallel the word order used in English. Signing Exact English (SEE II) is an outgrowth of SEE I. The purpose of this system is to maintain the syntactic structure of SEE I without making the system unintelligible for those using ASL. Linguistics of Visual English (LOVE) was established at approximately the same time that SEE II was initiated. Again, this was an attempt to refine another sign system aimed at approximating English. The vocabulary is more limited than that of SEE I and SEE II. It attempts to mirror spoken English by making signed movements that correspond to the number of syllables uttered in a spoken word. Yet LOVE is primarily a manual system identical to SEE II. The reader is urged to read the

Time   Car/Drive   Cry   Me

FIGURE 5.5 **Four iconic signs. The signs are visual images of the English words they represent.**
Source: Based on Riekehof (1978).

works of Scheetz (2001) and Vernon and Andrews (1990) for a historical and more detailed discussion of these systems.

Fingerspelling.   Another method of communicating manually is to have senders spell the words with their fingers. That is, instead of using pencil and paper, speakers spell their message in the air by using various hand shapes to represent the letters in the English alphabet. This mode of communication, fingerspelling, represents the 26 letters of the English alphabet by 22 hand shapes and two hand movements (see Figure 5.6). Collectively, these are also referred to as the manual alphabet. The letters *i* and *j* are produced by the same hand shape, with the *j* being produced by moving the hand in a hook or *j*-like motion. The letter *z* is made by moving a unique hand shape

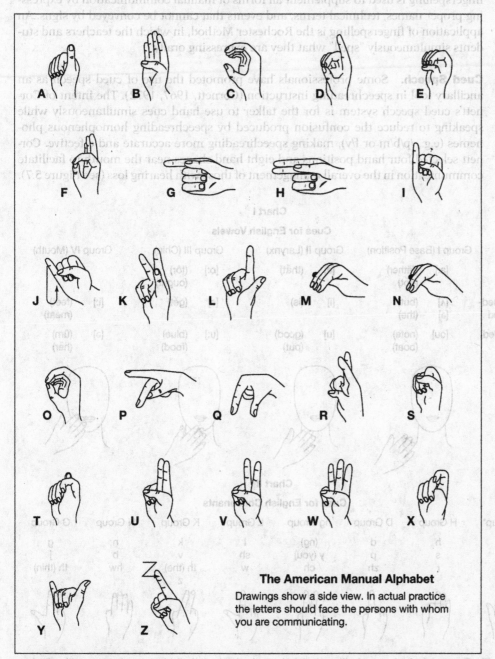

The American Manual Alphabet

Drawings show a side view. In actual practice the letters should face the persons with whom you are communicating.

FIGURE 5.6   **American manual alphabet. The hand positions are shown as they appear to the person reading them.**

Source: Courtesy of Gallaudet University Press, Washington, DC.

in the form of a *z*. Although fingerspelling is an exact and effective means of communication, it is the least efficient form of manual communication; each letter of each word must be produced, making it a relatively laborious means of communicating. Because no additional characters are included in the alphabet or digits in the numeric system, a person can learn to transmit a message via fingerspelling in a relatively short time. However, because of the rapidity with which one learns to "spell" a message and because of the similarity in the production of *e, o, m,* and *n* and between the letters *a* and *s*, the reception of fingerspelling requires considerable practice and concentration. As mentioned in the discussion of speechreading, the similarity among letters and sounds becomes more confounding during discourse than in isolation. But, as in every other form of communication, predictability mitigates this problem. Today, fingerspelling is used to supplement all forms of manual communication by expressing proper names, technical terms, and events that cannot be conveyed by signs. An application of fingerspelling is the Rochester Method, in which the teachers and students simultaneously "spell" what they are expressing orally.

Cued speech also has applications for speech therapy.

Cued Speech. Some professionals have promoted the use of cued speech as an ancillary tool in speechreading instruction (Cornett, 1967, 1972). The intent of Cornett's cued speech system is for the talker to use hand cues simultaneously while speaking to reduce the confusion produced by speechreading homophenous phonemes (e.g., /p/b/m or f/v), making speechreading more accurate and effective. Cornett selected four hand positions and eight hand shapes near the mouth to facilitate communication in the overall management of those with hearing loss (see Figure 5.7).

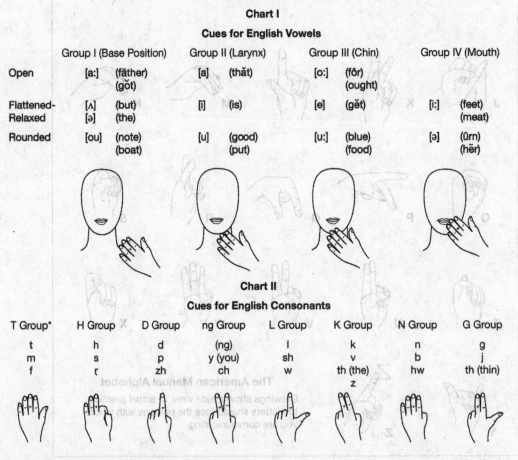

Chart I

Cues for English Vowels

	Group I (Base Position)		Group II (Larynx)		Group III (Chin)		Group IV (Mouth)	
Open	[a:]	(fäther) (gŏt)	[a]	(thăt)	[o:]	(fôr) (ought)		
Flattened-Relaxed	[ʌ] [ə]	(but) (the)	[i]	(is)	[e]	(gĕt)	[i:]	(feet) (meat)
Rounded	[ou]	(note) (boat)	[u]	(good) (put)	[u:]	(blue) (food)	[ə]	(ûrn) (hĕr)

Chart II

Cues for English Consonants

T Group*	H Group	D Group	ng Group	L Group	K Group	N Group	G Group
t	h	d	(ng)	l	k	n	g
m	s	p	y (you)	sh	v	b	j
f	ɾ	zh	ch	w	th (the)	hw	th (thin)
					z		

*Note: The T group cue is also used with an isolated vowel—that is, an individual vowel not run with a final consonant from the preceding syllable.

FIGURE 5.7 Hand positions and hand shapes used in cued speech.
Source: Based on Cornett (1967).

Summary Points

- Speechreading and the use of manual communication are two important aspects of audiologic rehabilitation that involve the use of vision by those with hearing loss.

- Speechreading is a complex process that involves a large number of variables associated with the speechreader and other components of oral communication.

- Speechreading assessment can be done with a variety of formal and informal test protocols, using vision-only or combined vision–hearing conditions.

- Intensive training in speechreading is not frequently done. When carried out, both analytic and synthetic skill development activities are included.

- Shorter forms of audiologic rehabilitation are frequently used that strongly encourage and assist those with hearing loss to maximize the use of the speechreading skills that they already have.

- Manual communication consists of sign language, sign systems, and fingerspelling.

- ASL is the language of the Deaf (see discussion of deaf and the Deaf in Chapter 7).

- Sign systems have been developed that modify ASL to make it more consistent with English. These systems are often used in educational programs.

- Fingerspelling, an adjunct to signing, uses the manual alphabet to spell out words in a message.

Supplementary Learning Activities

See www.isu.edu/csed/audiology/rehab to carry out these activities. We encourage you to use these to supplement your learning. Your instructor may give specific assignments that involve a particular activity.

1. Speechreading Activity: The website listed above includes an activity involving the use of the Utley Speechreading Test. As you will see, you have an opportunity to assess your own speechreading skills in this activity. There is also a great lipreading practice website at www.lipreadingpractice.co.uk.

2. Pick a favorite TV show of yours that involves actors engaged in dialogue. Try following what's taking place for a few minutes under two situations: (a) Turn off the audio signal, making you rely exclusively on your vision to follow what is occurring, and (b) turn down the audio a lot so that the signal is really not very audible and use that limited auditory signal plus speechreading in a combined manner and attempt to follow the show. You may realize that the vision-only mode is very challenging, while the combined mode makes it more possible to stay with the action.

3. Successful speechreading involves having to "fill in" missing information, just as it does with effective listening. The website above provides a learning activity involving visual and auditory closure that demonstrates how this closure skill, or filling in, works and how important it can be in the visual and auditory perception of speech in communication.

Recommended Reading

Alpiner, J., & McCarthy, P. (Eds.). (2000). *Rehabilitative audiology: Children and adults* (3rd ed.). Philadelphia: Lippincott Williams & Wilkins.

Lansing, C. (2013). Visual speech perception in spoken language understanding. In J. Montano & J. Spitzer (Eds.), *Adult audiologic rehabilitation*. San Diego, CA: Plural Publishing, 253–276.

Paul, P. (2001). *Language and deafness* (3rd ed.). San Diego, CA: Singular Publishing Group.

Tye-Murray, N. (Ed.). (1994). *Let's converse! A how-to guide to develop and expand the conversational skills of children and teenagers who are hearing impaired*. Washington, DC: Alexander Graham Bell Association for the Deaf.

Tye-Murray, N. (2015). *Foundations of aural rehabilitation* (4th ed.). Stamford, CT: Cengage Learning.

References

Albright, P., Hipskind, N., & Schuckers, G. (1973). A comparison of visibility and speechreading performance on English and Slurvian. *Journal of Communication Disorders, 6*, 44–52.

Alpiner, J. G. (1978). *Handbook of adult rehabilitative audiology*. Baltimore: Williams & Wilkins.

Alpiner, J. (1982). Evaluation of communication function. In J. Alpiner (Ed.), *Handbook of adult rehabilitative audiology*. Baltimore: Williams & Wilkins.

Berger, K. (1972a). *Speechreading: Principles and methods*. Baltimore: National Educational Press.

Berger, K. (1972b). Visemes and homophenous words. *Teacher of the Deaf, 70*, 396–399.

Bevan, R. C. (1988). *Hearing-impaired children: A guide for parents and concerned professionals*. Springfield, IL: Charles C. Thomas.

Binnie, C. (1973). Bi-sensory articulation functions for normal hearing and sensorineural hearing loss patients. *Journal of the Academy of Rehabilitative Audiology, 6*, 43–53.

Binnie, C. A., Jackson, P., & Montgomery, A. (1976). Visual intelligibility of consonants: A lipreading screening test with implications for aural rehabilitation. *Journal of Speech and Hearing Disorders, 41*, 530–539.

Boothroyd, A. (1988). Linguistic factors in speechreading. In C. L. DeFilippo & D. G. Sims (Eds.), New reflections on speechreading [Monograph]. *Volta Review, 90*(5), 77–87.

Boothroyd, A. (2008). CasperSent: A program for computer-assisted speech perception testing and training at the sentence level. *Journal of the Academy of Rehabilitative Audiology, 41*, 31–50.

Bruhn, M. E. (1929). *The Mueller-Walle method of lip reading for the deaf*. Lynn, MS: Nicholas Press.

Bunger, A. M. (1944). *Speech reading—Jena method*. Danville, IL: The Interstate Co.

Campbell, C., Polomeno, R., Elder, J., Murray, I., & Altosaar, A. (1981). Importance of an eye examination in identifying the cause of congenital hearing impairments. *Journal of Speech and Hearing Disorders, 46*, 258–261.

CHABA, Working Group on Communication Aids for the Hearing-Impaired. (1991). Speech-perception aids for hearing impaired people: Current status and needed research. *Journal of the Acoustical Society of America, 90*, 637–685.

Clouser, R. A. (1976). The effects of vowel consonant ratio and sentence length on lipreading ability. *American Annals of the Deaf, 121*, 513–518.

Cornett, R. (1967). Cued speech. *American Annals of the Deaf, 112*, 3–13.

Cornett, R. O. (1972). *Cued speech parent training and follow-up program*. Washington, DC: Bureau of Education for the Handicapped, Department of Health, Education and Welfare.

Craig, W. (1964). Effects of preschool training on the development of reading and lipreading skills of deaf children. *American Annals of the Deaf, 109*, 280–296.

Daly, N., Bench, J., & Chappell, H. (1996). Gender differences in speechreadability. *Journal of the Academy of Rehabilitative Audiology, 29*, 27–40.

Dancer, J., Krain, M., Thompson, C., Davis, P., & Glenn, J. (1994). A cross-sectional investigation of speechreading in adults: Effects of age, gender, practice and education. *Volta Review, 96*, 31–40.

DeFilippo, C., & Scott, B. (1978). A method for training and evaluating the reception of ongoing speech. *Journal of the Acoustical Society of America, 63*(4), 1186–1192.

Dodd, B., & Campbell, R. (1987). *Hearing by eye: The psychology of lip-reading*. London: Lawrence Erlbaum Associates.

Erber, N. P. (1971). Effects of distance on the visual reception of speech. *Journal of Speech and Hearing Research, 14*, 848–857.

Erber, N. P. (1974). Effects of angle, distance and illumination on visual reception of speech by profoundly deaf children. *Journal of Speech and Hearing Research, 17*, 99–112.

Feehan, P., Samuelson, R., & Seymour, D. (1982). *CLUES: Speechreading for adults*. Austin, TX: PRO-ED.

Fisher, C. G. (1968). Confusions among visually perceived consonants. *Journal of Speech and Hearing Research, 12*, 796–804.

French-St. George, M., & Stoker, R. (1988). Speechreading: An historical perspective. In C. L. DeFilippo & D. G. Sims (Eds.). New reflections on speechreading [Monograph]. *Volta Review, 90*(5), 17–31.

Gaeth, I. H. (1948). *A study of phonemic regression in relation to hearing loss*. Unpublished doctoral dissertation, Northwestern University, Evanston, IL.

Garstecki, D. (1977). Identification of communication competence in the geriatric population. *Journal of the Academy of Rehabilitative Audiology, 10*, 36–45.

Garstecki, D., & O'Neill, J. J. (1980). Situational cues and strategy influence on speechreading. *Scandinavian Audiology, 9*, 1–5.

Gibson, E. J. (1969). *Principles of perceptual learning and development*. New York: Appleton-Century-Crofts.

Giolas, T., Butterfield, E. C., Weaver, S. J. (1974). Some motivational correlates of lipreading. *Journal of Speech and Hearing Research, 17*, 18–24.

Hardick, E. J., Oyer, H. J., & Irion, P. E. (1970). Lipreading performance is related to measurements of vision. *Journal of Speech and Hearing Research, 13*, 92.

Hefler, K. (1998). Auditory and auditory–visual recognition of clear and conversational speech by older adults. *Journal of the American Academy of Audiology, 9*, 234–242.

Hutton, C., Curry, E., & Armstrong, M. (1959). Semi-diagnostic test material for aural rehabilitation. *Journal of Speech and Hearing Disorders, 24*, 319–329.

Jackson, P. L. (1988). The theoretical minimal unit for visual speech perception: Visemes and coarticulation. *Volta Review, 90*, 99–115.

Jackson, P. L., Montgomery, A. A., & Binnie, C. A. (1976). Perceptual dimensions underlying vowel lipreading performance. *Journal of Speech and Hearing Research, 19*, 796–812.

Jeffers, J., & Barley, M. (1971). *Speechreading*. Springfield, IL: Charles C. Thomas.

Johnson, D., Caccamise, F., Rothblum, A., Hamilton, L., & Howard, M. (1981). Identification and follow-up of visual impairments in hearing-impaired populations. *American Annals of the Deaf, 126*, 321–360.

Johnson, D., & Snell, K. B. (1986). Effects of distance visual acuity problems on the speechreading performance of hearing-impaired adults. *Journal of the Academy of Rehabilitative Audiology, 19*, 42–55.

Kinzie, C. E., & Kinzie, R. (1931). *Lipreading for the deafened adult*. Chicago: John C. Winston.

Kirk, K., Eisenberg, L., French, B., Prusich, L., Martinez, A., Ganguly, D., et al. (2011). *Development of the Multimodal Lexical Sentence Test for Children (MLST-C)*. Paper presented at the 13th Supervision on Cochlear Implant in Children, Chicago, IL.

Kleeman, M. (1996). *I see what you say*. San Luis Obispo, CA: Hearing Visions.

Kricos, P., & Lesner, S. (1982). Differences in visual intelligibility across talkers. *Volta Review, 84*, 219–255.

Lane, H., Hoffmeister, R., & Bahan, B. (1996). *A journey into the Deaf-world*. San Diego, CA: Dawn Sign Press.

Lesner, S., Sandridge, S., & Kricos, P. (1987). Training influences on visual consonant and sentence recognition. *Ear and Hearing, 8*, 283–287.

Lewis, D. (1972). Lipreading skills of hearing impaired children in regular schools. *Volta Review, 74*, 303–311.

Lovering, L., (1969). *Lipreading performance as a function of visual acuity*. Unpublished doctoral dissertation, Michigan State University, East Lansing.

Massaro, D. M. (1987). *Speech perception by ear and eye: A paradigm for psychology inquiry*. Hillsdale, NJ: Lawrence Erlbaum Associates.

McCaffrey, H. (1995). Techniques and concepts in auditory training and speechreading. In R. Roeser & M. Downs (Eds.), *Auditory disorders in school children* (3rd ed.). New York: Thieme.

Miller, G. A., & Nicely, P. E. (1955). An analysis of the perceptual confusions among some English consonants. *Journal of the Acoustical Society of America, 27,* 338–352.

Montgomery, A. (1994). WATCH: A practical approach to brief auditory rehabilitation. *Hearing Journal, 10,* 10–55.

Montgomery, A., & Houston, T. (2000). The hearing-impaired adult: Management of communication deficits and tinnitus. In J. Alpiner & P. McCarthy (Eds.), *Rehabilitative audiology: Children and adults* (3rd ed.). Philadelphia: Lippincott Williams & Wilkins, 377–401.

Montgomery, A. A., & Jackson, P. L. (1983). Physical characteristics of the lips underlying vowel lipreading performance. *Journal of the Acoustical Society of America, 73,* 2134–2144.

Montgomery, A. A., Walden, B. E., Schwartz, D. M., & Prosek, R. A. (1984). Training auditory–visual speech reception in adults with moderate sensorineural hearing loss. *Ear and Hearing, 5,* 30–36.

Myklebust, H., & Neyhus, A. (1970). *Diagnostic Test of Speechreading.* New York: Grune & Stratton.

National Technical Institute for the Deaf. (1987). *NTID speechreading videotapes.* Washington, DC: Alexander Graham Bell Association for the Deaf.

New York League for the Hard of Hearing. (1990). *Assessment of adult speechreading ability.* New York: Author.

Nitchie, E. B. (1912). *Lipreading: Principles and practice.* New York: Frederick A. Stokes.

O'Neill, J. J. (1951). An exploratory investigation of lipreading ability among normal-hearing students. *Speech Monographs, 18,* 309–311.

O'Neill, J. J., & Oyer, H. J. (1981). *Visual communication for the hard of hearing* (2nd ed.). Englewood Cliffs, NJ: Prentice Hall.

Pollack, D. (1964). Acoupedics. *Volta Review, 66,* 400.

Pollack, D. (1985). *Educational audiology for the limited hearing infant and preschooler* (2nd ed.). Springfield, IL: Charles C. Thomas.

Riekehof, L. (1978). *The joy of signing.* Springfield, MO: Gospel Publishing House.

Romano, P., & Berlow, W. (1974). Vision requirements for lipreading. *American Annals of the Deaf, 119,* 393–396.

Ross, M. (1982). *Hard of hearing children in regular schools.* Englewood Cliffs, NJ: Prentice Hall.

Russell, R. (1987). *Read my lips.* Oklahoma City, OK: Speechreading Laboratory, Inc.

Samar, V. J., & Sims, D. G. (1983). Visual evoked response correlates of speechreading performance in normal-hearing adults: A replication and factor analytic extension. *Journal of Speech and Hearing Research, 26,* 2–9.

Samar, V. J., & Sims, D. G. (1984). Visual evoked response components related to speechreading and spatial skills in hearing and hearing impaired adults. *Journal of Speech and Hearing Research, 27,* 23–26.

Sanders, D. A. (1993). *Aural rehabilitation* (3rd ed.). Englewood Cliffs, NJ: Prentice Hall.

Scheetz, N. A. (2001). *Orientation to deafness* (2nd ed.). Boston: Lenstok Press.

Schow, R. (2001). A standardized AR battery for hearing aid dispensers. *Hearing Journal, 54*(8), 10–20.

Sensimetrics. (2002). *Seeing and hearing speech.* Somerville, MA: Author.

Shepard, D. C. (1982). Visual–neural correlate of speechreading ability in normal-hearing adults: Reliability. *Journal of Speech and Hearing Research, 25,* 521–527.

Smith, R. (1964). *An investigation of the relationships between lipreading ability and the intelligence of the mentally retarded.* Unpublished master's thesis, Michigan State University, East Lansing.

Stokoe, W. C. (Ed.). (1978). *Sign and culture, a reader for students of American sign language.* Silver Spring, MD: Lenstok Press.

Stokoe, W., Casterline, D., & Croneberg, C. (1965). *A dictionary of American sign language on linguistic principles.* Washington, DC: Gallaudet College Press.

Summerfield, Q. (1992, January 29). Lipreading and audio–visual perception. *Philosophical Transactions of the Royal Society of London,* 71–78.

Tye-Murray, N. (1993a). *Cochlear implants: Audiological foundations.* San Diego, CA: Singular Publishing Group.

Tye-Murray, N. (1993b). *Communication training for hearing-impaired children and teenagers: Speechreading, listening and using repair strategies.* Austin, TX: PRO-ED.

Tye-Murray, N. (2002). *Conversation Made Easy.* Available through the Central Institute for the Deaf, St. Louis, MO.

Tye-Murray, N. (2009). *Foundations of aural rehabilitation* (3rd ed.). Clifton Park, NY: Delmar.

Tye-Murray, N. (2015). Foundations of aural rehabilitation (4th ed.). Stamford, CT: Cengage Learning.

Tye-Murray, N., & Geers, A. (2002). *The Children's Audiovisual Enhancement Test (CAVET).* St. Louis, MO: Central Institute for the Deaf.

Tye-Murray, N., Murray, M., & Spehar, B. (2007). The effects of age and gender on lipreading abilities. *Journal of the American Academy of Audiology, 18,* 882–893.

Tyler, R., Preece, J., & Tye-Murray, N. (1986). *The Iowa phoneme and sentence tests.* Iowa City: University of Iowa Hospitals and Clinics.

Utley, J. (1946). A test of lipreading ability. *Journal of Speech and Hearing Disorders, 11,* 109–116.

Vernon, M., & Andrews, J. F. (1990). *The psychology of deafness: Understanding deaf and hard-of-hearing people.* New York: Longman.

Walden, B., Erdman, S., Montgomery, A., Schwartz, D., & Prosek, R. (1981). Some effects of training on speech perception by hearing-impaired adults. *Journal of Speech and Hearing Research, 24,* 207–216.

Walden, B., Prosek, R., Montgomery, A., Scharr, C., & Jones, C. (1977). Effects of training on the visual recognition of consonants. *Journal of Speech and Hearing Research, 20,* 130–145.

Wayner, D., & Abrahamson, J. (1996). *Learning to hear again.* Austin, TX: Hear Again.

Wedenberg, E. (1951). Auditory training of deaf and hard of hearing children. *Acta Otolaryngology, 39*(Suppl. 94), 1–139.

Woodward, M., & Barber, C. (1960). Phoneme perception in lipreading. *Journal of Speech, Language and Hearing Research, 3,* 212–222.

Yoshinaga-Itano, C. (1988). Speechreading instruction for children. In C. L. DeFilippo & D. G. Sims (Eds.), *New reflections on speechreading* [Monograph]. *Volta Review, 90*(5), 241–254.

APPENDIXES

Appendix 5A: Utley—How Well Can You Read Lips?

This test, commonly referred to as the Utley test, consists of three subtests: Sentences (Forms A and B), Words (Forms A and B), and Stories accompanied by questions that relate to each of the stories. Utley (1946) demonstrated that the Word and Story subtests are positively correlated with the Sentence portion of the test. Therefore, these are the stimuli most often used and associated with the Utley test.

Utley evaluated her viewers' responses by giving 1 point for each word correctly identified in each sentence. A total of 125 words are contained in the 31 sentences on each form (Form A and B). Consequently, a respondent's score may range from 0 to 125 points. Utley suggested that homophenous words not be accepted when scoring the sentence subtest.

Utley administered the sentence subtest to 761 children and adults with hearing loss, and the following descriptive statistics summarize her findings:

	Form A	Form B
Range	0–84	0–89
Mean	33.63	33.80
SD	16.36	17.53

Practice Sentences

1. Good morning.
2. Thank you.
3. Hello.
4. How are you?
5. Goodbye.

Utley Sentence Test—Form A

1. All right.
2. Where have you been?
3. I have forgotten.
4. I have nothing.
5. That is right.
6. Look out.
7. How have you been?
8. I don't know if I can.
9. How tall are you?
10. It is awfully cold.
11. My folks are home.
12. How much was it?
13. Good night.
14. Where are you going?
15. Excuse me.
16. Did you have a good time?
17. What did you want?
18. How much do you weigh?
19. I cannot stand him.
20. She was home last week.
21. Keep your eye on the ball.
22. I cannot remember.
23. Of course.
24. I flew to Washington.
25. You look well.
26. The train runs every hour.
27. You had better go slow.
28. It says that in the book.
29. We got home at six o'clock.
30. We drove to the country.
31. How much rain fell?

Source: Based on Utley (1946).

Appendix 5B: The Denver Quick Test of Lipreading Ability

The Denver Quick Test is designed to measure adult ability to speechread 20 common everyday sentences. Sentences are presented "live" or taped by the tester and are scored on the basis of meaning recognition. No normative data are available to which individual scores may be compared; however, when the Quick Test was given without acoustic cues to 40 hearing-impaired adults, their scores were highly correlated (0.90) with their results on the Utley Sentence Test (Alpiner, 1982).

The Denver Quick Test of Lipreading Ability

1. Good morning.
2. How old are you?
3. I live in (state of residence).
4. I only have one dollar.
5. There is somebody at the door.
6. Is that all?
7. Where are you going?
8. Let's have a coffee break.
9. Park your car in the lot.
10. What is your address?
11. May I help you?
12. I feel fine.
13. It is time for dinner.
14. Turn right at the corner.
15. Are you ready to order?
16. Is this charge or cash?
17. What time is it?
18. I have a headache.
19. How about going out tonight?
20. Please lend me 50 cents

Source: Based on Alpiner (1982).

Appendix 5C: Craig Lipreading Inventory

The Craig Lipreading Inventory consists of two forms of 33 isolated words and 24 sentences. The vocabulary for these stimuli was selected from words used by children enrolled in kindergarten and first grade. A filmed version of the test is available. The test is usually presented "live" but may be videotaped by a clinician.

The viewer should be positioned eight feet from the speaker. Each of the isolated words is preceded by a contextually meaningless carrier phrase, "show me."

The respondent is provided with answer sheets that contain four choices for each stimulus. A single point is awarded for each of the words and sentences identified correctly. Consequently, maximum scores are 33 and 24 for the word test and sentence test, respectively.

Individual performances may be compared to the following mean scores obtained by Craig with deaf children:

	Preschool	**Nonpreschool**
Words	62.5–68%	68–69%
Sentences	52.5–62%	61.5–63%

Craig Lipreading Inventory

Word Recognition—Form A

1. white
2. corn
3. zoo
4. thumb
5. chair
6. jello
7. doll
8. pig
9. toy
10. finger
11. six
12. woman
13. fly
14. frog
15. grapes
16. goose
17. sled
18. star
19. sing
20. three
21. duck
22. spoon
23. ear
24. ice
25. goat
26. dog
27. cat
28. nut
29. milk
30. cake
31. eight
32. pencil
33. desk

Sentence Recognition—Form A

1. A coat is on a chair.
2. A sock and shoe are on the floor.
3. A boy is flying a kite.
4. A girl is jumping.
5. A boy stuck his thumb in the pie.
6. A cow and a pig are near the gate.
7. A man is throwing a ball to the dog.
8. A bird has white wings.
9. A light is over the door.
10. A horse is standing by a new car.
11. A boy is putting a nail in the sled.
12. A big fan is on a desk.
13. An owl is looking at the moon.
14. Three stars are in the sky.
15. A whistle and a spoon are on the table.
16. A frog is hopping away from a boat.
17. Bread, meat, and grapes are in the dish.
18. The woman has long hair and a short dress.
19. The boys are swinging behind the school.
20. A cat is playing with a nut.
21. A man has his foot on a truck.
22. A woman is carrying a chair.
23. A woman is eating an apple.
24. A girl is cutting a feather.

Craig Lipreading Inventory

Word Recognition

Name: _____

Age: _____   **Date:** _____   **School:** _____

Ex.	fish	table	baby	ball
1.	kite	fire	white	light
2.	corn	fork	horse	purse
3.	two	zoo	spoon	shoe
4.	cup	jump	thumb	drum
5.	hair	bear	pear	chair

Word Recognition			Page 2
6.	yoyo	hello	jello	window
7.	doll	ten	nail	suit
8.	pig	pie	book	pear
9.	two	toe	tie	toy
10.	flower	finger	fire	feather
11.	six	sing	sit	kiss

Word Recognition   Page 3

12.	table	apple	woman	rabbit
13.	fire	tie	fly	five
14.	four	frog	fork	flag
15.	grapes	airplane	tables	cups
16.	goose	tooth	shoe	school
17.	desk	sled	leg	nest

Word Recognition   Page 4

18.	dog	sock	star	car
19.	wing	sing	ring	swing
20.	three	teeth	key	knee
21.	duck	rug	truck	gun
22.	moon	school	spoon	boot
23.	ear	hair	eye	egg

Word Recognition			Page 5
24.	horse	house	ice	orange
25.	goat	gate	kite	girl
26.	dish	duck	desk	dog
27.	cat	cake	gun	coat
28.	nail	nut	nest	ten
29.	man	bat	milk	bird

Word Recognition Page 6

30.	egg	cake	key	car
31.	eight	egg	cake	gate
32.	pencil	picture	mitten	pitcher
33.	wet	dress	nest	desk

Language and Speech of the Deaf and Hard of Hearing

Kristina M. Blaiser, Gabriel A. Bargen

CONTENTS

Visit the companion website when you see this icon to learn more about the topic nearby in the text.

Learning Outcomes

After reading this chapter, you will be able to

- List the communication modes commonly used with children who are Deaf/Hard of Hearing (DHH)
- Identify how hearing loss can impact speech development
- Describe a Speechmap and identify the amplification goal when using a Speechmap with children who are DHH
- Describe the benefit of full-time use of a hearing assistive device with children who are DHH
- Identify assessments that can be used with children with hearing loss
- List three language characteristics of children who are DHH
- List three speech characteristics of children who are DHH

INTRODUCTION

One of the primary differences between the development of children with hearing loss and children with normal hearing is the ability to access the language around them. Historically, this reduced access has had a tremendous impact on the communication development of young children with hearing loss and their families. Today, increases in newborn hearing screening and advances in hearing technology have significantly changed the speech and language outcomes of children with hearing loss. One of the most important changes to the field of aural rehabilitation is the increased use of cochlear implants with young children. As of 2012, in the United States, over 38,000 children have received cochlear implants (National Institute on Deafness and Other Communication Disorders, 2014). Because of increased auditory access at younger ages, the speech and language outcomes of today's children are not limited by the degree of hearing loss, and even children with severe to profound hearing loss can develop age-appropriate speech and language skills. Today's intervention services often focus on helping children to develop speech and language skills close to the time that they were biologically intended (Cole & Flexer, 2016).

An important consideration for families of children with hearing loss is the language or communication modality that will match the family's goals for their child. When a hearing loss is diagnosed, families are introduced to the communication options available for children with hearing loss. It is the duty of audiologists, speech-language pathologists, and other early intervention professionals to follow recommendations for best evidence-based practices that support a family's right to a thorough, unbiased explanation of the communication options.

Language is a broad term to describe a system of symbols used as a social tool for the exchange of information.

COMMUNICATION OPTIONS FOR FAMILIES OF CHILDREN WHO ARE DEAF/HARD OF HEARING

It is important for families to be provided with nonbiased information related to their communication options. The website BEGINNINGS for Parents of Children Who Are Deaf/Hard of Hearing (www.ncbegin.org/communication-options) offers a summary of communication options and brief videos illustrating each of the approaches described below. Some communication options focus on developing spoken language as the child's first language by maximizing audition through hearing technology. Today, "auditory-verbal" and "auditory-oral" techniques are often combined under the label of "listening and spoken language." In contrast to auditory-based communication modalities, American Sign Language/English as a Second Language focuses on developing American Sign Language, a visual language with its own rules and syntax, as the child's first language. There are also communication approaches that utilize a combination of visual information (such as signs and hand shapes) and auditory information.

Systems Emphasizing Listening and Spoken Language

One form of listening and spoken language (LSL) is the *Auditory–oral approach*, which emphasizes the need for using residual hearing and consistent practice for developing spoken language. Full-time consistent use of amplification (hearing aids, FM systems) and/or cochlear implants is an essential feature, and parents are primarily responsible for establishing full-time use. Children enrolled in auditory–oral programs are typically educated in settings with peers with hearing loss. In these settings, children typically receive therapy targeting speech, language, and auditory development, and parents are given related home activities to support these goals. While speechreading is no longer explicitly taught in most auditory–oral programs, the use of these cues is not discouraged.

Family-centered intervention involves shared responsibility with the parents and caregivers for the child's intervention, with the family retaining the ultimate decision making regarding intervention goals and services. A major goal of family-centered intervention is to strengthen family functioning and communication, thus empowering the family to capitalize on its unique strengths when addressing the needs of the child who is Deaf/Hard of Hearing.

The *Auditory–verbal approach*, another form of LSL, also advocates the use of residual hearing for developing spoken language and is highly reliant on the use of amplification and/or cochlear implants. In this approach, auditory skills instead of visual cues are emphasized. Auditory–verbal therapy focuses on teaching parents how to integrate LSL activities into daily life. Parents and caregivers are responsible for establishing full-time use of devices and are expected to integrate listening and language activities into their everyday life (such as getting dressed, washing dishes) and family routines.

Manual–Visual Systems

The American Sign Language/English as a Second Language approach focuses on establishing *American Sign Language* (ASL), a distinct and natural language different from spoken English, as the child's first language. Use of amplification and/or cochlear implants is not critical to this approach; however, it remains an option. An essential element to successful acquisition of ASL is access to adults and community members fluent in ASL to provide fluent language models. If the parents are not fluent in ASL, then they need extensive training and opportunities to practice the language. English is developed later as a second language with an emphasis on reading and writing (i.e., rather than spoken language). In recent years, some educators have embraced a Bilingual–Bicultural (or Bi–Bi) approach for education of Deaf children. In this model, English is taught as a second language in written form, and the culture of Deaf individuals is emphasized in the curriculum.

> ASL is a form of manual communication used by culturally Deaf individuals in the United States and has a unique grammar that is not based on English.

Bilingual–Bicultural

Parents of children with hearing loss have a wide variety of communication options for their children. While some families choose to use a communication option focusing on LSL, others use ASL or a bilingual–bicultural (bi–bi) approach. This method is based on the premise that children will learn ASL as the first and primary language with English taught as a second language in written form. It is important to recognize that many communication approaches vary from family to family. While some families who choose a bi–bi approach use no spoken language, others choose to include supplementing a bi–bi approach with some component of speech training.

Case 6.1. BR

BR had meningitis at age 7 months, and a severe to profound hearing loss was subsequently identified. BR was immediately fitted with hearing aids, and home intervention based on Auditory–Verbal (AV) principles was initiated. At the age of 14 months, BR received a cochlear implant. At the age of 3, BR began receiving AV services through the public schools. BR is now 7 years of age, and he has been placed in a regular classroom in the public schools for kindergarten and first grade. While in school, he has received AV services from a teacher for the Deaf/Hard of Hearing and from a speech-language pathologist at an outpatient clinic. He has also had a classroom language facilitator, but there are plans to phase out this support provider in the upcoming school year. BR's mother is highly involved in his AV therapy and in fostering his educational success. She has integrated language stimulation and communication strategies into his everyday life. Her influence is judged to be an enormous factor in his overall success as an oral communicator. While he is delayed in receptive and expressive language, his speech is 100 percent intelligible. Current therapy goals include use of possessive and plural /s/ marker, use of *the* and *a*, and understanding telephone conversation from a disclosed topic.

Systems Combining Visual and Auditory Information

The *Total Communication* (TC) approach advocates the use of manually coded English, fingerspelling, speechreading, natural gestures, residual hearing, and speech. Use of amplification and/or cochlear implants is usually encouraged. In this modality, a combination of signs and oral communication are used. TC can range in terms of how it is presented from a model that is primarily sign based with the addition of spoken language to a model that is primarily spoken with an occasional sign used for clarification. The term *pidgin sign language* refers to signs or vocabulary from ASL used in English word order.

> *Cued speech* involves the use of hand positions and shapes to resolve some of the ambiguities associated with trying to speechread words that look alike on the lips. Unlike fingerspelling, which is based on letters, the hand supplements associated with Cued Speech are based on phonemes or sounds of a language.

The *Cued Speech* approach requires family members and therapists to learn and use cueing, a set of hand shapes and movements used to visually differentiate phonemes that look alike on the lips. Typically, this approach would also include the use of residual hearing and a goal of developing spoken language. Individuals communicating with the child would be expected to cue while speaking or use a transliterator.

> A transliterator uses cued speech to convey the information that is presented auditorily in English or another spoken language.

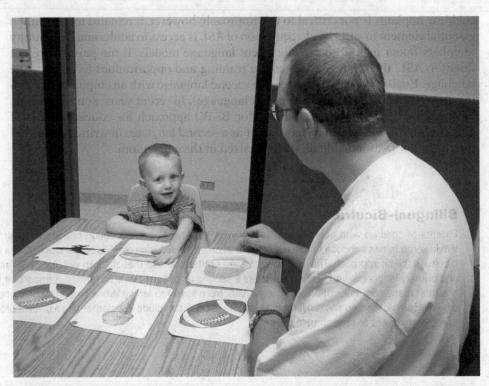

A young child works on communication skills in a therapy setting.

All communication options require extensive family involvement to be successfully generalized for the child's communication. It is important to remember that any of the communication options above can lead to successful language development. However, most options require therapeutic intervention, consistent use of appropriately fit hearing technology, and a commitment from the family.

Because over 90 percent of babies born with hearing loss have two hearing parents (Mitchell & Karchmer, 2004), many families are likely to choose an option focusing on spoken language development. In addition, because of newborn hearing screening and advanced hearing technology, there is a trend for more families choosing spoken language options now than ever before. In a North Carolina study, Brown (2006), from BEGINNINGS for Parents of Children Who are Deaf or Hard of Hearing, reported that in 1995, 40 percent of families chose spoken language options, whereas in 2005, 85 percent of families chose LSL options (i.e., auditory–verbal and/or auditory–oral approaches). The focus of this chapter is on characteristics and assessment of language and speech by children using spoken language. Sign language approaches are discussed in more detail in Chapter 5.

It is important to note that there are different terms based on hearing status and communication modality. *Deaf* (with a capital "D") signifies a person with a severe/profound loss who identifies with the Deaf culture and ASL, while *deaf* (with a lowercase "d") is representative of a severe/profound level of hearing loss without the cultural identity while making full use of residual hearing. The term *hard of hearing* is generally used when a person has a slight to mild to moderate hearing loss.

HEARING AS THE FOUNDATION FOR SPEECH AND LANGUAGE

Hearing allows for the development of speech perception. By 6 months of age, children with normal hearing have learned to discriminate the sounds of their native language. The critical importance of early hearing is also indicated by data that show the benefits of identifying and managing congenital hearing loss within the first 6 months. Children with hearing loss who have received appropriate management by

6 months of age often develop age-appropriate speech by age 5 (Downs & Yoshinaga-Itano, 1999).

In their often-cited study, Yoshinaga-Itano, Sedey, Coulter, and Mehl (1998) found the following:

- The first year of life, especially the first 6 months, is critical for children with hearing loss.
- Young children (1 to 3 years old at the time of this study) whose losses were identified by 6 months of age demonstrated significantly better receptive and expressive language skills than did children whose hearing losses were identified after the age of 6 months.

Technology use is a key issue when families choose a communication option that focuses on spoken language development. Infants and children with hearing loss may be fitted with hearing aids, FM systems, bone-anchored hearing aids, and cochlear implants. (Refer to Chapters 2 and 3 for further information on these devices). With hearing aid and FM systems, many pediatric audiologists now use real-ear probe tube verification measures to demonstrate that speech sounds are within the child's residual hearing range. It is essential that audiologists effectively communicate with parents, early interventionists, and speech-language pathologists about the proportion of speech (or the *speech banana*) and speech sounds that are audible with amplification/FM system use.

Speech banana: When the sounds of speech are graphed on an audiogram, they form a shape similar to a banana.

When deemed an appropriate intervention option, infants with hearing loss can and should be fitted with hearing aids within weeks of hearing loss diagnosis. Pediatric audiologists are key to successful hearing aid fittings for infants. Audiologists know about concerns and issues unique to pediatric fittings, such as the need for using estimated hearing level (eHL) thresholds based on auditory brainstem response findings, real ear to coupler difference (RECD) thresholds, and probe-tube real-ear verification measures, digital signal processing features, child-size earhooks, hearing aid retention devices, hearing aid insurance, childproof battery doors, frequent replacement of earmolds, ongoing hearing evaluation to further define hearing sensitivity, and the extensive parent support needed to establish full-time use of hearing aids. Newer signal processing strategies in digital hearing aids are of great benefit in the pediatric population, including feedback cancellation to allow for greater gain without feedback and frequency compression to bring high-frequency sounds that cannot be amplified into the audible range. In addition to ensuring optimal hearing aid amplification, the pediatric audiologist can also determine whether the fitting of an FM system may offer additional benefits.

The display that many audiologists now examine to verify pediatric amplification goals is the *Speechmap*, which is a graph of the child's hearing loss for one designated ear in decibels sound pressure level (dB SPL) near the eardrum (i.e., a value that is generally calculated based on threshold estimates from auditory brainstem evoked response measures or behavioral audiometric thresholds). Figure 6.1 displays a Speechmap; on this display, the decibel levels are plotted with the lowest intensities near the bottom of the graph in contrast to the standard audiogram. The curve connecting the circles displays hearing thresholds for the child's right ear in dB SPL near the eardrum. The darkened curve above the dark circle curve passes through short vertical lines that represent prescription targets. This shows that target gain is being achieved for a low-intensity speech passage on thresholds from 250 through 3000 Hz only. Since this fitting will not provide audibility above 3000 Hz, other strategies may be used to address this. On some test systems, this display can be plotted in decibels Hearing Level (dB HL), the decibel that is displayed on the audiogram, and that display might be more easily interpreted by those familiar with the audiogram.

Many parents have difficulty establishing full-time use of hearing aids or other hearing assistance devices. Full-time use is reached when children wear their amplification device during all waking hours of the day. Full-time use of hearing

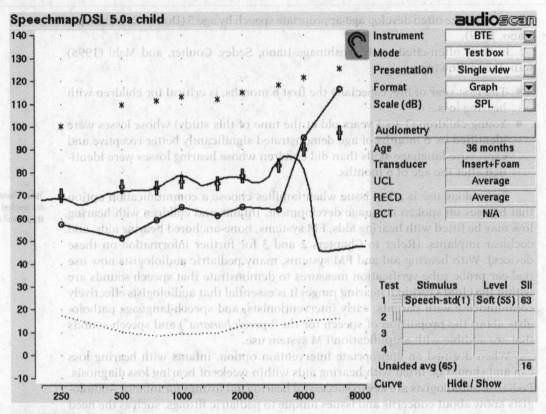

FIGURE 6.1 Speechmap.
Unaided hearing thresholds (curve through Os), real-ear aided response for 55 dB SPL speech (curve through short vertical lines).
Source: Used by permission of Etymotic Design Inc./Audioscan.

aids and/or cochlear implants is needed for brain development that allows for maximizing speech and language development. Professionals (i.e., audiologists, speech-language pathologists, and early intervention providers) need to work together to help parents understand the benefits of full-time use and develop strategies for their child's hearing aids and/or cochlear implants. Parents and professionals should communicate if there are barriers to full-time use of hearing technology. Audiologists can assist in ensuring that the device is programmed correctly or make the device more comfortable (e.g., modify or make a new earmold); early interventionists can provide parents with strategies for use in the home (e.g., child-friendly caps for the child who is pulling out hearing aids).

Ideally, most babies will be fitted with hearing aids by 3 months of age, and, in cases where limited hearing aid benefit is observed, consideration will be given for cochlear implantation. While U.S. Food and Drug Administration guidelines suggest that cochlear implant(s) are surgically placed around 12 months of age because of the benefits of early auditory stimulation, some children receive cochlear implants prior to 12 months of age (Nicholas & Geers, 2013; Waltzman & Roland, 2005). Once again, full-time use of the cochlear implant(s) is essential for maximizing speech and language development.

Children who are fitted with bone-anchored hearing aids or cochlear implants are using devices that do not produce amplified sound levels in the ear canal as hearing aids do. Thus, the aided verification results would be plotted on a standard audiogram or a familiar sounds audiogram, as illustrated in Figure 6.2. Regardless of the device (i.e., hearing aid, FM system, bone-anchored hearing aid, or cochlear implant), it is critical that speech audibility is verified and that the child consistently uses the device during waking hours.

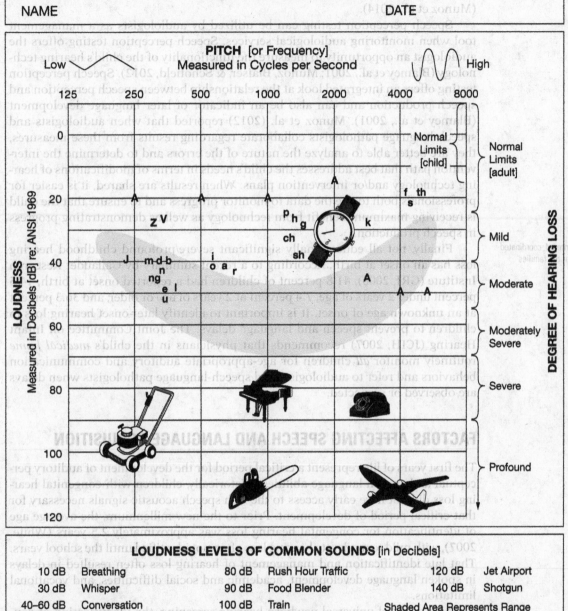

FIGURE 6.2   Aided thresholds (A) plotted on a familiar sounds audiogram.
Source: Used with permission of Etymotic Design Inc./Audioscan.

Several tools and resources are available to assist parents in establishing full-time use of amplification for their child who is deaf or hard of hearing. One tool available on most hearing aid technology is data logging which tracks the amount of use. Use of a data-logging tool can support behavior-change strategies that are necessary to support integration of recommendations into daily life (Glasgow et al., 1997), including the audiological recommendation of using hearing aids during all waking hours. Using data logging can assist with identification of barriers and opportunities to identify strategies with parents to increase consistency of hearing aid use (Munoz, Preston, & Hicken, 2014). Parents who are provided with objective feedback from data logging and ongoing individualized support from their audiologist, as well as other health care professionals on the management team, may integrate hearing aid management recommendations more consistently (Munoz et al., 2014).

Speech perception testing can be utilized by audiologists as a management tool when monitoring audiological services. Speech perception testing offers the audiologist an opportunity to measure the functionality of the child's hearing technology (Blamey et al., 2001; Munoz, Blaiser, & Schofield, 2012). Speech perception testing offers an integrated look at the relationship between speech perception and speech production and can also be an indicator of later language development (Blamey et al., 2001). Munoz et al. (2012) reported that when audiologists and speech-language pathologists collaborate regarding results from these measures, they are better able to analyze the nature of the errors and to determine the intervention path that best addresses the child's needs in terms of modifications of hearing technology and/or intervention plans. When results are shared, it is easier for professionals both to use the data to monitor progress and to ensure that the child is receiving maximum benefit from technology as well as demonstrating progress in speech production.

Finally, not all educationally significant severe/profound childhood hearing loss has an onset at birth. According to a recent summary by Gallaudet Research Institute (GRI, 2008), 41.8 percent of children had a reported onset at birth, 14.5 percent under 2 years of age, 7.4 percent at 2 years of age or older, and 36.3 percent at an unknown age of onset. It is important to identify later-onset hearing loss in children to prevent speech and language delays. The Joint Committee on Infant Hearing (JCIH, 2007) recommends that physicians in the child's *medical home* routinely monitor *all* children for age-appropriate auditory and communication behaviors and refer to audiologists and speech-language pathologists when delays are observed or suspected.

Medical home is family-centered, coordinated physician care ensuring that the families' needs are met.

FACTORS AFFECTING SPEECH AND LANGUAGE ACQUISITION

The first years of life represent a critical period for the development of auditory perceptual and spoken language abilities. Historically, children with congenital hearing loss did not have early access to the rich speech acoustic signals necessary for that critical period of development. Prior to the new millennium, the average age of identification for congenital hearing loss was approximately 2.5 years (White, 2007), with mild to moderate hearing loss often not identified until the school years. That late identification and management of hearing loss often resulted in delays in spoken language development, academic and social difficulties, and vocational limitations.

As a result of universal newborn hearing screening, the identification of congenital hearing loss now typically occurs within the first year of life. In fact, the average age of identification today is between 2 and 3 months (Harrison, Roush, & Wallace, 2003). Ideally, early intervention and technology options can be offered within weeks of identification. Early identification and intervention are key components to the development of age-appropriate speech and language skills. Ongoing family engagement in decision making and services forms the third key component in establishing a sound foundation for communication development. If a baby is identified early, managed appropriately, and part of an engaged family, then he or she is more likely to show communication abilities comparable to that of his or her normal-hearing peers (Cole & Flexer, 2016).

Early and appropriate intervention is the most effective strategy for developing normal speech and language in children with hearing loss (Downs & Yoshinaga-Itano, 1999).

If the hearing loss is identified by the target age of 3 months (JCIH, 2007), parents will be working with early interventionists and pediatric audiologists to make decisions about communication options and technology. These decisions can be impacted by other factors, such as the languages used in the home as well as cultural factors related to race and ethnicity. In a recent demographic summary (GRI, 2008), the most commonly used languages in homes of children with hearing loss were English in 82.5 percent, Spanish in 21.9 percent, and ASL in 3.8 percent. In that same summary (GRI, 2008), the most commonly reported race/ethnic categories reported were White (48.7%), African American/Black (15.9%), Hispanic/Latino (30.1%), and Asian or Pacific Islander (4.3%).

As of 2016, there were 43 states with statutes or other regulatory language related to universal newborn hearing screening for all babies born in the state, according to the National Center for Hearing Assessment and Management (NCHAM, 2016).

Case 6.2. FM

FM, a male child, and his twin brother were born at 26 weeks' gestation. While his brother was found to have normal hearing, FM was found to have severe to profound hearing loss and cerebral palsy. FM was aided at 5 months of age, and at 22 months of age FM received a cochlear implant. FM is now 28 months of age. He is showing signs of developing auditory awareness and is showing increased vocalizations. Evaluation at this point indicates that he is exhibiting a severe delay in both expressive and receptive language abilities. He receives services based on auditory–verbal therapy principles once a week at home through a state early intervention program and twice a week from a speech-language pathologist.

In addition to consideration of the family's cultural influences, it is important for early intervention providers to understand that the presence of other disabilities in the child may impact a child's communication development and outcomes. Approximately 40 percent of children with hearing loss have other disabilities, including 10.0 percent with learning disability, 9.1 percent with abnormal IQ, 6.6 percent with attention deficit, 4.5 percent with visual problems, 3.2 percent with cerebral palsy, 2.0 percent with emotional disturbance, and 13.3 percent with other conditions (GRI, 2008). The impact of other handicapping conditions is not fully known. However, cognitive disability has been found to have a significant negative impact on language development in children with hearing loss (Yoshinaga-Itano et al., 1998), and learning disability has also been documented to have a negative impact on auditory perception and linguistic competence in children with cochlear

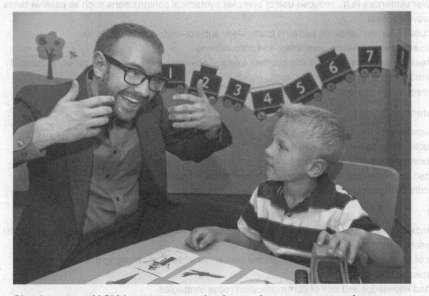

Sign language (ASL) is one communication option parents may choose.

implants (Isaacson, 1996). Findings from Yoshinaga-Itano et al. show language acquisition as a function of both age of identification and cognitive status:

- Children with higher cognitive skills, of course, do better in general.
- What was particularly stunning was the fact that early-identified children with lower cognitive levels achieved essentially the same language levels as late-identified children with higher cognitive skills.
- Children identified early who showed normal cognition showed a mean language quotient about 15 units higher than children with normal cognition skills identified later.
- Likewise, children with lower cognition identified earlier showed mean language quotients better by more than 30 units compared to lower cognition children identified later.

It is important for the early interventionist and pediatric audiologist to be aware of these factors and to present choices for communication options and technology in a manner that allows parents to make choices that reflect their goals and values.

Language Characteristics of Children with Hearing Loss

Delays in language can be a consequence of limited access to sound. A hearing loss can impact development of the *form* (*phonology, syntax, and morphology*), *content* (vocabulary and *semantics*), and *use* (*pragmatics*) of language. Even with advanced hearing technology, such as digital hearing aids and cochlear implants, the child with hearing loss may miss auditory and linguistic cues from the language models in his or her daily environment. The lack of opportunities to hear spoken language in its entirety can compromise the child's ability to develop the semantic, syntactic, morphologic, pragmatic, and phonologic aspects of language, which in turn may also increase the likelihood of subsequent reading and academic difficulties. Some common language characteristics of children with hearing loss are shown in Table 6.1.

Phonology is the study of sound systems used in languages.

Syntax is the aspect of language that governs the rules for how words are arranged in sentences.

Morphology is the study of the minimal units of language that are meaningful, such as *bug*, *-s* for plural nouns or third-person verb tenses, *-ing* for present progressive, and *-ed* for past tense.

Semantics is the study of word meanings and word relations.

Pragmatics refers to the functional use of language.

Important language acquisition information on the impact of hearing loss has arisen from research concluded over the past 60 years.

TABLE 6.1 Some Common Characteristics of Language Usage by Children with Hearing Loss

Form

Shorter sentences (reduced mean length of utterances [MLU])

Simpler sentences (e.g., reduced use of complex syntactical constructions such as passive tense and relative clauses)

Overuse of certain sentence patterns (particularly subject–verb–object patterns)

Infrequent use of adverbs, auxiliaries, and conjunctions

Decreased use of grammatical morphemes (plurals, possessive markers, verb tense, pronouns)

Incorrect word order

Incorrect usage of irregular verb tense

Content

Reduced expressive and receptive vocabulary

Reduced ability to produce category labels

Reduced understanding of object function

Limited understanding of metaphors, idioms, and other figurative language

Difficulty with multiple meanings of words (e.g., *row*, *run*)

Use

Restricted range of communicative intents (e.g., conversational devices, performatives, requests) in preschool children with hearing loss

Lack of knowledge regarding conversational conventions, such as changing the topic or closing conversations

Limited knowledge and use of communication repair strategies

Speech-language pathologists play an important role in a child's ability to develop and use spoken communication. Speech-language pathologists have knowledge related to language and speech development and disorders as well as assessment and intervention of individuals across the life span.

It is important that a speech-language pathologist does not assume that a child who is Deaf/Hard of Hearing will demonstrate all of these deficits. Children who have been identified early, have full-time use of appropriately fit hearing technology, and have above-average cognitive and linguistic processing skills and supportive learning environments can demonstrate little to no language delays with appropriate support and intervention (Gilbertson & Kamhi, 1995). At the other end of the spectrum, additional learning disabilities can exacerbate the language-learning difficulties of a child who is Deaf/Hard of Hearing. It is imperative that each child be evaluated without prior expectations of how children with hearing loss should or will perform in the language arena. Because language delay is prevalent in this population, full-time use of appropriate hearing technology and assistive listening devices (such as hearing aids, cochlear implants, and/or FM systems) and consistent speech-language therapy is often a necessity.

Impact of Hearing Loss on Language Components

Form.   According to Bloom and Lahey (1978), form is considered word order (syntax), word endings (morphology), and phonology. Syntactic and morphological difficulties have been documented in children with hearing loss (Geers, Nicholas & Sedey, 2003; Spencer, 2004). These include decreases in length of utterance, decreased use of articles (*a*, *the*), decreased use of auxiliary verbs (*is*, *are*), absence of morphological markers (*plural markers* and *verb tenses*), and incorrect use of pronouns (*he*, *she*, *his*, *her*). For example, research by Spencer (2004) examined the performance of 13 children with cochlear implants on the Clinical Evaluation of Language Fundamentals—Preschool (CELF-P; Wiig, Secord, & Semel, 1992). Children with cochlear implants demonstrated weaknesses in understanding and production of grammatical morphemes (such as pronouns, possessive markers, and verb tense).

Case 6.3. MW

MW is a child who was diagnosed at 2 years of age with a hearing loss that was believed to possibly have been progressive since birth. He has a moderate sensorineural hearing loss in the right ear and a moderate to severe sensorineural hearing loss in the left ear. Immediately following this diagnosis, amplification and auditory verbal therapy were initiated. From the onset, his parents were highly involved in maintaining effective amplification use and in offering home-based language stimulation. At age 6, MW was discharged from therapy because he had age-appropriate speech, language, and auditory skills. During kindergarten and first grade, he was fully mainstreamed in regular classrooms and received no support services. At the end of first grade, he was performing above grade level in reading and math. His speech is judged to be 90 to 100 percent intelligible. If his hearing loss continues to progress, he may become a candidate for a cochlear implant.

Clinical Applications.   It is important for clinicians to be aware of the specific grammatical and syntactic error patterns that are commonly found in the spoken language of Deaf/Hard of Hearing children. Intervention plans should focus on opportunities to practice these components of language through explicit teaching. It is important that this practice occurs under appropriate social (or pragmatic) conditions. Wilbur, Goodhart, and Fuller (1989) attribute many of the difficulties children with hearing loss have with linguistic structures to the practice of teaching them language through the use of sets of unrelated sentences. One technique parents and clinicians can use is *recasting*. Adults communicating with the child target syntactic–semantic structures for development. If and when the child uses incomplete or inappropriate forms during conversation, the adult recasts the utterance, maintaining the child's meaning but providing the appropriate form. For example, if the child says, "Daddy eated cookie," the parent responds, "Yes, daddy ate the cookie." The parent does not require the child to correct his or her original utterance. This technique has been found to facilitate language development in children with hearing loss. The clinician must also understand that some common errors (e.g., omission of plurals and possessives) could be due to a child's inability to hear high frequencies, and the clinician should collaborate with the child's audiologist to ensure that the child's hearing technology provides optimal benefit.

Content.   Content is considered vocabulary and word meanings (Bloom & Lahey, 1978). Children with hearing loss typically demonstrate delayed vocabulary skills relative to their age-matched normal-hearing peers. Mayne, Yoshinaga-Itano, Sedey, and Carey (2000) have provided normative data for the expressive vocabulary development of children who are deaf or hard of hearing. These investigators found that, on average, children whose cognitive quotients were 80 or greater (i.e., normal) and whose hearing loss had been identified by 6 months of age had a rate of vocabulary growth similar to children with normal hearing. Children whose hearing loss was identified after 6 months and/or whose cognitive status was compromised evidenced significant delays in their language acquisition rates. Hayes, Geers, Trieman, and Moog (2009) found that children with hearing loss using cochlear implants had lower receptive vocabulary scores than their age-matched normal-hearing peers. However, the children with cochlear implants demonstrated significant vocabulary gains over time. Specifically, children who were implanted at younger ages demonstrated more accelerated vocabulary growth than children who were implanted at later ages. Studies examining word learning in children with hearing loss have suggested that children with hearing loss need more exposures and louder presentations than their normal-hearing peers (Stelmachowicz, Pittman, Hoover, & Lewis, 2004).

Word meanings are often learned through daily routines in the child's life (Schirmer, 1994). The child, for example, experiences words through typical sequences of events and communication at dinnertime, bath time, and bedtime. Over time, the child stores and remembers a body of knowledge (called *schema*) about these events and forms (Yoshinaga-Itano & Downey, 1986). Children also learn about words and word meanings through "overhearing" routines and conversations. This is referred to as *incidental learning*. According to Beck and Flexer (2011), children learn approximately 90 percent of their information from incidental learning. For example, a child may hear the parents discussing what to have for dinner and then listing several options. This provides the child with a definition of *dinner* as well as some examples (pizza, chicken). A child with hearing loss may not have full access to these conversations and comments due to distance or reduced audibility. Children with hearing loss often demonstrate limited schema due to limited access to the incidental language used by parents and siblings during daily routines. Category labels, understanding object–function relationships, and the ability to answer questions logically are all examples of content that may be difficult for a child with hearing loss due to limited access to incidental language opportunities.

Clinical Applications.   Parents can narrate their thought process to give children direct access to the type of language that occurs in incidental language. For example, a parent may talk while she is creating a grocery list, saying, "I think we should have some vegetables. What kind of vegetables should we get? Broccoli, zucchini, or carrots?" Educators should also understand that repeated exposures to new words help children with hearing loss to master new vocabulary. Clinicians in school settings can *pre- and postteach vocabulary* in individual sessions to increase the child's experience with new words outside of class. Thematic units in school programs

Incidental learning is the learning that takes place through indirect or unplanned teaching, such as overhearing.

Pre- and postteaching vocabulary means that a clinician or educator will introduce and review vocabulary learned in the classroom setting in a quiet, individual context. This is helpful for students who are learning new words in what may be a noisy classroom setting.

are also helpful because the child is exposed to multiple repetitions of the new vocabulary throughout the day with books, activities, and projects. It is important to help parents understand the advantages of exposing children with hearing loss to sophisticated and varied vocabulary at home. Games (such as *"vocabulary bingo"*) that include category labels, object function, and descriptors also help to support the schema development and new vocabulary acquisition.

Use. Yoshinaga-Itano et al. (2011) reported that school-age children with hearing loss typically demonstrated delayed pragmatic skills compared to their age-matched hearing peers. Children with hearing loss were most likely to master the ability to make requests (e.g., "please" and "thank you"), express needs, and play roles with props. In general, by 7 years of age, children with hearing loss had not yet mastered the ability to provide information on request, repair incomplete sentences, interject, apologize, request clarification, ask questions to problem solve, or retell a story.

Nicholas and Geers (2003) examined communication samples from child–caregiver play interactions for a range of pragmatic functions (requesting, answering, calling attention to an event or action, directing, acknowledging, attempting to get information) in children with severe to profound hearing loss ranging in age from 1 to 4 years. When compared to normal-hearing peers, deaf children evidenced far fewer communicative acts, reduced utterance length, significantly reduced vocabulary use (words or signs), and significantly fewer informative functions (e.g., response, statement, question). The pattern of communication functions for deaf children was similar to that of younger normal-hearing children.

Clinical Applications. It is important to understand the role of pragmatics and social interaction for children with hearing loss, particularly as they enter mainstream settings at earlier ages. Clinicians should ensure that they support and coach parents to model communication functions beyond requesting and using polite forms (such as "please" and "thank you"). Luetke-Stahlman and Luckner (1991) point out that much of the success in teaching the pragmatic aspects of language will depend on the teacher's and caretaker's ability to create an abundance of meaningful language opportunities for the child to communicate in routine situations. Several environmental manipulation strategies are suggested to provide the child with opportunities to use language that has been mastered. One type of activity, for example, is to "violate" a routine event. For example, at the dinner table, set the table by placing the plates and silverware on the chairs, or forget to put the child's favorite food on the table. These *sabotaging activities* give children opportunities to initiate communication and to use language in a meaningful context. It is also important for parents and clinicians to monitor a child's social skills in a variety of settings (e.g., in classrooms, with peers, during lunch and recess) to ensure that the child is able to initiate and maintain communicative interactions with peers as well as adults. Examining performance in varying environments also provides information regarding how noise is impacting communication success.

Vocabulary bingo entails creating a bingo board with the target vocabulary. The child and the adult can take turns describing the objects and their functions/actions. This provides the child with increased access to not only the vocabulary labels but also the definitions and functions.

Sabotage activities provide motivation and opportunity for children to use and practice their emerging language skills. For example, a child may be presented with a desirable object that has been placed in a clear jar with a lid that is childproof. This increases the likelihood that the child will engage in communicative interaction with the caregiver, and the caregiver is provided with an opportunity to stimulate the child with the language needed to make a request for assistance, such as "open please."

Case 6.4. JF

JF is a child with mild autism whose mild sensorineural hearing loss was first identified at age 7. Use of an FM system was initiated at school, and use of personal hearing aids was implemented at home. JF's language abilities are age appropriate with the exception of pragmatics. He has difficulty in communicating effectively with children his age, but this has been related to his mild autism. JF's speech is fully intelligible, and no articulation or phonological problems were noted. However, JF tends to use breathy, whispered speech, and voice therapy was initiated to resolve that problem. There is evidence of prior vocal nodules, and a recurrence of nodules or some other vocal cord pathology is now suspected.

Phonologic skills: The development of speech sounds that are used in a rule-based way in everyday speech.

Preliteracy and Literacy Issues. The potential delays reviewed above can lead to weakness in literacy (reading and writing) development in children with hearing loss. Historically, low reading and writing proficiency skills for children with hearing loss have been related to limited oral language skills that serve as a base for literacy. Research by Geers and Hayes (2011) suggests that children with hearing loss have more difficulty with spelling and expository writing and poorer phonological skills than their hearing peers. However, due to early intervention and advanced hearing technology, more of these children are now developing reading skills commensurate with their age-matched peers.

An important precursor to reading ability is the development of phonological awareness. Phonological awareness is the ability to recognize that words consist of individual syllables, onsets and rhymes, and phonemes. Phonological awareness is related to the success with which children learn to read and spell. According to Miller (1997), prelingual deafness may inhibit phonemic awareness, although it does not preclude its formation. For a detailed review of the impact of hearing loss on literacy development see Moeller, Tomblin, Yoshinaga-Itano, Connor, and Jerger (2007).

Clinical Applications. It is important that children who are Deaf/Hard of Hearing are exposed to reading and writing from the start. Infants and toddlers see and are exposed to letters and words in pictures, traffic signs, toys, and books. It is also important to encourage parents to read books (both fiction and nonfiction) to their young children. Parents can incorporate reading and writing into daily activities (such as making lists and exposure to familiar print and symbols). Children should also be allowed the opportunity to draw pictures, trace letters, and watch their stories be written down by their parents. Literacy development and literacy facilitation activities are discussed in Schuele and van Kleeck (1987) and van Kleeck and Schuele (1987).

LANGUAGE ASSESSMENT

Measures used for assessing the language of children with hearing loss can be categorized as follows: (1) formal language measures, (2) communication checklists or criterion-referenced assessments, and (3) language sample and narrative analyses. Because of the advancements in the language development of Deaf/Hard of Hearing children, it is possible to use many of the assessments developed and standardized for use with children with normal hearing. Use of these assessments allows one to consider the language skills of children with hearing loss with reference to their age-matched hearing peers. One could determine, for example, that Johnny, age 7, who has hearing aids, has a vocabulary score typical of a 4.5-year-old child with normal hearing. While standard assessments typically indicate that spoken-language proficiency is usually delayed in children with hearing loss, an increasing body of literature suggests that children using LSL who are enrolled in intensive early intervention programs approach normal limits on standardized assessments.

Formal Language Measures

It is important to assess across domains of communication development: receptive and expressive vocabulary, receptive and expressive language, articulation/intelligibility, and pragmatics. Language measures standardized on children with normal hearing are often used to measure communication development of children with hearing loss. Assessments such as the Peabody Picture Vocabulary Test (PPVT; Dunn & Dunn, 1997), the Expressive One-Word Picture Vocabulary Test-Revised (EOWPVT-R; Gardner, 1990), the Preschool Language Scale—4 (PLS-4; Zimmerman, Steiner, & Pond, 2002), and the Clinical Evaluation of Language Fundamentals

(CELF; Wiig et al., 1992) can be administered to measure receptive and expressive vocabulary and language skills.

Assessments standardized on children with hearing loss can also be used to measure vocabulary and language development. These assessments are likely to be most available to clinicians working in settings with a caseload of children with hearing loss, particularly clinicians who work with children in settings using communication modalities, including sign language. A few language assessment tests have been developed for and normed on children with hearing loss (Table 6.2).

Implications of Using Formal Language Measures

It is critical that, prior to using standardized assessments, the evaluator checks to ensure the child's hearing aid(s) and/or cochlear implant(s) are working properly. Receptive language tests typically involve a spoken presentation of a word or sentence and require a picture-pointing response by the child. If a child with a hearing loss responds incorrectly, it is necessary for the speech-language pathologist to determine if the child does not understand the language concept or vocabulary item or if he or she was not able to hear the stimulus. A skilled professional will analyze assessment results and communicate with the audiologist if there are concerns regarding a child's ability to hear across frequencies.

Formal language measures offer an opportunity for speech-language pathologists to understand how a child with hearing loss using LSL is developing language compared to his or her age-matched hearing peers. They also provide clinicians with an excellent tool for measuring progress. It is important to give the assessments, as they have been standardized to ensure that the test provides reliable information over time.

Criterion-referenced assessments are checklists of skills that occur at certain ages or stages. They do not include normative information but can be helpful in assessing a child's progress over time.

There are also challenges in using a standardized assessment as the sole way of measuring the language development of a child with hearing loss. First, the standardized assessment may not provide a true measure of a child's linguistic skills in everyday conversations, in which the child has access to situational and linguistic cues to help decipher what is being said. Second, standardized assessments normed on hearing children may not be sensitive enough to pick up the language gaps that exist in children with hearing loss. For example, aggregate test scores, such as the CELF-Preschool Core Language score, include information about morphology and syntax but can be elevated by the addition of an Expressive Vocabulary score. When speech-language pathologists use standardized assessments for children who are Deaf/Hard of Hearing, it is important to use the item analysis features of the assessments to better determine the unique needs of the child. The need to combine formal and informal strategies for language assessment of children with hearing loss is delineated in an excellent book by Bradham and Houston (2014).

Communication Checklists or Criterion-Referenced Assessments

Another way to measure progress in the language development of children with hearing loss is to use checklists that compare specific skills. Criterion-referenced checklists, such as the Cottage Acquisition Scales for Listening, Language and Speech (CASLLS; Wilkes, 1999) and the Teacher Assessment of Spoken Language (TASL; Moog & Biedenstein, 1998), can be helpful for measuring progress and helping to inform parents about their child's current language skills and what skills to be expecting next developmentally. These checklists can be used for children with basic language (combination of two words) to complex language (13 or more words). Checklists are a particularly effective way of monitoring components of language form as a child's language becomes increasingly sophisticated.

TABLE 6.2   Language Assessment Tests Designed for Children with Hearing Loss

Test	Normed	Screening Version Available	Number of Subtests	Number of Versions	Format	Mode of Communication
Test of Syntactic Ability (TSA; Quigley, Steinkamp, Power, & Jones, 1978)	Normal hearing and hearing loss	Yes (2 different versions)	20	1	Paper and pencil	Written
Grammatical Analysis of Elicited Language (GAEL; Moog & Geers, 1979; Moog, Kozak, and Geers, 1983).	Hearing loss	No	0	3 (presentence, simple sentence, and complex sentence)	Props, modeled scripts, imitation	Oral, total communication
Teacher Assessment of Grammatical Structures (TAGS; Moog & Kozak, 1983)	Normal hearing	No	0	3 (presentence, simple sentence, complex sentence)	Teacher rates child using sentences in daily classroom activities	Oral, signed English
Spontaneous Language Analysis Procedure (SLAP; Kretschmer & Kretschmer, 1978)	Hearing loss	No	6	1	Child in conversation	Any
Carolina Picture Vocabulary Test (Layton & Holmes, 1985)	Hearing loss	No	0	1	Picture pointing	Any
Rhode Island Test of Language Structure (Engen & Engen, 1983)	Normal hearing and hearing loss	No	0	1	Picture pointing	Total Communication
Scales of Early Communication Skills (Moog & Geers, 1975)	Hearing loss	No	3	1	Demonstration and observation	Any
SKI*HI Language Development Scale (Tonelson & Watkins, 1979)	Hearing loss	No	2	1	Parent observation	Any

Language Sample and Narrative Analysis

Analysis of conversational and narrative skills is also important in reflecting the language abilities of children with hearing loss. The use of language samples can supplement information obtained from formal language assessments. Language samples can be completed as a diagnostic tool and also used periodically to measure development in spontaneous language. Clinicians can look at language used with peers, in individual therapy sessions, and in the classroom. If structured correctly, language samples can provide valuable information about the child's form, content, and use of language and supplement findings from formal evaluations (King, Olson, Shaver, & Blaiser, 2009). Conversational abilities typically are evaluated through video recording play interactions or natural conversations.

Narratives can be evaluated by asking children to review wordless picture books and then either tell the story (oral narration) or write the story (written narration). Analysis of conversational and narrative samples often includes consideration of syntactic and morphologic forms used, communicative functions, vocabulary, and length of utterances or sentences. Tur-Kaspa and Dromi (1998) found distinct differences between the spoken and written narratives of children with normal hearing and early identified children with severe to profound hearing loss. The children with hearing loss used less complex syntactic forms than the normal-hearing children.

Essential Conditions for Evaluating Language Abilities.   Several factors must be kept in mind when evaluating the language of a child with hearing loss. First, sensory devices, such as hearing aids or cochlear implants, should be checked for proper function prior to administering the test. Second, the test environment should be optimized by reducing noise and other environmental distractions. Third, assessments should not be modified when given to children with hearing loss. For example, a child with hearing loss normally should not be given multiple repetitions for a test item and then the answer is considered "correct." However, if multiple repetitions are required to elicit the correct response, that information should be noted in the evaluation report and considered as an educational adaptation. An extremely important factor in language evaluation is that persons administering language tests be proficient users of the child's primary communication mode and language, whether that be spoken language only, spoken language plus cued speech, spoken language plus signed English, or ASL. Otherwise, test results may well be invalid, reflecting misunderstanding of test instructions and desired responses rather than language ability.

Infant vocalizations: Sounds, such as crying, coughing, cooing, laughing, babbling, and vocables (word approximations), that precede spoken words.

SPEECH DEVELOPMENT IN CHILDREN WITH HEARING LOSS

Infants with hearing loss vocalize. However, findings from a few early studies suggested differences in babbling patterns for babies with hearing loss, specifically, fewer consonant-like sounds from 6 to 10 months of age and a delay in the onset of canonical (reduplicated) babbling (Oller & Eilers, 1988; Stoel-Gammon & Otomo, 1986). Advances in hearing aid technology and early identification and management allow for more acoustic information in the first year of life. If fitted and managed early, one would generally expect to observe the normal developmental sequence of sound productions (Oller, 1980): crying and vegetative sounds (burps, coughs, sneezes), cooing and laughing, reduplicated babbling (same consonant–vowel syllable in a string, *bababa*), and variegated babbling (change in consonant–vowel syllable in a string, *badabada*) with sentence-like intonation. Babies fitted early with more recent hearing aid technology often show vowel development comparable to that of children with normal hearing (Nelson, Yoshinaga-Itano, Rothpletz, & Sedey, 2007). Speech-language pathologists and early interventionists should understand normal speech development and milestones as well as how these milestones and productions can be impacted by a hearing loss. Providing audiologists with information on a child's speech development and/or concerns in a timely manner can help ensure that the child's hearing technology is appropriately fit.

However, early intervention does not eliminate all differences in early vocalizations between children with normal hearing and those with hearing loss. Even with early identification and management of hearing loss, 12-month-old children with hearing loss may produce fewer multisyllabic utterances with consonants and fewer fricatives and stops with alveolar–velar stop place and show more restricted tongue positions for vowels than children with normal hearing (McGowan, Nittrouer, & Chenausky, 2008). Normal hearing children and children with cochlear implants who are developing first words also differ in the accuracy of their consonant–vowel syllables, with the latter showing poorer production accuracy (Warner-Czyz, Davis, & MacNeilage, 2010). These differences may reflect the fact that no technological device can offer the speech acoustics offered by an ear with normal hearing. They also reflect the need for monitoring the early vocalizations of babies with hearing loss.

Speech Characteristics

Advances in early identification and management and in hearing aid, FM, bone-anchored hearing aid, and cochlear implant technologies offer children with hearing loss greater access to speech acoustic cues than ever before. Historically, children with mild to moderate degrees of hearing loss often had intelligible speech with the predominant speech errors being either the misarticulation of single consonants (Elfenbein, Hardin-Jones, & Davis, 1994) or consonant blends (Cozad, 1974). Sounds most commonly in error were the affricates, fricatives, and blends (Elfenbein et al., 1994). Given these types of errors, the use of standard articulation tests is appropriate.

Children with early-onset severe to profound hearing loss who do not utilize advanced hearing technology often demonstrate significant deficits in speech production. Speech and language difficulties can include the production of consonants

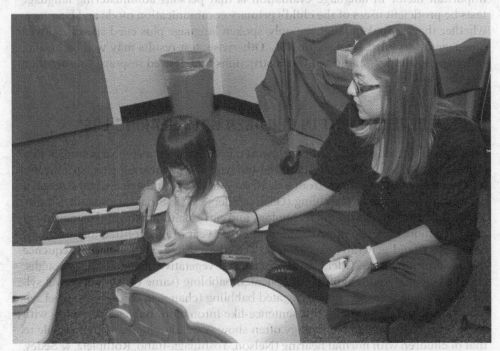

Age-appropriate activities in therapy or in real life can be helpful for improving speech and language skills.

Case 6.5. EF

EF is the 3-year-old sister of JF. Her mild to moderate sensorineural hearing loss was identified at age 3 when her hearing was tested after the identification of her brother's hearing loss. She was immediately fitted with powder-pink hearing aids. EF is highly communicative, and her language abilities are within the normal range. Her primary deficit is in the area of articulation, and she is receiving speech therapy to address that.

and vowels as well as problems with speech breathing, *resonance*, and the production of *suprasegmental features*, such as duration and fundamental frequency changes across an utterance. Specific difficulties include problems with speech breathing, such as not taking in enough breath to produce a phrase and/or allowing too much air out across the phrase and then running out of breath at the end (Cavallo, Baken, Metz, & Whitehead, 1991; Hutchinson & Smith, 1976). These breathing patterns result in children stopping and breathing before each phrase or during phrases or children continuing to speak with little breath support and sounding strained because they ran out of air before the end of the phrase. Difficulties with resonance (i.e., hyponasality and hypernasality) have also been observed in this population. Reduced speaking rate (one and a half to two times slower than normal) has been observed in individuals who are deaf (Tye-Murray, 1992) and attributed, in part, to lengthy pauses and prolongation of individual speech sounds. Historically, excessive pitch variation and limited pitch variation also have been observed in those with severe hearing loss of early onset (Formby & Monsen, 1982).

With the advances in access to hearing technology, degree of hearing loss is often not as important a factor for outcomes in speech development (Cole & Flexer, 2016). Children with profound hearing loss and cochlear implants can develop similar speech to children with mild hearing loss or normal hearing. Research suggests that age of implantation (or amount of auditory experience) is an important predictor of speech development and that children continue to demonstrate progress in speech development over time (Chin & Kaiser, 2000; Connor, Craig, Raudenbush, Heavner, & Zwolan, 2006; Flipsen, 2011). Carter, Dillon, and Pisoni (2002) reported on the speech production abilities in a group of school-age children, most of whom had hearing loss identified before 6 months of age (i.e., 19 of 24 children) and who had been using a cochlear implant for approximately 3½ to 6½ years. This group of children was found to be much more successful at producing correct syllable number (64% average accuracy) and primary stress (61% average accuracy) than overall accuracy (5% average accuracy), which reflected their speech sound errors. While cochlear implantation appears to offer greater acoustic access, some children with cochlear implants may produce unusual speech errors, such as the production of non-English sounds. Teoh and Chin (2009) offered a tutorial on narrow phonetic transcription methods to capture those unusual types of speech errors. Work by Flipsen (2011) suggests that children with cochlear implants may well develop speech sounds in a similar time line as hearing peers, as proposed by Shriberg (1993).

Some individuals acquire hearing loss at older ages, or after they have developed speech and language. This is called *postlingual* hearing loss. The speech skills of children with postlingual hearing loss can be maintained if the hearing loss is identified early and well managed with hearing technology. A wide variation of speech production abilities has been observed in this population. Kishon-Rabin, Taitelbaum, Tobin, and Hildesheimer (1999) found specific errors in the speech of postlingually deafened adults that included (1) decreased vowel space due to centralization of the first two formants, (2) inaccurate production of high-frequency sounds /s/ and /sh/, (3) similar voice onset time values for voiced and voiceless plosives, (4) substitution of /r/ with /w/, and (5) a tendency to omit consonants in

Resonance: Vibration of air in the throat, oral cavity, and/or nasal cavity; resonance problems include hypernasality and hyponasality.

Suprasegmental features: Variations in intensity, fundamental frequency, and duration of syllables and pauses across an utterance; problems with suprasegmentals include overall slow speaking rate, within-phrase pauses, excessive fundamental frequency variation, and less-than-normal fundamental frequency variation.

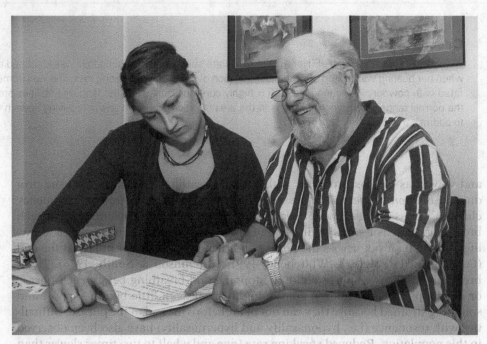

Adults who experience postlingual hearing loss can be helped to maintain their speech skills.

the final positions of words. Kishon-Rabin et al. also reported that after receiving cochlear implants, postlingually deafened adults showed significant improvements in speech and voice quality over a two-year period.

Speech Assessment

Two main categories of tools have been used to evaluate the speech production abilities of children with hearing loss: (1) traditional articulation and phonology tests and (2) measures of overall speech competence or intelligibility (i.e., the proportion of a child's speech that is understood by others). The more familiar approach to assessing speech production is with the use of articulation and phonological tests developed for normal-hearing children. In the new millennium, the target goal is to develop age-appropriate speech, and use of traditional articulation and phonological tests is appropriate. Recent research (Chin & Kaiser, 2000; Flipsen, 2011) examining performance on articulation tests normed for hearing children (e.g., the Goldman-Fristoe Test of Articulation [GFTA]; Goldman & Fristoe, 2002) demonstrated that the majority of the children using cochlear implants were within normal limits compared to their normal-hearing peers.

Speech intelligibility: Proportion of speech understood by a listener.

One way to reflect the proportion of spoken words that can be understood by other listeners is to measure the child's *speech intelligibility*. Speech intelligibility measures typically are based on recorded speech samples with two different ways to obtain the intelligibility rating. One or more listeners can be asked to write down the words they hear, and the examiner can determine the percentage of words accurately identified (e.g., 80% intelligible or accurately identified words). Alternatively, listeners can be asked to listen to the entire speech passage and rate how recognizable the words are in the passage (e.g., speech is completely intelligible). Intelligibility scores for connected speech (i.e., sentences or passages) are not closely related to scores on traditional word-based articulation tests and can offer an important index of overall speech competence (Ertmer, 2010; Huttunen & Sorri, 2004).

Clinical Applications. The development of intelligible speech in children with prelingual hearing loss is possible with technological advances and early identification but can still be a challenge. Monitoring and training accurate speech production must be included in the realm of establishing overall communicative competence. Robbins suggested six guidelines for achieving this: (1) integrate auditory and speech goals, (2) follow a "dialogue" or conversational approach to intervention rather than "tutorial" format, (3) use bridging activities to promote real-world carryover and generalization, (4) practice communication sabotage, (5) use contrasts in perception and production, and (6) select speech goals that enhance communicative competence. One enjoyable and meaningful way to develop and practice speech sound discrimination and production is to establish associations between familiar toys or actions and their sounds. Srinivasan (1996) provided a chart for clinicians and parents (see Table 6.3). The child can listen to family members "moo" when playing with the toy cow and be encouraged to "moo" also. (For sample speech activities, see Estabrooks, 1994; Robbins, 1994.)

TABLE 6.3 **Listening Sounds List**

Sound	Associated Object	Associated Action	Associated Phrase
ah	airplane (high pitch) truck (low pitch)		
oo	train (*woo woo*), owl (*hoot hoot*), ghost (*boo!*), cow (*moo*), dog (*woof woof*)		"Oops!"
ee	mouse (*ee ee ee*), bird (*cheep cheep*),	sweep down the slide ("Whee!")	
ai			"Hi!" "Bye bye!"
au	cat (*meow*),	down, around	"Ouch!"
o	rabbit (*hop hop*),	hop	hot, pop, "All gone!" knock (on the door)
oe		open, roll over	"Row, row the boat" "Roll (the ball)"
ay	horse (*neigh*)		"Hooray!"
a	duck (*quack*) sheep (*baaa*)		
u	up	run	"Uh oh!"
oi	pig (*oink*)		
m	ice cream (*Mmm!*)		"Mama," more, "Yumm! Yumm!"
n		knock	"No!"
w		walk, wind, wash, wipe	
b	bubbles, bus (*buh buh buh*)		"Bye! Bye!"
p	pop boat (*putt putt*)	pour, pat, pull/push	
t	clock (*tick tock*)	turn, tiptoe	
d	hammer (*duh duh duh*)		
k		cut	
g		go, drinking (*guh guh guh*)	
sh		sleeping (*shh!*)	
s	snake (*sss*)		
f		off (take ___ *off*)	
l		lalling to a tune (*lah lah lah . . .*)	
z	bee (*zzzz*)		
h	witch (*hee hee hee*)	laughing ("Ha! Ha! Ha!")	"It's hot!"
y	yo yo		"Yuk," yes

Source: From Pratibha Srinivasan, Practical aural habilitation: for speech-language pathologists and educators of hearing-impaired children, 1996. Courtesy of Charles C Thomas Publisher, Ltd., Springfield, Illinois.

Several considerations should be kept in mind while working on speech development with children who are Deaf/Hard of Hearing. First, use auditory feedback cues to draw the child's attention to the phoneme that is being targeted. When the child is using appropriately fit hearing technology, he or she should have acoustic access to the target phoneme; however, some children may need additional visual, tactile, and/or kinesthetic cues to supplement audition.

Second, the clinician must be familiar with the child's hearing capabilities with hearing aids and/or cochlear implants. This information can be gained by plotting the child's aided hearing thresholds on a familiar sounds audiogram (see Figure 6.2) and understanding how patterns of errors (e.g., placement errors such as *k* for *t*) may be related to the child not having acoustic access to that frequency/frequency range. When a child cannot hear a specific sound or phoneme, accurate production of that phoneme is not likely. Consequently, regular communication should take place between the speech-language pathologist and the audiologist.

Third, the clinician should be familiar with the impact of coarticulation since speech sounds change when paired with different speech sounds. Consequently, training on isolated speech sound productions should be limited and instead should move quickly to the production of sounds in meaningful words and phrases. For children with hearing loss in the birth to 3-year age range, Cole (1992) advocates use of the following guidelines:

1. Selecting and sequencing the child's speech targets based on normal developmental information.
2. Maximizing and ensuring optimal residual hearing.
3. Having parents and clinicians target spoken language goals during normal everyday activities (p. 74).

Summary

The audiologist, speech-language pathologist, teacher of the Deaf/Hard of Hearing, and family members will all have a role in the communication development of the child with hearing loss. All have complementary and sometimes overlapping contributions toward speech and language. The audiologist will have the greatest expertise in monitoring the child's hearing loss, establishing and ensuring that sensory devices are providing the maximum amount of speech acoustic cues, and communicating to others about the aspects of speech that may be inaudible to the child. The speech-language pathologist will have the strongest background and training in current speech and language intervention techniques, including ways to establish and maintain family-centered intervention. The teacher of the Deaf/Hard of Hearing will ensure that the child is making progress not only in communication development but across all domains of development (academic and cognitive). The family is the constant in the child's life (Crais, 1991); as such, the family's needs and choices are critical to the success and carryover of language and speech intervention.

When they are identified early and managed appropriately, children with hearing loss have the potential to develop speech and language skills commensurate with their hearing peers. Educational providers and parents must work together to maintain high expectations and educational plans to maximize communication outcomes.

Summary Points

- The presence of hearing loss in children does not preclude age appropriate speech and language development, particularly if it is identified early and managed consistently; however, hearing loss can have a serious impact on the child's overall language competence.

- Children with hearing loss need full-time use of appropriately fitted hearing technology to fully develop semantic, syntactic, pragmatic, and phonologic aspects of spoken language.

- Although there are several language measures specifically designed for children with hearing loss, the clinician will most likely use assessment tools that were designed and standardized with children who have normal hearing to assess speech and language development of children using LSL.

- A combination of focused practice and natural conversational language is necessary to maximize speech and language development.

- Early identification and intervention are essential to optimize the child's chance of developing age-appropriate speech and language skills.

- Because hearing is the foundation for speech development, hearing aid and/or cochlear implant use must be implemented as soon as possible to provide children with hearing loss access to speech acoustic information.

- The development of speech in children with congenital hearing loss can best be promoted when hearing loss identification, early intervention, and hearing technology are provided within the first 6 months of life.

Supplementary Learning Activities

See www.isu.edu/csed/audiology/rehab to carry out these activities. We encourage you to use these to supplement your learning. Your instructor may give specific assignments that involve a particular activity.

1. Hands and Voices is a parent support and resource for families of children who are Deaf/Hard of Hearing. A primary mission of this organization is to help provide nonbiased information about communication options. Watch the video "Lost and Found" (www.handsandvoices.org/resources/video/index.htm).

2. Google "cochlear implant simulation" and listen to what cochlear implants sound like. As you listen to the simulations, see how many words you can understand with the varying number of channels. Think about how more or fewer channels would impact speech and language development.

3. Tele-intervention, the provision of early intervention services via teleconferencing technology, is increasing in popularity as a viable method to provide services for families of children who deaf and hard of hearing. Go to the NCHAM website (www.infanthearing.org) and watch the introductory level course "Tele-Intervention 101 for Providers" to see how to implement tele-intervention and engage families.

Recommended Reading

Berg, F. S. (2008). *Speech development guide for children with hearing loss*. San Diego, CA: Plural Publishing.

Bradham, T. S., & Houston, K. T. (2014). *Assessing listening and spoken language in children with hearing loss*. San Diego, CA: Plural Publishing.

Cole, E. B., & Flexer, C. (2016). *Children with hearing loss developing listening and talking* (3rd ed.). San Diego, CA: Plural Publishing.

Estabrooks, W., Mac-Iver Lux, K., & Rhoades, E. A. (2016). *Auditory-verbal therapy for young children with hearing loss and their families, and the practitioners who guide them*. San Diego, CA: Plural Publishing.

Houston, K. T. (2013). *Telepractice in speech-language pathology*. San Diego, CA: Plural Publishing.

LaSasso, C., Crain, K. L., & Leybaert, J. (2010). *Cued speech and cued language for deaf and hard of hearing children*. San Diego, CA: Plural Publishing.

Mayne, A. M., Yoshinaga-Itano, C., Sedey, A. L., & Carey, A. (2000). Expressive vocabulary development of infants and toddlers who are deaf or hard of hearing [Monograph]. *Volta Review, 100*(5), 1–28.

Moeller, M. P., Tomblin, B., Yoshinaga-Itano, C., Connor, C. M., & Jerger, S. (2007). Current state of knowledge: Language and literacy of children with hearing impairment. *Ear and Hearing, 28*, 740–753.

Yoshinaga-Itano, C. (2003). From screening to early identification and intervention: Discovering predictors to successful outcomes for children with significant hearing loss. *Journal of Deaf Studies and Deaf Education, 8*(1), 11–30.

Recommended Websites

Alexander Graham Bell Association for the Deaf and Hard of Hearing:
http://www.agbell.org

Free videos and library on oral deaf education:
http://www.oraldeafed.org

Resources for families of children with hearing loss:
http://www.handsandvoices.org
http://www.hearingfirst.org
http://www.ncbegin.org
http://www.raisingdeafkids.org
http://www.cdc.gov

Resources for deaf educators and speech-language pathologists:
http://www.auditoryoptions.org
http://www.asha.org
http://www.infanthearing.org

References

Beck, D., & Flexer, C. (2011). Listening is where hearing meets brain . . . in children and adults. *The Hearing Review, 18*(2), 30–35.

Blamey, P. J., Sarant, J. Z., Paatsch, L. E., Barry, J. G., Bow, C. P., Wales, R. J., et al. (2001). Relationships among speech perception, production, language, hearing loss, and age in children with impaired hearing. *Journal of Speech, Language, and Hearing Research, 44*, 264–285.

Bloom, L., & Lahey, M. (1978). *Language development and language disorders.* New York: Wiley.

Bradham, T. S., & Houston, K. T. (2014). *Assessing listening and spoken language in children with hearing loss.* San Diego, CA: Plural Publishing.

Brown, C. (2006, June). *Early intervention: Strategies for public and private sector collaboration.* Paper presented at the 2006 convention of the Alexander Graham Bell Association for the Deaf and Hard of Hearing, Pittsburgh, PA.

Carter, A. K., Dillon, C. M., & Pisoni, D. B. (2002). Imitation of nonwords by hearing impaired children with cochlear implants: Suprasegmental analyses. *Clinical Linguistics and Phonetics, 16*(8), 619–638.

Cavallo, S. A., Baken, R. J., Metz, D. E., & Whitehead, R. L. (1991). Chest wall preparation for phonation in congenitally profoundly hearing-impaired persons. *Volta Review, 12*, 287–299.

Chin, S. B., & Kaiser, C. L. (2000). Measurement of articulation in pediatric users of cochlear implants. *Volta Review, 102*(4), 145–156.

Cole, E. B. (1992). Promoting emerging speech in birth to three-year-old hearing-impaired children. *Volta Review, 94*, 63–77.

Cole, E. B., & Flexer, C. (2016). *Children with hearing loss developing listening and talking* (3rd ed.). San Diego, CA: Plural Publishing.

Connor, C., Craig, M., Raudenbush, S., Heavner, K., & Zwolan, T. (2006). The age at which young deaf children receive cochlear implants and their vocabulary and speech-production growth: Is there an added value for early implantation? *Ear and Hearing, 27,* 628–664.

Cozad, R. L. (1974). *The speech clinician and the hearing-impaired child.* Springfield, IL: Charles C. Thomas.

Crais, E. R. (1991). Moving from "parent involvement" to family-centered services. *American Journal of Speech-Language Pathology, 9,* 5–8.

Downs, M. P., & Yoshinaga-Itano, C. (1999). The efficacy of early identification and intervention for children with hearing impairment. *Pediatric Clinics of North America, 46*(1), 79–87.

Dunn, L., & Dunn, L. (1997). *Peabody Picture Vocabulary Test—Revised (PPVT-3).* Circle Pines, MN: American Guidance Service.

Elfenbein, J. L., Hardin-Jones, M. A., & Davis, J. M. (1994). Oral communication skills of children who are hard of hearing. *Journal of Speech and Hearing Research, 37,* 216–226.

Engen, E., & Engen, T. (1983). *Rhode Island Test of Language Structure.* Austin, TX: PRO-ED.

Ertmer, D. J. (2010). Relationships between speech intelligibility and word articulation scores in children with hearing loss. *Journal of Speech, Language and Hearing Research, 53,* 1075–1086.

Estabrooks, W. (1994). *Auditory–verbal therapy for parents and professionals.* Washington, DC: Alexander Graham Bell Association for the Deaf.

Flipsen, P. (2011). Examining speech sound acquisition in children with cochlear implants using the GFTA-2. *Volta Review, 111*(1), 25–37.

Formby, C., & Monsen, R. B. (1982). Long-term average speech spectra for normal and hearing-impaired adolescents. *Journal of the Acoustical Society of America, 71,* 196–202.

Gallaudet Research Institute. (2008, November). *Regional and national summary report of data from the 2007–08 Annual Survey of Deaf and Hard of Hearing Children and Youth.* Washington, DC: Author.

Gardner, M. E. (1990). *Expressive One-Word Picture Vocabulary Test—Revised.* Novato, CA: Academic Therapy Publications.

Geers, A. E., & Hayes, H. (2011). Reading, writing, and phonological processing skills of adolescents with 10 or more years of cochlear implant experience. *Ear and Hearing, 32*(1), 49S–59S.

Geers, A. E., Nicholas, J. G., & Sedey, A. L. (2003). Language skills of children with early cochlear implantation. *Ear and Hearing, 24*(1), 46S–58S.

Gilbertson, M., & Kamhi, A. G. (1995). Novel word learning in children with hearing impairment. *Journal of Speech, Language, and Hearing Research, 38,* 630–642.

Glasgow, R. E., La Chance, P. A., Toobert, D. J., Brown, J., Hampson, S. E., & Riddle, M. C. (1997). Long-term effects and costs of brief behavioural dietary intervention for patients with diabetes delivered from the medical office. *Patient Education and Counseling, 32*(3), 175–184.

Goldman, R., & Fristoe, M. (2002). *Goldman Fristoe Test of Articulation, second edition.* Circle Pines, MN: American Guidance Service.

Harrison, M., Roush, J., & Wallace, J. (2003). Trends in age of identification and intervention in infants with hearing loss. *Ear and Hearing, 24,* 89–95.

Hayes, H., Geers, A., Treiman, R., & Moog, J. (2009). Receptive vocabulary development in deaf children with cochlear implants: Achievement in an intensive auditory-oral education setting. *Ear and Hearing, 30,* 128–135.

Hutchinson, J. M., & Smith, L. L. (1976). Aerodynamic functioning during consonant production by hearing-impaired adults. *Audiology and Hearing Education, 2,* 16–24.

Huttunen, K., & Sorri, M. (2004). Methodological aspects of assessing speech intelligibility among children with impaired hearing. *Acta Otolaryngolica, 124,* 490–494.

Isaacson, S. L. (1996). Simple ways to assess deaf or hard-of-hearing students' writing skills. *Volta Review, 98*(1), 183–199.

Joint Committee on Infant Hearing. (2007). Year 2007 position statement: Principles and guidelines for early hearing detection and intervention programs. *Pediatrics, 120,* 898–921.

King, E., Olson, E., Shaver, J., & Blaiser, K. (2009). *Preschool children with hearing loss: Trends in spoken language.* Paper presented at the American Speech-Language-Hearing Association Convention, New Orleans, LA.

Kishon-Rabin, L., Taitelbaum, R., Tobin, Y., & Hildesheimer, M. (1999). The effect of partially restored hearing on speech production of postlingually deafened adults with multichannel cochlear implants. *Journal of the Acoustical Society of America*, *106*(5), 2843–2857.

Kretschmer, R. R., & Kretschmer, L. W. (1978). *Language development and intervention with the hearing impaired.* Baltimore: University Park Press.

Layton, T. L., & Holmes, D. W. (1985). *Carolina Picture Vocabulary Test.* Austin, TX: PRO-ED.

Luetke-Stahlman, B., & Luckner, J. (1991). *Effectively educating students with hearing impairments.* New York: Longman.

Mayne, A. M., Yoshinaga-Itano, C., Sedey, A. L., & Carey, A. (2000). Expressive vocabulary development of infants and toddlers who are deaf and hard of hearing [Monograph]. *Volta Review*, *100*(5), 1–28.

McGowan, R. S., Nittrouer, S., & Chenausky, K. (2008). Speech production in 12-month-old children with and without hearing loss. *Journal of Speech, Language, and Hearing Research*, *51*, 879–888.

Miller, P. (1997). The effect of communication mode on the development of phonemic awareness in prelingually deaf students. *Journal of Speech, Language, and Hearing Research*, *40*, 1151–1163.

Mitchell, R. E., & Karchmer, M. A. (2004). Chasing the mythical ten percent: Parental hearing status of deaf and hard of hearing students in the United States. *Sign Language Studies*, *4*, 138–163.

Moeller, M. P., Tomblin, B., Yoshinaga-Itano, C., Connor, C. M., & Jerger, S. (2007). Current state of knowledge: Language and literacy of children with hearing impairment. *Ear and Hearing*, *28*, 740–753.

Moog, J., & Biedenstein, J. (1998). *Teacher Assessment of Spoken Language.* St. Louis, MO: Moog Center for Deaf Education.

Moog, J. S., & Geers, A. E. (1975). *Scales of early communication skills for hearing impaired children.* St. Louis, MO: Central Institute for the Deaf.

Moog, J. S., & Geers, A. E. (1979). *Grammatical analysis of elicited language—Simple sentence level.* St. Louis, MO: Central Institute for the Deaf.

Moog, J. S., & Kozak, V. J. (1983). *Teacher assessment of grammatical structures.* St. Louis, MO: Central Institute for the Deaf.

Moog, J.S., Kozak, V.J. and Geers, A.E. (1983). *Grammatical Analysis of Elicited Language—Pre-Sentence Level.* Central Institute for the Deaf, St. Louis, MO.

Munoz, K., Blaiser, K., Schofield, H. (2012). Aided speech perception testing practices for three-to-six year old children with permanent hearing loss. *Journal of Educational Audiology*, *18*, 53–60.

Munoz, K., Preston, E., & Hicken, S. (2014). Pediatric hearing aid use: How can audiologists support parents to increase consistency? *Journal of the American Academy of Audiology*, *25*, 380–387.

National Center for Hearing Assessment and Management. (2016). State EHDI/UNHS mandates: Summary table. Retrieved from http://www.infanthearing.org/legislative/summary/index.html

National Institute on Deafness and Other Communication Disorders. (2014). *Cochlear implants.* Retrieved from https://www.nidcd.nih.gov/health/cochlear-implants

Nelson, R., Yoshinaga-Itano, C., Rothpletz, A., & Sedey A. (2007). Vowel production in 7- to 12-month-old infants with hearing loss. *Volta Review*, *107*(2), 101–121.

Nicholas, J. G., & Geers, A. E. (2003). Hearing status, language modality, and young children's communicative and linguistic behavior. *Journal of Deaf Studies and Deaf Education*, *8*(4), 422–437.

Nicholas, J. G., & Geers, A. E. (2013). Spoken language benefits of extending cochlear implant candidacy below 12 months of age. *Otology and Neurotology*, *34*(3), 532–538.

Oller, D. K. (1980). The emergence of speech sounds in infancy. In G. Yeni-Komishan, J. Kavanaugh, & C. A. Ferguson (Eds.), *Child phonology: Vol 1. Production* (pp. 93–112). New York: Grune and Stratton.

Oller, D., & Eilers, R. E. (1988). The role of audition in infant babbling. *Child Development*, *59*, 441–449.

Quigley, S. P., Steinkamp, M., Power, D., & Jones, B. (1978). *The Test of Syntactic Abilities*. Beaverton, OR: Dormac.

Robbins, A. M. (1994). Guidelines for developing oral communication skills in children with cochlear implants. *Volta Review*, *96*(5), 75–82.

Schirmer, B. R. (1994). *Language and literacy development in children who are deaf*. New York: Maxwell Macmillan International.

Schuele, M. A., & van Kleeck, A. (1987). Precursors to literacy: Assessment and intervention. *Topics in Language Disorders*, *7*(2), 32–44.

Shriberg, L. D. (1993). Four new speech and prosody-voice measures for genetics research and other studies in developmental phonological disorders. *Journal of Speech and Hearing Research*, *36*, 105–140.

Spencer, P. (2004). Individual differences in language performance after cochlear implantation at one to three years of age: Child, family and linguistic factors. *Journal of Deaf Studies and Deaf Education*, *9*, 395–412.

Srinivasan, P. (1996). *Practical aural rehabilitation for speech–language pathologists and educators of hearing-impaired children*. Springfield, IL: Charles C. Thomas.

Stelmachowicz, P. G., Pittman, A. L., Hoover, B. M., & Lewis, D. L. (2004). Novel word learning in normal hearing and hearing-impaired children. *Ear and Hearing*, *25*, 47–56.

Stoel-Gammon, C., & Otomo, K. (1986). Babbling development of hearing-impaired and normally hearing subjects. *Journal of Speech and Hearing Disorders*, *51*, 33–41.

Teoh, A.P., & Chin, S. B. (2009). Transcribing the speech of children with cochlear implants: Clinical application of narrow phonetic transcriptions. *American Journal of Speech Language Pathology*, *18*, 388–401.

Tonelson, S., & Watkins, S. (1979). *SKI*HI Language Development Scale*. Logan, UT: Hope, Inc.

Tur-Kaspa, H., & Dromi, E. (1998). Spoken and written language assessment of orally trained children with hearing loss: Syntactic structures and deviations. *Volta Review*, *100*(3), 186–203.

Tye-Murray, N. (1992). Articulatory organizational strategies and the roles of auditory information. *Volta Review*, *94*, 243–260.

van Kleeck, A., & Schuele, C. M. (1987). Precursors to literacy: Normal development. *Topics in Language Disorders*, *7*(2), 13–31.

Waltzman, S. B., & Roland, J. T., Jr. (2005). Cochlear implantation in children younger than 12 months. *Pediatrics*, *116*(4), e487–e493.

Warner-Czyz, A. D., Davis, B. L., & MacNeilage, P. F. (2010). Accuracy of consonant-vowel syllables in young cochlear implant recipients and hearing children with the single-word period. *Journal of Speech, Language, and Hearing Research*, *53*, 2–17.

White, K. (2007). Early intervention for children with permanent hearing loss: Finishing the EHDI Revolution. *Volta Review*, *106*(3), 237–258.

Wiig, E., Secord, W., & Semel, E. (1992). *Clinical Evaluation of Language Fundamentals—Preschool*. San Antonio, TX: The Psychological Corporation, Harcourt Brace.

Wilbur, R., Goodhart, W., & Fuller, D. (1989). Comprehension of English modals by hearing-impaired students. *Volta Review*, *91*, 5–18.

Wilkes, E. M. (1999). *Cottage Acquisition Scales for Listening, Language, and Speech*. San Antonio, TX: Sunshine Cottage School for Deaf Children.

Yoshinaga-Itano, C., & Downey, D. M. (1986). A hearing-impaired child's acquisition of schemata: Something's missing. *Topics in Language Disorders*, *7*(1), 45–57.

Yoshinaga-Itano, C., Sedey, A., Baca, R., Goberis, D., Abrisch, A., & Dolpes, M. (2011). *The development of pragmatics in children with hearing loss*. Paper presented at the Early Hearing Detection and Intervention Conference, Atlanta, GA.

Yoshinaga-Itano, C., Sedey, A. L., Coulter, D. K., & Mehl, A. L. (1998). Language of early- and later-identified children with hearing loss. *Pediatrics*, *102*, 1161–1171.

Zimmerman, I., Steiner, V., & Pond, R. (2002). *Preschool Language Scale—4*. San Antonio, TX: The Psychological Corporation.

Psychosocial Aspects of Hearing Loss and Counseling Basics

Kris English

CONTENTS

Visit the companion website when you see this icon to learn more about the topic nearby in the text.

Learning Outcomes

After reading this chapter, you will be able to

- Distinguish between the terms *deaf* and *Deaf*
- Explain how a child's self-concept may be adversely affected by hearing loss
- Describe what hearing aid effect refers to
- List the main components of the grief cycle often experienced by the parents of a child born with hearing loss
- Identify at least five common psychoemotional reactions experienced by adults to hearing loss
- Define counseling and list the key steps associated with the counseling process

INTRODUCTION

Adjusting to hearing loss and accepting recommendations regarding audiologic rehabilitation can be a difficult process for many individuals as well as for their families. This chapter describes a range of psychological, social, and emotional difficulties frequently experienced by persons with hearing loss across the life span. In addition, a description of basic counseling concepts is provided to demonstrate how professionals can help individuals with hearing loss contend with the problems of living with hearing loss and identify and assume ownership of their individual solutions.

PSYCHOSOCIAL ASPECTS OF HEARING LOSS

No hearing loss is exactly like another, but there are some ways to organize our understanding. First to be recognized is the distinction between the terms *deaf* and *hard of hearing*. As mentioned in Chapter 1, more than 32 million individuals in the United States have some degree of hearing loss, and more than 95 percent of these persons can be described as being *hard of hearing*, that is, having a mild, moderate, or severe hearing loss and some ability to understand speech with the use of hearing aids or other amplification. The remaining persons with hearing loss have a bilateral profound hearing loss

deaf: Profound degree of hearing loss,
whereas Deaf connotes a pride in associating
with a group who share the same culture (i.e.,
the Deaf community).

and would be described as being *deaf*, whereby even with powerful hearing aids, speech generally is not perceived in auditory-only perceptual situations. Another important distinction is needed between the concepts of being deaf (having bilateral profound hearing loss) and being Deaf. The latter phrase, with the capital "D," refers to a cultural identification with the Deaf community; this distinction and the unique concerns of cultural Deafness are reviewed in a later section.

Initially, however, we consider some general psychosocial and emotional implications of living with hearing loss, first among children and adolescents (i.e., growing up with hearing loss) and then among adults (acquiring hearing loss). This first section expands on the CORE model described in Chapter 1. Specifically, we will consider how hearing loss affects and is affected by Overall Participation Variables (psychoemotional and social) and Related Personal Factors.

Growing Up with Hearing Loss

The most significant consequence of growing up with a hearing loss is the difficulty in perceiving others' words because this limitation has a direct effect on the ability to develop one's own words and subsequent language skills. Even a mild degree of hearing loss can adversely affect vocabulary development and the subtle intricacies of language use. When language development is delayed, there is a cascading effect on many aspects of a child's psychosocial development, including self-concept, emotional development, family concerns, and social competence.

Self-concept or self-image: How one sees
oneself.

Self-Concept. Individuals are not born with their *self-concepts* intact; rather, self-concept is learned by absorbing the input, feedback, and reactions from those around us. Children typically internalize such reactions without question and allow others' attitudes to define themselves to themselves. Children are likely to think these thoughts: "I see myself the way you tell me you see me. If you see me as loved or unlovable, capable or not capable, a delight or a trial—this is how I see myself."

It appears that children with hearing loss are at risk for developing a relatively poor self-concept, most likely from negative reactions regarding their communication difficulties and also from being perceived differently as hearing aid users. For example, Cappelli, Daniels, Durieux-Smith, McGrath, and Neuss (1995) collected information from 23 hard of hearing children, ages 6 to 12, as well as from 23 children with no hearing loss, matched by sex and classroom. From the Self-Perception Profile for Children, it was found that children with hearing loss perceived themselves as less socially accepted than their non–hearing-loss peers. Another study (Bess, Dodd-Murphy, & Parker, 1998) asked more than 1,200 children with mild hearing loss to answer questions such as this: "During the past month, how often have you felt badly about yourself?" Overall, children with mild hearing loss exhibited significantly higher dysfunction in self-esteem than children without hearing loss (self-esteem or self-regard being an evaluative component of self-concept). The researchers concluded that "even mild losses can be associated with increased social and emotional dysfunction among school aged children" (p. 350).

Children who grow up with hearing loss receive negative feedback and reactions not only because of their communication difficulties but also because of the cosmetic issue of looking different. Our society has yet to accept hearing aids as a neutral technical device; instead, there tends to be a negative association with hearing aid use, with biased assumptions of reduced abilities, attractiveness, and intelligence. Many studies have examined this phenomenon, often called the *hearing aid effect* (Blood, Blood, & Danhauser, 1977), by showing subjects a set of pictures of individuals, some wearing visible hearing aids and some not. All characteristics were identical except for the presence of hearing aids, yet when the instruments were visible, individuals were given lower scores in almost every category of intelligence, personality, attractiveness, and capability. It appears that the very presence of a hearing aid can cause overall negative reactions.

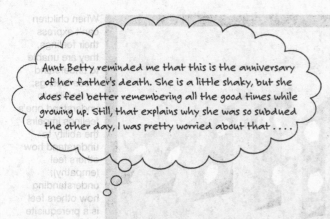

FIGURE 7.1 Missing out on adult conversations about emotions.

Aunt Betty reminded me that this is the anniversary of her father's death. She is a little shaky, but she does feel better remembering all the good times while growing up. Still, that explains why she was so subdued the other day, I was pretty worried about that . . . .

It is encouraging to note that preschool children seem less likely to hold these negative and preconceived notions (Riensche, Peterson, & Linden, 1990) and that teens may be becoming more accustomed to and accepting of hearing aids among their peers (Stein, Gill, & Gans, 2000). But, in general, if the appearance of a device on or in the ears creates a negative reaction among people who see it, their reaction is likely to be perceived by the hearing aid user, and this can adversely affect the user's self-concept. We would do a disservice to children growing up with hearing loss to dismiss society's reactions to hearing aids as a nonissue or to downplay it as "only the other person's problem." (To experience the *hearing aid effect* firsthand, college students [with normal hearing] are frequently assigned to wear a very visible pair of hearing aids for a full day around their community and record their subjective impressions of those around them as well as their own reactions.)

Acquiring language is essential for the development of self-concept, so it follows that a delay in language acquisition would adversely affect the development of self. This correlation, in fact, has been demonstrated in several studies, described in the next section.

Hearing aid effect: A psychological reaction to the presence of a hearing aid; the viewer has negative assumptions about the hearing aid user.

Emotional Development.   An individual uses language to describe, interpret, and ultimately understand the abstract nature of his or her emotions. Because of concomitant language deficits, children growing up with hearing loss may have limited experience in self-expression and a subsequent delay in awareness and understanding of their own emotions as well as the emotions of others. By virtue of having a hearing loss, they frequently miss overhearing adults and older children talk about and verbally manage their feelings about situations (see Figure 7.1).

Researchers have shown that children with hearing loss are often less accurate in identifying others' emotional states than children without hearing loss and have a poorer understanding of affective words. Understanding *affective vocabulary* has been positively related to personal adjustment (Greenberg & Kusche, 1993), so these findings reinforce our understanding of the contributions of communication to self-understanding. (For further information about the importance of general emotional development, see Goleman, 2006.) Figure 7.2 shows how these issues adversely affect a child's emotional and social development.

Hoffman, Quittner, and Cejas (2015) suggest that, without active intervention, deficits in one area of development have cascading effects on other areas. For example, when children can't express their feelings, they are unable to understand those feelings; an inability to understand one's feelings impairs the ability to understand how others feel (empathy); understanding how others feel is a prerequisite for friendship development..

Affective vocabulary: Words and phrases that describe feelings or emotional reactions (e.g., discouraged, elated, bored, upset).

Family Concerns.   More than 95 percent of children with hearing loss are born into families with at least one normal-hearing parent (Mitchell & Karchmer, 2004). The vast majority of these parents have little or no experience with hearing loss, so the diagnosis of hearing loss is devastating news, a moment frozen in time that they

FIGURE 7.2 Hearing loss in children can have a "domino effect."

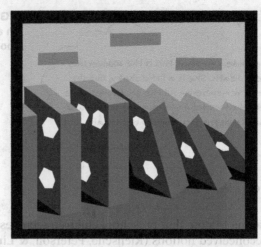

When children can't express their feelings, they are unable to understand those feelings; an inability to understand one's feelings impairs the ability to understand how others feel (empathy); understanding how others feel is a prerequisite for friendship development.

never forget. Even if parents have suspected hearing loss for some time before the diagnosis, they still report experiencing sadness, as well as relief, for having their suspicions confirmed. From their reports, it appears that most parents experience emotional reactions consistent with the stages or phases of the "grief cycle" (Kübler-Ross, 1969). The grief cycle includes a progressive set of emotional reactions, starting with *shock* because the information generally was not expected, and *denial* because the information does not reconcile with one's dreams for the future. When the reality of the situation begins to sink in, parents in grief may find themselves feeling *depressed* or helpless for a time while they attempt to cope with the implications of the diagnosis. The final stage of this cycle is *acceptance*, but more than one parent has been heard to say that they feel the term *resignation* is more accurate. Other reactions include depression, sorrow, confusion, and vulnerability, and they have been known to resurface at unexpected times in the family's development. Luterman (2008) reminds us that it is inappropriate for a professional to expect families to be "over their grief by now"; families have the right to feel the way they feel, and professionals must refrain from passing judgment. It is important to keep in mind that we do not predictably "march through" stages of grief and ultimately recover to be the same person as before. Parents report moving back and forth within these emotional reactions during different stages of their child's development, and often they find themselves almost as grieved by a new event as when they first received the diagnosis of hearing loss.

Case 7.1. Ms. Carlow

Ms. Carlow had been surprised but not worried when she had been told that her new daughter did not pass a hearing screening—after all, no one in the family had any hearing problems. So, when the audiologist told her that the more advanced tests indicated hearing loss in both ears, she was stunned. She held her baby close while the audiologist talked, but she couldn't pay attention. Her mind immediately jumped to her husband: He will say the test results must be wrong, that they must get a second opinion. That is always a good idea anyway, right? She picked up isolated words as the audiologist talked, something about more appointments and—what else? Impressions—of what? And why was she talking about fruit? A year later, Ms. Carlow realized, at a moment when all she wanted to do was hold her baby and think, that the audiologist had been explaining the "speech banana."

Over time, parents work their way past their own anticipated self-concept of being parents of a "perfect" child to the new reality of being parents of a child who has a hearing loss, and this process can be harder for some parents than for others.

Kricos (2000) writes about professionals' perceptions of parents who are struggling with acceptance:

> Parents in the denial stage may appear to clinicians to be blocking efforts to initiate the intervention program. However, it should be remembered that this initial reaction to the diagnosis may provide a time for parents to search for inner strength and accumulate information. The goal for clinicians during this stage of grieving is to find ways of not merely tolerating parental denial but accepting it, while still offering, to the best of their abilities, the services the child needs. Unfortunately, parents who appear to be denying their child's hearing impairment are often perceived by clinicians as foolish and stubborn, when they should be perceived as loving parents who, for the time being, cannot accept the professional's diagnosis of such a severe disability in their child. (pp. 279–280)

Even as parents work through their emotional reactions, difficulties may persist, again because of communication. Several studies have described a tendency in mother–child interactions to be more rigid and more negative when the child has a hearing loss. Verbal exchanges are briefer and more directive and include less praise compared to mothers whose children have normal hearing (Pipp-Siegel & Biringen, 2000). Without intervention, these communication styles can have an impact on the quality of parent–child attachment.

Professionals may inadvertently contribute to parental confusion or stress by emphasizing issues that are not at the forefront of parents' concerns. For example, on first fitting hearing aids on a child, professionals are likely to intone these instructions: "Mrs. Tomas, you will want to make sure that Isabella wears these hearing aids every waking hour. That way, she will have the best conditions to develop speech and language." Although an accurate statement, this clinical approach may miss the mark for many parents; it might be more helpful to "speak their language" by "saying the same thing differently." For example,

> Mrs. Tomas, the more Isabella wears her hearing aids, the more she will learn from your voice how much you love her and cherish her; the more she will learn when you are teasing and when you are serious about obeying you; the more she will be a part of family jokes and family lessons and family history.

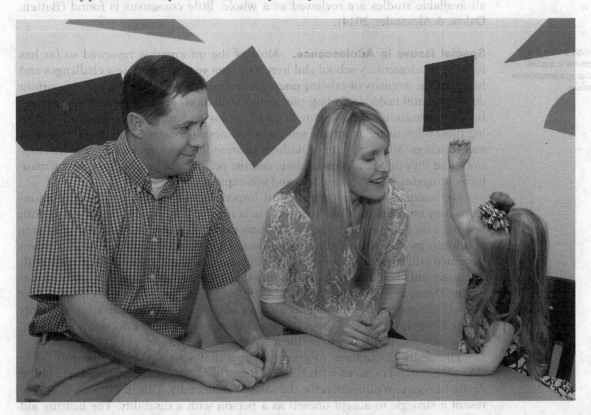

Family counseling can assist in establishing successful parent–child attachment.

At the time that all this is happening, Isabella will also have optimal conditions to develop speech and language, but it has been presented in a context that families can understand and use. In addition, the undue pressure of "pleasing the professional" has been removed; instead, the parent has been acknowledged as a competent adult who has a lot to manage and who will do her best for her child as her energy level allows.

Social competence: Skills for successful and satisfying personal relationships.

Social Competence.

As children grow up, their social world expands to include same-age peers. Here, too, difficulties have been observed among children with hearing loss: because of their delay in developing communication skills, children with hearing loss have fewer opportunities for peer interactions, making it difficult to learn social rules associated with communication, such as turn taking, eye gaze, and responding (Paasch & Toe, 2014).

> Poor and limited communication results in poor social competence, which includes these skills (Greenberg & Kusche, 1993):
>
> - Capacity to think independently
> - Capacity for self-direction and self-control
> - Understanding the feelings, motivations, and needs of self and others
> - Flexibility
> - Ability to tolerate frustration
> - Ability to rely on and be relied on by others
> - Maintaining healthy relationships with others

It is possible that children with hearing loss are at risk in developing these social competencies (Fellinger, Holtzinger, Sattel, & Laucht, 2008), although when all available studies are reviewed as a whole, little consensus is found (Batten, Oakes, & Alexander, 2014).

Peer groups or relationships provide safe environments for adolescents to practice important life skills, including communication, cooperation, and compromise.

Special Issues in Adolescence.

Most of the information reviewed so far has focused on elementary school children. The teen years present new challenges and heighten the intensity of existing ones. Adolescence is a stage of life with important developmental tasks, including *peer group* affiliation, identity formation, occupational preparation, and adjustment to physiologic changes (Kunnen, 2014). During these often turbulent times, self-consciousness increases, as do uncertainty and mood swings. All teens, with or without hearing loss, may feel besieged with emotions that they find hard to articulate, and the presence of hearing loss can increase teens' struggles for self-awareness and self-expression.

Peer relationships take paramount importance for teens, yet these relationships may be strained when hearing loss is involved. Being with other teens with hearing loss may be more important than expected when we consider how peer relationships help teens define themselves. In one study, most of the 220 mainstreamed students indicated that they preferred to spend most of their time with other students with hearing loss, finding these relationships deeper and more satisfying (Stinson, Whitmore, & Kluwin, 1996). Since most teens with hearing loss attend their neighborhood schools and are likely to be one of only a few students with hearing loss in their school (National Center for Special Education Research, 2011), they might struggle to define an identity in a vacuum.

The desire to conform to group expectations seems to peak in ninth grade (Merrell, 2007). For teens with hearing loss, this desire will probably include the desire to reject amplification for the sake of conformity. This desire may also represent a struggle to accept oneself as a person with a disability. The hearing aid effect is probably still in play, although there is some evidence that the magnitude of negative effect has lessened (Stein et al., 2000). Overall, however, it is agreed that being different is generally not valued during the teen years.

During these years, students need to develop appropriate social or interpersonal skills to advocate for their needs as they transition as young adults into college, work settings, and the health care system. This developmental task frequently is not supported, resulting in high school graduates who move on without learning how to describe and request the services that they need to succeed (English, 2012; Pajevic & English, 2014). Professionals who serve adolescents face the challenge of helping with the here-and-now issues of self-identity as well as concerns of the imminent future, and the former may seem so paramount that the latter is overlooked.

Summary.   This section described a range of possible psychosocial and emotional difficulties that might occur as a result of growing up with a hearing loss. Self-concept can be affected because of communication limitations as well as parental attachment, emotional development, and social competency. Interventions are available to help to reduce these effects, and they should be used when concerns arise (Luckner & Sebald, 2013). The following section considers how similar psychosocial issues can affect persons who acquire hearing loss in their adult years.

Acquiring Hearing Loss as Adults

Although relatively few children are born with hearing loss, most individuals, if they live long enough, acquire some degree of hearing loss as part of the aging process. Occasionally, adults also acquire hearing loss as a side effect of some medications or as a result of head injury or noise exposure. Adults are not immune to the psychological, emotional, and previous social effects described with respect to children. Parallel categories will be considered here as they apply to adults: self-concept, psychoemotional reactions, and family and social concerns.

Self-Concept.   It has long been noted that adults can be reluctant to admit to having a hearing loss and to take steps toward remediation. When people seek help from an audiologist, they have usually waited an average of seven years from the time that they first noticed hearing problems. During these years, they may attempt to dismiss the problem as the fault of others (e.g., accusing people of mumbling) or using other avoidance techniques. Another indicator that adults have a difficult time adjusting to their self-concept of a person with hearing loss is the fact that only about 30 percent of the population who have hearing loss actually obtain and use hearing aids (Abrahms & Kihm, 2015). Those not using hearing aids indicate cosmetic concerns as second only to the cost of hearing aids (Kochkin, 2012). Unlike other health issues related to aging (e.g., arthritis), hearing loss is complicated by perceived stigma of embarrassment, handicap, diminished capacity, and "defectiveness" (Wallhagen, 2010). Patients who express reservations about acknowledging and dealing with their hearing problems need careful counseling to help them recognize the barriers they have created and find the confidence to put "hearing better" as a higher priority than "what other people think."

To underscore the effect of hearing aids on self-concept, consider the following study: A group of older women with hearing loss was divided in half, but only the women in one group were fitted with hearing aids (Doggett, Stein, & Gans, 1998). All subjects then interacted with unfamiliar same-age peers who later rated them on attractiveness, friendliness, confidence, and intelligence. The subjects who wore the hearing aids were rated as less confident, less friendly, and less intelligent than the subjects not wearing hearing aids. The remarkable point about this study is that the raters did not even notice the hearing aids and so were not responding to their appearance! The authors surmised that the subjects wearing the hearing aids displayed less confidence, friendliness, and intelligence

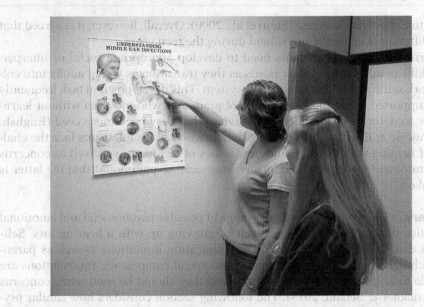

Helping the person to understand the underlying basis for a hearing loss facilitates adjustment to it.

because they projected a negative self-image. Again, as with children, ignoring the hearing aid effect with adults is akin to ignoring the proverbial elephant standing in the middle of the living room. It would be naive to assume that, because they are self-confident adults in most other aspects of their lives, they are invulnerable to this undeniable cosmetic concern.

Psychoemotional Reactions. In addition to avoidance and worry about cosmetics, adults have reported a full range of other emotions and psychological reactions to hearing loss, including anger ("Why is this happening?"), anxiety and insecurity ("What will this mean about my future?"), stress (especially before the effects of the hearing loss are well understood, such as in understanding speech in restaurants), resentment, depression, and grief. See Table 7.1 for a list of typical emotional reactions to hearing loss. The grief cycle was mentioned earlier with respect to parents and the diagnosis of hearing loss in children, but adults also experience a type of grief when their suspicions about deteriorating hearing have been confirmed. Its expression can be very subtle, as depicted in the following scenario.

Case 7.2

A 92-year-old man sought a hearing evaluation to address recent listening difficulties. Test results confirmed that he had a mild to moderate hearing loss, and hearing aids were recommended to help him meet his listening goals. On hearing this, he lowered his head, sighed deeply, and said, "I've always thought of hearing aids as only for old people." His audiologist waited with him quietly, and in less than one minute he raised his head, shook himself slightly, and asked, "Well, what do we do first?" That moment was a very brief but real expression of grief: "I am vulnerable, mortal, getting farther and farther away from my youth."

Paranoia: The perception that others are talking about us.

When we are excluded from a conversation, it is human nature (because we are naturally egocentric) to suspect that the conversation is about us. Adults with hearing loss struggle regularly with conversational exclusion, which can lead to behaviors that would suggest paranoia. However, it is vital that we do not confuse these reactions with the paranoia associated with schizophrenia and other mental health problems; this kind of *paranoia* is actually a natural reaction to the situation. At the same time, such reactions should not be dismissed as unimportant: If

TABLE 7.1   Common Psychoemotional Reactions to Hearing Loss

Alienated	Angry	Annoyed	Anxious	Bewildered	Bitter
Cheated	Confused	Denial	Depressed	Disturbed	Drained
Enraged	Fearful	Frustrated	Guilty	Hopeless	Impatient
Insecure	Lonely	Lost	Nervous	Overwhelmed	Panicked
Sad	Skeptical	Suspicious	Tense	Upset	Vulnerable
Weary	Withdrawn	Worried			

persons with hearing loss feel actively ignored or talked about or excluded, they may not have associated these reactions with the existence of hearing loss and may experience an undefined sense of disquiet or confusion.

Family Concerns.   Family members take the brunt of the stress while a member is coming to accept the fact that his or her hearing is changing. They are blamed for not speaking clearly or for purposefully leaving the person with hearing loss out of the conversation. Because communication is difficult, families do tend to talk around the patient or, if asked to repeat something, to minimize the effort by responding, "Never mind, it wasn't really important." Significant others (particularly spouses) often assume the responsibility of "hearing" for the family member by explaining what was missed, covering up for miscommunications, taking responsibility for all telephone contacts, or worrying about possible social embarrassment when a response is unrelated to the comment made. In half jest, adults with hearing loss have been known to introduce their spouses this way: "Have you met my hearing aid?"

The person with the hearing loss usually does not realize the burden that this spouse carries. When the patient and spouse take identical surveys to describe the effects of the hearing loss on their lives, the spouse usually reports greater problems before a hearing aid fitting and greater benefit after the hearing aid fitting than the patient does. These reports tell us a great deal about the stress of the hearing loss on the normal-hearing spouse or significant other.

Other family members may experience frustration and disappointment when communication by phone or in person is ineffective, and the person with the hearing loss may internalize these problems as a rejection of him- or herself rather than of the communication problems. A downward spiral can occur: "It's too hard to talk to Dad, so I'll keep the details to a minimum." Dad resents the limitation and contributes even less to the communication efforts.

Social Concerns.   When communication becomes gradually more difficult, our social world can constrict accordingly. The adult with hearing loss may opt out of favorite activities because the listening challenges are too stressful. When efforts are made to interact as if no hearing loss exists, misunderstandings typically occur (believing a comment was a joke when it was meant to be serious or completely misunderstanding a comment); this may result in embarrassment, possible blame directed to the communication partner, and eventually the use of *avoidance techniques*. Regular attendance at religious, family, and leisure activities becomes curtailed, often with excuses about losing interest rather than recognizing the root of the problem. This social withdrawal has been shown to lead to depression. It is not uncommon to find adults not making the connection between the change in their lifestyles and their gradual hearing loss.

Avoidance techniques: Strategies used to postpone acknowledgment of a difficult situation.

Summary.   Acquiring hearing loss in adulthood is usually a gradual, insidious process and is usually recognized by family and friends before being recognized by the person whose hearing is diminishing. Before, during, and after confirmation of hearing loss, adults may experience many of the same psychosocial difficulties that children do.

About Being Deaf

So far, we have considered the psychosocial and emotional effects of hearing loss in general. Several studies have noted that the more severe the hearing loss, the more severe the psychosocial and emotional problems can be (Warren & Hasenstab, 1986). These kinds of severe difficulties have been described by Meadow (1976), who reported how deaf children and adults have been characterized as *impulsive*, compulsive, egocentric, and rigid. Deficits in empathy have been described (Bachara, Raphael, & Phelan, 1980), as have higher-than-expected levels of anxiety (Harris, Van Zandt, & Rees, 1997). It must be understood that these kinds of psychological difficulties are not caused by the hearing loss per se but rather by the communication problems that result from hearing loss. If these kinds of concerns present themselves, a referral to a qualified psychologist or other counselor is in order.

Being Deafened.   The previous paragraphs focused on issues of individuals who were born deaf. Persons who become deafened in their adult years (late-onset deafness) have a uniquely stressful situation because they have no preestablished ties to the Deaf community yet also face challenges in maintaining their ties to the hearing world. Communication may be limited to writing notes or speechreading, neither procedure being very conducive to spontaneous or lengthy conversation. A sense of isolation is likely to occur, as are anger, frustration, denial, or depression (Barlow, Turner, Hammond, & Gailey, 2007).

Depression may result not only from the difficulties in communication, however. Speech communication occurs at a "symbolic" level of hearing, as defined by Ramsdell (1960). But there are other levels of hearing as well, including the *warning* or environmental level and the *primitive* level, which means that hearing sounds is so basic to our lives that we are not even aware of their occurrence. Virtually every action we make, every activity in our environment, produces a sound to which we react, often unconsciously. Persons who suddenly lose their hearing frequently report that the world has become "dead" to them. For example, to see a door shut forcefully and not hear the anticipated slam tends to make deafened people feel they are no longer interacting with the world around them. Even more distressing may be the absence of sound produced by the self, such as one's own footsteps or voices. Ramsdell (1960) stressed that the depression of a deafened person occurs because he "is not aware of the loss he has suffered at the primitive level. . . . He is unaware that there is such a thing as this primitive level in the first place" (p. 464).

Fortunately, hearing aids and cochlear implants often provide much psychological relief to many deafened adults. Recovering some degree of sound perception, even if only at the primitive level, can result in reduced anxiety and depression.

Deafness with a Capital "D"

About 1 million people in the United States not only have a profound hearing loss and derive no benefit from hearing aids (i.e., being audiologically deaf) but also identify themselves as members of the *Deaf community* (being culturally deaf). This cultural affiliation is described by Vernon and Andrews (1990):

> Membership in the deaf community involves identification with deaf people, shared experiences in school and work, and active participation in group activities with other deaf people. . . . Most notably, deaf community members share frustrating experiences trying to communicate in the hearing world. . . . [S]ome hearing individuals, such as educators, counselors, and spouses, can be "courtesy" members. However, only deaf persons can really know what deafness means. Neither social class nor sex nor religion are important attributes for membership; the most distinguishing criteria are communication skill and preference. (pp. 7–8)

Impulse disorder: Having difficulty controlling one's initial reactions or impulses; acting without considering consequences.

Deaf community: A group of individuals who share cultural similarities in language (American Sign Language, or ASL), mores, traditions, and values.

Communication within the Deaf community is based on the use of American Sign Language (ASL), a manual language with its own syntax and rules of use (with roots in French and English) (see Chapter 5). Deaf theater and Deaf poetry thrive across the country, notably at Gallaudet University in Washington, D.C., the only liberal arts university for the Deaf in the world. In addition to having its own language, like other cultures the Deaf community has its own traditions, mores, and values. The passing on of these values and traditions and even ASL is not accomplished through the more common vertical *enculturation process* from parent to child because only about 5 percent of deaf children are born to deaf parents (a phrase usually shortened as "deaf of deaf"). Instead, the transference of culture has occurred horizontally, among peers in residential schools or in postsecondary settings, such as colleges or communities.

Deaf persons tend to marry other Deaf persons and often prefer to have children who also have profound hearing loss like themselves (see the following case study). Connections to the Deaf community are usually lifelong, and elderly Deaf individuals typically maintain friendships established in their childhood (Becker, 1980; Leigh, Andrews, & Harris, 2016).

Enculturation process: Shaping or raising children according to values defined by a culture.

Case 7.3. Tony

The topic for the day in Audiology 101 was the early identification of hearing loss. A young man named Tony sat in the front of the class to follow the sign language interpreter. He raised his hand and explained with both speech and sign language, "This topic is particularly important to me because my wife and I just had a baby last Saturday." The class applauded, and he continued, "Yes, because both she and I are deaf, they tested our baby's hearing. Unfortunately, he didn't pass the test." The class responded with silent nods of the head to show they were sorry. But he wasn't done—with a twinkle in his eye, he added, "Yes, he can hear." The collective jaw of the entire class dropped, and a few students laughed uncomfortably. Even though it was said teasingly, he wanted the class to understand that their preference would have been for a child who was deaf as they were, and the fact that the baby had normal hearing was a type of "failed test" to them.

The psychological, emotional, and social development of Deaf individuals will be influenced by all the same variables as those who are not culturally Deaf. Are they raised in families that accept them for who they are? Is communication easy to establish and sustain? Is the ability to express oneself and be understood and accepted part of one's experience? The topic of "being Deaf" is far too complex to cover in depth here; for more information about the psychology of deafness, refer to the Recommended Reading at the end of this chapter. Readings on the phenomenon of Deaf culture are also provided.

"KNOWING IS NOT ENOUGH": COUNSELING BASICS

Having an understanding of the psychological, social, and emotional effects of living with hearing loss ("knowing" about its effects) satisfies one level of professional development. However, persons with hearing loss expect more from the professionals who serve them: They expect active support as they adjust to their situation and have consistently expressed disappointment that, in general, they do not receive it (Glass & Elliot, 1992). Clearly, then, "knowing" about these concerns is not enough. The next step in professional development is to advance from "knowing" to "know-how," as in knowing how to provide the personal adjustment support that our patients and their families need and expect. Extensive materials are available on developing this know-how, but this section provides only highlights on counseling basics. Readers are strongly encouraged to seek formal course work in counseling as it relates to their disciplines, both in their training program and in informal training throughout their professional careers.

FIGURE 7.3 Important distinctions.

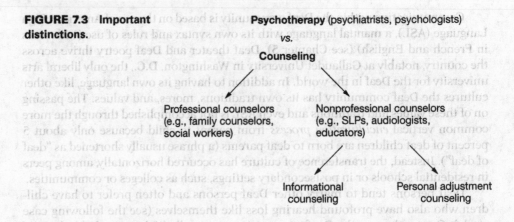

Important Distinctions

Before proceeding, we must be clear about the following terms. When we refer to counseling, we are not referring to psychotherapy or psychoanalysis, whereby mental health professionals (i.e., psychiatrists and psychologists) use their professional training to help clients find ways to solve pervasive life problems. Psychotherapy helps patients explore unconscious behavior patterns in order to alter ways of relating and functioning by examining and challenging personal history and by analyzing the meanings of one's responses (Cormier, 2014; Crowe, 1997). Psychotherapy generally views the patient as being ill and searches for the cause of a person's problems, which might be rooted in family relationships or childhood trauma.

Counseling, in comparison, is designed to help people to develop "here-and-now strategies" for coping with life, decision making, and current problems. Social workers, school counselors, ministers, and other spiritual leaders are professional counselors. Whereas psychotherapy attempts to effect major personality changes, counseling focuses on supporting personal adjustments to situations by helping a person understand his or her feelings and engage in problem solving (see Figure 7.3).

Nonprofessional counseling may not be as familiar a concept, but it occurs routinely: A financial planner will counsel on tax problems, a teacher will counsel on test-taking strategies, an *audiologist* will counsel on hearing conversation, and so on (Kennedy & Charles, 2001). These examples involve content or *informational counseling*, which is one facet of nonprofessional counseling, but all professionals on occasion will work with clients or students facing emotional crises as well (e.g., the stress associated with financial risk or the despair and discouragement from failing an important exam). When the emotional crisis is related to the professional's specialty, *nonprofessional personal adjustment support* becomes a second facet of nonprofessional counseling.

Professional boundaries must be respected, of course. Nonprofessional counselors must define relationships by boundaries that clarify the roles and functions of individuals in the relationship (Stone & Olswang, 1989). When a professional begins to feel uncomfortable with either the content or the intensity of the interaction, he or she can assume that a boundary is being approached, and it is probably an appropriate time to refer the patient or parent to a professional counselor.

What We May Think Counseling Is

Counseling is often narrowly perceived as *explaining*: A professional talks while a patient or parent listens to information about the audiogram, the anatomy of the ear, the benefits and limitations of hearing aids and cochlear implants, and the range of communication options. Undoubtedly, explaining is an essential aspect of service delivery because patients, parents, and family members want and need information. Providing this information is called *content counseling* or *informational counseling* and is vital to audiologic rehabilitation.

Non-professional audiologic counseling: Helping patients "own their hearing loss" and advance to problem solving.

Professional boundaries: Notable distinctions between professions as they approach common areas of concern.

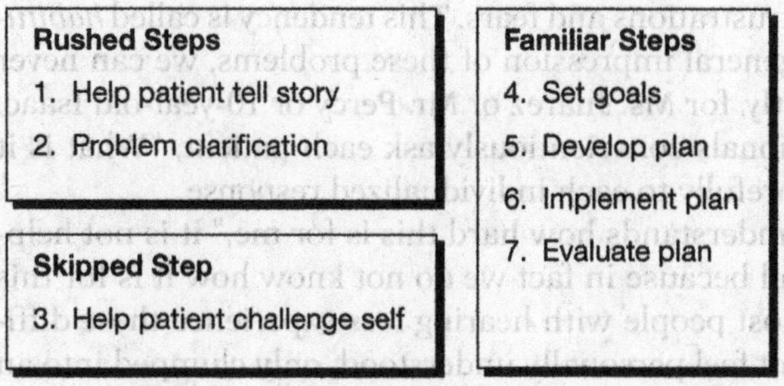

Rushed Steps

1. Help patient tell story
2. Problem clarification

Skipped Step

3. Help patient challenge self

Familiar Steps

4. Set goals
5. Develop plan
6. Implement plan
7. Evaluate plan

FIGURE 7.4 The counseling process as it might be applied to some audiologic rehabilitation situations.

The primary characteristic of content counseling is its tendency to become a one-way direction of communication (i.e., the professional talks, and the patient or parent listens). If a patient or parent wants to talk about any of the psychosocial or emotional concerns discussed previously, how is he or she to interact with this one-way stream of information? It isn't possible, so when personal adjustment issues present themselves, another direction in communication needs to be made available, a two-way conversation in which the parent or client can talk more and the counselors talk less. This two-way direction of interaction is a key component of personal adjustment counseling.

What Counselors Say Counseling Is

The counseling profession describes this kind of two-way conversation as a facilitative process, whereby the patient is given room, time, and permission to "tell his story." Stone, Patton, and Heen (2010) call this process "developing a learning conversation." In our context, we encourage the patients or parents to teach us what life with hearing loss is like for them and what their concerns are at that moment. This approach respects patients and parents as the experts of their lives and requires us to drop our assumptions that we somehow know how they feel.

The Counseling Process

The facilitative or counseling process (Figure 7.4) involves the following steps (adapted from Egan, 2014):

1. Help patients tell their story.
2. Help patients clarify their problems.
3. Help patients take responsibility for their listening problems (challenge themselves).
4. Help patients establish their goals.
5. Develop an action plan.
6. Implement the plan.
7. Conduct ongoing evaluation.

Readers will notice that the CARE model described in Chapter 1 includes these steps under "C" (counseling). Without care and reflection, audiologic rehabilitation may rush through steps 1 and 2, bypass step 3, and pick up again at step 4; in other words, the professional may assume that he or she already knows the patient's story and begin setting goals immediately (taking over the rehabilitation or adjustment process rather than developing a partnership with the patient).

Long-term success in adjusting to hearing loss may ultimately depend on the effective management of the first three steps because they usually involve an understanding of the psychological and emotional impact of living with a hearing loss. This chapter concludes with a discussion of how to incorporate these steps in audiologic rehabilitation.

Help Patients (or Parents) Tell Their Story. Every patient and every parent has a unique perspective on living with a hearing loss. There is an inherent danger for professionals to assume that "we've heard it all before" and therefore that we truly understand their struggles and frustrations and fears. This tendency is called *habituation*. While we surely have a general impression of these problems, we can never know what it is really like, exactly, for Ms. Juarez or Mr. Percy or 10-year-old Isaac. It is essential first that professionals conscientiously ask each patient, "What is it like for you?" and then listen carefully to each individualized response.

If a patient says, "No one understands how hard this is for me," it is not helpful to say that we do understand because in fact we do not know how it is for this patient. A response such as "Most people with hearing loss experience these difficulties" does not help the patient feel personally understood, only clumped into an impersonal category of "others." A response that focuses only on the patient, such as "You are having a tough time right now," gives the patient the message that he or she was heard and understood.

Using a *self-assessment* instrument can be very helpful in providing the opportunity for a patient to tell his or her story. While a patient takes the time to consider and describe his or her communication problems (part of step 2), that person is also provided the opportunity to expand on the items that are of particular concern. Describing one's communication difficulties is an act of personal self-disclosure that may make a patient feel uncomfortable; however, the exercise of reading and talking about a standardized, neutral set of questions can take the pressure off because both patient and professional are looking at the instrument rather than at each other. Many examples of self-assessments are provided in this text. See the Appendix at the end of this chapter for a version designed for teenagers with hearing loss.

Self-assessments: Paper-and-pencil questionnaires or surveys to help persons describe their listening problems to themselves and others.

Help Patients Clarify Their Problems. Because the development of hearing loss in adults can occur slowly over several years, because parents of children with hearing loss have a complicated life to juggle, or because children with hearing loss have limited experience in expressing their feelings and concerns, considerable time is needed to help individuals describe and clarify their actual communication problems as well as their emotional reactions to them and the psychosocial ramifications. Earlier, self-assessment instruments were mentioned as a strategy to help patients tell their stories—and, as they tell their stories, not only are they being heard, but they are also getting clear in their minds what these problems are. Many instruments are available. For example, the Abbreviated Profile of Hearing Aid Benefit (APHAB;Cox & Alexander, 1995) poses 24 statements in the areas of ease of communication and communicating in adverse conditions (background noise, reverberation, etc.). An example of such a statement is "I have trouble hearing a conversation when I am with family at home." The patient describes his or her perception from "Always" to "Never" and receives the opportunity to recognize that such difficulties are a common aspect of living with a hearing loss. Many instruments open the door to a discussion about psychosocial reactions to hearing loss; for example, the Self-Assessment of Communication (SAC; Schow & Nerbonne, 1982) asks this question: "Does any problem or difficulty with your hearing upset you?" Responses range from "Almost always" to "Almost never," and it is up to the patient to decide whether he or she is comfortable with this kind of self-disclosure.

Formal self-assessment measures are not the only way to help patients to clarify their problems; conversation and carefully selected questions can also provide this opportunity. The point here is that patients need to understand their problems before they can develop solutions for them.

Help Patients Take Responsibility for Their Listening Problems. Once patients clarify their communication and/or interpersonal problems, it might be assumed that they are ready to solve them. However, we have already learned that the psychosocial and emotional aspects of hearing loss can interfere with logical problem solving (using hearing aids to their best advantage etc.). There is a real risk at this stage for the professional to take over and tell the patient or parent what to do: obtain and use hearing aids, learn sign language, or enroll in speechreading classes, for example. But like any other personal problem, the patient has to accept responsibility for the

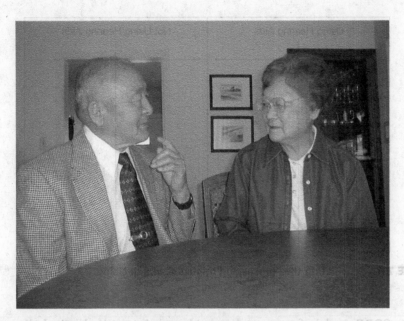

Good communication is vital in understanding the impact of hearing loss.

problem in order to commit him- or herself to the solution. Far too often, patients agree to purchase hearing aids but with no personal commitment or sincere intention to use them. It is possible that there are more hearing aids in drawers than on ears.

Another behavior that indicates that patients are not yet assuming the responsibilities of living with hearing loss is the common complaint that communication breakdowns occur because other people speak too softly or mumble or children speak too quickly and with high voices. As long as the patient insists that everyone else should just speak more clearly, he or she is shirking his or her own role in successful communication. To help patients move past this stage of inaction, audiologic rehabilitation must take its cue from other helping professions and place *responsibility for successful rehabilitation* squarely on the patient. Once the problems have been clarified, we must ask, "And now, what are *your* listening goals? As you identify them, I will support you in attaining these goals."

This may be the point where the adult patient says, "I want to hear my grandchildren when they visit—but I won't wear hearing aids." He has identified two goals, and (for the purpose of our discussion), unfortunately, they are incompatible. The ultimate decision is still his: He won't be able to hear his grandchildren without amplification, so what does he want to do about that? No amount of persuading will make a genuine difference; the patient has to find the internal resources to commit to his decision.

Not all adults struggle with the cosmetics of hearing aids, but, if they do, they can be encouraged to conduct a type of cost–benefit analysis: that is, compare the social costs of hearing aid use to the listening benefits that they seek. Which provides the outcome more valuable to them? If the listening benefits are perceived as greater, they might be more willing to tolerate the social costs of hearing aid appearances. Figure 7.5 gives an example of this activity.

Another way to describe this thought process is called "substituting *and* for *but*," that is, trading the word *but* for the word *and*. Initially, an adult may believe, "I want to hear my grandchildren better, *but* I dislike how these hearing aids look." This way of thinking pits one condition against the other, and they mutually exclude each other. The adult could be asked to try thinking in these terms: "I want to hear my grandchildren better, *and* I dislike how these hearing aids look." Including the possibility of both conditions coexisting at the same time gives the adult another way to look at the situation, one that could move her past a mental block to one that could help her to meet her goals (Kelly, 1992).

Patients must assume responsibility for their hearing problem before they will genuinely engage in the effort to improve their situation.

Some amplification goals can be accomplished with assistive devices when hearing aids are not accepted.

Using Hearing Aids		Not Using Hearing Aids	
+	−	+	−

FIGURE 7.5 Articulating the "pluses and minuses" of a decision.

The CORE model of assessment considers patient attitudes, including readiness for change. Professionals must appreciate that some patients struggle with change and would rather avoid it if possible. An empathetic, nonjudgmental attitude on our part can help patients face their fears and consider "taking the plunge."

When to Refer

It is not uncommon for patients to present with difficulties that cannot be accounted for by the hearing loss alone. Marital problems, family dissension, parenting dilemmas, financial or legal stress, fragile emotional and mental health—all these situations can be made worse by the presence of hearing loss, but treating the hearing loss will not resolve the fundamental problems.

Harvey (2008) provides some helpful guidelines regarding the referral process:

1. Be prepared and develop a list of qualified professionals before a need arises. Confirm that these colleagues understand the implications of hearing loss and its effects on social isolation, self-efficacy, and depression.
2. Rehearse a few ways to broach the subject, such as "What you are discussing right now is beyond my area of expertise. I do know someone who is qualified to help you; I'd like to give you that phone number."
3. Normalize (destigmatize) the referral and "humanize" mental health professionals ("I've known Dr. B for years; he is very kind and helpful").

There is no easy answer to the question "When should I refer to a professional counselor?"; however, the answer is apparent when the professional sees a situation outside his or her expertise and scope of practice. It is strongly recommended that a referral system be established in advance so that when the need to refer arises, a phone contact is immediately provided to the patient. This preparation will suggest to the patient that an outside referral is not rare and that the professional is aware of and is adhering to his or her professional boundaries.

DOES COUNSELING MAKE A DIFFERENCE?

Research indicates that counseling as described here makes a positive difference in a patient's progress. Effective counseling helps the audiologist develop common ground with the patient and enhance trust building. Not surprisingly, the degree to which patients trust health care providers is directly related to their decision to follow our recommendations (Zolnierek & DiMatteo, 2009). In other words, the more patients trust their audiologists, the more likely they will consider hearing aids, accept hearing aid limitations, use communication repair strategies, protect their hearing from noise, and listen to other provider recommendations. Patients often struggle with audiologic rehabilitation and may abandon the struggle if they don't experience genuine trust with the audiologist, so our efforts to earn and keep that trust are an investment in their success.

Concluding Remarks

The second half of this chapter takes the reader beyond an awareness of patients' psychosocial difficulties with hearing loss to an awareness of how the professional's interactions with patients can support (or hinder) their adjustment process. The basic concepts were these: listen carefully as the patient tells her story, help her identify her listening problems, and help her assume ownership for her problems so that she can commit to the solutions. If a professional finds herself wondering, "If this patient didn't want these hearing aids, why did she come for an evaluation in the first place?" the professional did not spend time in the beginning to hear the patient's story (i.e., her perception of her problems) and whether she was ready to take on the challenge of adjusting to hearing aid use. Following the counseling process through each step will lead to a deeper and more accurate understanding between patient and professional and facilitate the development of a therapeutic relationship with mutual goals.

Summary Points

- Many persons with hearing loss experience a range of psychological, social, or emotional difficulties, although it is impossible to know exactly how a hearing loss affects a particular individual unless he or she specifically tells us.

- Because of resultant language delays, children with hearing loss may experience difficulties with self-expression and self-awareness, which can affect their ability to empathize with others and to achieve age-appropriate social skills.

- Adults who acquire hearing loss may also experience problems as they adjust to the consequences of the disability, including the acceptance of hearing aids and a sense of stigma.

- The Deaf culture sees hearing loss not as a disability but rather as a difference in abilities. Like other communities, its members share core values and traditions and also share the use of a common language (ASL).

- Counseling techniques are often used to help patients accept and develop solutions for their listening problems.

- Self-assessment questionnaires give patients an opportunity to tell their story and clarify their problems.

- Patients are more likely to accept recommendations if they feel they have been listened to and respected.

Supplementary Learning Activities

See www.isu.edu/csed/audiology/rehab to carry out these activities. We encourage you to use these to supplement your learning. Your instructor may give specific assignments that involve a particular activity.

1. Empathy exercise: view a video created by the Cleveland Clinic.
   Title: Empathy: The Human Connection to Patient Care
   URL: https://www.youtube.com/watch?v=cDDWvj_q-o8

   Then ask someone close to you to view it as well and discuss it. Would you describe the video as impactful, and, if so, why? What memories did it trigger; what insights did you both glean?

2. Figure 7.5 is an empty grid that helps people sort out the pluses and minuses of making a decision. Sketch out this grid on a blank piece of paper. Put yourself in the "shoes" of a woman, age 55, who works as a nurse of the post-op floor of a typical hospital. She has a bilateral moderate hearing loss but has not yet decided to get hearing help. Fill out the grid as she might fill it out. If either column is significantly longer than the other, keep thinking. When we genuinely empathize with others, we will see more concerns through their eyes than we see with our own.

3. Ask a study partner to role-play a 14-year-old male with a hearing loss who has decided not to use his hearing aids anymore. The study partner then completes the Self-Assessment of Communication—Adolescent (see Appendix). Discuss the answers. What did you and the study partner not consider before? If this teen indicated "almost never" to most situations, what does that tell us?

Recommended Reading

Audiologic Counseling

Clark, J., & English, K. (2014). *Counseling-infused audiologic care*. Boston: Allyn & Bacon.

Flasher, L., & Fogle, P. (2011) *Counseling skills for speech-language pathologists and audiologists* (2nd ed.). New York: Thomson/Delmar Learning.

Luterman, D. M. (2008). *Counseling persons with communication disorders and their children* (5th ed.). Austin, TX: PRO-ED.

Psychology of Deafness

Harvey, M. (2003). *Psychotherapy with deaf and hard of hearing persons: A systemic model* (2nd ed.). Mahwah, NJ: Lawrence Erlbaum Associates.

Leigh, I. (2009). *A lens on Deaf identities: Perspectives on Deafness*. Oxford: Oxford University Press.

Shirmer, B. (2001). *Psychological, social, and educational dimensions of deafness*. Boston: Allyn & Bacon.

Deaf Culture

Dirkson, H., Baumann, L., & Murray. J. (Eds.). (2014). *Deaf gain: Raising the stakes for human diversity*. Minneapolis: University of Minnesota Press.

Greenberg, J. (1970). *In this sign*. New York: Holt, Rinehart and Winston.

Holcomb, R. (2011). *Deaf culture our way* (4th ed.). San Diego, CA: Dawn Sign Press.

Leigh, I., Andrews, J., & Harris, R. (2016). *Deaf culture: Exploring deaf communities in the United States*. San Diego, CA: Plural Publishing.

Matlin, M. (2002). *Deaf child crossing*. New York: Simon & Schuster.

Oliva, G. (2004). *Alone in the mainstream: A Deaf woman remembers public school*. Washington, DC: Gallaudet University Press.

Padden, C., & Humphries, T. (2005). *Inside deaf culture*. Cambridge, MA: Harvard University Press.

Preston, P. (1995). *Mother father deaf: Living between sound and silence*. Cambridge, MA: Harvard University Press.

Recommended Websites

Association of Late Deafened Adults:
http://www.alda.org

Hands and Voices:
http://www.handsandvoices.org

Hearing Loss Association of America:

http://www.hearingloss.org

Ida Institute:

http://idainstitute.com

National Association of the Deaf:

http://www.nad.org

Gallaudet University:

http://www.gallaudet.edu

References

Abrahms, H. B., & Kihm, J. (2015). An introduction to MarkeTrak IX: A new baseline for the hearing aid market. Hearing Review, 22(6), 16.

Bachara, G., Raphael, J., & Phelan, W. (1980). Empathy development in deaf preadolescents. *American Annals of the Deaf, 125*, 38–41.

Barlow, J., Turner, A., Hammond, C., & Gailey, L. (2007). Living with late deafness: Insight from between worlds. *International Journal of Audiology, 46*(8), 442–448.

Batten, G., Oakes, P., & Alexander, T. (2014). Factors associated with social interactions between deaf children and their hearing peers: A systematic literature review. *Journal of Deaf Studies and Deaf Education, 19*(3), 285–304.

Becker, G. (1980). *Growing old in silence.* Berkeley: University of California Press.

Bess, F. H., Dodd-Murphy, J., & Parker, R. (1998). Children with minimal sensorineural hearing loss: Prevalence, educational performance, and functional status. *Ear and Hearing, 19*(5), 339–355.

Blood, G. W., Blood, M., & Danhauser, J. L. (1977). The hearing aid "effect." *Hearing Instruments, 20*, 12.

Cappelli, M., Daniels, T., Durleux-Smith, A., McGrath, P. J., & Neuss, D. (1995). Social development of children with hearing impairments who are integrated into general education classrooms. *Volta Review, 97*, 197–208.

Cormier, S. (2014). *Counseling strategies and interventions for professional helpers* (9th ed.). Boston: Allyn & Bacon.

Cox, R., & Alexander, O. (1995). The Abbreviated Profile of Hearing Aid Benefit. *Ear and Hearing, 16*, 176–186.

Crowe, T. (1997). Approaches to counseling. In T. Crowe (Ed.), *Applications in counseling in speech-language pathology and audiology* (pp. 80–117). Baltimore: Williams & Wilkins.

Doggett, S., Stein, R., & Gans, D. (1998). Hearing aid effect in older females. *Journal of the American Academy of Audiology, 9*(5), 361–366.

Egan, G. (2014). *The skilled helper* (10th ed.). Belmont, CA: Brooks/Cole.

Elkayam, J., & English, K. (2003). Counseling adolescents with hearing loss with the use of self-assessment/significant other questionnaires. *Journal of the American Academy of Audiology, 9*(14), 485–499.

English, K. (2012). Self-advocacy for students who are deaf and hard of hearing. Retrieved from http://gozips.uakron.edu/~ke3/Self-Advocacy.pdf

Fellinger, J., Holtzinger, D., Sattel, H. & Laucht, M. (2008). Mental health and quality of life in deaf pupils. *European Child and Adolescent Psychiatry, 17*, 414–423.

Glass, L., & Elliot, H. (1992). The professional told me what it was but that was not enough. *Shhh, 13*(6), 26–28.

Goleman, D. (2006). *Emotional intelligence: Why it can matter more than IQ.* New York: Bantam Books.

Greenberg, M. T., & Kusche, C. A. (1993). *Promoting social and emotional development in deaf children: The PATHS project.* Seattle: University of Washington Press.

Harris, L. K., Van Zandt, C. E., & Rees, T. H. (1997). Counseling needs of students who are deaf and hard of hearing. *School Counselor, 44*, 271–279.

Harvey, M. (2008). How to refer patients successfully to mental health professionals. Retrieved from http://www.hearingreview.com/2008/07/how-to-refer-patients-successfully-to-mental-health-professionals

Hoffman, M., Quittner, A., & Cejas, I. (2015). Comparisons of social competencies in young children with and without hearing loss: A dynamic systems framework. *Journal of Deaf Studies and Deaf Education, 20*(2), 115–124.

Kelly, L. J. (1992). Rational-emotive therapy and aural rehabilitation. *Journal of the Academy of Rehabilitative Audiology, 25,* 43–50.

Kennedy, E., & Charles, S. (2001). *On becoming a counselor: A basic guide for non-professional counselors and other helpers* (3rd ed.). New York: Crosswords Publishing.

Kochkin S. (2012). MarkeTrak VIII: The key influencing factors in hearing aid purchase intent. *Hearing Review, 7*(3), 12–25.

Kricos, P. B. (2000). Family counseling for children with hearing loss. In J. Alpiner & P. A. McCarthy (Eds.), *Rehabilitative audiology: Children and adults* (3rd ed., pp. 275–302). Philadelphia: Lippincott Williams & Wilkins.

Kübler-Ross, E. (1969). *On death and dying.* New York: Macmillan.

Kunnen, E. S. (2014). Identity development in deaf adolescents. *Journal of Deaf Studies and Deaf Education, 19*(4), 496–507.

Leigh, I., Andrews, J., & Harris, R. (2016). *Deaf culture: Exploring deaf communities in the United States.* San Diego, CA: Plural Publishing.

Luckner, J., & Sebald, A. (2013). Promoting self-determination of students who are deaf or hard of hearing. *American Annals of the Deaf, 158*(3), 377–386.

Luterman, D. L. (2008). *Counseling persons with communication disorders and their families* (5th ed.). Austin, TX: PRO-ED.

Meadow, K. (1976). Personality and social development of deaf persons. *Journal of Rehabilitation of the Deaf, 9,* 3–16.

Merrell, K. W. (2007). *Strong teens, grades 9–12: A social and emotional learning curriculum.* Baltimore: Paul H. Brookes.

Mitchell, R., & Karchmer, M. (2004). Chasing the mythical ten percent: Parental hearing status of deaf and hard of hearing students in the United States. *Sign Language Studies, 4*(2), 138–163.

National Center for Special Education Research. (2011). *The secondary school experiences and academic performance of students with hearing impairments: Facts from the National Longitudinal Study 2 (NLTS-2).* Washington, DC: U.S. Department of Education.

Paasch, L., & Toe, D. (2014). A comparison of pragmatic abilities of children who are deaf or hard of hearing and their hearing peers. *Journal of Deaf Studies and Deaf Education, 19*(1), 1–18.

Pajevic, E., & English, K. (2014). Teens as health care consumers: Planned transition and empowerment. *Audiology Today, 26*(6), 14–18.

Pipp-Siegel, S., & Biringen, Z. (2000). Assessing the quality of relationships between parents and children: The Emotional Availability Scales [Monograph]. *Volta Review, 100*(5), 237–249.

Ramsdell, P. (1960). The psychology of the hard of hearing and the deafened adult. In H. Davis & S. Silverman (Eds.), *Hearing and deafness* (pp. 459–473). New York: Holt, Rinehart and Winston.

Riensche, L., Peterson, K., & Linden, S. (1990) Young children's attitudes toward peer hearing aid wearers. *Hearing Journal, 43*(10), 19–20.

Schow, R., & Nerbonne, M. (1982). Communication screening profile: Use with elderly clients. *Ear and Hearing, 3,* 135–147.

Stein, R., Gill, K., & Gans, D. (2000). Adolescents' attitudes toward their peers with hearing impairment. *Journal of Educational Audiology, 8,* 1–6.

Stinson, M. S., Whitmore, K., & Kluwin, T. N. (1996). Self perceptions of social relationships in hearing-impaired adolescents. *Journal of Educational Psychology, 88*(1), 132–143.

Stone, D., Patton, B., & Heen, S. (2010). *Difficult conversations: How to discuss what matters most* (2nd ed.). New York: Viking.

Stone, J. R., & Olswang, L. B. (1989). The hidden challenge in counseling. *Asha, 31,* 27–31.

Vernon, M., & Andrews, J. (1990). *The psychology of deafness: Understanding deaf and hard of hearing people.* New York: Longman.

Wallhagen, M. I. (2010). The stigma of hearing loss. *Gerontologist, 50*(1), 66–75.

Warren, C., & Hasenstab, S. (1986). Self-concept of severely to profoundly hearing impaired children. *Volta Review, 88,* 289–296.

Zolnierek, K. B., & DiMatteo, M. R. (2009). Physician communication and patient adherence to treatment: A meta-analysis. *Medical Care, 47*(8), 826–834.

APPENDIX

Self Assessment of Communication—Adolescent (SAC-A)*

Judy Elkayam, AuD, and Kris English, PhD (2003)

The purpose of this questionnaire is to identify problems you may be having because of your hearing loss. We will talk about your answers. That conversation may help us understand the effect the hearing loss is having on you. It may also give us ideas to help you manage those problems. The information you give will not affect your grades in school.

Please circle the most appropriate answer for each of the following questions. Select only one answer for each question. If you usually use hearing aids or cochlear implants, answer each question in a way that describes your experiences with the technology on. If you do not usually use hearing aids or cochlear implants, answer each question in a way that describes your experiences without the technology.

Student Name _____ Date _____

TECHNOLOGY USE

I usually do/do not use hearing aid(s). I usually do/do not use cochlear implant(s).

HEARING AND UNDERSTANDING AT DIFFERENT TIMES

1. Is it hard for you to hear or understand when talking with only one other person?
   1 = almost never 2 = occasionally 3 = about half the time 4 = frequently 5 = almost always

2. Is it hard for you to hear or understand when talking with a group of people?
   1 = almost never 2 = occasionally 3 = about half the time 4 = frequently 5 = almost always

3. Is it hard for you to hear or understand TV, the radio ,or CDs?
   1 = almost never 2 = occasionally 3 = about half the time 4 = frequently 5 = almost always

4. Is it hard for you to hear or understand if there is noise or music in the background or other people are talking at the same time?
   1 = almost never 2 = occasionally 3 = about half the time 4 = frequently 5 = almost always

5. Is it hard for you to hear or understand in your classes?
   1 = almost never 2 = occasionally 3 = about half the time 4 = frequently 5 = almost always

6. Do you hear better when using your hearing aids or cochlear implants?
   1 = almost never 2 = occasionally 3 = about half the time 4 = frequently 5 = almost always

FEELINGS ABOUT COMMUNICATION

7. Do you feel left out of conversations because it's hard to hear?
   1 = almost never 2 = occasionally 3 = about half the time 4 = frequently 5 = almost always

8. Does anything about your hearing loss upset you?
   1 = almost never 2 = occasionally 3 = about half the time 4 = frequently 5 = almost always

9. Do you feel different from other kids when you are wearing your hearing aids or cochlear implants?
   1 = almost never 2 = occasionally 3 = about half the time 4 = frequently 5 = almost always

* Modified, with permission, from Self Assessment of Communication (Schow & Nerbonne, 1982).

OTHER PEOPLE

10. Do strangers or people you don't know well notice that you have a hearing loss?
   1 = almost never 2 = occasionally 3 = about half the time 4 = frequently 5 = almost always

11. Do other people become frustrated when they talk to you because of your hearing loss?
   1 = almost never 2 = occasionally 3 = about half the time 4 = frequently 5 = almost always

12. Do people treat you differently when you wear your hearing aids or cochlear implants?
   1 = almost never 2 = occasionally 3 = about half the time 4 = frequently 5 = almost always

Audiologic Rehabilitation Services in the School Setting

Kris English

CONTENTS

Visit the companion website when you see this icon to learn more about the topic nearby in the text.

Learning Outcomes

After reading this chapter, you will be able to

- List the key components of the Individuals with Disabilities Education Act
- Describe what the "least restrictive environment" implies for educating children with hearing loss
- Identify the common placement options utilized in educating children with hearing loss (which is the most frequently used?)
- Describe what an Individualized Education Plan and Individualized Education Plan Committee are and explain their relevance in educating a child with hearing loss
- Define and distinguish between the oral-aural communication and total communication options (Listening and Spoken Language, or LSL)
- Describe the influence that classroom acoustics can have on the education of those with hearing loss
- Distinguish between personal and sound field FM systems
- List at least four out of twelve common behaviors frequently exhibited by children with auditory processing disorders
- List four key areas of responsibility typically carried out by an educational audiologist

INTRODUCTION

Research has confirmed that when a hearing loss is identified early and when amplification and early intervention are in place by 6 months of age, a child is much more likely to acquire age-level language and learning milestones (Moeller, Carr, Seaver, Stradler-Brown, & Holzinger, 2013). This kind of aggressive management is just the start of many years of audiologic rehabilitative (AR) services as a child progresses through the educational system. Readers are encouraged to relate this chapter's content to the two rehabilitation models discussed in Chapter 1. For example, education is one of the variables included in the "O" in CORE (for Overall Participation Variables), and in both the CORE and the CARE models, the "E" (Environment) is addressed when considering classroom acoustics.

This chapter examines school-based audiologic rehabilitative (AR) services by addressing three questions:

- *Why* are AR services required in school settings?
- *What* AR services are provided in schools?
- *Who* is responsible for AR services in the school environment?

WHY AR SERVICES ARE REQUIRED IN SCHOOL SETTINGS: THE EDUCATIONAL CONSEQUENCES OF HEARING LOSS

Hearing loss is considered to be an educationally significant disability. Unless immersed at home and at school in a signing environment, children learn language through the auditory system. If the auditory input is distorted or inconsistent, the child can experience a variety of difficulties in language development, such as reduced vocabulary development, delayed syntax development, and inappropriate use of morphological markers and figurative speech (Trussell & Esterbrooks, 2016).

deaf: Having a bilateral profound hearing loss. Deaf: Having a cultural identification with the Deaf community and a bilateral profound hearing loss.

Because most academic success depends on a competent use of language, these deficits in a child's language development can have a direct effect on cognitive development (learning). Children with hearing loss have often been found to have depressed math scores and reading levels (Moeller, 2007). In the twenty-first century, our futures depend on the ability to acquire and use a broad information base; thus, children with hearing loss start out with a marked disadvantage. AR services are needed now more than ever to help children stay competitive in school and in the marketplace.

Hearing Loss and Learning

Minimal hearing loss: When a child cannot hear sounds that are greater in intensity than 20 dB HL.

There is a strong relationship between the degree of hearing loss and the degree of educational impact: The more severe the loss, the more difficult learning can be. However, it would be a mistake to assume that a slight hearing loss would have little or no impact on learning; even a *minimal* or mild loss can put a child at risk for academic failure (McFadden & Pittman, 2008). A study of 1,218 children with minimal hearing loss showed that 37 percent had failed a grade (Bess, Dodd-Murphy, & Parker, 1998). In addition, a statistically high number had poorer communication skills than children with no hearing loss, and, as a group, they exhibited more problems in stress, social support, and self-esteem. We are learning that any type of hearing loss presents the risk of academic failure and psychosocial difficulties, and no loss can be discounted as insignificant (Moeller, 2007).

We cannot even assume that children with hearing loss in only one ear, with normal hearing in the other ear (unilateral hearing loss), are not experiencing academic difficulties (Lieu, 2004). It was once thought that one normal ear was sufficient; however, it has been found that children with unilateral hearing loss are 10 times more likely to fail a grade by age 10 compared to normal-hearing children (Bess, Klee, & Culbertson, 1986; English & Church, 1999; Yoshinaga-Itano, Johnson, & Brown, 2008).

> While the degree of hearing loss is an important variable to consider, it would be a mistake to use it by itself as a predictor of academic achievement or as a determiner of the level of support provided by a school.

The exact prevalence rate depends on how hearing loss is defined; for example, some states include in their census children with unilateral hearing loss or mild conductive hearing loss, while others do not. Some states consider hearing loss to be present when a child does not respond to a pure tone at 15, 20, or 25 dB HL. Depending on the screening methods and definitions of hearing loss, studies have described incidence rates ranging from 3 to 15 percent (Johnson, 2000). If a conservative estimated prevalence rate of 3 to 4 percent is used, this would mean that among the 50 million schoolchildren in the United States, at least 1.5 million to 2 million children have some degree of hearing loss.

Mandated by Law

Because hearing loss is an educationally significant disability, by federal law these children are entitled to a free appropriate public education (FAPE), which means access to "special education and related services which are provided at public supervision and direction, and without charge" (Individuals with Disabilities Education Act [IDEA], 34 CFR § 300, 4[a]). In other words, the services needed to support the education of a child with hearing loss are paid for by public funds rather than by parents. The term *appropriate* is intentionally left undefined with the understanding that each child's educational plan will be based on individual requirements. Some of the related services include a range of AR services, to be discussed in a subsequent section.

The law under discussion is IDEA. It was first enacted in 1975 as the Education for All Handicapped Children Act (Public Law [PL] 94-142). Before PL 94-142 was passed, parents who had children with disabilities were frequently denied the right to enroll their children in the public school system. The passage of PL 94-142 was a milestone in ongoing efforts to protect the rights of all persons with disabilities. The actual law can be located in Volume 34 of the Code of Federal Regulations (CFR), found in all law school libraries and many general university and public libraries as well as on the Internet. The volume is divided into sections, designated with the "§" symbol. Readers are encouraged to refer to this original source as they develop a background in special education issues.

IDEA (Individuals with Disabilities Education Act): Guarantees educational rights to children with disabilities.

The mandate of a free appropriate public education (FAPE) was described earlier as a key component of this law. A second mandate, directly related to our discussion of AR services, can be found in 34 CFR § 300.113: "Each public agency must ensure that hearing aids . . . and external components of surgically implanted medical devices are functioning properly." This requirement has often been the door opener to AR services in school settings. If a parent asks, "How is your school meeting this requirement?," the school (the "public agency") must demonstrate that it has a program in place to monitor and check hearing aid and classroom amplification systems.

The U.S. Congress is required to reauthorize this law every few years, allowing for the opportunity to refine, update, and possibly expand on the original version. The first reauthorization occurred in 1986, when the Education of the Handicapped Amendments (PL 99-457) were passed. All educational services, including audiologic rehabilitation, were expanded to include children from birth to 5 years of age. This development formally brought audiologic rehabilitation into the area of early intervention services for infants and toddlers and their families.

The next reauthorization occurred in 1990. At this time, the law (PL 101-476) was renamed the Individuals with Disabilities Education Act (IDEA). This law used

People-first language: An identification of an individual before the mention of a disability.

the term "disability" rather than "handicap" and substituted the term "children with disabilities" for "handicapped children," codifying the use of *people-first language*. Persons with disabilities asked for this change, preferring to be considered persons first who also happen to have a disability. Terms such as "autistic children" or "the hearing impaired" are now revised to say "children with autism" or "individuals with hearing loss."

Amendments to IDEA were passed in 1997, and the changes included requirements to make educational goals as functional as possible (i.e., related to classroom performance and classroom expectations). It also required programs to provide progress reports at least as often as parents are informed of the progress of children without disabilities and to include the general education teacher in meetings to ensure integration of special education goals into the general education curriculum.

In 2004, IDEA was again reauthorized and is now officially known as the Individuals with Disabilities Education Improvement Act (IDEIA). For consistency, it is typically referred to as IDEA 2004 (Wright, 2004). Its amendments align special education law with the 2001 No Child Left Behind Act, which requires teachers to use scientifically proven instructional practices and requires each student's progress to be measured and reported. By law, IDEA will continue to be reexamined every four or five years to ensure that children with hearing loss and other disabilities receive an appropriate education. A time line of these legislative events can be found in Table 8.1.

Key Components of IDEA

Throughout these reauthorizations, three critical components have remained constant. The first was the guarantee of a FAPE, which was discussed previously. The other two components are these:

- The FAPE is to be provided in the least restrictive environment
- A child's education plan will be documented with the use of the Individualized Education Program (IEP)

Least Restrictive Environment

LRE (least restrictive environment): Where the child has most access to academic, social, and emotional support.

The concept of *least restrictive environment* (LRE) is often considered synonymous with *mainstreaming*, or educating children with disabilities in a local public school among children without disabilities. However, it is important to note that IDEA does not mandate mainstreaming per se but simply the consideration of the LRE for the most appropriate education. Therefore, LRE is essentially open to interpretation and consequently remains imprecise.

Educational Options. To help schools make educational placement decisions, the Code of Federal Regulations (CFR) states the following: "Each public agency shall insure that a continuum of alternative placements is available to meet the needs

TABLE 8.1 Time Line of Special Education Legislative Acts

Year	Law
1975	PL 94-142: Education of All Handicapped Children Act
1986	PL 99-457: Education of Handicapped Act Amendments (birth to age 5)
1990	PL 101-476: Individuals with Disabilities Education Act (IDEA)
1997	PL 105-71: IDEA 1997 Amendments
2004	PL 108-446: Individuals with Disabilities Education Improvement Act (IDEIA)

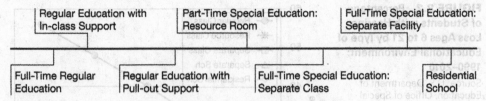

FIGURE 8.1   Continuum of educational placements.

of children with disabilities for special education and related services" (34 CFR § 300.551[a]). Placement options include variations of the following settings:

- Full-time regular education classroom in the child's neighborhood school.
- Regular education with in-class support, such as instruction from a speech-language pathologist or teacher of children who are deaf or hard of hearing
- Regular education, with pull-out sessions held in another classroom.
- Part-time regular education classroom and part-time special education in a resource room.
- Full-time special education in a separate or self-contained classroom held by a teacher of children with hearing loss, with a small number of other children with hearing loss, often in the child's general neighborhood.
- Full-time special education in a separate facility (often called a *center-based program*), not necessarily in the child's neighborhood.
- Residential school, with a large number of children with hearing loss and many teachers of children with hearing loss. Some children live on campus during the week; some attend as day students.

The LRE continuum is represented in Figure 8.1.

In the first 15 years of special education, placement decisions considered the concept of mainstreaming as a move from special education to regular education. That is, children with hearing loss would most likely be placed in a special education environment, and as the child demonstrated grade-level competencies in math or in reading, he or she would gradually spend more time in a regular education classroom. In the past three decades, there has been a reconsideration of this concept, and now the philosophy of *inclusion* is being applied, resulting in the primary placement of the child in a regular education program and the provision of supports or special services as needed to help the child succeed in this placement. Only when it is clear that individualized or small-group instruction is necessary is the child taken from the class and provided help in resource room instruction or other educational placements.

LRE continuum: A range of educational options, from regular education in one's neighborhood to a residential school.

Case 8.1. Laurie

Laurie is 5 years old and has a severe bilateral hearing loss, identified before her first birthday. She has received a range of services from that time, wears two hearing aids all day, is currently enrolled in a kindergarten program in her neighborhood, and is also receiving therapy consistent with an auditory–verbal approach (i.e., a strong emphasis on developing listening skills) in a private clinic. Her language development is delayed but measurably improving, and her social skills are age appropriate. Her mother has been told by school officials that the first-grade placement should be at a specialized program, which would involve a bus ride of over an hour both ways. This placement would use sign language in its instruction, but Laurie's parents have been committed to an auditory–verbal approach for four years. They are therefore opposed to this placement recommendation because of the distance and because of the communication methods used. They will have to meet with the school administrators to make their case, and because they have learned their rights, they expect their understanding of the term "least restrictive environment" to carry the day.

FIGURE 8.2 Percentage of Students with Hearing Loss Ages 6 to 21 by Type of Educational Environment: 1990–2010

Source: U.S. Department of Education, Office of Special Education Programs.

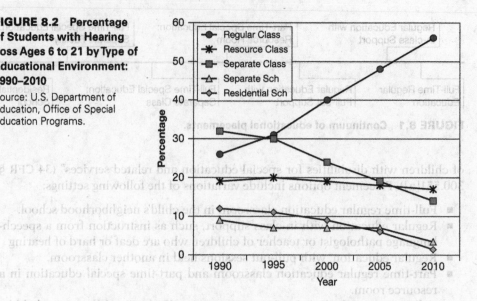

"Other environments" includes separate school, residential school, homebound/hospital environment, correctional facilities, and parentally placed in private schools.

Figure 8.2 gives the distributions of students with hearing loss across a variety of educational placements (U.S. Department of Education, 2015). It shows a steady trend toward placing children with hearing loss in regular education classrooms. Research supports the effectiveness of inclusive classroom placements, but the concept is not without its dissenters. Interpreters of this regulation repeatedly caution that it is not appropriate to generalize about LRE among children with hearing loss. *The determination of the LRE for each child must be made on an individual basis.*

LRE for a Child with Hearing Loss. For a child with a hearing loss, the preceding interpretation of least LRE may not be appropriate. A child with a mild to moderately severe hearing loss may succeed in a regular education classroom if full support is provided to address the variety of language and listening needs that can impede learning. Because so much learning (social as well as academic) is language based, it is impossible to generalize about the appropriate environment for individuals who are hard of hearing.

The appropriate environment becomes a more complicated issue for the child who is deaf (Kreisman & John, 2010). The Commission on Education of the Deaf (1988) held that placement of a deaf child in a regular classroom, even with an interpreter, may be more restrictive than placement in a fully signing environment with deaf peers. Because of communication difficulties, a deaf child may experience unique academic, social, and emotional complications in the regular classroom. If such is the case, the regular classroom is not the LRE for a deaf child: "Placing a deaf child in the regular classroom without the language needed to function as a participant seriously impedes, if not precludes, the child from receiving any worthwhile education in the class" (p. 33).

Case 8.2. Carlos

Carlos was identified as having a bilateral profound hearing loss at age 6 months. His family decided against cochlear implants, choosing total communication as his primary mode of communication. He began to attend sign classes offered by the Early Intervention program. He attended a preschool that included many other deaf children and developed several friendships there. By the time he was ready for kindergarten, most of his family members were fairly fluent in sign, and Carlos was developing early reading skills.

Because his preacademic skills were near age level, it was decided that Carlos would attend his neighborhood school with a sign language interpreter. He was to be the only deaf child in the school, but he was friendly and gregarious, and it was assumed that he would "fit right in." His new teacher spent the summer learning sign language to achieve as much direct communication as possible.

Everyone was surprised that it took Carlos several months to acquire the skills needed to use an interpreter effectively. Even more surprising was the difficulty his classmates had in adjusting to the presence of the interpreter. Although he tried to be inconspicuous, most of Carlos's classmates did not feel comfortable communicating with Carlos through the interpreter. Their initial attempts were to speak to Carlos directly and, when that failed, to mime their intentions. Eventually, the role of the interpreter was understood, but both he and the classroom teacher noted that communication between Carlos and his peers was restricted to the essentials: providing abbreviated directions, one- or two-word answers, and so on. The natural interaction that had occurred in the preschool environment was missing here. Because of the communication limitations, Carlos was effectively alone in a room full of people. When asked if he would like to go to a kindergarten with his signing deaf friends from preschool, he looked happier than he had all year. It became clear that, for Carlos, the regular education environment was more, not less, restrictive.

In response to these concerns, the U.S. Department of Education issued "policy guidance" to states and school districts regarding the LRE for children with severe to profound hearing loss (*Federal Register*, 57[211], October 30, 1992, 49274–49276). Noting that "the communicative nature of the disability is inherently isolating" (p. 49274), the Department of Education advised that the LRE provisions of IDEA may be incorrectly interpreted for children who are deaf. The following factors are of paramount importance when determining the LRE for a child who is deaf:

- Communication needs and the child's and family's preferred mode of communication
- Linguistic needs
- Severity of hearing loss and potential for using residual hearing
- Academic level
- Social, emotional, and cultural needs of the child, including opportunities for peer interactions and communications

The Department of Education reminded educators that "the provision of FAPE is paramount, and the individual placement determination about LRE is to be considered within the context of FAPE" (p. 49275). In other words, no interpretation of LRE is meant to override the provision of an appropriate education (Marschark & Hauser, 2012; Shaver, Marschark, Newman, & Marder, 2014).

The Individualized Education Plan

The services to be provided to a child with a hearing loss are described in a document called an *individualized education plan* (IEP). It has been said that the IEP is not only a collection of forms but also a *process*; that is, a group of interested persons (parents, teachers, school administrators, and related service providers, such as audiologists, speech–language pathologists, school nurses, etc.), referred to as the individualized education plan committee, spend considerable time reviewing a child's current level of skills and decide on reasonable goals for the upcoming year. The process involves a great deal of sharing, learning, and ultimately agreeing on how to implement the child's education plan. Parents can request a revisit of this process at any time to consider changes in the child or other variables.

IEP (individualized education plan): A written report describing a child's current level of performance, annual goals, and procedures used to meet these goals.

As mentioned earlier, services are available to families as soon as a disability has been identified. From birth to age 3, services are tailored to the needs of the child within the context of the family (rather than the need of the child alone), so the document used to describe these services is called the individualized family service plan.

Types of Communication Modalities

Perhaps the most important consideration regarding classroom placement is the communication method used. By the time children with hearing loss enter school, their families have usually decided on a mode of communication. However, families do occasionally change their minds and will need unbiased and complete information about alternative methods. If the communication mode depends on amplification, school-based audiologists can contribute that component to their knowledge base. Students of audiologic rehabilitation will want to have a working knowledge of the issues; however, the choice of approach ultimately lies with parents, and professionals do not serve parents well by persuading them to adapt an approach that does not fit with their family.

The communication options include an Oral–Aural approach (i.e., using speech and hearing), a combination of signing with speech and hearing (Total Communication), a system called Cued Speech, and the use of sign only. Each approach is briefly described here.

Listening and Spoken Language. Listening and spoken language (LSL) emphasizes speech communication (oral), optimal use of amplified residual hearing (aural), and the development of speechreading (also known as lipreading) while discouraging the use of sign language. This approach was originally referred to as the Oral–Aural method and was espoused by Alexander Graham Bell (1847–1922), who, in addition to his other accomplishments, was a skilled speech teacher. Supporters of the LSL approach feel that "with spoken language, opportunities for higher education are less restricted, a more extensive range of careers is open, and there is greater employment security. Those who can talk also face fewer limitations in the personal and social aspects of their lives" (Ling, 1990, p. 9).

A refinement of the oral–aural approach is the *Auditory–Verbal approach*. The primary difference between these approaches is that the auditory–verbal approach makes a concerted effort during aural rehabilitation therapy to remove visual cues, encouraging the child to develop the auditory system with directed listening practice. Speechreading is used as a secondary rather than primary teaching strategy. To stimulate auditory development, the therapist reduces or eliminates visual information by covering most of his or her face while presenting the speech stimuli (Estabrooks, 2012).

Approximately 53 percent of the schoolchildren with moderate to severe hearing loss in the United States are instructed in spoken language (LSL) only (Gallaudet Research Institute, 2011).

Total Communication. To capitalize on the visual information provided by sign language, *Total Communication* (TC) was introduced in the 1960s. TC incorporates the use of many modalities at once: signing, speech, listening, and speechreading as well as the contributions of nonverbal communication (body language and facial expressions). The nature of the signing depends on the background of the educator, who may use American Sign Language (ASL), a sign system such as Signed Exact English (SEE), or a combination of ASL and SEE called Pidgin Sign, described in Chapter 5. Briefly, ASL is recognized as a legitimate language with a rich lexicon and a fully developed linguistic structure. Its roots are in French Sign Language, and it has been in existence for over 200 years. Because fewer than 5 percent of deaf children are born of deaf parents, ASL is typically learned from deaf friends, teachers, interpreters, and other adults rather than from family (Kushalnagar et al., 2010). In spite of this limited access to ASL, supporters feel that it should be the language of instruction for all children who are deaf.

Whereas ASL has evolved as a natural *sign language*, SEE is a *sign system* (i.e., a way to sign English words) created in the 1960s to address concerns regarding low reading and writing skills. SEE uses manual markers for linguistic concepts (e.g., plurality and tense) to correspond directly to the structures of the English language and follows the exact word order of English. SEE is just one of several artificial systems; readers of historical records will come across references to many versions. The use of these systems has diminished since the 1980s, for the most part being replaced with Pidgin Sign.

Sign system: Not a language but rather a method of depicting an oral language like English with manual symbols.

Like other pidgin languages, Pidgin Sign combines elements of different languages, in this case a manual language (ASL) and a spoken language (English). In an exchange, a hearing person communicating with Pidgin Sign is likely to omit articles such as *the* or *a/an* or the *-ing* endings of gerund verbs, as done in ASL. The word order, however, is usually identical to English, while in ASL the word order could be quite different (e.g., adjectives following rather than preceding nouns, as in *shoes brown*).

A combination of sign with speech is used in about 21 percent of classroom instruction for children with hearing loss (Gallaudet Research Institute, 2011).

Cued Speech. Another approach developed in the 1960s is called *Cued Speech*. Cued Speech is not a language but a visual support system to facilitate speechreading. Hand shapes made close to the face represent phonemes, which helps the speechreader discriminate between similar phonemes. For example, the phonemes /k/ and /g/ require distinct handshapes (/k/ as if pointing to the throat with the index and middle fingers, while the /g/ points with all five fingers), thus providing the speechreader with a visual cue to the voiced or unvoiced component of the phonemes. Cued Speech can be found in concentrated areas across the United States but in only about 1 percent of classroom instruction (Gallaudet Research Institute, 2011).

Cued Speech: A set of handshapes to help with speechreading sounds that look virtually identical (compare "Friday" to "fried egg").

Using Sign Only. Approximately 11 percent of children with hearing loss are instructed only in sign language (Gallaudet Research Institute, 2011). About 1 percent receive instruction with sign using a "bilingual–bicultural" (or "bi–bi") approach, which advocates teaching ASL as a child's first language and written English as a second language (Gárate, 2012). Speech production and listening skills are not emphasized. The bi–bi approach requires teachers to be native or highly fluent users of ASL, and, as one might expect, not many teachers are so qualified.

Summary. The numbers above indicate a major shift from TC to the LSL/speech-only approach. As indicated by the significant changes (20% to 30%) that have occurred in recent data related to both placement and communication modalities used in the education of children with hearing loss, there has been a strong trend to move them into regular classrooms and utilize listening and spoken language as the communication mode for their education. This trend may well be linked with an increased use of cochlear implants among infants with severe to profound hearing loss.

Readers are encouraged to visit these websites for more information on communication methods:

- American Sign Language and bilingualism (https://www.gallaudet.edu/Documents/Clerc/FAQ-ASL-SpokenEnglish.pdf)
- Listening/spoken language (http://www.agbell.org/Landing.aspx?id=476)
- Cued speech (www.cuedspeech.org)

AR SERVICES PROVIDED IN SCHOOLS

This section describes a range of school-based AR services (Educational Audiology Association, 2009):

- Screening and assessment of hearing loss
- Management of amplification
- Direct instruction and indirect consultation
- Hearing conservation
- Evaluation and modification of classroom acoustics
- Transition planning to postsecondary placements

Ideally, these services are provided by an audiologist. However, statistics presented later in this chapter indicate this often is not the case. As noted in Chapter 1, when audiologists provide these services, there are five times as many children with hearing loss served and two-and-a-half times more hearing aids and other forms of amplification in use as compared to when others (speech-language pathologists, school nurses, aides) provide the services (Downs, Whitaker, & Schow, 2003).

Screening and Assessment

Early Identification of Hearing Loss. Most children are now screened for hearing loss at birth. When newborns do not pass the screening, their parents are referred to a hospital or clinic for a comprehensive assessment. If a hearing loss is confirmed, parents are referred to their local early intervention program. That program will provide auditory training, speech and language therapy, and also other supports (e.g., physical therapy) if needed.

Screening in Kindergarten Through Grade 12. Schools are usually required by law to screen all school-age children at select grades to determine the existence of unidentified hearing loss (e.g., in kindergarten, grades 1 through 3, and grade 12). Because more and more children are demonstrating mild hearing loss in the high frequencies (most likely due to high levels of noise exposure), these screening programs have become more valuable than ever in identifying hearing problems that may not be evident to parents, teachers, or the child.

In addition to screening, children with *known* hearing loss must have an annual hearing assessment to determine the stability of the loss and to reconsider the appropriateness of the child's hearing aids and other amplification systems. Assessment information should include conventional hearing test information, speech recognition and speechreading abilities in quiet and in noise, and functional performance with amplification.

Management of Amplification/Audition

Managing amplification is a critical AR service. Amplification or audition includes personal hearing aids, personal FM systems, cochlear implants, sound field amplification, and assistive devices. Educational audiologists have agreed that, given the

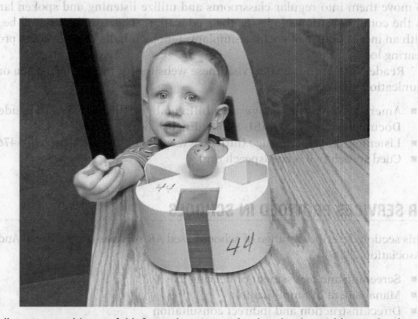

Play audiometry provides useful information concerning hearing loss with preschoolers. This child is being conditioned for the test.

high and unacceptable likelihood of malfunction, a monitoring program should be established, consisting of a daily visual inspection and listening check and at least one electroacoustic analysis every semester for each hearing aid and FM device (Johnson & Seaton, 2012). When such a program is rigorously applied, the malfunction rate can decrease from 50 percent to 1 percent (Langan & Blair, 2000). Given the importance of amplification to a child's academic success, a zero tolerance for malfunction rates should be established in each school.

The day-to-day management of amplification depends primarily on teachers, classroom aides, and speech-language pathologists. The audiologist must appreciate that these professionals' days are already crowded with countless responsibilities. The request to include yet another task might be received with skepticism, doubt, or worry. The technical aspects of the request also can be intimidating: Typically, classroom professionals have little or no background in amplification, and they might worry that they will break something. Therefore, the audiologist must consider strategies that will not only train but also motivate school professionals to provide consistent amplification management. In developing an in-service, the audiologist should remember that active learning is more likely to effect changes than traditional lecture (Naeve-Velguth, Hariprasad, & Lehman, 2003). Whether training is formal or informal, procedures should be reviewed on a regular basis to confirm that details are not forgotten or misapplied. Every time the student changes teachers, of course, the process needs to be repeated.

The audiologist should combine classroom records with his or her own (e.g., in chart or spreadsheet format) to document that the program is doing everything possible to help the student hear well, then share these data with parents and administrators while giving full credit to the classroom professionals. This public acknowledgment will help classroom professionals perceive the value of their role in this long-term effort.

Direct Instruction and Indirect Consultation

When children have hearing loss, they usually need direct instruction in developing their listening skills, speech production, and use of language. These supports may be provided within the classroom, one-on-one, or in small groups, or children may leave the classroom to join a teacher, speech-language pathologist, or audiologist in another (resource) room.

If a child's needs are not very involved or if personnel are not available for direct support, indirect consultation may take place among teachers and related service providers. As mentioned earlier, an audiologist may train the teacher how to do a daily hearing aid check because it is not possible for the audiologist to do it him- or herself every day, or a speech-language pathologist may provide an informal in-service on how to develop language skills within the curriculum rather than work with the child directly.

Hearing Conservation

Because society is becoming increasingly noisy and because children are being exposed to ever-higher noise levels, the incidence of high-frequency noise-induced hearing loss in children is on the rise. Noise exposure comes from toys, snowmobiles, and other engines but most often from music through headphones. The output from personal radio systems through headphones can exceed 115 dB SPL. The hearing loss caused by this noise trauma is permanent and entirely preventable; therefore, school programs are required to develop educational training programs to teach all children about hearing health and hearing loss prevention.

The World Health Organization (2015) has reported that approximately *1.1 billion youth* are at risk of permanent hearing loss due to unsafe recreational noise levels. Health textbooks typically do not cover this topic, so it is usually left to

Hearing conservation: Teaching children how to protect their hearing from high noise levels.

the communication disorders specialist (audiologist, speech-language pathologist, teacher of children with hearing loss) to develop age-appropriate lessons. Programs typically include a description of the auditory system, the effects of noise on this system, and a review of preventive measures. These programs have proved to be very effective (Bennett & English, 1999; Griest, Folmer, & Martin, 2007), but they are also time intensive and are often considered a luxury item on the menu of services delivered. The school audiologist may also need to monitor fluctuating hearing levels of children who are taking ototoxic drugs or experiencing difficult-to-treat otitis media.

Evaluation and Modification of Classroom Acoustics

Classroom acoustics is a key element in AR services in schools. There are three variables that can affect the acoustic environment of a classroom: noise levels, reverberation, and distance between teacher and student.

The *noise level* of the typical classroom can be very high, often louder than the teacher's voice. Children talk while working in small groups, feet shuffle on linoleum floors, heat and air-conditioning systems turn on and off, computers hum, and so on. The higher the noise level, the harder it is for children with hearing loss to hear oral instruction. In fact, when the noise level is just slightly higher than the teacher's voice, a child with hearing loss will understand very little of what he or she says. Unfortunately, most classrooms currently have background noise levels that exceed acceptable levels.

Even if a room is quiet, it can still have problems with *reverberation*. Reverberation is another word for *echo* and refers to the prolongation of sound as sound waves reflect off the hard surfaces in a room. Excessive reverberation occurs when floors have linoleum or tile instead of carpet or the walls and ceilings are covered with plaster instead of acoustic tile. Reverberation interferes with speech perception by overlapping with the energy of the direct signal of the teacher's voice. A child with hearing loss cannot interpret this distorted speech quickly enough, so reverberation is as much a problem as high noise levels. *Reverberation time* (RT) is a value used to indicate the amount of time it takes for a sound to decay 60 dB from its initial onset. For optimal perception of speech, it has been recommended that the RT in a classroom not exceed 0.3 second; however, the RT for most classrooms typically ranges from 0.4 to 1.2 seconds (Crandell, Smaldino, & Flexer, 2005).

Reverberation is the prolongation of sound due to hard surfaces. Reverberation time (RT) ideally is 0.3 second or less.

The third variable to consider with respect to classroom acoustics is the *distance* between teacher and student. Teachers move around the room most of the day, so the distance between teacher and student will vary from one minute to the next. The distance will affect the perceived sound level of the teacher's voice: The sound level for most conversational speech is approximately 60 dB SPL measured from six feet away, but this level drops as the distance between speaker and listener increases. When teachers stand a distance away, their voices may become too soft for most children with hearing loss to hear and understand, even with good hearing aids.

FM: A frequency modulated radio signal that carries the speaker's voice directly to a receiver.

Hearing aids are limited not only by distance but also by their nonselective amplification of all sounds in the classroom. Background noise sources, such as overhead fans, buzzing fluorescent lights, and shuffling feet, all contribute to the auditory input, and it can be very difficult to discriminate speech from this noise. An ideal solution to these listening challenges is the use of wireless *FM* amplification systems. There are two kinds of FM systems: *personal* systems used by individual students and *sound field* systems designed to amplify the teacher's voice throughout the entire classroom (i.e., the sound field).

Personal FM Systems.   Personal FM systems have two components. The first is the teacher's microphone and transmitter unit, which picks up and transmits the teacher's voice. The microphone may be attached to a lapel or worn on a neck loop or headset.

The second component of the system is the student's unit, a device that picks up the FM signal carrying the teacher's voice, amplifies it, and delivers it to the student's ears. This receiver can be an attachment to a personal hearing aid or built into the hearing aid itself (see Chapter 2).

With an FM system, the teacher's voice is transmitted by an FM signal to the student's receiver, which works very much like a personal radio station. The teacher's mouth is approximately six to eight inches away from the microphone, and, because the teacher's voice is transmitted by FM signal rather than airwaves, the student perceives this voice as if the teacher were always speaking six to eight inches away from his or her hearing aid microphone (overcoming the limitation of distance). Reception stays consistent up to a distance of 200 feet. With an FM system, the problem of direction of the speaker is also eliminated. The clarity of the teacher's voice is not affected as he or she turns away from the listener (changing directions).

In addition to overcoming the problems of distance and direction, FM systems also address the problem of hearing in noise. FM systems are designed to amplify and transmit the teacher's voice at intensity levels well above the environmental noise, creating a favorable signal-to-noise listening condition. Controls are available to receive input from the FM microphone only (e.g., to listen to a lecture when the teacher is the only one talking), hearing aid plus FM input together (to hear both teacher and classroom conversation), or hearing aid microphone only (to hear class discussion only when the teacher is working with other students).

These factors combine in what is called the *FM advantage* (Flexer, Wray, & Ireland, 1989). The FM advantage consists of overriding the negative effects of noise by increasing the teacher's voice as well as eliminating the adverse effects of distance and direction.

> FM advantage: Amplifying a speaker's voice above background noise while not being affected by distance or direction.

Sound Field FM Systems and Looping/Telecoils.   Another way of improving classroom acoustics is to amplify the teacher's voice for the entire classroom with the use of sound field amplification, usually recognized as a type of PA system. By amplifying the teacher's voice via loud speakers placed around the classroom, the problems with background noise and distance can be reduced. With a sound field system, the teacher wears a wireless microphone (an FM transmitter), his or her voice is transmitted to an FM receiver and amplifier, and one or more speakers are placed around the room. The teacher is free to move as before, but, regardless of his or her position, the teacher's voice will be amplified to all corners of the room. *Sound field amplification* has been found to enhance academic performance not only for children with hearing loss but also for children whose first language is not English, who have language disorders, or who have mild mental disability (Larson & Blair, 2008).

> Sound field amplification: Amplifying an entire area (the sound field), such as a classroom or an auditorium.

A variation of the concept of amplifying the whole classroom is to amplify the small area around the student. Desktop speakers are used with students who change rooms across the day; they take both the microphone and the book-sized speaker with them as they move from math to science class, for example.

Another hearing assistive technology used in classrooms is called "looping." When children have telecoils in their hearing aids, they can pick up a signal from the teacher's microphone transmitted to a loop of wire run along the perimeter of the classroom. The wire converts the teacher's signal to electromagnetic energy.

The t-coil converts that energy back to acoustic energy for the user to hear. This option is very cost effective and can be moved to another classroom easily.

It is important to note that amplifying the sound field (the classroom area) does not completely overcome reverberation problems, so a classroom would still need to be evaluated to determine how to reduce the amount of hard surfaces. The usual first modifications are to carpet the floor and to install acoustic tile on the ceiling.

Why the strong interest in classroom acoustics? Because the overall record of poor acoustic environments has attracted the interest of the federal government as an issue of access for persons with disabilities. Just as restaurants are required to provide menus in Braille and government offices must have restroom facilities that can accommodate wheelchairs, so it is reasoned, the acoustics of a school should allow full *acoustic access* to oral instruction. Acoustic standards have been developed and can be found on the website for the Federal Architecture and Transportation Access Board (www.quietclassrooms.org). The evaluation of classroom acoustics will be an increasing responsibility for persons providing AR services in the school setting and an exciting opportunity to positively affect the education of children with hearing loss. And as mentioned at the beginning of this chapter, attention paid to a student's classroom environment addresses both of the Es described in the CORE and CARE models.

Transition Planning to Postsecondary Placements

ITP (Individualized Transition Plan): A long-term plan to arrange for further education or job training after high school.

Ultimately, AR services are expected to support a child through to a successful high school graduation, but even here planning for the future is required. Once students graduate, the special education safety net is no longer in place for students with hearing loss. To prepare for the transition to placements after high school (college, vocational training, and work settings), students are required to meet with teachers and parents to develop an *Individualized Transition Plan* (ITP). If the student plans on attending a particular college, a representative of the college should attend this meeting; likewise, representatives from vocational training programs or work settings should provide input, as deemed necessary. The purpose of this transition planning is to ensure that the student has time to prepare for the requirements needed to enter college or vocational training or for job placement. The law requires that each student's IEP, beginning no later than age 16 (and at an earlier age, if deemed appropriate), include a statement of each public agency's and each participating agency's responsibilities, linkages, or both before the student leaves the school setting (34 CFR § 300.43).

This transition planning is especially important when we consider college placements. Although students with hearing loss enter college programs at the same rate as students without hearing loss, their attrition or dropout rate is much higher (61% compared to 35%) (Boutin, 2008; National Center for Special Education Research, 2011). It would appear that college career success depends as much on the ability to develop a social support system and to obtain and use support systems (interpreters, note takers, FM systems) as on the ability to earn good grades. Materials are available to help students to prepare for college, particularly in the area of being one's own advocate for supports and services (DuBow, 2015; English, 2012).

Deaf students may be particularly interested in attending colleges with an emphasis in Deaf culture, such as Gallaudet University (the only liberal arts college for the Deaf in the world) in Washington, D.C., or the National Technical Institute for the Deaf in Rochester, New York. On the West Coast of the United States, California State University at Northridge also has a large Deaf student enrollment. Transition to these environments requires planning as well, and students need a great deal of support during this process. Many universities provide interpreter and other support services for the deaf, which also allows students to attend near their homes.

How Services Are Provided

Although these AR responsibilities are carefully described, they are not implemented as widely as one would expect. Earlier it was mentioned that at least 1.5 million to 2 million schoolchildren are estimated to have some degree of hearing loss; however, according to annual data collected by the U.S. Department of Education (2015), fewer than 10 percent of children with hearing loss receive the audiologic services to which they are entitled. The reasons why children with hearing loss are underserved vary from one region to the next, but a common reason seems to be that parents are not fully aware of their rights to these services.

Another reason is the fact that most hearing loss falls in the slight to moderate range. If we envision a pyramid representing all children with hearing loss, the peak would represent the small number of children with profound loss, and the base would represent the majority with slight to moderate loss. Because children with slight to moderate loss tend to demonstrate (relatively) less obvious learning problems, they often appear to have fewer concerns and are assigned less support. Additionally, schools face the harsh reality of dwindling resources and increasing challenges. Children with many kinds of disabilities are underserved simply because the "pie" (tax-based funding) cannot cover all needs. As advocates for children with hearing loss, however, audiologists continue to put a spotlight on the subtle challenges of learning with all kinds of hearing loss and find creative ways to provide services using a team approach, as described in the next section.

AR SERVICE PROVIDERS IN SCHOOL SETTINGS

School-based AR services are provided in a team approach, with the following professionals working as team members.

Teachers

Not too long ago, most children with hearing loss were taught in small, self-contained classes run by teachers specially trained to teach them. This model still exists, but now, because of the movement toward inclusion (discussed earlier), many of these teachers may be assigned to several schools to provide support to children as they attend their neighborhood schools. Support may consist of direct instruction, individually or in small groups, or indirect consultation with the general classroom teacher. This collaboration is essential since most regular education teachers receive little training about hearing loss. Information on adapting curriculum, verifying hearing aid function, and the like is shared, as are reports on student progress.

Audiologists

School-based audiologists have developed a specialty called educational audiology, often considered to be audiology *plus*, that is, clinical audiology skills *plus* an understanding of the school culture, legal mandates, and the roles and responsibilities unique to the school setting (Johnson & Seaton, 2012). A primary limitation to the provision of these services has been the relatively small number of audiologists hired to serve children in schools. The American Speech-Language-Hearing Association (2002) has conservatively estimated the need for one audiologist for every 10,000 schoolchildren. This 1:10,000 ratio would necessitate hiring at least

One audiologist is needed for every 10,000 children.

One-on-one speech therapy focused on articulation.

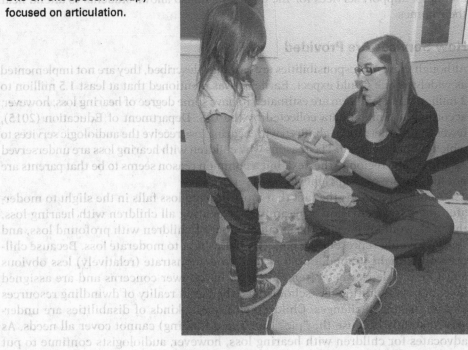

5,000 audiologists, but for over two decades only about 1,300 educational audiologists have been employed by schools. Because of this hiring shortage, provision of services may be shared by any of the following professional colleagues. As noted earlier, audiologists are much more effective in providing these services.

Speech-Language Pathologists

Speech-language pathologists (SLPs) are the professionals most likely to provide speech and language therapy and auditory training. They may be the persons responsible for ensuring that a child's hearing aids are functioning, troubleshooting basic problems, and reporting any problems to the audiologist. Speech-language pathologists usually provide support to the classroom teacher by describing how to provide visual cues, promote speechreading opportunities, control for acoustic problems, and so on. They also often conduct hearing screening programs.

Because audiologists are underemployed in the schools, speech-language pathologists are more likely to provide audiologic services.

Related Support Personnel

Approximately 30 to 40 percent of children with hearing loss have additional disabilities, such as vision loss, autism, and learning disabilities (Gallaudet Research Institute, 2011). Therefore, associated AR services are also provided by the following (as well as others):

- School nurses, for medications and other health concerns, as well as hearing screening
- School psychologists, for assessment of verbal and nonverbal intellectual abilities
- Adaptive physical education teachers, for large motor and balance development
- Mobility and orientation specialists, for children with visual disabilities
- Itinerant teachers (educators assigned to several schools who provide individualized instruction to a caseload of students per their IEPs)
- School counselors, for support with family challenges and social concerns, such as bullying (Squires, Spangler, Johnson, & English, 2013)

It is not at all unusual for these professionals to have a limited background in the area of hearing loss, which makes it all the more important to take a team approach in providing services.

SERVICES FOR CHILDREN WITH AUDITORY PROCESSING PROBLEMS

Up to this point, we have considered AR services only for children with hearing loss. However, in the past few years, increased attention is being paid to children who have normal hearing sensitivity but deficits in their ability to understand what they hear. We can appreciate the depth of this problem when we realize that the vast majority of a school day requires a child to listen to his or her teacher's instruction, understand it, remember it, and respond to it. Imagine a classroom teacher giving the following instructions: "Class, I want you to take out your yellow math book and turn to page 197. Do only the even-numbered problems and then leave your paper on my desk. When you are done, you may do some silent reading until 10:40." A child with an auditory processing problem might be easily confused with this long set of instructions, or he or she might sufficiently understand until other children start making noise as they reach for their books, pencils, and paper. Such a child may look distracted or "off task" as he or she looks around trying to figure out what to do, and to a teacher the child's behaviors might appear hyperactive or immature.

Because auditory processing (listening) is an invisible behavior, it may be difficult for teachers to realize that it involves instantaneous complex cognitive activity, specifically, receiving, symbolizing, comprehending, interpreting, storing, and recalling auditory information or, put more simply, "what we do with what we hear" (Lasky & Katz, 1983, p. 5).

The American Speech-Language-Hearing Association (2005) described auditory processing disorders (APD) to include problems in several listening domains, including these three:

- *Monaural discrimination*, or the ability to perceive degraded words or words in competition when signal and competition are present in one ear
- *Understanding binaural acoustic information*, such as a signal in one ear, by ignoring competition in the other, or different *(dichotic) information*, when both parts are useful and heard in two ears at once
- *Temporal aspects of hearing or pattern recognition*, or the ability to rapidly and accurately sequence auditory information

---

When a child has problems with one or more of these listening domain areas, he or she may have an *auditory processing disorder* (APD). The term *central auditory processing disorder* (CAPD) has also been used, and while both terms continue to be used, some professionals now prefer a hybrid form—(C)APD (American Academy of Audiology, 2010).

The overall impression of a child with APD is one who seems generally inattentive, "out of it," restless, forgetful, or impatient or acts socially inappropriately. Listening difficulties often surface in third grade, when classroom instruction becomes less directed, and this has been recommended as a good time for screening these children. Such difficulties may even be apparent from the first days of formal schooling because listening is the mode by which a prereader acquires information.

The overall impression of a child with APD is one who seems inattentive.

Diagnosis/Assessment of APD

As of now, there is no general consensus on how to diagnose this condition, except that the three domains listed above are generally evaluated. The Multiple Auditory Processing Assessment (MAPA) is one method for assessment of these three domains and is described in Chapter 9. Screening instruments such as the S.I.F.T.E.R. (Anderson, 1989), found in the Appendix, and the Scale of Auditory Behaviors (SAB; Schow & Seikel, 2007; Schow, Seikel, Brockett & Whitaker, in press), may be used by audiologists to determine that a child's listening behaviors are outside normal limits.

As mentioned, secondary behaviors that arise as a consequence of listening problems provide us with clues to the possible presence of APD. Both the SAB and S.I.F.T.E.R. have cutoff levels that can be used for referral purposes.

There are 12 behaviors used as items in the SAB; when this scale is used by teachers and parents, it can be helpful in identifying children who can benefit from more extensive diagnostic testing. These items are listed below:

1. Difficulty hearing or understanding in background noise
2. Misunderstands, especially with rapid or muffled speech
3. Difficulty following oral instructions
4. Difficulty in discriminating and identifying speech sounds
5. Inconsistent responses to auditory information
6. Poor listening skills
7. Asks for things to be repeated
8. Easily distracted
9. Learning or academic difficulties
10. Short attention span
11. Daydreams, inattentive
12. Disorganized

There are 12 common behaviors associated with children with APD.

It is important to remember that the types of behaviors listed previously are seen in all children at some time, depending on general health and energy levels, personal worries or other distractions, a variety of other learning disabilities, or the presence of temporary hearing loss due to ear infections and allergies. However, when these behaviors are persistent at a level that reaches the screening cutoff, a referral is indicated.

There is no specific count of the number of children who have auditory processing problems. Approximately 8 million to 12 million schoolchildren in the United States have learning disabilities, and many of them have APD. It appears that more boys have APD than girls, and many have a positive history of chronic ear infections (Whitton & Polley, 2012). APD is typically considered a learning disorder, although it is not clear whether the disorder is one aspect of a more complex language-learning disorder (Kahmi, 2011), a problem with attention (Moore, Ferguson, Edmonson-Jones, Ratib, & Riley, 2010), or a combination of difficulties with selective attention, working memory, motivation, and context (Musiek & Chermak, 2016). As noted before, the three kinds of processing problems are (1) monaural competition problems, (2) binaural competition problems, and (3) temporal problems.

The first two of these involve difficulties attending to speech with competing signals in the background (important when we consider the usual noise level in classrooms) compounded by difficulties hearing the differences in sounds and words (an essential skill for phonetic reading and spelling).

In the third, temporal problems, there is evidence that some children's auditory systems are not as efficient in identifying different timing aspects of transmission (slower neural activity). For example, it may take longer than normal for signals to travel from the outer ear to the brain. If a delay like this is occurring, it could be said that a child cannot listen as fast as a teacher is talking (Bellis, 2002).

Remediation of APD

After APD diagnosis, providers of AR services in schools may be called on to provide three forms of remediation (Educational Audiology Association, 2015):

1. One form of remediation is *Direct Therapy* in one or more of the three domain areas. Traditional auditory training techniques have been successfully applied to help children with normal hearing develop better listening skills, such as learning to discriminate temporal or pattern differences in long versus short tones or high versus low tones as well as the sounds in words. Computer games have been designed to help a child to listen and discriminate between these kinds of sounds (see website information in "Recommended Resources" at the end of the chapter). If a child has difficulties ignoring background noise, many listening activities are presented while a tape of white noise or cafeteria noise is played as a method of desensitization. Activities are also provided to develop auditory memory and to help a child "listen faster" or hear temporal differences by presenting stimuli with increasing speed or different interval times. An innovative program called Fast ForWord has been designed to help children improve temporal auditory skills: By logging onto the Internet, a child uses a computer to work through a series of games that are individualized to work on processing speed. Speech sounds are electronically altered and are made increasingly more challenging to perceive. Scores are entered into the Fast ForWord mainframe, and subsequent games are modified to increase or decrease the level of difficulty as needed. Readers are referred to "Recommended Resources" at the end of the chapter for website information.

The research on these products has been mixed, however. The U.S. Department of Education analyzes research on a range of educational strategies, and its 2009 report for an older program called Earobics (no longer commercially available) identified only two studies that met its quality standards (http://ies.ed.gov/ncee/wwc/pdf/wwc_earobics_011309.pdf). However, its 2013 analysis of Fast ForWord could include seven studies that met its scientific qualifications, so its conclusions were more favorable (http://ies.ed.gov/ncee/wwc/pdf/intervention_reports/wwc_ffw_031913.pdf).

A different approach to remediation is being tested by the National Acoustic Lab (NAL) in Australia, based on results gleaned from a test called Listening in Spatialized Noise—Sentences Test (LiSN-S). The test evaluates the listener's ability to use directional cues while listening in background noise, much like the conditions children face in classrooms. The associated auditory training software (LiSN and Learn) uses video games to help the listener (under headphones) learn how to focus on speech delivered from different directions.

The NAL is systematically evaluating listener outcomes (http://capd.nal.gov.au/lisn-learn-about.shtml). As in clinic settings, audiologists in school environments must critically evaluate the efficacy of all available remediations (DeBonis, 2015).

Fast Forword and LiSN and Learn are two different forms of APD direct therapy.

2. In addition to direct therapy, a second form of APD remediation involves *Environmental Modifications*. This includes minimizing the negative effects of noise by eliminating unnecessary noise sources (replacing buzzing fluorescent lightbulbs or placing carpet on the floor to absorb chair and feet noise) and increasing the "signal" of a teacher's voice by installing classroom amplification.

Case 8.3. Kim

Kim is 8 years old and is in third grade. His classmates had been acquiring beginning reading skills for some time, but he did not understand the teacher's instructions about "letter sounds," and he was getting farther and farther behind. He was discouraged and struggling with his self-perception of "being stupid." He had been seeing a reading tutor for two months and was not making any progress. His motivation to learn was almost nonexistent.

After confirming Kim's hearing sensitivity was normal, the audiologist diagnosed him as having an auditory processing problem, specifically with not being able to hear the subtle pattern differences in sounds. Using several modalities (visual cues, kinesthetic cues, etc.), he was taught first to recognize and describe the differences between long and short tones on a keyboard and between low and high frequencies. He was taught to perceive the differences between similar consonants and vowels and consonant–vowel combinations.

In the beginning, he was not eager to "work on listening." However, he enjoyed the one-on-one interaction and soon changed his attitude about learning. By the end of the 12-week session, he had learned how to translate these listening games to reading skills and was dismissed from the program.

3. The third form of APD treatment involves teaching *Coping and Problem-solving Strategies*, such as learning how to make lists and use calendars, pretutoring key vocabulary and concepts, and using a "study buddy" (Bellis, 2003).

Children with APD can usually improve their listening skills and become actively engaged in communication and learning. However, after experiencing repeated failure and fatigue from effort, children with APD can present motivational problems, creating a downward spiral of discouragement even when they try hard. Remediation must include opportunities to promote and reward a student's efforts to persist when faced with a difficult task.

> Children with APD can present motivational problems, creating a downward spiral of discouragement even when they try hard.

"A DAY IN THE LIFE" OF AN EDUCATIONAL AUDIOLOGIST

Introduction: Educational audiologists address a variety of rehabilitation concerns in the school setting. The following account is an example of a so-called typical workday.

Martha Jones, AuD, arrives at her office at 8:00 a.m. to pick up portable testing equipment and student files. This morning, she trains school nurses on hearing screening protocols, and she needs the equipment for demonstration purposes. Later that morning, she drives to a school across town to meet a student new to the district. After checking this fourth grader's cochlear implants and setting her up with a personal FM system, Dr. Jones sits in the back of the classroom and evaluates the classroom acoustics with some apps on her smartphone while observing the child's listening skills and the teacher's instructional style. She usually finds it necessary to help the teacher with some basic communication techniques (using Clear Speech, getting the child's attention before speaking, writing page numbers on the board, etc.). She always brings her calendar, so before leaving, she schedules an in-service with the teacher later in the month where she will bring some written materials to help teach these concepts.

Back in the office, she completes several reports needed before next week's IEP meetings and then spends 30 minutes putting the final touches on a presentation she will give to a 10th-grade science class on hearing and audiology. She moves on to the sound booth for two hours, testing children's hearing and troubleshooting their hearing aid problems. She ends the day working on a research project that she will present at a local conference: the role of the audiologist in helping children with hearing loss learn to read (since reading depends on perception of speech sounds).

She takes her calendar home to prepare for the next day since each day is always different. She has professional autonomy, personal satisfaction helping children do well in school, and professional support from a local group of fellow audiologists who collaborate on various projects. But for now, she needs to organize more materials: Tomorrow she supervises an audiology student, and together they will meet with a physical education teacher and demonstrate how using an FM system will help a child with hearing loss understand instructions in a noisy gym.

Summary Points

- Hearing loss has educational significance, and children with hearing loss are entitled to AR services to support their education plans.

- AR services include testing, amplification management, modified instruction, and consideration of classroom acoustics.

- Classroom acoustics can adversely affect learning, especially when there are high levels of noise and reverberation. Federal standards have been developed to help programs improve classroom acoustics.

- To reduce listening challenges, technologies such as personal and group FM systems are used to amplify the teacher's voice and deliver that signal directly to students' ears.

- AR services are documented in a child's IEP and are intended to provide a free appropriate public education (**FAPE**) in the least restrictive environment (**LRE**).

- Children with normal hearing and auditory processing problems benefit from many of the same AR services.

- AR services in school settings are provided to children by a team of professionals, primarily teachers, audiologists, and speech-language pathologists.

Supplementary Learning Activities

See www.isu.edu/csed/audiology/rehab to carry out these activities. We encourage you to use these to supplement your learning. Your instructor may give specific assignments that involve a particular activity.

1. This chapter describes why we must confirm that children's hearing aids are working while at school. Design a monitoring program to meet this mandate. Who will check hearing aids, FMs and cochlear implants and how often? Who will train these individuals? How will the checks be documented? Will there be backup systems (extra batteries and hearing aids), and, if so, how will those be managed? See Johnson and Seaton (2012) for guidance.

2. This chapter also briefly discussed the risk of noise exposure to young ears and the application of hearing loss prevention programs. Take time to explore the material on the website DangerousDecibels.org and select a component to present on in class. What teaching techniques do the designers use to engage the learner?

3. Review the materials in APD on the text website (see instructions) and prepare a short one-page summary describing briefly the research that you find there on the basic strategy for diagnosis (involving three areas) and remediation of APD (three areas).

Recommended Reading

Bellis, T. J. (2002). *When the brain can't hear: Unraveling the mysteries of auditory processing disorder.* New York: Pocket Books.

Estabrooks, W. (2012). *101 frequently asked questions about auditory verbal practice.* Washington, DC: Alexander Graham Bell Association.

Johnson, C. D., & Seaton, J. B. (2012). *Educational audiology handbook* (2nd ed.). Clifton Park, NY: Cengage Delmar Learning.

Oliva, G. (2004). *Alone in the mainstream: A deaf woman remembers public school.* Washington, DC: Gallaudet University Press.

Recommended Resources

Software

Fast ForWord: An Internet-based auditory training program designed for children with auditory processing problems. http://www.scienticlearning.com

Johnson, C. D., & Seaton, J. B. (2012). *Educational audiology handbook* (2nd ed.). Florence, KY: Cengage Delmar Learning. This text gives an in-depth review of the roles and responsibilities of the audiologist in school settings. It comes with a CD with more than 500 pages of forms to help document services and provides a standardized method of service delivery.

Websites

Acoustics Standards Update:
http://www.ncef.org

Educational Audiology Association:
http://www.eduaud.org

IDEA Amendments:
http://idea.ed.gov

Supporting Success for Children with Hearing Loss:
http://successforkidswithhearingloss.com

References

Academic Therapy Publications. (2017). Navato, CA.

American Academy of Audiology. (2010). *Diagnosis, treatment, and management of children and adults with central auditory processing disorders.* Reston, VA: Author.

American Speech-Language-Hearing Association. (2002). *Guidelines for audiology service provision in and for the schools.* Rockville, MD: Author.

American Speech-Language-Hearing Association. (2005). (Central) auditory processing disorders: The role of the audiologist [Position statement]. Retrieved from http://www.asha.org/members/deskref-journals/deskref/default

Anderson, K. (1989). Screening Instrument for Targeting Educational Risk (SIFTER). Retrieved from http://www.hear2learn.com

Bellis, T. J. (2002). *When the brain can't hear: Unraveling the mysteries of auditory processing disorder.* New York: Pocket Books.

Bellis, T. J. (2003). *Assessment and management of central auditory processing disorders in the educational setting: From science to practice* (2nd ed.). Clifton Park, NY: Delmar Thomson Learning.

Bennett, J. A., & English, K. (1999). Teaching hearing conservation to school children: Comparing the outcomes and efficacy of two pedagogical approaches. *Journal of Educational Audiology, 7,* 29–33.

Bess, F. H., Dodd-Murphy, J., & Parker, R. A. (1998). Children with minimal sensori-neural hearing loss: Prevalence, educational performance, and functional status. *Ear and Hearing, 19*(5), 339–354.

Bess, F., Klee, T., & Culbertson, J. L. (1986). Identification, assessment, and management of children with unilateral sensorineural hearing loss. *Seminars in Hearing, 7*(1), 43–50.

Boutin, D. (2008). Persistence in postsecondary environments of students with hearing impairments. *Journal of Rehabilitation, 74*(1), 25–41.

Commission on Education of the Deaf. (1988). *Toward equality: Education of the deaf.* Washington, DC: U.S. Government Printing Office.

Crandell, C., Smaldino, J., & Flexer, C. (2005). *Sound field amplification: Applications to speech perception and classroom acoustics.* Clifton Park, NY: Thomson Delmar Learning.

DeBonis, D. (2015). It is time to rethink central auditory processing disorder protocols for school-aged children. *American Journal of Audiology, 24,* 124–136.

Downs, S. K., Whitaker, M. M., & Schow, R. L. (2003). *Audiological services in schools that do and do not have an audiologist* (paper presented at the Educational Audiology Association Summer Conference, St. Louis, MO).

DuBow, S. (2015). *Legal rights: The guide for deaf and hard of hearing people* (6th ed.). Washington, DC: Gallaudet University Press.

Educational Audiology Association. (2009). Recommended professional practices for educational audiology. Retrieved from http://www.edaud.org/position-stat/6-position-05-09.pdf

Educational Audiology Association. (2015). Auditory processing assessment. Retrieved from http://www.edaud.org/advocacy/16-advocacy-10-15.pdf

English, K. (2012). Self-advocacy skills for students who are deaf and hard of hearing. Retrieved from http://gozips.uakron.edu/~ke3/Self-Advocacy.pdf

English, K., & Church, G. (1999). Unilateral hearing loss in children: An update for the 1990s. *Language, Speech, and Hearing Services in Schools, 30,* 26–31.

Estabrooks, W. (2012). *101 frequently asked questions about auditory verbal practice.* Washington, DC: Alexander Graham Bell Association.

Flexer, C., Wray, D., & Ireland, J. (1989). Preferential seating is NOT enough: Issues in classroom management of hearing impaired students. *Language, Speech, and Hearing in Schools, 20,* 11–21.

Gallaudet Research Institute. (2011). *Regional and national summary of data from the 2009–2010 annual survey of deaf and hard of hearing children and youth.* Washington, DC: Author.

Gárate, M. (2012). *ASL/English bilingual education: Models, methodologies, and strategies* (Research Brief No. 8). Washington, DC: Visual Language and Visual Learning Science of Learning Center.

Griest, S., Folmer, R., & Martin, M. (2007). Effectiveness of "Dangerous Decibels," a school-based hearing loss prevention program. *American Journal of Audiology, 16,* S165–S181.

Johnson, C. D. (2000). Management of hearing in the educational setting. In J. Alpiner & P. McCarthy (Eds.), *Rehabilitative audiology: Children and adults* (3rd ed.). Baltimore: Lippincott Williams & Wilkins, 226–274.

Johnson, C. D., & Seaton, J. B. (2012). *Educational audiology handbook* (2nd ed.). Florence, KY: Cengage Delmar Learning.

Kahmi, A. (2011). What speech-language pathologists need to know about auditory processing disorder. *Language, Speech and Hearing Services in Schools, 42,* 265–272.

Kreisman, B., & John, A. (2010). A case law review of the Individuals with Disabilities Education Act for children with hearing loss or auditory processing disorders. *Journal of American Academy of Audiology, 21*(7), 426–440.

Kushalnagar, P., Mathur, G., Moreland, C. J., Napoli, D. J., Osterling, W., Padden, C., et al. (2010). Infants and children with hearing loss need early language access. *Journal of Clinical Ethics, 21*(2), 143–154.

Langan, L., & Blair, J. C. (2000). "Can you hear me?" A longitudinal study of hearing aid monitoring in the classroom. *Journal of Educational Audiology, 8,* 24–26.

Larson, J., & Blair, J. (2008). The effect of classroom amplification on the signal-to-noise ratio in classrooms while class is in session. *Language, Speech, and Hearing Services in Schools, 39,* 451–460.

Lasky, E. Z., & Katz, J. (1983). *Central auditory processing disorders: Problems of speech, language, and learning.* Baltimore: University Park Press.

Lieu, J. E. (2004). Speech-language and educational consequences of unilateral hearing loss in children. *Archives of Otolaryngology and Head and Neck Surgery, 130,* 524–530.

Ling, D. (1990). Advances underlying spoken language development: A century of building on Bell. *Volta Review, 92*(4), 8–20.

Marschark, M., & Hauser, P.C. (2012). *How Deaf children learn.* Oxford: Oxford University Press.

McFadden, B., & Pittman, A. (2008). Effect of minimal hearing loss on children's ability to multitask in quiet and in noise. *Language, Speech, and Hearing Services in Schools, 39*(3), 342–351.

Moeller, M. P. (2007). Current state of knowledge: Language and literacy of children with hearing impairment. *Ear and Hearing, 28,* 740–753.

Moeller, M. P., Carr, G., Seaver, L., Stradler-Brown, A., & Holzinger, D. (2013). Best practices in family-centered early intervention for children who are deaf or hard of hearing: An international consensus statement. *Journal of Deaf Studies and Deaf Education, 18*(4), 429–445.

Moore, D., Ferguson, M., Edmonson-Jones, A. M., Ratib, S., & Riley, A. (2010). Nature of auditory processing disorder in children. *Pediatrics, 126*(2), e382–e390.

Musiek, F., & Chermak, G. (2016). Perspectives on central auditory processing disorder. *Audiology Today, 28*(1), 24–30.

Naeve-Velguth, S., Hariprasad, D., & Lehman, M. (2003). A comparison of lecture and problem-based instructional formats for FM inservices. *Journal of Educational Audiology, 11,* 5–14.

National Center for Special Education Research. (2011). *The post-high school outcomes of young adults with disabilities up to 6 years after high school.* Washington, DC: U.S. Department of Education.

Schow, R., Seikel, A., Brockett, J., & Whitaker, M. (in press). Multiple Auditory Processing Assessment-2. Novato, CA: Academic Therapy Publications.

Schow, R. L., & Seikel, J. A. (2007). Screening for (C)APD. In F. Musiek & G. Chermak (Eds.), *Handbook of (central) auditory processing disorder* (Vol. 1, pp. 137–161). San Diego, CA: Plural Publishing.

Shaver, D., Marschark, M., Newman, L., & Marder, C. (2014). Who is where? Characteristics of deaf and hard-of-hearing students in regular and special schools. *Journal of Deaf Studies and Deaf Education, 19*(2), 203–219.

Squires, M., Spangler, C., Johnson, C., & English, K. (2013). Bullying is a safety and health issue: How pediatric audiologists can help. *Audiology Today, 25*(5),18–26.

Trussell, J., & Esterbrooks, S. (2016). Morphological knowledge and students who are deaf or hard-of-hearing: A review of the literature. *Communication Disorders Quarterly.* doi:10.1177/1525740116644889

U.S. Department of Education. (2015). *Thirty-seventh annual report to Congress on the implementation of the Individuals with Disabilities Education Act.* Washington, DC: U.S. Government Printing Office.

Whitton, J., & Polley, D. (2012). Ear infection today, "lazy ear" tomorrow? *Audiology Today, 24*(4) 33–37.

World Health Organization. (2015, February). 1.1 billion people at risk of hearing loss: WHO highlights serious threat posed by exposure to recreational noise. Retrieved from http://www.edaud.org/position-stat/6-position-05-09.pdf

Wright, P. (2004). The Individuals with Disabilities Education Improvement Act of 2004: Overview, explanation and comparison. Retrieved from http://www.wrightslaw.com/idea/idea.2004.all.pdf

Yoshinago-Itano, C., Johnson, C. D., & Brown, A. S. (2008). Outcomes of children with mild bilateral hearing loss and unilateral hearing loss. *Seminars in Hearing, 29*(2), 196–211.

APPENDIX

S.I.F.T.E.R.

by Karen L. Anderson, EdS, CCC-A

STUDENT _____ TEACHER _____ GRADE _____

DATE COMPLETED _____ SCHOOL _____ DISTRICT _____

The above child is suspect for hearing problems that may or may not be affecting his/her school performance. This rating scale has been designed to sift out students who are educationally at risk possibly as a result of hearing problems. Based on your knowledge from observations of this student, circle the number best representing his/her behavior. After answering the questions, please record any comments about the student in the space provided on the reverse side.

ACADEMICS

1. What is your estimate of the student's class standing in comparison of that of his/her classmates?	UPPER				MIDDLE			LOWER
	5		4		3		2	1
2. How does the student's achievement compare to your estimation of his/her potential?	EQUAL				LOWER			MUCH LOWER
	5		4		3		2	1
3. What is the student's reading level, reading ability group or reading readiness group in the classroom (e.g., a student with average reading ability performs in the middle group)?	UPPER				MIDDLE			LOWER
	5		4		3		2	1

ATTENTION

4. How distractible is the student in comparison to his/her classmates?	NOT VERY				AVERAGE			VERY
	5		4		3		2	1
5. What is the student's attention span in comparison to that of his/her classmates?	LONGER				AVERAGE			SHORTER
	5		4		3		2	1
6. How often does the student hesitate or become confused when responding to oral directions (e.g., "Turn to page . . .")?	NEVER				OCCASIONALLY			FREQUENTLY
	5		4		3		2	1

Used with permission of Karen L. Anderson. Preschool, Elementary, and Secondary S.I.F.T.E.R. checklists can be downloaded from http://successforkids with hearingloss.com/tests

COMMUNICATION

7. How does the student's comprehension compare to the average understanding ability of his/her classmates?	ABOVE		AVERAGE				BELOW	
	5	4	3		2		1	
8. How does the student's vocabulary and word usage skills compare with those of other students in his/her age group?	ABOVE		AVERAGE				BELOW	
	5	4	3		2		1	
9. How proficient is the student at telling a story or relating happenings from home when compared to classmates?	ABOVE		AVERAGE				BELOW	
	5	4	3		2		1	

CLASS PARTICIPATION

10. How often does the student volunteer information to class discussions or in answer to teacher questions?	FREQUENTLY		OCCASIONALLY				NEVER	
	5	4	3		2		1	
11. With what frequency does the student complete his/her class and homework assignments within the time allocated?	ALWAYS		USUALLY				SELDOM	
	5	4	3		2		1	
12. After instruction, does the student have difficulty starting to work (looks at other students working or asks for help)?	NEVER		OCCASIONALLY				FREQUENTLY	
	5	4	3		2		1	

SCHOOL BEHAVIOR

13. Does the student demonstrate any behaviors that seem unusual or inappropriate when compared to other students?	NEVER		OCCASIONALLY				FREQUENTLY	
	5	4	3		2		1	
14. Does the student become frustrated easily, sometimes to the point of losing emotional control	NEVER		OCCASIONALLY				FREQUENTLY	
	5	4	3		2		1	
15. In general, how would you rank the student's relationship with peers (ability to get along with others)?	GOOD		AVERAGE				POOR	
	5	4	3		2		1	

Teacher Comments

Has this child repeated a grade, had frequent absences, or experienced health problems (including ear infections and colds)? Has the student received, or is he/she now receiving, special services? Does the child have any other health problems that may be pertinent to his/her educational functioning?

The S.I.F.T.E.R. Is a Screening Tool Only

Any student failing this screening in a content area as determined on the scoring grid below should be considered for further assessment, depending on his/her individual needs as per school district criteria. For example, failing in the Academics area suggests an educational assessment, in the Communication area a speech–language assessment, and in the School Behavior area an assessment by a psychologist or a social worker. Failing in the Attention and/or Class Participation area in combination with other areas may suggest an evaluation by an educational audiologist. Children placed in the marginal area are at risk for failing and should be monitored or considered for assessment depending upon additional information.

Scoring

Sum the responses to the three questions in each content area and record in the appropriate box on the reverse side and under Total Score below. Place an **X** on the number that corresponds most closely with the content area score (e.g., if a teacher circled 3, 4, and 2 for the questions in the Academics area, an **X** would be placed on the number 9 across from the Academics content area). Connect the **X**s to make a profile.

CONTENT AREA	TOTAL SCORE	PASS	MARGINAL	FAIL
ACADEMICS		15 14 13 12 11 10	9 8	7 6 5 4 3
ATTENTION		15 14 13 12 11 10 9	8 7	6 5 4 3
COMMUNICATION		15 14 13 12 11	10 9 8	7 6 5 4 3
CLASS PARTICIPATION		15 14 13 12 11 10 9	8 7	6 5 4 3
SOCIAL BEHAVIOR		15 14 13 12 11 10	9 8	7 6 5 4 3

part **2**

Comprehensive Approaches to Audiologic Rehabilitation

Comprehensive Approaches to Audiologic Rehabilitation

Audiologic Rehabilitation for Children

Assessment and Management

Mary Pat Moeller, Ronald L. Schow, Mary M. Whitaker

CONTENTS

Visit the companion website when you see this icon to learn more about the topic nearby in the text.

Learning Outcomes

After reading this chapter, you will be able to

- List five principles of family-centered practice
- Identify the three relationships involved in home-based early intervention
- Identify four areas of specialized knowledge needed by aural rehabilitation specialists
- Identify six roles the audiologic rehabilitation specialist can activate during early intervention sessions
- List and describe the management aspects of the audiologic rehabilitation therapist during the school years
- Describe the potential hearing assistive technology that may be used by school-age children
- Describe the role of the audiologic rehabilitation therapist in managing the hearing assistive technology
- Describe basic assessment and management of auditory processing skills for school-age children

INTRODUCTION

This chapter provides a comprehensive discussion of audiologic rehabilitation for children as provided at two major levels: (1) parent–infant/preschool and (2) the school years. Before specific components that constitute the rehabilitation process are addressed, however, the reader will get a brief overview of prevalence and service delivery statistics, applicable definitions and terms, a general profile of the client, typical rehabilitation settings at various age levels, and the identification and assessment process.

PREVALENCE OF LOSS AND LEVEL OF SERVICE

Of all audiologic rehabilitation efforts, those focusing on the child are probably the most frequently applied.

There are 10 to 40 in every 1,000 children (1% to 4%) who can be considered to be permanently hard of hearing in both ears at levels poorer than 20 dB HL in the speech range, and there is a much less consistent rate of service for children who are hard of hearing as compared to children who are deaf.

Up to 2 million school-age youngsters in the United States are seriously hard of hearing.

This estimate would suggest that up to 2 million school-age youngsters in the United States are seriously hard of hearing. However, when we include minimal hearing loss with levels poorer than 15 dB HL, unilateral, and high-frequency losses, we add another 3 million to 5 million children. Conductive losses add at least another 1 million to 2 million. Inclusion of the younger population (0 to 5 years) could put the total at 10 percent or more, or as many as 10 million children in the United States with hearing loss (National Institute on Deafness and Other Communication Disorders [NIDCD], 2005; Porter & Bess, 2011; Tharpe, 2011). Slightly higher and lower estimates have been reported, but the above numbers represent a reasonable estimate (Downs, Whitaker, & Schow, 2003; Niskar et al., 1998).

Study of minimally hard of hearing children in Tennessee shows that they experience excessive grade repetition (Porter & Bess, 2011). When hearing loss in the Iowa public schools was studied extensively, the rate of mild to moderate sensorineural and mixed losses was relatively constant in school-age children from grades K through 12. Conductive, temporary losses decreased as the children got older, but high-frequency, noise-induced types of losses increased (Shepard, Davis, Gorga, & Stelmachowicz, 1981). The level of services (the percentage of youngsters receiving rehabilitation help) reported in Iowa for youngsters having sensorineural and mixed losses varied by the degree of loss. Specifically, there was only a 27 percent level of service for the mildest losses but up to a 92 percent level for the losses of greatest severity. Although Iowa was then considered to have exemplary services (70 school audiologists, 500 speech-language pathologists, 100 teachers of the deaf/hard of hearing) for its school-age children with hearing loss, the state was still found to be serving only 46 percent of all such youngsters with some kind of special placement or itinerant service. Also, slightly less than 50 percent of children in the overall sensorineural–mixed group were amplified. While numbers vary depending on the criteria used, it is commonly reported that there are approximately 50,000 youngsters who are deaf in the U.S. educational system (about 1 in every 1,000 children), and the majority of them receive special services.

There are approximately 50,000 youngsters who are deaf in the U.S. educational system (about 1 in every 1,000 children).

These data indicate a clear need to address, in a more comprehensive fashion, the needs of children with hearing losses of all types and degrees. More recent investigations have focused on examining factors affecting early intervention for children who are hard of hearing. Harrison et al. (2015) conducted a survey of 122 early intervention professionals and 131 parents. Results suggest that home-based services promote family involvement. Further, early intervention professionals who had more children who are deaf or hard of hearing in their caseloads reported higher levels of comfort in serving this population than those professionals whose caseloads contained a limited number of children who are deaf or hard of hearing. Hands-on experience from professional preparation programs or from caseloads composed of a large number of children who are deaf or hard of hearing contributes to professional comfort. Investigators are continuing to explore this important dimension of personnel preparation and home-based services for children who are deaf or hard of hearing.

Contemporary Efforts to Strengthen the Evidence Base in Audiologic Rehabilitation (AR)

Advances in hearing technology, earlier hearing loss identification, and implementation of longitudinal, multi-center studies have not only changed the landscape of service provision but also supported the critical need to examine longitudinal outcomes in children who are deaf and hard of hearing.

Contemporary efforts to strengthen the evidence base in audiologic rehabilitation for children with cochlear implants and hearing aids have expanded in the past several years, with a goal of understanding the impact of earlier service delivery as well as factors that lead to risk or resilience in children's outcomes. The Early Development of Children with Hearing Loss Project (Nittrouer, 2010) and the National Early Childhood Assessment Project (Yoshinaga-Itano, 2015) are examples of multistate projects examining outcomes of children with hearing loss. Several longitudinal research projects have exclusively examined the outcomes of children with cochlear implants (Fink, Wang, Visaya, & CdaCI Investigation Team, 2007; Geers, Tobey, & Moog 2011; Niparko et al., 2010).

Empirical evidence remains limited, especially for the group of children who are hard of hearing (Moeller, Tomblin, Yoshinaga-Itano, Connor, & Jerger, 2007). One specific longitudinal study is highlighted in this chapter because of its focus on this historically underserved group of children. The Outcomes of Children with Hearing Loss (OCHL) Study is a multi-site, longitudinal study that was implemented with funding from National Institute on Deafness and Other Communication Disorders (NIDCD) to investigate the outcomes of children with mild to severe hearing losses. The Outcomes of Children with Hearing Loss Study (OCHL) was a collaboration of the University of Iowa, Boys Town National Research Hospital, and University of North Carolina at Chapel Hill. Three hundred and seventeen children with hearing loss were enrolled, along with a comparison group of over 117 children with normal hearing. The study focused on children who had bilateral, permanent, mild to severe hearing loss who used hearing aids (or no hearing aid in the case of seven children with mild loss). Thirty-eight percent of the children had slight or mild hearing loss, 40 percent had moderate losses, and 22 percent had moderately severe or severe hearing losses. This study was unique in the comprehensive nature of the measures of outcomes (e.g., audiological, speech/language, psychosocial, academic, family) and the effort to examine a wide range of factors contributing to success (e.g., aided audibility, intervention characteristics, family background characteristics, device type, usage consistency). Comprehensive methods, results, and implications from this study were published in a supplementary volume of *Ear and Hearing* (open access at http://ochlstudy.org). Primary conclusions from that study (as reported by Moeller, Tomblin, & the OCHL Collaboration, 2015) were as follows:

1. Children with mild to severe hearing loss are at risk for delays in language development, and the level of risk increases with the severity of hearing loss.
2. Provision of well-fit hearing aids provides some degree of protection against child language delays. Greater audibility is associated with better language outcomes for preschoolers.
3. A substantial proportion (more than half) of children's hearing aids were not fit optimally. When the actual boost provided by hearing aids did not match target values, aided audibility was negatively impacted. Early hearing aid provision was associated with better early language outcomes, but later-fit children demonstrated accelerated growth patterns after longer durations of hearing aid use.
4. Children with consistent hearing aid use demonstrated better language and auditory development outcomes.
5. Caregivers' use of directive language was negatively associated with child language outcomes, supporting the importance of qualitative features of caregiver–child interaction.

6. Children's receptive language abilities and their aided audibility contributed to functional auditory and speech recognition skills. Because some domains of language depend on access to fine acoustic details in the input, children who are hard of hearing appear to be at particular risk for delays in morphology.

7. Norm referenced scores may overestimate the performance of children who are hard of hearing which may result in underestimating the needs of this group of children.

The OCHL team tested three factors that were hypothesized to influence the relationship between degree of hearing loss and children's outcomes. The results demonstrated the influential effects of the three factors: (1) aided audibility, (2) duration and consistency of hearing aid use, and (3) characteristics of the language environment.

The second study to be highlighted is a large-scale outcome study conducted through the National Acoustics Laboratory in Australia (see www.outcomes.nal .gov.au). Unlike the previous study, this study included children who used hearing aids or cochlear implants and children with additional disabilities. This research team explored outcomes in 451 participants, including 317 children with hearing aids and 134 children with cochlear implants (52 bilateral). Within this sample, 19 percent of the participants had mild hearing loss, 33 percent moderate, 18 percent severe, and 32 percent profound. There were 44 children identified with auditory neuropathy, and 107 children identified with additional disabilities. Like the U.S. team, these researchers explored the effects of provision of early access to interventions and the multiple factors that influence outcomes for individual children. Ching et al. (2013) showed the following:

1. Children whose hearing loss was identified early received earlier auditory and educational intervention.

2. Earlier diagnosis was associated with higher levels of maternal education and socioeconomic status.

3. Children with more severe hearing loss received earlier auditory and educational intervention.

4. While early hearing aid fitting was not significantly associated with outcomes, age at which a first cochlear implant was received was associated with outcomes at 3 years of age.

5. Additional disabilities are associated with decreased outcomes at 3 years of age.

6. Higher maternal education was associated with better outcomes for children at 3 years of age.

7. On average, the children's performance in expressive and receptive language, speech production, and social and auditory functional abilities were at or one standard deviation below the normative mean.

TERMS AND DEFINITIONS

As noted in Chapter 1, a rigid distinction between habilitation and rehabilitation is not being made in this book. Although some prefer to use the word *habilitation* when working with children having prelingual hearing loss, we use the term *audiologic rehabilitation* (AR) because of its generic usage in the profession.

AR for the child may be viewed best as an advocacy in which the rehabilitation professional works with the parents and the child to identify needs in relation to the hearing loss and subsequently arranges to help meet those needs. Needs resulting from hearing loss are detailed in the chapters on amplification/audition (Chapters 2 and 3), auditory and visual skill development (Chapters 4 and 5), speech-language communication (Chapter 6), and psychosocial (Chapter 7) and school issues (Chapter 8), all of which are contained in the first section of this book. AR includes both assessment and management (see discussion in Chapter 1). While all these AR needs are important, they should be approached differently for various children, depending, among other variables, on the degree and time of onset of the hearing loss and the age of the child. Consequently, in order to be meaningful, a discussion of AR should be seen in the context of a profile of possible clients. The following section specifically focuses on severity and type of hearing loss, age of child, and other disabilities.

PROFILE OF THE CLIENT

Hearing Loss

Deafness categories for children include *congenital* (present at birth), *prelingual*, and *postlingual*. Youngsters with congenital deafness should generally be served through early intervention programs, which include parent–infant and preschool programs. As soon as the loss is identified (preferably by 3 months of age or before), parent–infant services and the individualized family service plan (IFSP) should start. Preschool programming typically begins when the child is about 3 years of age. Ideally, children continue with such programs until AR services are provided in connection with school placement. Youngsters with prelingual deafness, with onset after birth, will generally receive similar treatment. Children with postlingual deafness, however, will be served in a variety of settings, depending on technological intervention and geographic area.

> *Congenital* refers to hearing loss present at birth. *Prelingual* refers to the onset of hearing loss prior to the acquisition of spoken language. *Postlingual* refers to the onset of hearing loss after spoken language has been acquired.

A variety of children who are hard of hearing also participate in AR. Youngsters with milder losses are sometimes identified early and receive AR through early intervention. Other youngsters with slight or mild losses are not identified and/or do not receive assistance until after they start school. Indeed, some losses are progressive and reach significant dimensions only as the child gets older. One type of slight to mild loss involves middle ear infections, which result in conductive hearing problems. Frequently, such losses are of a transient nature, but in other cases they persist over a long period and require rehabilitation assistance. These conductive problems can have an educational impact on children even if the loss is only on the order of 15 dB HL.

> The individualized family service plan (IFSP) is required by special education law to guide birth to age 3 services. It is developed in collaboration with the family to identify family and child strengths and needs and family priorities and to identify outcomes for the early intervention program.

Since many more children are hard of hearing than are deaf, most AR work should be performed with children who are hard of hearing (although AR should not be neglected with either group) (see Table 1.2). Today, many children with severe and profound hearing losses receive cochlear implants. According to the NIDCD, more than 28,000 children in the United States have received them (www.nidcd.nih.gov/health/hearing/coch.asp). The AR program for children with cochlear implants focuses on developing listening skills and maximizing use of the device(s) in the development of spoken language skills. In this chapter, we describe the various types of rehabilitative efforts without precisely distinguishing between service models for children who are deaf and those for children who are hard of hearing. Although this approach involves some loss of specificity, it is necessary in order to avoid excessive duplication. There is, naturally, much in common in AR services regardless of the degree of hearing loss or the mode of communication used. Thus, the reader must selectively apply AR techniques consistent with the individual child's needs.

> LSL = Listening and Spoken Language

Age

If the assumption is made that children become adults somewhere between 18 and 21 years of age, graduation from high school provides a natural line of demarcation between childhood and adulthood. In that case, we may separate the years from birth to age 18 into two basic divisions: those before school years (0 to 5) and the school years themselves (5 to 18+). In addition, we may make a number of other subdivisions, including the years of infancy and toddlerhood (0 to 3), the preschool years (3 to 5), and the kindergarten, grade school, junior high, and high school years (5 to 18).

In this chapter, we use the two-way division (0 to 5 and school years) since children who are deaf or hard of hearing generally undergo a major adjustment of rehabilitation services when they enter regular school programming. Before that, AR includes parent–infant and preschool programs. When kindergarten begins, the school personnel will generally take over rehabilitation responsibilities from the early intervention–preschool professional. These age ranges are general; consequently, some children progress through intervention programs more quickly than others. Services are not time locked but rather sequential, depending on the child's progress.

Other Disabling Conditions

A multidisciplinary approach involves a team of specialists from a variety of disciplines in the child's care.

Youngsters with hearing loss often have other disabling conditions, such as visual loss, motor disabilities, or intellectual disabilities. The percentage is on the order of 30 to 40 percent based on data from national surveys of young children with hearing loss (Eze, Ofo, Jiang, & O'Connor, 2013; Gallaudet Research Institute, 2011; Palmieri et al., 2012) (see also Chapters 6 and 8). Improvements in medical science have resulted in the survival of more children with multiple disabilities. This underscores the need for a multidisciplinary approach to rehabilitation in which important professionals coordinate all services to ensure integrated treatment of the child. (See Chapter 11, Case 1, for an example in working with such a youngster.)

REHABILITATION SETTINGS AND PROVIDERS

AR settings and providers are determined to a great extent by the child's age, the severity of the hearing loss, and the presence of other disabilities. Typically, services start as family-centered programs in the home coordinated by a parent advisor (sometimes called a parent–infant teacher or specialist) and progress through preschool programs up through the formal school years. Throughout the rehabilitation process, the services of many professional disciplines are called on in addition to continued strong parental involvement. Figure 9.1 contains an overview of the AR process as it relates to the roles of clinical audiologists, educators, and medical personnel.

IDENTIFICATION AND ASSESSMENT PROCEDURES WITH CHILDREN

Early identification of children with hearing loss or who are at risk for hearing loss is critical for successful rehabilitation. Also, proper diagnosis requires precise and appropriate screening and assessment instruments, administered, scored, and interpreted by skilled professionals. The following sections will present prevailing trends in these areas as well as implications for amplification and the overall AR process.

Early Identification

Two tests used in early identification programs are otoacoustic emissions (OAE) and auditory brain stem response (ABR).

As indicated previously, audiologists are frequently involved in early identification of hearing loss. Naturally, early AR efforts cannot be initiated until the presence of hearing loss is known. Identification of hearing loss soon after birth can be determined through the use of two tests, otoacoustic emissions (OAE) and auditory brain stem response (ABR). The National Institutes of Health & National Institute on Deafness and Other Communication Disorders, (1993), the Joint Committee on Infant Hearing (JCIH, 2000, 2007), and the American Academy of Pediatrics (1999) endorsed the practice of universal screening of hearing in newborns, a majority of

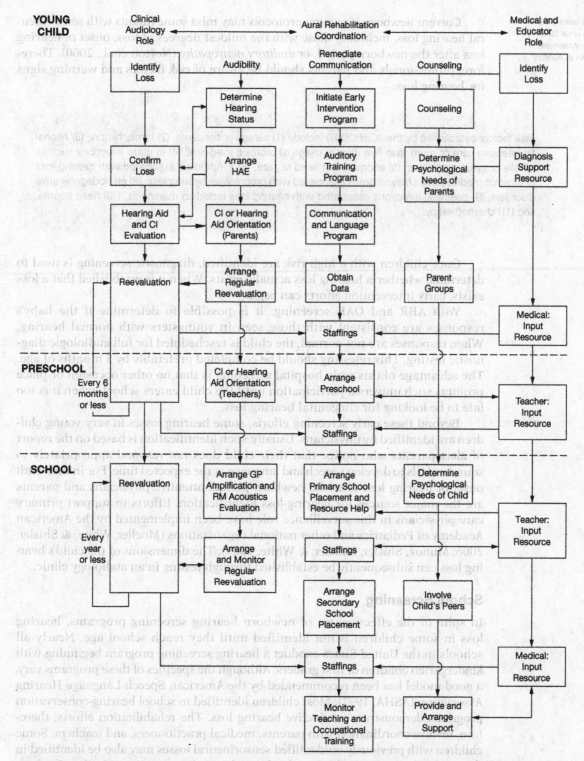

FIGURE 9.1   Overview of the AR process. Note that the CARE model is shown here in this flowchart in that (C)ounseling, (A)udibility, (R)emediate Communication, and (E)nvironmental Coordination are key elements shown at the top.

states across the nation have enacted legislation, and all states have initiated screening programs. Current newborn hearing screening procedures have been found to be more effective than previously used high-risk screening programs (Norton et al., 2000). These initiatives allow for proactive management by identifying the majority of hearing losses early in life.

Auditory neuropathy: a hearing loss in which sound information is not faithfully transmitted to the *auditory nerve* and *brain* properly. Also known as Auditory Dys-synchrony.

Current newborn screening protocols may miss some infants with sensorineural hearing loss, including those with the mildest degrees of loss, onset of hearing loss after the newborn period, or *auditory neuropathy* (Norton et al., 2000). Therefore, professionals and parents should be aware of risk factors and warning signs for hearing loss.

Risk factors established by the JCIH (2007) include (1) caregiver concerns, (2) family history, (3) neonatal intensive care of more than five days or usage of ototoxic medicine, (4) in utero infections such as rubella or cytomegalovirus, (5) anomalies of head or face, (6) syndromes associated with hearing loss or ototoxic medications, (7) syndromes associated with progressive hearing loss, (8) neurodegenerative disorders, (9) postnatal infections associated with hearing loss including meningitis, (10) head trauma, and (11) chemotherapy.

Once children with a high risk are identified, diagnostic screening is used to determine whether a hearing loss actually exists. When it is established that a loss exists, early intervention efforts can begin.

With ABR and OAE screening, it is possible to determine if the baby's responses are consistent with those seen in youngsters with normal hearing. When responses are not normal, the child is rescheduled for full audiologic diagnostic testing. This retesting should be completed preferably by 3 months of age. The advantage of this early hospital screening is that no other occasion or place prompts such universal participation until the child enters school, when it is too late to be looking for congenital hearing loss.

Beyond these early screening efforts, some hearing losses in very young children are identified by physicians. Usually, such identification is based on the report of alert parents who notice that their child does not respond appropriately to sound or fails to develop speech and language at the expected time. For infants with onset of hearing loss after the newborn period, attentive physicians and parents are the major sources for hearing-loss identification. Efforts to support primary care physicians in this surveillance role have been implemented by the American Academy of Pediatrics and other national organizations (Moeller, White, & Shisler, 2006; Munoz, Shisler, Moeller, & White, 2009). The dimensions of the child's hearing loss can subsequently be established through testing in an audiology clinic.

School Screening

In spite of the effectiveness of newborn hearing screening programs, hearing loss in some children is not identified until they reach school age. Nearly all schools in the United States conduct a hearing screening program beginning with kindergarten children or first graders. Although the specifics of these programs vary, a good model has been recommended by the American Speech-Language-Hearing Association (ASHA, 1997). Most children identified in school hearing-conservation programs demonstrate conductive hearing loss. The rehabilitation efforts, therefore, involve coordination with parents, medical practitioners, and teachers. Some children with previously unidentified sensorineural losses may also be identified in these school programs. This may be due to later onset or progressive hearing loss, mild losses that were undetected by early screening measures, or lack of follow-up from newborn screening. In such cases, medical referral is indicated to clarify the medical aspects of the loss, followed by AR assistance provided by educational audiologists or other personnel.

Medical and Audiologic Assessment

Before AR is initiated, the child should undergo a medical examination as well as a basic hearing assessment. Complete, definitive results are not always available on very young children. When the child is old enough, results from such assessments

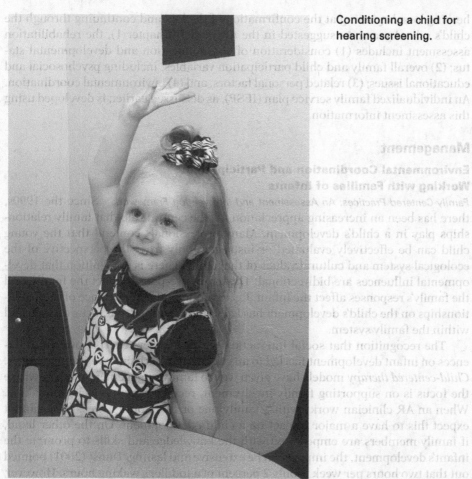

Conditioning a child for hearing screening.

should include information on both ears, giving (1) otoscopic findings, (2) degree and configuration of loss, (3) type of loss and cause, (4) speech recognition ability (clarity of hearing), (5) most comfortable level (MCL), (6) threshold of discomfort (TD), and (7) hearing aid performance (verification) and audibility measures. Functional skills in the areas of academic achievement, language, and amplification systems should also be evaluated using standardized speech-language assessments, teacher and parent questionnaires, and audiologic procedures, including speech perception testing.

Medical consultation is necessary to determine the need for a genetic evaluation, obtain clearance for amplification usage, receive any indicated medical treatments, and maintain contact with the medical home. After initial hearing aid fitting, regular assessments should take place for children with sensorineural losses. Temporary conductive loss may occur and complicate the hearing situation, especially in young children. Audiologic data should be obtained on a regular basis so that, if necessary, amplification or other dimensions of the rehabilitation program can be changed. From birth to age 3 years, children should be seen for audiologic assessment at three-month intervals and at six-month intervals during the preschool years. After that, they should be clinically tested at least once a year.

ASPECTS OF AR: EARLY INTERVENTION FOR PARENT–INFANT AND PRESCHOOL

Rehabilitation Assessment: Individualized Family Service Plan (IFSP)

With children, the extensive rehabilitative assessments that generally precede management are integrated with management more than with adult clients. Thus, we outline here an ongoing assessment approach to the AR of the young child with hearing loss, beginning at the confirmation of the loss and continuing through the child's school years. As suggested in the AR model (Chapter 1), the rehabilitation assessment includes (1) consideration of communication and developmental status; (2) overall family and child participation variables, including psychosocial and educational issues; (3) related personal factors; and (4) environmental coordination. An individualized family service plan (IFSP), as discussed earlier, is developed using this assessment information.

Management

Environmental Coordination and Participation: Working with Families of Infants

Family-Centered Practices: An Assessment and Intervention Framework. Since the 1990s, there has been an increasing appreciation for the central role that family relationships play in a child's development. Many professionals contend that the young child can be effectively evaluated or instructed only from the perspective of the ecological system and cultural values of the family. There is recognition that developmental influences are bidirectional: The infant's responses affect the family, and the family's responses affect the infant. Recognition of the importance of these relationships on the child's development has led to interventions that focus on the child within the family system.

The recognition that social interaction with caregivers exerts powerful influences on infant development has led to an evolution in early intervention practices. *Child-centered therapy* models have given way to family-engagement models, where the focus is on supporting family involvement, reciprocity, and decision making. When an AR clinician works with a family one or two hours a week, one cannot expect this to have a major impact on a child's development. On the other hand, if family members are empowered with the knowledge and skills to promote the infant's development, the impact can be extensive and lasting. Dunst (2001) pointed out that two hours per week is only 2 percent of a toddler's waking hours. However, diapering, feeding, and playing happen at least 2,000 times before the first birthday. If caregivers optimized just 10 interactions per waking hour in everyday activities, a toddler would have more than 36,000 learning opportunities between the ages of 1 and 2 years. This is why early intervention practices have shifted away from child-focused therapy to techniques that support quality relationships and interactions between infants and their family members.

Family-centered practice includes a focus on family-identified needs and priorities, efforts to form partnerships with parents to address child needs, and empowerment of families as the primary decision makers for their child. *Child-centered therapy* refers to an intervention that provides direct service for the child, with limited direct involvement of the parent in intervention.

Some major principles of family-centered practice include the following:

1. The primary goal of early intervention is to support care providers in developing competence and confidence in helping the infant learn (Hanft, Rush, & Sheldon, 2004).

2. Family-identified needs should drive the intervention agenda, and professionals should adapt to the unique values, culture, and goals of each family.

3. Family members are recognized as the constant in the child's life and experts on the child's development. Professionals draw on the expertise of the family to address needs.

4. Families are equal team members. Professionals seek to establish balanced partnerships with family members in the intervention process.

5. Professionals respect the decision-making authority of the family. As noted by McWilliam (2010), the "current concept of early intervention places a high value on the family's decision making authority" (pp. 4–5).

Consistent with the concept of family-centered practice, federal legislation (Part C of IDEA) also requires the provision of early intervention services in *natural environments*. Although this term has been interpreted in a variety of ways, the intention is that infants and their families should receive services in the home or in routinely accessed community settings rather than in clinics or center-based programs. This concept of providing service only in *natural environments* sometimes conflicts with the values of providing ideal acoustic environments (Cole & Flexer, 2016) and/or access to native language models (e.g., for children who use sign language). A Fact Sheet on Natural Environments for children who are deaf or hard of hearing and their families was developed to clarify these issues (ASHA & Council on Education of the Deaf, 2006). It is important to keep in mind that the intent of the natural environments concept is to promote the application of learned strategies by practicing them in meaningful contexts that occur regularly in the family with the child. This avoids the need for parents to generalize a concept practiced in a toy-based activity to their regular parent–child interactions. For example, when parents learn to respond to the infant's communicative attempts during diapering, feeding, or other common routines, it fosters natural incorporation of the strategy throughout routines all day long. In contrast, if the skill is taught with a toy brought by the clinician, it may not be as easy for families to generalize the technique to everyday interactions. In other words, if home-based visits focus on child-directed therapy with clinician-provided toys, the intent of teaching in natural contexts is missing.

> *Natural environments* are promoted in federal early intervention laws. The term is used to promote the provision of services in the home or in community settings that families routinely access.

The purpose of early intervention, then, is to support and assist families in providing learning opportunities for their infant within the activities, routines, and events of everyday life. One contemporary model of family centered practice is called Routines-Based Early Intervention In this approach, typical routines engaged in by family members and the children are identified by the family. These are then used as contexts for supporting and promoting the child's development in partnership with the family This approach includes transdisciplinary (collaborative) models of service delivery, support-based home visits, and integration of services in day care settings, as appropriate (McWilliam, 2010).

Family-centered practice models are considered current best practice in response to universal newborn hearing screening programs (ASHA, 2008). As a result of early screening efforts, infants are identified much earlier in development than they were previously. This requires that the content of early intervention shift to focus on the parent–infant relationship in ways that support attunement to the infant's affect and signals, joyful interactions, turn taking, and contingent responding. The professional works together with the family to promote a nurturing and responsive social and communicative environment. Some professionals prefer the term *early development* rather than *intervention* to characterize this work. The concept of *development* captures the joint goals of nurturing infant growth through parent–infant interaction and of supporting the growth of parenting skills. Professionals need to cultivate the skills of being sensitive and responsive to family-identified needs in order to implement such programs.

> Parent–professional partnerships involve family members collaborating with professionals to identify needs and implement strategies to encourage infant development.

Shifting Roles and Strategies in the AR Program. The principles of family-centered practice require reconceptualization of professional roles. AR professionals now work with families who have very young infants; a child-focused model simply does not fit this scenario. There is work to be done to ensure that early intervention is family centered in its focus. Past survey studies indicate that many programs lack substantial family participation and tend to implement child-centered approaches (Roush, Harrison, & Palsha, 1991). Furthermore, Brinker, Frazier, and Baxter (1992) stressed the need for programs to examine how family-centered care can best be approached with families who have limited resources. Brown and Nott (2006) stressed the importance of cultural competence in early intervention, which requires adaptation of approaches to address cultural differences. They add that providers of family-centered practice focus on the following key ingredients: (1) understanding the family routines and important events (which will vary by culture), (2) keeping the intervention focused around these, (3) directing intervention at the capacities of the parents to interact appropriately with their child during these activities, (4) understanding next steps in development, and (5) having skills in teaching parents effective scaffolding techniques (pp. 139–140).

Early intervention also has been conceptualized as "relationship-focused." Mahoney (2009) describes relationship-focused intervention as an approach that fosters child development by encouraging parents to engage in *highly responsive interactions* throughout natural daily routines with the child. In the experience of the first author of this chapter, there are at least three relationships involved in the home-based early intervention: (1) the relationship between parents and child (which should be the primary focus), (2) the relationship between the parents and the AR provider (which ideally takes the form of a balanced partnership), and (3) the relationship between the infant/child and the provider (which is secondary to the parent–infant relationship and includes ongoing developmental observation to guide next steps in intervention).

While focusing on the parent–infant relationship, the AR specialist promotes parental ability to use strategies that are known to facilitate auditory and language development for all children. However, because the child is deaf or hard of hearing, parents will be encouraged to do all the things one would typically do with a young child but in a manner that is consistent, strategic, adaptive, and informed. *Consistent* refers to embedding language and auditory learning opportunities during authentic, natural interactions all day long. It also means learning the characteristics of a language- and auditory-rich environment (described further below) and working to provide those. *Strategic* means that parents/caregivers "engineer" additional meaningful opportunities for language and auditory exposure or practice. For example, the infant might just be learning to alert to her name. As the mother approaches to take her baby out of the car seat, she calls her by name ("Molly!"). She notices that Molly stops kicking her legs and becomes still, as if listening. Mother gets a little closer and says her name again, just outside the baby's visual field. Molly turns toward the voice, and Mom smiles and says, "You heard me! I said Molly. That's you!" Although this might take a little more time for the parent than just removing the infant from the car seat, the parent has strategically promoted auditory learning and observed that this practice is bringing about results. *Adaptive* means that family members are attuned to changes in the infant's development, and they adjust their strategies to promote further developmental change. For example, while sharing books with the toddler, the parent might observe that the child is beginning to point to various pictures when the object name is mentioned. The parent supports this skill by selecting books that offer additional opportunities and by inviting the child to comment on pictures and then expanding the child's response. The term *informed* suggests that the parent is aware of the importance of strategies that support the child's turn taking and communication. Although many positive parenting behaviors may happen instinctively, early intervention programs do not leave that to chance. They work with families to ensure that caregivers know why they are using the strategy and its importance for the child's development.

These goals are approached through parent–professional collaborations on home visits. A team of experienced AR professionals (Stredler-Brown, 2005; Stredler-Brown, Moeller, Gallegos, Cordwin, & Pittman, 2004) contends that there is both an art and a science to early intervention conducted in the home with families. The *science* is the special knowledge of deafness, infancy, and families that the parent–infant educator brings to the task. These skills are critical for cultivating early listening and vocal and visual behaviors in the context of responsive, reciprocal communication. On the other hand, the *art* is the human side. It has to do with how we are joining with families in a manner that conveys respect, builds trust, and establishes effective partnerships. Through partnerships, parents and professionals listen to one another and seek joined perspectives. Specialized skills that AR clinicians need for serving families in the birth to age 3 period are summarized in Table 9.1 (Stredler-Brown et al., 2004).

TABLE 9.1 **Specialized Knowledge and Skills Required of AR Specialists in Early Intervention**

Science: Specialized Knowledge and Skills	Art: Skills for Interaction with Families
■ Infant development ■ Family systems, values, and culture ■ Impact of hearing loss in development ■ Communication, auditory, speech, language, cognitive, social-emotional development, and techniques for enhancing skill of parents and infants in natural contexts ■ Communication approaches and fluency in the selected approach(es) ■ Amplification technologies (hearing aids, cochlear implants, FM systems) ■ Promoting listening skills as a foundation for spoken language development ■ Assistive technology ■ Appropriate developmental expectations ■ Infant–family assessment skills ■ Cultural competence	■ Creates an atmosphere of trust, experimentation, learning from one another ■ Active listener who conveys understanding, empathy, acceptance ■ Responds to feelings, moving away from "what ought to be" ■ Paces the work effectively ■ Navigates ambiguity and contradiction ■ Acts as a nonjudgmental sounding board ■ Recognizes the role of grief in healthy adjustment ■ Enhances self direction/independence ■ Prioritizes needs ■ Recruits and accepts parents' interpretations, perceptions, advice, and predictions about infant ■ Adapts to the individual family constellation, culture and needs

Contributors: A. Stredler-Brown, M. P. Moeller, R. Gallegos, P. Pittman, J. Cordwin, and M. Condon.

Source: Adapted from Stredler-Brown et al. (2004).

Further analysis of the behaviors of skilled providers revealed several roles and techniques that promote collaboration with families on home visits. These were called "tools of the trade" by the authors, and they include the following:

1. *Information resource.* Although this role may be obvious, it takes skill to adapt to the learning needs of individual families, to provide information in objective ways, and to share information-gathering responsibilities so that families become independent advocates and learners. Professionals work with families to access a variety of sources of information and experiences to build an objective information base (see Figure 9.3). This knowledge base aids families in the decision-making process. The process of timing of the information is also critical. Professionals are sensitive to the overwhelming experience of being a new parent who may be adjusting to an unexpected diagnosis and work to share information in manageable ways. Parents may be accessing information from a wide variety of sources (e.g., Internet, social networking), which can be overwhelming in some cases. This suggests the need for professionals to effectively pace the work, which requires sensitivity to family needs.

2. *Coach/partner role.* Coaching in this sense does not mean directing parents in their actions. Rather, it is a mind-set for interaction that shifts the focus away from expert-driven ideas toward "learner-focused" techniques (Hanft et al., 2004). Adults (parents and clinicians) are the learners, but parents are in the "driver's seat," and the clinician is literally on the sidelines, providing tips or guidance that support the integration of skills by the parent. Coaching provides opportunities for family members to integrate new skills within their typical interactions with the child. The clinician uses skills of observation, well-timed input, and outcome analysis to support and guide the interaction. The shaded box on page 262 contrasts a clinician-directed response with a partnership and a coaching-oriented response.

3. *Joint discoverer.* This is a key ingredient in a partnership process. Family members learn that any question can be addressed as an "experiment" (Moeller & Condon, 1994). This prepares families to try techniques with the child and evaluate how they work. It allows clinicians to maintain balance in the relationship. Instead of telling the parent what to do (expert driven), the idea can be proposed as an experiment (learner focused). As an example, the clinician

might observe that the parent is having trouble getting the baby's auditory attention because there is an attractive stuffed toy captivating her imagination. The clinician can pose an experiment by asking, "I wonder what would happen if you set the toy to the side and called her name before you start talking. I wonder if that will help her listen." This is a subtle but important distinction. It is likely that the suggested adaptation will work, but it will be the parents who bring about the success in engaging their baby's attention. The role of joint discoverer also means that the AR clinician and the parents are becoming skilled observers of the child's successes and of what works to promote success. The process of evaluation is integrated in each session, as this becomes the guide or road map for future sessions.

4. *News commentator (Moeller & Condon, 1994).* This technique also promotes partnership and the process of basing decisions on ongoing evaluation of what works. The news commentator role is one of providing objective, descriptive feedback about key behaviors (e.g., "I notice that each time she vocalizes, you vocalize right back to her. Then she takes another turn. That keeps communication going between the two of you."). This strategy points out to families what is working well. It demonstrates that the adults are figuring out what to do based on observing the child's responses to the family. The clinician often comments on what the child is doing, which typically prompts the family to give an interpretation. These experiences help families learn the strategy of observing to figure out what works. Brandwein (2010) emphasizes that professionals can provide feedback in ways that are confidence building. Given that a primary goal of early intervention is to promote parental confidence, this is a skill professionals want to cultivate. For example, suppose a parent is struggling with a toddler who constantly removes the hearing aid. This is a situation that potentially can undermine parental confidence ("No matter what I do, he will not leave it in!" which might translate to, "I can't do this."). Suppose the parent expresses, "Sometimes I feel like giving up, but then I just try again." The AR provider might respond, "You persist in the face of challenges. That takes strength." Suppose another parent decides to give the hearing aid a brief "rest" after a tug-of-war with the toddler. The AR provider could say, "You know what works with your child. You trust your judgment." In another scenario, the parent chuckles to herself after the child takes the device out for the tenth time. The provider could say, "You've got a sense of humor about this." These nonjudgmental descriptive responses point out resilient characteristics and may promote confidence. It is tempting to address the events (what is happening with the hearing aid), but it is important to acknowledge and support parental responses to these events. These are examples of practicing compassion instead of correction.

5. *Partner in play.* Sometimes it is useful for the clinician to demonstrate a strategy or new skill for parents. However, parents should then have immediate opportunities to "try the skill on for size" so that both parties can see if the technique works in the parents' hands. Practicing in a context of playful interactions with the infant promotes comfort with the new skill.

6. *Joint reflector and planner.* At the end of each session, partners work together to list key observations and successes from the time together. What did we get out of today's session? What did we learn? This brings ongoing concerns into focus and sets agendas for the next session. Collaborative questions, such as "So what should we do next time?" and "Who else would you like to join our work and how will we involve them?," promote planning.

Figure 9.2 illustrates a model for home visit planning. Stredler-Brown et al. (2004) described a rubric for home visits that included the steps of (1) reconnect and review (discuss with the family how things have gone over the past week), (2) address priorities (identify and address parental concerns and focus on the skills

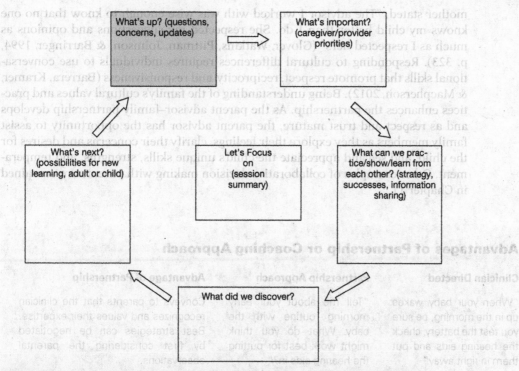

FIGURE 9.2   **A Home Visit Planning Guide. This model represents some of the experiences and sources of support that can be brought together in partnership with families to facilitate intervention planning and decision making.**

and strategies parents and professional partners will jointly address in this visit), (3) share the craft (partners try out and practice relationship-focused strategies for communicating during natural routines), (4) assess and evaluate (partners observe the child's and parents' responses to various strategies and determine what is working), and (5) reflect on the home visit (summarize what was learned today, comment on strengths, and summarize implications for next steps). This rubric was adapted by Carotta, Kline, and Brennan (2014) into a guide for professionals who are working to implement routine-based interventions in the home setting. The questions posed in this model (Figure 9.2) guide the thought process of the professional throughout each session. By addressing these process-oriented questions, the professional engages in a mental exercise that leads to appropriate focus and accountability for session planning and outcomes. It is critical to keep in mind that the focus is on relationships and that the professional is also using the skills of sensitivity and active listening to provide psychosocial support for the family.

Guiding Families in Decision Making.   One of the most dramatic role shifts occurring in AR as a result of family-centered practice goals is that decision-making authority is to rest with family members. Professionals are challenged to help parents gain the skills and knowledge to be effective advocates and decision makers for their child. Previously, professionals made many of the decisions regarding the habilitative management of the child. Now professionals are being challenged to work as partners with families in assessing needs, implementing practices, and developing the knowledge base to support decision making. So, for example, in the parent advisor–family partnership, both partners contribute expertise and at the foundation is a trusting relationship built on mutual respect. Family members know the child's likes, dislikes, time schedules, favorite toys and activities, food preferences, and many other matters that the parent advisor cannot be expected to know. One

Professionals need to shift their traditional roles and ensure that families are placed in the role of primary decision makers for the child.

mother stated, "The advisor I worked with was wise enough to know that no one knows my child better than I do. She respected my suggestions and opinions as much as I respected hers" (Glover, Watkins, Pittman, Johnson, & Barringer, 1994, p. 323). Responding to cultural differences requires individuals to use conversational skills that promote respect, reciprocity, and responsiveness (Barrera, Kramer, & Macpherson, 2012). Being understanding of the family's cultural values and practices enhances the partnership. As the parent advisor–family partnership develops and as respect and trust mature, the parent advisor has the opportunity to assist family members as they explore their feelings, clarify their concerns and desires for the child, and see and appreciate the child's unique skills, strengths, and temperament. Other examples of collaborative decision making with parents are contained in Chapter 11.

Advantages of Partnership or Coaching Approach

Clinician Directed	Partnership Approach	Advantage of Partnership
"When your baby wakes up in the morning, be sure you test the battery, check the hearing aids and put them in right away."	"Tell me about your early morning routine with the baby. What do you think might work best for putting the hearing aids in?"	Conveys to parents that the clinician recognizes and values their expertise. Best strategies can be negotiated by first considering the parental observations.

Clinician Directed	Coaching Approach	Advantage of Coaching
"You need to give her a chance to communicate about the picture before you turn the page of the book."	"I wonder what will happen if you pause a moment before turning the page?" "Oh, when you waited, he took a turn. He used his voice. That worked for you."	The clinician-directed example leaves the professional in the role of expert. In the coaching example, the same idea is posed as a question or experiment, and the parent is the one who is successful with the technique.

Transdisciplinary teamwork refers to a process in which team members collaborate and are interdependent. Rather than each member separately working with the child and sharing viewpoints, team members work together and integrate their perspectives.

A second major shift in service delivery influences the teamwork roles of the AR professional/hearing specialist. In order to meet comprehensive family and child needs, professionals must employ *transdisciplinary teamwork*. No one discipline has all the knowledge and expertise to adequately address the comprehensive nature of most cases. The AR clinician in a parent advisor role has a particularly critical role on the team. Because the parent advisor has frequent contact with the family in their home (e.g., one to two times per week), this professional is often in a good position to gain a full understanding of the family's strengths and priorities and to work with the parent to implement strategies to achieve these priorities. The parent advisor may also serve in a role of case coordination with the assistance of a service coordinator.

The parent advisor–AR clinician can and should draw on the resources of a community-based team of professionals, depending on the needs that present themselves. Parent advisors need to cultivate the skills for collaborative consultation and teamwork in order to effectively serve families. Idol, Paolucci-Whitcomb, and Nevin (1986) state, "Collaborative consultation is an interactive process that enables teams of people with diverse expertise to generate creative solutions to mutually defined problems. The outcome is enhanced and altered from the original solutions that any team member would produce independently" (p. 9).

Supporting Families in Decision Making. Newborn hearing screening has brought about a paradigm shift in the ways AR clinicians and educators work with families. In earlier decades, parents may have noted their child's lack of or inconsistent responses to sound. When hearing loss was diagnosed, this news was difficult but also confirmed the parents' suspicions in many cases. Today, hospital personnel or audiologists are telling parents who have no reason to suspect a problem that their newborn may have a hearing loss. This information is delivered at a time of tremendous personal adjustment (to the birth of a baby). Luterman (2004) states, "This presents a very different counseling paradigm than the parent-initiated model where the audiologist is often seen as an ally confirming that parent's suspicion." Luterman advocates for increased training in counseling in the preparation of audiologists/ AR professionals.

On diagnosis of hearing loss, families are met with a host of decisions about communicating with the infant, about technologies, about educational programs, and about parenting this baby in the context of the family. At a consensus conference on early intervention for infants who are deaf and hard of hearing (Marge & Marge, 2005), professionals unanimously agreed that parents should have access to objective information about all communication, technological, and educational options for the child. Few would disagree with this notion. However, much is to be learned about the best ways to provide this information to families who are in the process of adjusting to the birth of a new baby. In some cases, programs provide written brochures explaining various options. In other cases, families have opportunities to meet with other parents, visit programs, search the Internet, or explore other sources. In reality, each family should have an approach that is tailored to its individual needs. This requires of the AR professional both sensitivity and the establishment of effective partnerships with families.

Decision making is not a reading activity—it is a *process*. Within that process, family members (1) get to know their infant as well as the infant's unique abilities and needs, (2) become skilled at observing the baby and figuring out what strategies are successful for making communication connections in the family, (3) clarify the goals they have for themselves and their child, (4) have opportunities for parent-to-parent contact and other supports, and (5) and learn about various options in education, technology, and communication. This entire process typically does not happen in the few weeks after diagnosis. For many families, the process unfolds over several months, and opinions about what to do change as the family gains relevant experiences, support, and knowledge. It is important to recognize that the "learning about options part" is one of five steps! It is not sufficient to give parents reading materials and ask that they decide. Instead, families benefit from a variety of supports and experiences as they make decisions for the infant. The role of the AR professional is to help families clarify which supports may be helpful at different times and to assist families in accessing these. Some possible sources of support and information are visualized in Figure 9.3. This could be thought of as a puzzle. The pieces that will fit together to make a whole picture will be unique for each individual family. The AR clinician seeks to be a facilitator and sounding board as the family builds its system of supports. The "art" in this process involves the AR clinician sensitively supporting the family in identifying which supports are most helpful at what times in the process. The AR clinician may find that a family initially states that they do not want to meet other parents who have deaf or hard of hearing children. By revisiting that issue a few months later, the clinician discovers not only that the parents want that experience but also that they benefit greatly from it. The process needs to be adaptive to the changing values and perceived needs of the family.

A national parent organization called Hands and Voices provides perspectives and information that are helpful to parents and professionals alike (see www.handsandvoices.org). They acknowledge that making choices for the child is a process that is flexible, ongoing, and changeable. Many families do not make "one choice" on their communication journey with the child. They often adapt and choose a variety of tools and approaches as the child's needs evolve. DesGeorges (2004a)

Collaborative consultation comes about when team members contribute diverse expertise to creatively solve intervention problems.

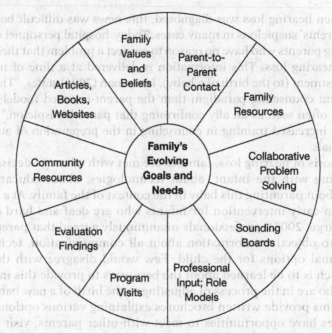

FIGURE 9.3 This model represents some of the experiences and sources of support that can be brought together in partnership with families to facilitate decision making.

published a "wish list" from parents for audiologists that supports many of the points raised so far. Selected excerpts are shown in the following box.

Parent Wish List for Audiologists

- Provide us with the information we need to make well-informed decisions.
- If we ask a question and you don't have the answer, help us find the resources where we can find the answer.
- Be connected to community resources.
- As children and parents grow, their choices and need for information grow and change.
- Respect the choices that families make. Let us, the parents, make the final decision.
(DesGeorges, 2004a)

An aspect of decision making that sometimes gets overlooked concerns the resources that are needed within the family system to support the communication or technology approach. Families should not only understand the features of various methodologies but also consider what the particular approach will require of them as a family. This type of information is covered in program materials from *Beginnings for Families* (www. http://ncbegin.org). Current options for communication are described along with family responsibilities that come along with the approach. Video samples are provided that illustrate key features of various communication development programs. Such information is another helpful piece of the puzzle.

Implications of Family-Centered Care for Intervention. Family-centered parent–infant programs, then, focus on family members as the primary interventionists. The AR specialist provides guidance and coaching to the family in several key content areas: (1) fitting and adjustment to full time use of amplification, cochlear implants, and other devices; (2) auditory learning (use of residual hearing); and (3) techniques for optimizing communicative development (whether the family is using auditory, auditory-visual, or visually based approaches). Another vital content area for the program is helping the family meet its support needs and providing activities that promote psychosocial well-being. Once the child is of preschool age (around 3 years old), services typically shift to center-based models where the child attends a preschool and/or individual listening and spoken language sessions. These services are commonly provided in a regular preschool setting with support services, a setting that integrates children who are typically developing with those who have hearing loss, or a self-contained preschool for children who are deaf or hard of hearing. Some self-contained programs also integrate peers with typical hearing. Wherever the service delivery or whatever the model, family-centered practices continue to be vital. Families learn at the parent–infant level to be knowledgeable advocates for their children. They become intricately involved in influencing the child's success. It would be a mistake to "graduate" the child into a center-based program and minimize the contributions family members can make. Instead, programs should continue to address family needs, family support, and family guidance into the preschool years. In the next sections, we describe approaches in each of the key content areas at the parent–infant and preschool levels.

Audibility, Amplification, and Assistive Device Issues

Hearing Aid Fitting. Once preliminary medical and audiologic findings are available on the child, the selection of amplification, when appropriate, becomes an early goal in the rehabilitative program. Experts agree that hearing aids are extremely important tools in early intervention programs in helping children develop their residual hearing and their speech and language abilities. Unfortunately, as previously noted, some youngsters with hearing loss do not have and/or do not consistently use amplification. Consequently, the efforts of the AR clinician may need to be directed toward achieving those goals. The hearing aid fitting will be performed by an audiologist who may also be providing other rehabilitative services (see Figure 9.1). If the AR professional does not perform the fitting, he or she will want to review its adequacy. Children should be fit using a data-driven formula and that fitting verified in order to achieve the highest levels of speech recognition ability and comfort in noise. The Desired Sensation Level (DSL) or the National Acoustics Laboratories (NAL) fitting formulas have been documented to provide a quality listening experience for individual children in real-world environments. Many important considerations in fitting hearing aids in children are contained in a Pediatric Amplification Protocol (AAA, 2013). Although hearing aid fitting is a first priority, other hearing assistive technology should also be considered.

The Desired Sensation Level (DSL) and the National Acoustic Laboratories fitting formulas are data-driven formulas used to maximize speech recognition ability and comfort levels for children using hearing assistive technology (HAT).

Pediatric and school-age amplification should focus on personal amplification devices but not exclude personal or classroom FM systems and other hearing assistance technology (HAT) (American Academy of Audiology, 2008).

HAT = Hearing assistive technology and hearing assistance technology both have the same acronym and can be used interchangably. These terms have a broad meaning which includes hearing aids, cochlear implants, hearing assistive devices and various forms of amplification.

Fitting protocols should include ongoing evaluation, verification, and validation of the child's performance with all devices. Evaluation should be used to confirm and monitor actual or fluctuating hearing levels. Verification of the devices' appropriateness can be completed using real ear measures, such as real ear to coupler difference and speech mapping. Validation of performance should include measures that document whether the child has access to the speech of others and is able to clearly monitor his or her own speech. All measures should be completed with consideration of the ever-changing auditory needs of preschool and school-age children. Functional assessment measures such as checklists and questionnaires can be used to validate and document individual performance in individual and natural listening environments. Parents and teachers can provide valuable input using some of these instruments, which are designed for use by individuals in the child's life. A review of these tools can be found in the Pediatric Amplification Protocol (AAA, 2013), and specific tools can be accessed on the text website.

In addition to hearing aids, hearing assistive technology, like FM systems for use in noisy environments (e.g., classrooms), should be considered.

Type and Arrangement of Aid. The type of aid and the arrangement (monaural, binaural, or other special fitting, such as a direct input feature or integrated FM capability) need careful attention and review in the AR process. Behind-the-ear (BTE) aids are used by most children from infancy through the teenage years (AAA, 2013). Some children, especially teenagers, use in-the-ear or-canal aids. While requiring special adjustment, these are feasible for use by certain individuals. (See a discussion of various hearing aid issues in Chapter 2, which covers hearing aid fitting procedures.) From a rehabilitative standpoint, binaural fittings are nearly always the rule since children who are deaf or hard of hearing require every educational advantage possible.

If children are found to have little usable residual hearing or serious progressive loss, cochlear implants should be considered (see Chapter 3). Promising results with children who have been implanted are leading to an increased use of these implants, which have now been used for over 38,000 U.S. children (NIDCD, 2016) since the U.S. Food and Drug Administration approved such use beginning in June 1990. When children are implanted, extensive AR follow-up is needed. Children who use cochlear implants may have the following configurations of fittings: (1) unilateral, (2) unilateral with a hearing aid in the other ear, (3) bilateral with surgeries happening sequentially, and (4) bilateral with simultaneous surgeries. Many centers provide access to cochlear implants around 12 months of age, and some centers provide the surgery prior to 12 months of age.

> Cochlear implants may be considered for children with deafness who have received limited benefit from hearing aids.

Hearing Aid Features

1. *Earmold fit and gain setting of aid.* With very young or fast-growing children, the earmold will need to be changed frequently to ensure a well-fitting mold and to provide adequate gain without feedback, even though feedback is less of a problem now with the new technology. Turning the gain down will help eliminate the feedback, but it is an unacceptable long-term solution. The therapist should not rely entirely on the clinical audiologist or the dispenser for this assessment but should personally monitor the earmold condition on each rehabilitation visit. In some situations, the AR clinician is trained to make ear impressions. This can be a valuable asset to the program, especially considering the frequency of mold changes in an adequate program (see Table 9.2).

2. *Real-ear measures.* Precise information on aided results can be obtained with real-ear measures, which provide accurate and complete information (see Chapter 2). They make it possible to evaluate and verify benefit from the aids thoroughly without requiring more than passive cooperation from the child.

3. *Electroacoustic assessment of aid.* An electroacoustic check of a hearing aid should provide information on the frequency response, the gain, the Ouput Sound Pressure Level (OSPL), and the distortion of the instrument (see Chapter 2 for a description of this process). These data can help uncover inadequacies in the amplification that can otherwise be devastating to the child's progress in the rehabilitation program. Electroacoustic checks are particularly helpful in the case of distortions, which are not found in the real-ear tests, and when biologic listening checks do not reveal a distortion problem.

4. *Six-sound test of aid.* In connection with hearing aid adjustment, it may be helpful for the AR clinician to use the six-sound test described by Ling (1989). According to Ling, the sounds /u/, /a/, /i/, /ʃ/, /s/, and /m/ can be used to determine the effectiveness of an aid. With the infant, visually reinforced audiometry can be used to determine if the child can hear these sounds. Older children can simply indicate they hear the sounds by imitating or giving a detection or repetition response.

TABLE 9.2 Average Months per Set of Earmolds for Children Whose Molds Were Replaced at the First Evidence of Feedback Difficulty[a]

Degree of Loss (dB)	Average Months per Mold	
	2 ½-Year-Old Child (N = 25)	2 ½- to 5-Year-Old Child (N = 27)
Mild (30–55)	3.0	5.2
Moderate (56–75)	2.7	4.1
Severe (76–90)	2.5	5.6
Profound (91–110)	2.0	4.6

[a]Also included are average loss and gain values for children in total project (N = 52) with properly fitting molds. Mean loss pure-tone average (PTA), 75 dB HL; mean aided loss, 44 dB HL; mean gain, 31 dB.

Source: Reprinted by permission: SKI-HI data.

Hearing Instrument Orientation.   It is essential for parents, teachers, and other involved professionals to be knowledgeable about hearing aids or cochlear implants so that they can help monitor use. This information can be provided in home visits, in clinic counseling sessions, in parent groups, and through in-service training in the school setting. (See suggestions in Chapters 2 and 3.)

At first, the benefit of these devices may not be readily obvious to parents or teachers, especially in cases where spoken language is minimal. The purposes of the device may include some or all of the following: verbal communication, signal or warning function, and environmental awareness. Parents must recognize why their child is wearing the device since with younger children, parents have the major responsibility for maintaining them and ensuring that they are used regularly. If parents understand hearing aids and their benefits for the child's development, they will be encouraged to help their child form good habits of use.

These devices will be more acceptable to the child when they function properly, but the procedures for obtaining accessories, repairs, or loaners will vary with local conditions. The AR provider should be aware of these conditions in order to be an effective resource person.

Monitoring Cochlear Implants.   Cochlear implants were discussed in Chapter 3 in this text. The AR clinician has a role in ensuring that the child's device(s) is worn consistently and works properly. Parents should be asked about any challenges they may be having with the child bonding to the cochlear implant for full-time use. Many children wear their cochlear implants full waking hours, and this should be the expectation. However, if a child is rejecting the device in certain situations or times of the day, it is important to work closely with the cochlear implant team to determine the nature of the concern and create a plan for increasing device use. In some cases, programming will be done again to ensure that the child's map is set appropriately. Comprehensive guidelines for daily visual and listening checks for cochlear implants are provided by Ertmer (2005) and described in more detail later in this chapter. Parents and AR clinicians should be vigilant about conducting these checks to ensure that malfunctions do not interrupt children's auditory experiences. Over time, parents and the AR clinician will become quite familiar with the child's typical responses at close and far range. This observational history is helpful in determining when a child's response to the device(s) is atypical. This is another situation where consultation with the cochlear implant team is warranted. For comprehensive guidance in working with children who have cochlear implants, the reader is referred to Eisenberg (2009b).

Remediation of Communication Activity: Auditory Learning and Development with Hearing Aids and Cochlear Implants

Auditory Learning: Naturalistic Approaches at the Parent–Infant and Preschool Levels.   The tools of newborn hearing screening and improved/advanced hearing technologies provide infants who are deaf or hard of hearing with earlier and better access to auditory experience than ever before. This supports the need for an integrated approach to auditory/linguistic learning and communication. Listening "lessons" are not separate activities but are embedded in meaningful communication interactions between parent and child.

Within this approach, parents and family members are guided to be vigilant about the listening environment (e.g., reducing background noise that would compete with the baby's attention, positioning themselves in proximity to the baby), including ensuring that the child's hearing assistive technology is in excellent working order each day and that the infant wears devices during full waking hours. Although this is important for all children using amplification, recent research (Moeller, Hoover, Peterson, & Stelmachowicz, 2009) suggests that not all families are successful in achieving full-time use with toddlers for a variety of reasons. It is possible that the fidelity of intervention around promoting consistent device use varies across programs; more research is needed, as this variable is likely to exert influence on child outcomes.

Cole and Flexer (2016) describe a developmental approach to auditory linguistic learning. The process they outline involves four phases of infant auditory learning: (1) being aware of sounds, (2) connecting sound with meaning, (3) understanding simple language through listening, and (4) understanding increasingly complex language through listening (in both quiet and in noise).

Auditory learning activities for infants should focus on observing and promoting natural listening opportunities throughout natural daily routines.

There are many natural opportunities in the home setting for exposing the child to auditory development opportunities. Current technologies (digital hearing aids, cochlear implants) provide most children with hearing loss greater access to spoken language than in the past. This suggests the need to have high expectations and a systematic approach to listening development that promotes auditory learning, regardless of the communication approach. Once the child is fitted with appropriate hearing assistive technology, the parents and clinician work to provide meaningful and frequent listening opportunities to encourage the child to rely on his or her residual hearing. For many children, systematic introduction to spoken language through listening alone during the early years will have a positive impact on language learning. Effective stimulation of residual hearing is critical to the development of spoken communication. Early auditory learning should consist of observing and strategically promoting the child's listening experiences in many meaningful daily activities.

Using an early developmental framework, Cole and Flexer (2016, Appendix 3, pp. 347–360) provide a comprehensive listing of targets for auditory/linguistic learning. This is a helpful guide for AR clinicians that provides skill sets, indicators or examples of the target behavior, and a checklist for monitoring changes. Such a framework can be used to guide the process of auditory/linguistic learning with children who have hearing aids and/or cochlear implants. Skills at Phase I (becoming aware of sound) include such behaviors as responding to auditory stimulation by alerting, lateralizing, localizing, sustaining attention, or demonstrating a learned response (e.g., showing surprise, pointing to ear). Once little ones are well aware of sound and have the requisite communicative abilities, they may also let adults know when hearing aids or cochlear implants are not functioning. To exemplify how these behaviors are addressed "naturally," consider a mother singing to her baby while rocking her to calm her before naptime. She might be strategic by (1) initiating the song before the movement and watching for the child to respond, (2) stopping the song and action briefly (watch for a reaction), and (3) starting up the song again and then the rocking. She might see that the baby notices when the song stops. Perhaps the baby will look to Mom as if to say, "I want more singing." As this comforting routine is repeated over a time period, the child's signals that demonstrate listening behaviors may become very clear. For example, the baby might vocalize when the song starts, or she might start a rocking motion as soon as she hears the singing. Parents are guided to read these signals and appreciate that they are demonstrations of the child's budding listening skills.

The skills reinforced at Phase II (Cole & Flexer, 2016) help the child connect sound with meaning. Now the child is not just alerting and attending to the presence of sound. Rather, the child is learning to respond in meaningful ways to sound. This might include behaviors like smiling or turning when spoken to or called, using body movements in anticipation of what comes next in a fingerplay, producing increasingly speechlike vocalizations (babbling), searching for novel sounds, and engaging in vocal turn taking. Auditory as well as spoken language behaviors provide evidence that listening skills are developing.

Within the framework described by Cole and Flexer (2016), Phase III involves developing early language skills through listening. Many programs have borrowed from the strategies of listening and spoken language specialists (LSLS) (see http://agbell.org) to incorporate "learning to listen" sounds (Estabrooks, 1998) as a way to promote initial sound–meaning associations. Sound–toy associations (*aaaaa* for airplane, *meow* for kitty) or sound–event associations (*uh-oh* when things fall) are used systematically to promote the child's perception and production of speech sounds. "Learning to listen" sounds and phrases vary acoustically in ways that allow parents and clinicians to provide the baby with key auditory contrasts. As Cole and Flexer explain, these associations can contrast variations in (1) intonation contours (*uh-oh* vs. *mmmmm* vs. *oh no!*), (2) loudness (*shhh!* vs. *boo!*), (3) rhythmic patterns (*mmm* for smells good vs. *yuck* for smells awful), (4) specific vowel contrasts (*hop* vs. *peek*), and (5) specific consonant contrasts (*pop* vs. *walk-walk*). Parents are encouraged to use the sound–event or sound–toy associations whenever the event occurs or the child plays with the toy. This leads to very natural assignment of meaning by the child (Cole & Flexer, 2016). These auditory learning contrasts are intended to be embedded in natural conversation and everyday routines. For example, one could easily use contrasts like *mmmm* and *uh-oh* during feeding routines. This stage also includes a variety of word and phrase identification skills, increasing abilities to imitate target words and phrases through audition alone, follow simple directions, answer simple questions, and engage in basic conversations. Phase IV in Cole and Flexer's framework involves increasing complexity of auditory/linguistic challenges. This stage incorporates practice at recognizing and comprehending everyday expressions through audition alone, demonstrating evidence of learning by overhearing others, responding to familiar language at a distance, following complex directions, answering a variety of questions, retelling stories after listening, or answering questions after listening to a story. Rotfleisch (2009) also describes auditory development processes that are taught to enable the meaningful use of sound by young children.

For preschoolers and older children who are still developing listening skills, structured listening sessions may be needed, particularly if the child demonstrates delays in auditory/linguistic development. Some children may receive a cochlear implant after 3 years of age, and structured listening sessions may be useful for teaching the child to rely on new auditory abilities provided by the technology. Some children receive sequential bilateral cochlear implants. This means that the child has used a single implant for a period of time and receives a cochlear implant on the other side. Children typically require a period of acclimatization to the second cochlear implant. Some AR clinicians report that they devote a portion of the listening session to using the new device alone and then both devices together. Clinics vary in their use of this practice, but in general, it represents an effort to support the child's auditory learning with the new device.

A variety of materials have been developed that describe auditory skill development. Erber (1982) developed a particularly useful model that distinguishes between levels of detection, discrimination, identification, and comprehension (a complete discussion of Erber's model is contained in Chapter 4). Erber's initial hierarchy is at the foundation of many approaches to developing listening skills. However, in contemporary practice, the model has been expanded and viewed not as discrete steps but rather as skill levels that are adapted to meet specific needs. For example, a child might produce the word *cat* when she meant to say *cats*. The AR clinician might present *cats* auditory only, prompting the child to focus on and detect the missing "s." Another choice is to provide a discrimination level prompt, saying, "Is it cat or cats?" An identification-level prompt might involve presenting photos of one cat versus several and prompting auditory only to find "cats, cat, cat, cats, etc." If the child's auditory skills were advanced, prompts might include comprehension level responses, presented auditory only, such as, "One time you and I read your favorite book about some little animals that lost their mittens. What was the name of that story? What is that about?" The AR clinician uses the auditory levels adaptively to fine-tune the child's skills and to constantly promote advancement in auditory-linguistic abilities. Other auditory skills, such as hearing at a distance, auditory self-monitoring, auditory memory, and localization, are typically included in a child's auditory development plan. All of these skill areas are important as a part of diagnostic/functional assessments and AR therapy.

Koch (1999) applies Erber's classic model in an approach to auditory development that integrates listening, producing speech, and developing language concepts. In each AR session, she includes four basic components of listening therapy: (1) auditory attention, (2) perception/production, (3) sound/object association, and (4) language and listening integration (Table 9.3). The first component (auditory attention) is comparable to Erber's level 1 in Table 9.3. The goal of training at this

TABLE 9.3 Auditory Skill Development Sequence

Auditory Skills	Child's Behavior	Stimulation Skills
1. Auditory awareness (detection) and attending	Child learns to spontaneously alert to meaningful environmental sounds and speech; child selectively attends to speech.	Encourage parent to use child's name to get his or her attention. Draw child's attention to meaningful sounds in the environment (e.g., "I hear the phone.... Oh listen, that's the microwave.... Listen, Daddy is calling your name").
2. Listening from a distance	Child responds to sounds from increasing distance and at various locations.	This skill can be incorporated whenever working on awareness; simply present the meaningful stimulus from greater distance. This helps children strengthen selective attention to auditory signals/speech.
3. Locating	Child searches for or locates sound or vocal sources in the environment. Localization skills help child associate sound sources with their meanings.	Create natural opportunities for child to search for the source of sound. Involve children in "hide-and-seek" games in the home, where Mom or Dad calls the child, and the child searches to find the parent.
4. Discrimination	Child perceives similarities and differences between two or more sounds/words. Child learns to respond when he notices that a sound is different or has changed.	Play peek-a-boo with the family and young child. Encourage child to listen to familiar expressions ("Where's Joey? Where's Joey?") and respond only when the sound changes (e.g., "Peek-a-boo"—child pulls blanket down). Encourage parents to play motor games where family members move slowly to a slow stimulus (walk-walk-walk) and rapidly to a fast one (hippity hop). When children are older, same/different tasks can be used to clarify identification or comprehension errors ("Listen, are cat/sat the same or different?").
5. Identification	Child can reliably associate a sound with its source and eventually name it ("That's the telephone"). Child is able to label words heard by imitating or pointing to objects/pictures.	In early stages, children play games that develop association between high-contrast sounds (*beep-beep*; *uuuuuuuup*) with familiar toys (car vs. airplane). As the child's skills develop, clinician and family present finer contrasts in the words presented during naturalistic activities. While sitting in mom's lap, the child finds pictures that she names in the storybook. Dad says a familiar nursery rhyme ("Itsy Bitsy Spider"), and the child uses the associated gestures.
6. Comprehension	Child understands the meaning of spoken language by answering a question, following a direction, making an inference, or joining in a conversation.	Family is guided to give children opportunities to listen and respond to cognitively challenging questions (e.g., "The airplane goes up. What else goes up?"). Emphasis is placed on strengthening attention and remembering (e.g., listening to a simple story and being expected to "tell it in your own words" or act it out with toys). Family members help children listen and relate information in books to their own experiences (e.g., "The bumble bee is frustrated. Can you remember a time when you were frustrated?")

level is to develop a child's ability to spontaneously alert to the presence of speech and environmental sounds. It also provides the clinician an opportunity to determine if the child is responding to amplification devices in his or her usual manner. Koch's second component (perception/production) involves the child's actively listening through audition alone and imitating the spoken model. Such activities incorporate elements of Erber's concepts of discrimination and identification (levels 4 and 5 in Table 9.3). The goal is to provide systematic and frequent opportunities for a child to discover the connection between speech/phoneme perception and production. The third therapy component (word/object association) incorporates elements covered by level 5 in Table 9.3. The clinician presents closed set listening tasks that are strategically adapted to challenge the child. Factors that are adjusted include content and presentation. For example, the clinician adjusts the content by manipulating (1) the familiarity of the language (e.g., *cat* vs. *kangaroo*), (2) the set size (3 vs. 6 vs. 12 items), (3) the acoustic contrast (*pea/banana* vs. *pea/bee*), and (4) the number of critical elements of meaning (*hat* vs. *soft striped hat*). Presentation can be adjusted by manipulating the following factors: (1) speaking rate, (2) use of acoustic highlighting (*Can you find the CAR?*), (3) number of repetitions provided, and (4) use of visual cues. Koch's fourth component of each AR session involves embedding the listening skills into natural communication activities to promote carryover of listening and learning in daily routines. This component, called language and listening integration, incorporates Erber's concept of comprehension (level 6 in Table 9.3). Activities are designed to challenge the child's listening in the context of a natural conversation or language lesson. By systematically incorporating all four components, children are challenged to work on perceptual skills and to immediately apply these skills in a conversational context.

Many new curricular guides are available for promoting auditory learning in infants and young children who are deaf or hard of hearing. Although many have been developed to address the needs of children with cochlear implants, the strategies have broad application for children with hearing aids as well. Although the list is not exhaustive, the following box highlights some excellent curricular and assessment resources.

- *101 Frequently Asked Questions About Auditory-Verbal Practice* (Estabrooks, 2012). Resource providing information about Auditory–Verbal practice.

- *Bringing Sound to Life: Principles and Practices of Cochlear Implant Rehabilitation* (Koch, 1999). Videotape and guidebooks for developing an integrated approach listening and language development using Auditory–Verbal strategies (see Table 9.4 for an outline of the therapy components that Koch includes in each AR session to promote an integration of language, speech, and listening skills).

- *Cottage Acquisition Scales for Listening, Language and Speech* (CASLLS). www.sunshinecottage. org/Products/CASLLS/Default. Promotes an integrated approach to listening, language and speech, and tracking of progress.

- *Contrasts for Auditory and Speech Training* (CAST; Ertmer, 2003). Linguisystems, East Moline, IL. An analytic listening assessment/training program for older children.

- John Tracy Clinic Correspondence and Distance Learning Courses for Parents of Young Deaf Children. Parents of children with hearing loss, ages 5 and under, are able to enroll in this guidance course from anywhere in the world. The course is available in English or Spanish and can be accessed via the Internet or through regular mail. www.jtc.org/parent-child-services/distance-education-courses-parents

- *My Baby and Me: A Book About Teaching Your Child to Talk* (Moog-Brooks, 2002). A family-friendly, highly readable guide for families about encouraging development of listening and talking.

- *Listening Games for Littles* (Sindrey, 1997). Specific auditory–verbal activities for developing language-based listening skills in infants and young children.

TABLE 9.4 Four Basic Components of Auditory Rehabilitation Sessions for Children

- **Auditory Attention:** The development of auditory awareness and the ability to attend to various environmental sounds.
- **Syllable Approximation:** The ability to imitate what is heard through the integration of speech perception and speech production.
- **Sound-Object Association:** The development of a connection between what is heard and what it represents.
- **Listening and Language Integration:** The integration of auditory skills as a foundation for understanding and processing new information through spoken language.

Source: Koch (1999).

- *The Listening Room.* www.advancedbionics.com/CMS/Rehab-Education/The-Listening-Room. Has free downloadable activities from Dave Sindrey each week. Provides activity examples for toddlers and for older children.

- *The Listening Tree.* www.Listening_Room.com. This is a subscription-based program that offers archival access to a two-year curriculum of 208 activities (104 preschool and 104 school age). Also has a Spanish version and Spanish instructional videos.

- *Listen, Learn and Talk* (Cochlear Corp., 2003). Resources written to encourage parents in their roles of daily auditory and language stimulation for the infant. http://www.cochlear.com/wps/wcm/connect/in/home/support/rehabilitation-resources/early-intervention/listen-learn-and-talk

- *Auditory Speech and Language* (AuSpLan; McClatchie & Therres 2009). A manual for professionals working with children who have cochlear implants or amplification. This is a valuable resource for evaluating and guiding auditory progress. Available from Advanced Bionics Tools for Schools at www.advancedbionics.com/-content/dam/ab/Global/en_ce/documents/libraries/AssessmentTools/3-01066-D-2_AuSPLan%20Supplement-FNL.pdf

- *SKI*HI Curriculum* (Watkins, 2004). This curriculum has been used for many years by early intervention programs to guide their work in families in a number of developmental areas, including listening. This resource has a wealth of resources for working with families.

- *Speech Perception and Instructional Curriculum Evaluation* (SPICE; Moog, Bildenstein, & Davidson, 1995). A curriculum for systematic auditory skill development for children 3 years of age and above. www.cid.edu/ProfOutreachIntro/EducationalMaterials.aspx

- *Tune Ups.* A resource that seamlessly weaves music and spoken language together in the therapy sessions. This resource was created through a collaboration of music therapist Chris Barton and speech-language pathologist Amy McConkey Robbins. http://amymcconkeyrobbins.com/tuneups.html

Adaptive auditory skill development refers to the continual monitoring of a child's responses and adjustment of the level of difficulty of the task to bring about success or further challenge.

Teachers and clinicians in the preschool setting can also take advantage of natural opportunities to encourage the children to rely on their residual hearing. It is common for clinicians in preschool settings to integrate auditory challenges throughout curriculum lessons. Rather than specifying a "listening lesson" or "listening time," clinicians integrate auditory learning as a process that pervades all activities. This can be challenging in a total communication (TC) program (sometimes referred to as simultaneous communication programs), where visual learning opportunities may take precedence over auditory opportunities. Some professionals in TC programs assume that if they are simultaneously speaking and signing, then the child is receiving sufficient auditory stimulation. However, it cannot be assumed that simultaneous exposure provides the child specific and focused opportunities to develop his or her auditory skills. Children may be in TC programs because it has been documented that they need visual supports to enhance language learning. However, the goal of their parents and clinicians may be to increase their auditory and spoken language skills (see A to V Continuum Model in Chapter 11, Case 2). If this is the goal, then it is imperative that the program include numerous focused opportunities to work on auditory learning through auditory-only stimulation. In

TC programs, AR clinicians may begin challenging the child's auditory abilities using familiar language and routines. If the child struggles, visual supports can be given, and then auditory challenges are repeated. The key point is that clinicians in TC settings need to make a conscious effort to provide realistic auditory challenges to the child in support of other communicative goals (see Case 2 in Chapter 11). Erber's (1982) concept of *adaptive auditory skill development* is very useful at the preschool level. This concept implies that a clinician constantly is monitoring a child's level of success with a particular auditory contrast or task and adjusting the task as necessary to bring about successive approximation to the goal.

It is important for AR clinicians to fit auditory skill development within a conceptual model of speech and language learning. For many children with hearing loss, the auditory channel is viable for language learning, given appropriate hearing assistive technology and stimulation. Boothroyd (1982) and Ling (1989) stress the primacy of the auditory channel for speech and language learning. Throughout the course of development, the AR clinician should closely integrate listening goals with those of speech and language learning. For example, a young child learning to discriminate and identify temporal patterns should also be working on production of the appropriate number of syllables in simple word approximations. The child learning to detect sounds should have opportunities to answer in a socially appropriate manner when his or her name is called. A child with residual hearing benefits from auditory-only or auditory-first correction when a speech error is made. Ling (1989) stresses the importance of helping the child establish an auditory feedback loop. That is, auditory skills need to develop to the point where the child can self-monitor his or her speech productions through audition. These goals are realistic for the majority of children with appropriate hearing assistive technology. Language, audition, and phonological acquisition are intricately related processes that should be addressed in an integrated fashion. Rather than "auditory training," the notion is "auditory learning" or "auditory communication." A comprehensive discussion of phonological development strategies is beyond the scope of this chapter. The primacy of auditory learning as a foundation for phonological development is emphasized with this population of children, unless the child has minimal auditory access. When that is the case, other sensory channels are recruited in support of speech development.

Documentation of learning rates in audition is useful in selecting intervention approaches and in ascertaining the need for additional sensory aids. Several tools have been developed to assist AR clinicians in monitoring auditory development in infants and young children. Some examples are shown in the following box.

Tools for Monitoring Audiologic Development

- Auditory Skills Checklist (ASC; Anderson, 2004)
- *Auditory-Verbal Ages and Stages of Development* (Estabrooks, 1998)
- *Early Listening Function* (ELF; Anderson, 2000) Downloadable at http://successforkidswith hearingloss.com/uploads/ELF_Questionnaire.pdf
- *Listening Skills Scale for Kids with Cochlear Implants* (Estabrooks, 1998)
- *Infant-Toddler Meaningful Auditory Integration Scale* (IT-MAIS; Robbins, Zimmerman-Phillips, & Osberger, 1998)
- *Early Speech Perception Test* (ESP; Moog & Geers, 1990)
- *Functional Auditory Performance Indicators* (FAPI; Stredler-Brown & Johnson, 2004)
- *Little Ears Auditory Questionnaire* (Tsiakpini et al. 2004)
- *Open-and Closed-Set Task* (O & C; Ertmer, 2008)
- *Mr. Potato Head Task* (Robbins, 1993); *Parent's Evaluation of Auditory/Oral Performance of Children* (PEACH; Ching & Hill, 2007)
- *Targets for Auditory-Verbal Learning* (Cole & Flexer, 2016)

Communication and Language Stimulation: Parent–Infant. At the same time that auditory learning is being initiated in the home, the clinician helps parents build on their communication strategies with the child. Effective interaction between parent and child is fundamental to the process of language acquisition. The communicative interaction between the child and family members is a primary focus of parent–infant rehabilitation.

When parents and professionals team together in a partnership, intervention can proceed in a fashion of joint discovery (Moeller & Condon, 1994). During home intervention sessions, family members engage the infant in stimulating routines, and the parent and clinician actively monitor the child's responses and adjust techniques as necessary. Family members also receive guidance, information, and support during home visits. Components of a home-based program are shown in Figure 9.4.

An outstanding curriculum guide for working with families was developed by Karen Rossi, longtime parent–infant educator and auditory–oral school director. The program, titled *Learning to Talk Around the Clock*, is intended to guide the content of home visits conducted in natural settings. Rossi (2003) identified *signature*

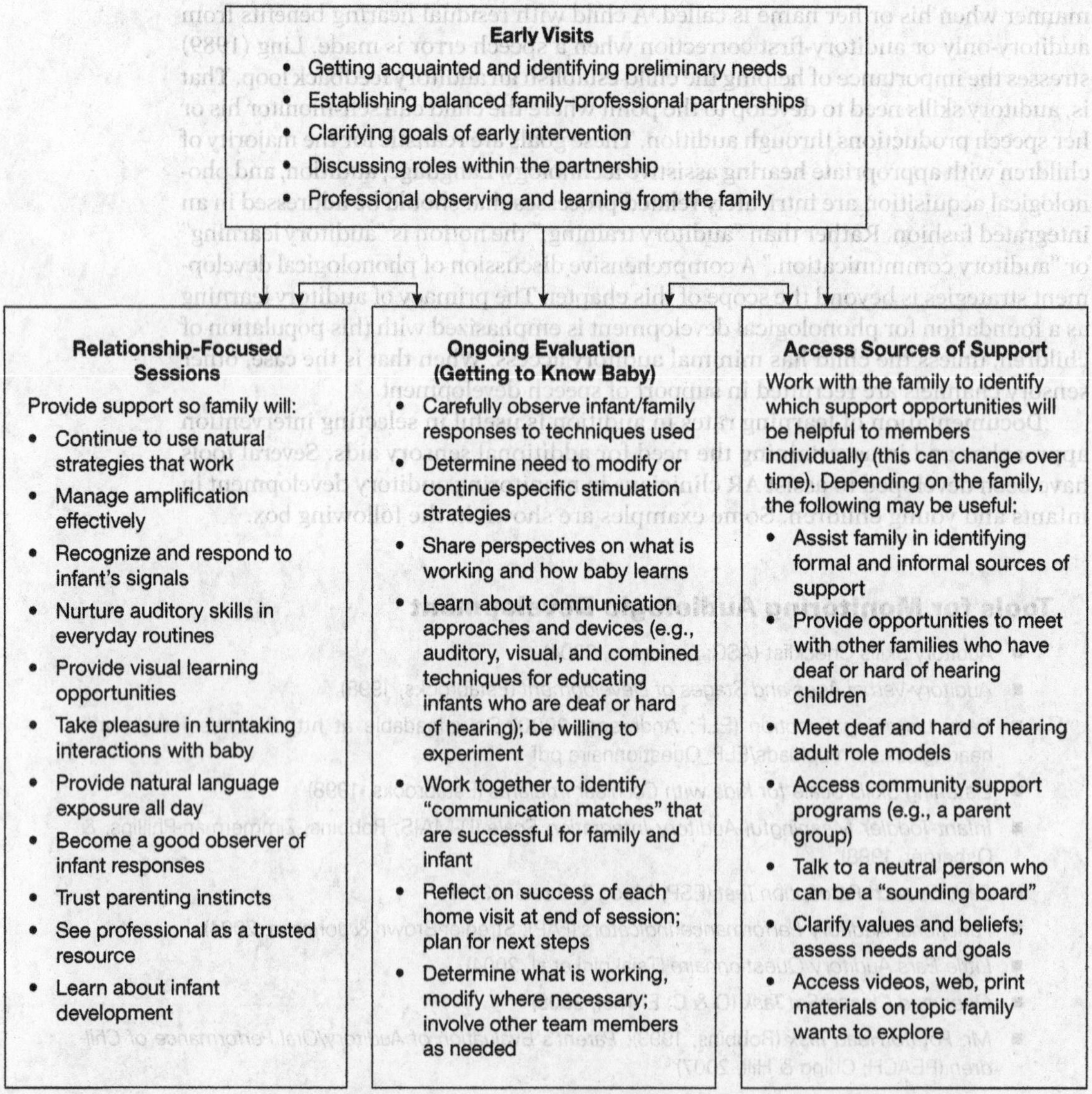

Early Visits

- Getting acquainted and identifying preliminary needs
- Establishing balanced family–professional partnerships
- Clarifying goals of early intervention
- Discussing roles within the partnership
- Professional observing and learning from the family

Relationship-Focused Sessions

Provide support so family will:

- Continue to use natural strategies that work
- Manage amplification effectively
- Recognize and respond to infant's signals
- Nurture auditory skills in everyday routines
- Provide visual learning opportunities
- Take pleasure in turntaking interactions with baby
- Provide natural language exposure all day
- Become a good observer of infant responses
- Trust parenting instincts
- See professional as a trusted resource
- Learn about infant development

Ongoing Evaluation (Getting to Know Baby)

- Carefully observe infant/family responses to techniques used
- Determine need to modify or continue specific stimulation strategies
- Share perspectives on what is working and how baby learns
- Learn about communication approaches and devices (e.g., auditory, visual, and combined techniques for educating infants who are deaf or hard of hearing); be willing to experiment
- Work together to identify "communication matches" that are successful for family and infant
- Reflect on success of each home visit at end of session; plan for next steps
- Determine what is working, modify where necessary; involve other team members as needed

Access Sources of Support

Work with the family to identify which support opportunities will be helpful to members individually (this can change over time). Depending on the family, the following may be useful:

- Assist family in identifying formal and informal sources of support
- Provide opportunities to meet with other families who have deaf or hard of hearing children
- Meet deaf and hard of hearing adult role models
- Access community support programs (e.g., a parent group)
- Talk to a neutral person who can be a "sounding board"
- Clarify values and beliefs; assess needs and goals
- Access videos, web, print materials on topic family wants to explore

---

FIGURE 9.4 Model showing major components of a home-based early intervention program.

behaviors in language and listening that foster the development of spoken language. Signature behaviors represent a hierarchy of skills parents can master to provide a language-rich environment for the child. The program includes thematically based lesson ideas and educational handouts for parents. Principles of family-centered practice are integrated throughout this developmentally appropriate material. It provides substantive direction for guiding families in a coaching-based approach.

Language and auditory development techniques need to be incorporated into natural parenting routines.

A primary focus of the intervention program is promoting nurturing and effective interactions between the parents and the infant. Although mothers of children who are deaf have been described as being overly controlling in interactions with their children, there are many examples in clinical practice of parents who interact in highly facilitative ways with their infants who are deaf and hard of hearing. Family-centered programs work in collaboration with families to optimize the communication and auditory input from the earliest ages. It is likely that these practices are resulting in much different characterizations of maternal and paternal interaction styles, and more research is needed in this area. Some parents will need direct guidance to develop facilitative styles with their infants. However, the parent advisor should not assume this to be the case. There may be many existing strengths in the parent–child interaction that can be built upon.

During home intervention sessions, the parents and parent advisor work together to implement nondirective language stimulation approaches. Some primary techniques include the following:

1. Ensuring that family members recognize the infant or toddler's prelinguistic communication signals (e.g., gestures, vocalizations, eye gaze, crying, pointing) and support these by responding in developmentally appropriate ways.

2. Supporting parents to interpret communication signals as conversational "turns" and then provide semantically appropriate responses, such as comments or expansions. For example, if the child reaches for the bottle and vocalizes, does the parent recognize that this was a complex signal? How does the parent respond? Optimally, the parent will interpret the child's intention and put the child's idea into words (e.g., "Oh, you want more milk. Here's your bottle.").

3. Facilitating the establishment of conversational turn taking between primary interactants and the child. Are family members following the child's interest and conversational lead? How does the child respond when family members follow his or her lead? What activities promote extended turn taking?

4. Supporting parents consider the need to strategically engineer developmentally appropriate opportunities for the child to respond to auditory stimuli in the environment. When the child responds to meaningful sounds, how does the family react? Do they comment on the child's observation and give the sound a name? Do they take the child to the sound and reinforce that it is the source of the sound?

5. Guiding the parents in taking advantage of everyday occurrences to expose the child to relevant language concepts. What language concepts occur naturally and are of interest to the child? What is the child curious about? Primary language targets become evident from observing typical interactions and also from following the child's interest lead.

6. Guiding family members to provide the words for what a child is trying to express. This involves helping family members to be accurate interpreters of the child's message and then providing the verbal model for that message.

7. Supporting family members in developing positive ways to engage the child in joint attention/engagement. This involves securing and maintaining the child's interest and attention. Joint attention on objects is positively correlated with vocabulary acquisition in young children (Saxon, 1997). Some evidence suggests that hearing mothers may not always use the most facilitative strategies for securing joint attention on objects. Deaf mothers of children who are deaf

have been observed to implement effective strategies in this regard. Further study of approaches by parents who are deaf would provide useful input for working with parents with normal hearing.

8. Guide family members in the use of contingent expansions and parallel talk strategies that describe what the child is doing, seeing, or thinking while experiencing an event.

9. Guiding parents in strategies for encouraging cognitive and sensorimotor play skills within communicative routines. Parents should learn to encourage the early pretend skills of the toddler, mapping language onto these accomplishments.

A summary of selected skills for establishing effective parent–child communication is included in Table 9.5.

TABLE 9.5   Some Methods for Parents to Establish Effective Communication with Their Child Who Is Deaf or Hard of Hearing

Identify the child's early use of signals and respond interactively	Understand the importance of early communication and how babies learn to communicate. Identify child's early communicative attempts. Respond to child's early communication. Tune in to the child's temperament and pace talk and interactions in synchrony with the child. There needs to be a "goodness of fit" with the parent adjusting to the child's temperament. Promote interactive turn taking. Respond appropriately to child's cry. Encourage smiling and laughing in early interactions. Give child choices. Utilize daily routines for communication.
Optimize daily communication in the home	Minimize distracting noises. Get close to child and on child's level. Create natural opportunities for listening and language. Establish joint attention and engagement with the child. Use pauses to invite the child to take a turn. Provide a safe, stimulating communication environment. Communicate frequently with child each day.
Optimize parent communication with child in early interactions	Understand how parents communicate to babies and young children. Use natural gestures, voice, and touch to attract the child's attention and interest. Increase the "back and forth" exchanges in turn taking. Encourage vocalization in communicative interactions; imitate the baby's vocalizations. Use facial expressions and characteristics of child-directed speech (parentese) in communicative interactions. Talk about what interests the child. Describe what the child sees, feels, or experiences. Introduce the child to book sharing on a daily basis. Interact with child about meaningful here-and-now experiences; make an experience book.

Source: Adapted from Watkins, S. (2004). *The SKI-HI model: A resource manual for family-centered home-based programming for infants, toddlers, and pre-school children with hearing impairments* (p. 262).

In addition to Rossi's (2003) material described above, several resources are useful in helping family members implement an indirect language stimulation approach. One was developed at the Hanen Early Language Resource Centre in Toronto for children with speech and language delay. The program provides in-service training to professionals and distributes a parent guidebook titled *It Takes Two to Talk* (Pepper & Weitzman, 2004) and many other guides and resources for guiding families in language stimulation (see www.hanen.org/Home.aspx). Training in this intervention program can be very useful to clinicians in encouraging developmentally appropriate interactions with infants. Curricular materials for guiding parents and professional training are also available from the Infant Hearing Resource (Parent/Infant Communication; Schuyler & Sowers, 1998) and from Project SKI-HI (Watkins, 2004).

Families involved in signing programs (especially those with a bilingual–bicultural emphasis) often desire and benefit from opportunities to learn about Deaf culture. Furthermore, many parents are seeking resources and support for learning American Sign Language (ASL). The SKI-HI Institute has developed and tested the Deaf Mentor Programming, which enables family members to learn ASL and to learn about Deaf culture. The program utilizes the services of adults who are Deaf as mentors and models of the language and culture of the Deaf. These Deaf mentors make regular visits to the home, interact with the child using ASL, show family members how to use ASL, and help the family understand and appreciate deafness and Deaf culture. Meanwhile, the family continues to receive visits from a parent advisor who focuses on helping the parents promote English acquisition in the young child who is deaf. In this way, the family and child use both English and ASL and participate comfortably in both the hearing and the deaf worlds. A variety of Deaf mentor materials have been developed at the SKI-HI Institute, including guides for teaching families ASL, information on Deaf culture, and Deaf Mentor Program operation guides. An array of data has been obtained on the children and families receiving Deaf mentor programming. These data were compared with data on children who were not receiving Bilingual–Bicultural programming. Children receiving this early Bilingual–Bicultural (bi–bi) Deaf mentor programming made greater language gains during treatment time, had considerably larger vocabularies, and scored higher on measures of communication, language, and English syntax than the matched children who did not receive this programming Data on program operation, service satisfaction from persons involved in the program, and cost-effectiveness also were obtained (Watkins, Pittman, & Walden, 1996).

Motherese or *parentese* are terms used to describe ways parents typically talk to a young infant. Adults make a number of modifications to their speech (e.g., shorter, simpler ideas with higher pitch and varied intonation) that are believed to support infants' language development.

Shared Reading Project

An innovative and practical program developed by David Schleper (1996) at Gallaudet University has supported hearing parents who want to incorporate ASL and/or visual principles into their communication with young children. The Shared Reading Project (SRP) is designed to support deaf children's literacy development through the provision of fluent models of storytelling. Deaf individuals are trained to go into family homes and coach the parents in visual methods for sharing books with their young children. This innovative program has been implemented through support from Gallaudet in several states across the United States. A most innovative application has been developed in the state of Washington through the efforts of Nancy Hatfield and Howie Seago. In this application, the SRP is brought to families throughout the state through videoconferencing technology. Information on this approach may be found at www.gallaudet.edu/clerc-center/our-resources/shared-reading-project.html.

Hatfield and Humes (1994) also describe a parent–infant program that has incorporated a Bilingual–Bicultural model, and Busch and Halpin (1994) describe an approach to incorporating Deaf culture into the early intervention program. Many professionals and Deaf persons stress the importance of considering the natural ways that ASL, a visual-spatial language, is organized and the potential advantages this language organization may have for the young learner who is deaf. Some families

Fluency of sign refers to the smoothness, accuracy, and flow of movement from one sign to the next. *Prosody* relates to the ways a signer segments thought units and stresses certain ideas in the message.

enroll their children in a bilingual–bicultural approach and also elect for the child to receive a cochlear implant. When this is the case, it is important for the child to receive focused opportunities for learning through audition. More information about working with cochlear implant s in a Bilingual–Bicultural approach may be accessed at the Gallaudet Clerc Center for Deaf Education (www.gallaudet.edu/clerc_center/information_and_resources/cochlear_implant_education_center.html).

Parent–Infant and Preschool Language. In contemporary practices, many children with hearing aids or cochlear implants and their families have derived significant benefit from the services provided in the birth-to-age-3 intervention program. Some of these children will enter preschool programs with age-appropriate speech and language abilities or perhaps only mild delays in their communicative abilities. They may be served in typical preschool settings, with support services from a professional with expertise in serving deaf or hard of hearing children. Other children, for various reasons, including additional disabilities, may enter preschool with many communicative delays and challenges that must be addressed within the preschool curriculum. A comprehensive discussion of various approaches to preschool programs is beyond the scope of this chapter. Our focus is to provide some key principles and considerations that will support the ongoing provision of a language-rich environment that promotes children's language, listening, and literacy skills. Given the diversity in children's skills at the preschool level, it is paramount that instruction is supported by ongoing evaluation so that professionals have guidance in adapting intervention goals to meet the child's individual needs. Evaluations include formal and informal measures of speech, language (including sign language, as appropriate), listening, pragmatic communication skills, and early literacy and learning (e.g., executive function). Another critical aspect of assessment is the process of setting realistic and specific goals for each intervention session and measuring the child's responses to intervention during each session. This information allows the clinician to adjust strategies as needed to bring about eventual success on the selected goals. Comprehensive evaluation of the child's overall abilities paired with intervention data serve as a road map that guides the clinician and the family in promoting development.

When children are participants in typical preschool settings, the role of the AR clinician may extend to ensuring that the acoustic environment supports the child's needs. Cole and Flexer (2016) provide guidelines for evaluating the acoustic and listening environment for a child who is enrolled in a typical preschool setting. These guidelines include determining if the room acoustics and teacher strategies support the child's learning and that professionals in the environment carefully monitor the child's technology. Importantly, they stress that the child enrolled in a typical preschool setting may continue to have individual language learning needs that must be addressed by a professional with expertise in working with children who are deaf or hard of hearing.

See the following box for some general principles and strategies for promoting language and learning.

Preschool Language Stimulation Strategies

1. *Children should be regarded as active learners, not passive recipients of information.* Clinicians need to recognize that children bring to tasks past experiences, knowledge, and assumptions that contribute to learning. By exploiting children's background knowledge during lessons, clinicians help children to construct new knowledge in a mentally active manner. This can happen through provision of choices, teacher-guided questioning, and opportunities to solve problems (for further discussion, see Moeller & Carney, 1993). Ertmer (2005) notes that clinician-directed activities are sometimes necessary for older children with language deficits. But for many preschool children with access to early interventions and current technologies, language facilitation may be best addressed in the context of naturally occurring conversations and the typical rich curricular approaches that are commonly used with young

Children are not passive learners. They actively construct meaning by testing out ideas, manipulating materials, asking questions, and making discoveries.

children. This includes the provision of a curriculum and individual lessons that are language rich, cognitively interesting, and focused on building on the foundation of knowledge the child brings to the task.

2. Some *children who are deaf or hard of hearing typically benefit from a systematic approach to vocabulary development.* Typically developing children access word meanings and experiential knowledge through direct exposure and through overhearing the conversations of others. Some children with hearing loss may have less access to overhearing in some circumstances for developing word and world knowledge. Therefore, vocabulary development approaches that seek to expand world knowledge and build connections between new and established words are useful with this population. Yoshinaga-Itano and Downey (1986) describe a schema-based approach to building word and world knowledge. Within the overall goal of providing a language-rich environment, professionals strive to include opportunities to expand word, concept, and world knowledge as an integral part of hands on activities and lessons.

3. *Developmentally appropriate practices should be at the foundation of any program serving preschoolers.* Guidelines from the National Association for the Education of Young Children (NAEYC) are included in Table 9.6 (Bredekamp, 2009). This includes a focus on language, preliteracy skills (like phonological awareness, print knowledge, and exposure to rich children's literature), and verbal reasoning.

4. *Question asking should be a priority goal with children who are deaf and hard of hearing.* For all children, language serves as a powerful tool for accessing information and making discoveries about the world. One of the most frequent verbalizations of a 4-year-old is "Why?" Children who are deaf or hard of hearing are equally curious. If children with hearing loss are encountering difficulty forming questions, they benefit from supportive contexts, modeling, and multiple opportunities to participate in question asking. Activities and routines that purposely provoke curiosity are ideal.

5. *Question understanding is also a priority so that children benefit from classroom discourse routines that guide thinking.* In quality preschool programs, many teachers use collaborative learning methods within learning centers. During explorative activities, teachers use questions to elicit observations and guide children's thinking and discovery. A useful classroom discourse model for developing children's ability to respond to questions of increasing abstraction was developed by Blank, Rose, and Berlin (1978). Emphasis on answering increasingly abstract questions helps to develop children's verbal reasoning skills. Within this model, the authors describe four levels of cognitive abstraction that teachers use to guide children's thinking. They include the following: (1) matching perception—this is the simplest level of abstraction, where the child matches language to the here and now context ("What is that?");

TABLE 9.6   Guidelines for Developmentally Appropriate Practices (NAEYC, 2009)

1. **Decision making needs to be informed by knowledge.** This includes research-based knowledge about child development and about learning. An effective professional also takes into account what is known about the child as an individual. This will allow the professional to adapt to the individual needs, interests, temperament, and abilities of the individual child. Professional decision making also is guided by what is known about social and cultural influences and how they impact child development. Effective educators think about typical development, which serves as a general framework for planning effective activities and interaction contexts. Modifications are made based on each child as an individual and consideration of the social and cultural context of the child's family. The clinician or teacher prepares the learning environment and plans activities to promote discoveries and exploration.

2. **Goals are both challenging and achievable.** It is suggested that children may learn best when activities build on what they know already but also challenge them to stretch to gain new skills or knowledge. The professional is engaged in a cycle of presenting appropriate challenges, monitoring the child's mastery of the new skills, and reflecting on what goals should be addressed next. This cycle promotes developmentally appropriate advancement of knowledge and skills.

3. **Teaching needs to be both intentional and effective.** This suggests that professionals know why they are doing what they are doing, whether in setting up a classroom, planning lessons, assessing outcomes, or implementing activities with children. The professional has a purpose for each action and is thoughtful about directing the teaching toward well-defined goals.

4. **High-quality learning experiences are provided.** The NAEYC has defined five key areas in which there are guidelines for developmentally appropriate practices. The specific guidelines may be found at www.naeyc.org/dap. The key areas are (1) creating a caring community of learners, (2) teaching to enhance development and learning, (3) planning curriculum to achieve important goals, (4) assessing children's development and learning, and (5) establishing reciprocal relationships with families.

(2) selective analysis of perception—this involves attention to one or two characteristics of a perceived object or event in answering questions responding to language, such as "Name something that is an animal." "Can you think of something else salty that we have tasted?"; (3) reordering perception—this involves thinking about the object or event from a different perspective, as in a requirement to identify similarities, such as "How are a cow and a mouse the same?"; and (4) reasoning about perception—this might involve the child being asked to form a solution and consider the perspective of others. It requires reliance on verbal reasoning skills. Here the child might be told, "The girl cannot find her other shoe. What should she do?" In a language-rich environment, professionals are constantly aware of the need to challenge the child's language and thinking skills. These levels of abstraction are helpful in analyzing what skills are emerging in the child's repertoire so that he or she can be challenged. High expectations for performance are a key to promoting these skills.

6. *Quality preschool programs recognize that language (whether oral, signed, or written) is a tool for conveying meanings and for communicating purposefully.* Language "lessons," then, need to be integrated in pragmatically appropriate contexts that have communicative value. As much as possible, children should be engaged in rich conversations about hands-on activities that engage their curiosity and promote their developmental strengths.

7. *Thematic or literature-based units can be a useful way to present concepts and vocabulary in an organized manner with relevant topical links.* Themes should be developmentally appropriate, interesting, and relevant to the child's communicative needs. Many preschool programs incorporate concepts from Emergent Curriculum. In such approaches, units emerge from responsiveness to children's interests and learning needs. Rather than predefined traditional thematic units, professionals create units that build on their observations of children's interests. Quality children's books are then selected to build on these interest-based areas of focus. In addition, intervention goals should be integrated into the natural contexts and routines presented in the preschool setting. This approach is referred to as Activity-Based Intervention (Pretti-Frontczak & Bricker, 2004). It means that professionals think about how target goals can be embedded in authentic learning contexts to promote the child's utilization of the skills and knowledge being taught. Table 9.7 shows an example of a session planning guide (Carotta et al., 2014) that facilitates professional thinking about how to incorporate the key goals into each activity, so that learning will occur in authentic contexts.

8. *Opportunities for exploration through play should be provided regularly.* Children learn thinking, language, and social skills through playful exploration. Adults can guide children's learning during play by using thought-provoking questions, by pointing out or instigating problems in need of solution, and by helping the child to make and express choices. Children benefit from a play process that includes (1) opportunities to learn to verbally plan prior to playing; (2) support from adult play partners in the form of descriptive comments, problem-solving opportunities, and questions; and (3) a period devoted to verbally recalling what happened during play (Hohmann, Banet, & Weikart, 1979).

9. *Children benefit in many ways from exposure to quality children's literature.* Storytelling should be a daily curricular component. Exposure to stories helps children expand on event knowledge (scripts), develop a notion of story grammar, and prepare for future literacy tasks. There are many indications in the literature that children who are read to with regularity at home become the most literate. Parents should be actively involved in the storytelling program.

Children learn best when activities build on what they know already but also challenge them to gain new skills.

Children should be involved in rich conversations that engage their curiosity and promote their strengths.

TABLE 9.7 Activity-Based Planning Guide

Activity	Goals	Monday	Tuesday	Wednesday	Thursday	Friday
Opening	Concept(s)					
	Language					
	Auditory					
	Speech					
Story time	Concept(s)					
	Language					
	Auditory					
	Speech					

Source: Based on Carotta et al. (2014).

10. *Children at the preschool level benefit from exposure to early literacy opportunities.* These include reading books and being read to, demonstrating knowledge about books (e.g., book handling, reading pictures, recognizing environmental print), developing phonological awareness skills through listening, beginning to recognize simple print forms, being exposed to functional uses of print, and having opportunities to explore with written symbols.

Counseling and Psychosocial Aspects. During the early years of the child's life, hearing families who have a child who is deaf or hard of hearing require both informational and adjustment counseling (ASHA, 2008). Adjustment counseling is not a separate activity or lesson; rather, it is a set of skills (active listening, responding to emotional needs) that are an integral part of the AR process. The ASHA Guidelines on Adjustment Counseling describe adjustment to hearing loss counseling as the support professionals provide to families as they learn of their child's hearing loss and strive to recognize, acknowledge, and understand the realities of having a child with hearing loss. Ongoing emotional support from the professional can assist the family in adjusting to the various emotional challenges that arise throughout the child's development. This process requires a parent–professional relationship that is founded on mutual respect and trust. Parenting, itself, is a developmental process that typically is challenging for most new fathers and mothers. The added responsibility of having a child with hearing loss can be overwhelming at first for many families. The rehabilitative relationship can be a context in which parents' natural reactions and feelings can be acknowledged with understanding and support.

Needs of Parents. Psychosocial (emotional) support is vital for the parents of infants who are deaf or hard of hearing. Mindel and Vernon (1987) wrote that "unless parents' emotional needs are attended to, the programs for young children who are deaf or hard of hearing have limited benefit" (p. 23). Munoz et al. (2015) emphasize the importance of supporting parents in their journey toward successful management of their child's hearing loss. Parents need comprehensive audiologic care for their child and an opportunity for support as they navigate the typically unfamiliar areas of hearing loss, hearing aid management, and the emotional challenges associated with the same.

During the child's early years, the parent advisor is often the key person in enabling families to understand hearing loss and deal creatively and positively with the child. Because over 90 percent of children who are deaf or hard of hearing have parents with normal hearing, these parents typically have had little or no experience with deafness. Although family members may not know much about deafness, they have hopes and dreams for their child, and they have many concerns and questions. Often, family members are confused and surprised by the variety of emotions they experience by having a family member who is deaf or hard of hearing. The competent parent advisor is able to listen to family members sensitively and provide needed support, information, and skills.

It is important to keep in mind that families now experience screening and diagnosis at much earlier stages in the infant's life than in past years. Although newborn hearing screening provides a distinct set of advantages, the process can present emotional challenges for families (see ASHA, 2008). Prior to newborn hearing screening, parents often experienced many months of observing the child, noticing inconsistent responses or expressing concerns for communication delays. Diagnosis was often a shock, yet it often confirmed parental suspicions and observations. In the case of newborn hearing screening, parents describe "needing to trust the equipment." They do not have a history of interacting with the baby and observing typical responses. In the case of the baby with mild to moderate hearing loss, they may see responses to sound that appear to contradict "what the equipment says." One mother in this circumstance reported, "It was very confusing to see her reactions and to know that

When parents have to accept that their child has a hearing loss, it can be helpful if they watch the hearing tests and observe firsthand the sounds their children can hear and cannot hear. Noisemakers may be used to obtain a functional response, which must be confirmed with more precise methods.

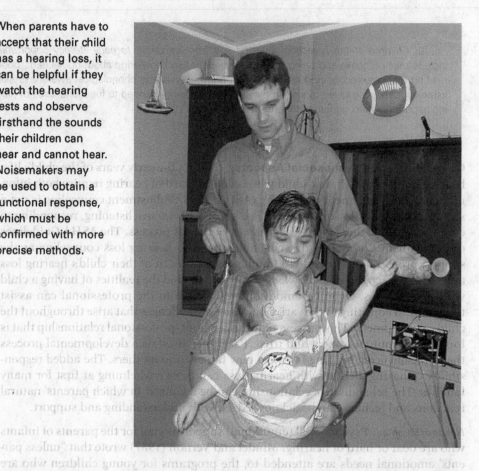

the doctors and the audiologists were saying she had hearing loss. At first when the school district offered services, I turned them down because I thought maybe there was something wrong with the test. After a few months, we realized we had to get our head around this and believe in what the audiologist was saying so that we could do the best for our daughter." In addition, parents are receiving screening results during a time of intense family adjustment to the birth of a baby. This suggests that the period from screening to diagnosis to entry in an early development program needs to be handled sensitively by professionals. The ASHA (2008) guidelines are particularly helpful in addressing this goal, and the reader is urged to read those guidelines, available online at www.asha.org/policy/GL2008-00289.htm.

Young and Tatersall (2007) interviewed parents about their experiences following newborn hearing screening, and their report provides useful insights about counseling and guiding families. Importantly, these authors found that AR specialists need to exercise caution in making statements that appear to "promise" typical rates of development just because the child was identified early. There remains a range in individual outcomes for children with hearing loss, even when diagnosis is early, which promotes the need for *cautious* optimism with families.

In the SKI*HI resource guide (Watkins, 2004), Janet DesGeorges describes in more detail some of the common emotional responses parents encounter in the days, months, and years following diagnosis. An early reaction is one of shock, which parents have described as a feeling of numbness or disbelief (*this cannot be happening to us*). During strong reactions like this, it is very hard for parents to absorb informational content. This is why the parent advisor needs to listen "beneath the words" with sensitivity in order to give support rather than information that could overwhelm. DesGeorges adds that denial is another common response and that parents may be denying the hearing loss, its permanence, or its potential effect on the child. A key point is that these are natural human responses to an unexpected diagnosis, particularly one involving a family's child. They serve as a buffer, giving parents some time to regroup and find the energy and resources to address the needs of the child and family (DesGeorges, 2004b).

Another common response described by DesGeorges (2004b) is protest, which may be expressed as sorrow, panic, anger, and endless searching for information. Such responses may occur as parents feel a strong sense of responsibility to do something for the child, but they lack the information and resources to act. This can be overwhelming, especially when they encounter a wealth of information on the Internet, some of which may be contradictory. This phase may propel a parent to learn and discover resources, but it may invoke feelings of fear about the child's future and inadequacy for the journey ahead. DesGeorges further explains that families may experience periods of disorganization that include depression, guilt, lack of hope, and isolation from others. These are challenging human emotions that need to be met with understanding and acceptance from the professional. A willingness to listen in a nonjudgmental fashion is key to providing support. Rather than trying to fix or minimize the pain, professionals can offer a safe context where the parents can express hurtful or frightening feelings, with the trust that they will be understood and accepted. DesGeorges (2004b) stresses that parents gradually reorganize their thoughts and feelings, which leads to adjustment. They may develop personal meanings or explanations for their experience of having a child who is deaf or hard of hearing. They develop new perspectives about the child, including his or her strengths and resilience. With support, they develop similar perspectives about themselves and their family.

It is not possible to predict how any individual family may react to the diagnosis of hearing loss (English, 2010). However, natural human responses include feelings like shock, anxiety, guilt, doubt, powerlessness, grief, and a sense of vulnerability (English, 2010; Luterman, 2008). Janet DesGeorges (2004b) states, "Some parents feel guilty about the hearing loss, feel angry with themselves for wishing it would go away, and feel depressed and helpless in the face of the unknown" (pp. 203–204). She describes the adjustment and grief process as a complex family journey that does not progress in linear, discrete steps from shock to acceptance. Rather, she states that families may react to events throughout the child's life (e.g., school transitions, anniversaries, milestones) that trigger earlier feelings, and these reactions prompt continual reorganization with gradual adjustment over time. Parents typically develop skills for coping with various responses, yet grief reactions may be chronic and revisited in unexpected ways (ASHA, 2008). This makes it incumbent on the AR clinician to be responsive to parental concerns and feelings in a manner that supports the ongoing process of adjustment.

Support for Parents and Family-to-Family Support. Parent advisors and AR clinicians will be of support to families by cultivating their active listening and adjustment counseling skills. In the early stages following diagnosis, often characterized by confusion and denial, the parent advisor or AR clinician establishes contact with the family and begins the process of developing a supportive relationship. The professional offers emotional support and, over time, supports the family in developing hopefulness about their abilities to parent within this unexpected circumstance.

There is truly an *art* to being a sensitive listener who provides support in response to a range of parental concerns and emotions. English (2010) notes that professionals need to avoid "mismatches" in our responses. She notes that mismatches occur when families describe how they feel, and the professional provides informational content. As an example, a parent might say, "I just wish my mother would accept that Julie needs to wear her hearing aid." A content-oriented response might be "Yes, wearing the hearing aid full time is important to promote her language development." It denies some challenging feelings the parent may be indirectly expressing. A more supportive response can be something as simple as "Tell me more about that." This invites the parent to share more about her concerns, and it avoids any quick assumptions about what the mother feels about this situation.

An invaluable way of providing family support is to link families with veteran parents who have had similar experiences. "There is probably no greater gift that a professional can give to families than to provide them with a support group. Groups are marvelous vehicles for learning and emotional support" (Luterman, 1987, p. 113). Today, many family-to-family support efforts have been established by parents. An excellent example is the Hands and Voices organization that was started in Colorado and is now implemented across the United States and in other nations. The Hands and Voices program initiated a guide by your side program (GBYS) that is designed to offer parent-to-parent support at the time of diagnosis and in the next few months in the home visit setting. This effective model has been implemented successfully in a number of states.

Effective programs typically offer formal and informal opportunities for families to interact with other families who have children who are deaf or hard of hearing. In some programs, these may take the form of weekly meetings facilitated by a professional. Other formats blend informational presentations with opportunities for informal discussion and support or informal gatherings that promote parent-to-parent exchange. Key to such approaches is for the AR specialist to act as a facilitator, not an instructor (ASHA, 2008). Family-to-family support programs are often effective when they address family-identified needs, may be family led, and provide ample opportunities for networking with other families. A content-dense program designed and led by the professional can reduce the chances of meeting this goal. Other family support models include weekend workshops where families and children come together to meet one another, learn from veteran parents and their children, and participate in social interactions and selected informational sessions. Luterman (1987) described the benefits of support group interactions: (1) they enable members to recognize the universality of their feelings; members come to appreciate that others in the group have similar feelings; (2) they give participants the opportunity to help one another; and (3) they become a powerful vehicle for imparting information.

Parents are great sources of help and comfort to other parents. In attending support group meetings, professionals are constantly impressed with the amount of help and moral support parents give each other. Inclusion of adults who are deaf or hard of hearing in support groups is highly recommended. Such adults can describe their experiences of being deaf and answer questions about deafness that professionals with normal hearing simply cannot do. In addition, parents report that they benefit from meeting older children who are deaf or hard of hearing. Such experiences can assist parents in understanding what their own child's future may hold, and it may support families in increasing their expectations for their child's outcomes.

Consultation between Counselor and AR Professional. Some parents may experience ongoing challenges that may be beyond the expertise of the AR clinician. Such issues may present themselves in the form of ongoing unrealistic expectations for the child, overprotection, or extended mental health issues, such as depression. The AR clinician should be familiar with local and community resources so that referrals for professional counseling can be made when the student or family needs exceed the therapist's expertise or comfort level. Families may experience problems with general child-rearing practices, such as discipline and sibling rivalry. The parent advisor may benefit from consultation from counselors or social workers in dealing with these types of problems.

Needs of and Support for the Child. Successful resolution of parental anxieties, warm acceptance of the child who is deaf or hard of hearing, and establishment of communication with the child promote normal psychosocial development. However, the child may also present social, emotional, or psychological problems. Consequently, the AR clinician must have knowledge of what to expect in these developmental areas from the child who is deaf or hard of hearing. In some cases, referral of the child for counseling support services may be needed. Throughout development, families should be encouraged to promote prosocial behaviors, positive self-esteem, and socialization opportunities for the child.

Development scales established by Vincent et al. (1986) and others enable professionals to know what behaviors a child should exhibit at a particular age (see text website, www.isu.edu/csed/rehab). The AR clinician observes the child's behaviors and determines what age levels they typify. In addition to developmental scales, the therapist should arrange for appropriate developmental and psychosocial assessments for the child. These tests should be administered by competent psychologists who are familiar with children who are deaf or hard of hearing. According to Davis (1990), this may be difficult since "most psychologists receive little or no training in testing or working with hearing-impaired children" (p. 36).

If the child is lagging in a specific area, the AR clinician can seek help from other professionals, such as speech-language pathologists, child development specialists, psychologists, social workers, occupational and physical therapists, pediatricians, and nurses.

ASPECTS OF AR: SCHOOL YEARS

Rehabilitation Assessment: Individualized Education Plan

Public law stipulates that primary and secondary school placements must be based on assessments of the child, which are reviewed in an individualized education plan (IEP) meeting (see Chapter 8). The IEP meetings serve to develop, review, or revise educational program goals for the student. The AR clinician is responsible for completing an appropriate assessment prior to the IEP meeting. The AR clinician working with the school-age student may be an educational audiologist, an educator of the deaf or hard of hearing, a speech-language clinician, or some other professional charged with the responsibility of coordinating components of the child's educational support services.

> An individualized education plan (IEP) is a document developed for each student receiving special education services in the schools. Required by law, this document includes specific objectives and progress indicators.

Assessment of the school-age child includes the four general areas described in the AR model presented in Chapter 1:

1. Communication status, including audiologic and amplification issues, receptive and expressive language, and social communication skills
2. Overall participation variables of academic achievement, psychosocial adaptation, and prevocational and vocational skills
3. Related personal factors
4. Environmental factors

In many cases, multidisciplinary input is valuable in gaining a comprehensive understanding of student needs. Assessment guidelines are available in Alpiner and McCarthy (2000) and Ertmer (2005). Consistent with the goal of ecologically valid assessment practices, it is useful to include a classroom observation and/or teacher questionnaires regarding the student's performance in that setting. As the section on communication rehabilitation stresses, classroom communication behaviors are unique and complex. Many standardized tests do not reflect the kinds of language skills that are required in the classroom setting. Therefore, observations in that setting and teacher impressions offer invaluable insights for the IEP. The S.I.F.T.E.R. (Screening Instrument for Targeting Educational Risk) (see Chapter 8 Appendix and the resource website) is an example of an efficient tool for recruiting teachers' impressions of the student's performance in relation to her peers. A member of the assessment team or a representative of the team who is familiar with the results of the assessment (often the AR clinician) must attend the IEP meeting along with the teacher, parents, and student, as appropriate. Based on the educational recommendations from the child's IEP, the AR clinician proceeds to arrange for or provide the needed services. Excellent guidelines for comprehensive service provision have been published by ASHA (2002).

Management

Environmental Coordination and Participation.   As a part of the overall coordination in management, the therapist is responsible for maximizing the child's learning environment (classroom), assisting in securing ancillary services, promoting development of social skills, teaching hearing conservation and self-advocacy, and arranging for special college preparation or occupational training. If the primary educational programming is delivered by someone other than the AR clinician (e.g., the teacher), the therapist needs to assume a supporting role and assist the teacher in these areas.

Child Learning Environment (Classroom Management).   School placement alternatives are necessary so that the best educational setting can be selected. For the older child, additional placement options are available beyond those listed for the preschool child.

The AR clinician is responsible for informing the child's teachers of the conditions that will optimize learning, that is, seating, lighting, visual aids, and reduction of classroom noises. In addition, the therapist should ensure that an appropriate student–teacher ratio is maintained to the degree possible.

The AR clinician should also promote home and school coordination. Cooperation can be facilitated by regular conferences between parents and teachers, periodic visits to the home by the teacher, notes, newsletters, and special student work sent home to the parents, telephone conversations, and allowing parents to participate in classroom activities.

Ancillary Services.   The therapist also needs to help set up ancillary services required for the child who is deaf or hard of hearing. Services such as otologic assessments and treatment, occupational or physical therapy, medical exams and treatment, social services, and neurologic, ophthalmologic, and psychological services are important components for the welfare of a child who is deaf or hard of hearing. Finally, secondary students who are deaf or hard of hearing in public school programs may require the services of note takers or interpreters.

Placement Options

The range of options includes (1) inclusive mainstream setting in the public schools with ancillary services like speech therapy; (2) day school or day classes for students who are deaf or hard of hearing; (3) resource rooms where the child who is deaf or hard of hearing learns communication skills to keep pace with academic requirements and is integrated into regular classrooms for less language-oriented subjects, such as math and physical education; (4) residential school placement; and (5) a co-teaching model where inclusive classroom is instructed jointly by a regular education teacher and a teacher of the deaf or hard of hearing. (See Chapter 8 on school placement alternatives for a discussion of these options.)

Development of Social Skills.   Several authors report on the high incidence of social problems, pragmatic language, and peer acceptance difficulties of children with hearing loss (Batten, Oakes, & Alexander, 2014; DeLuzio & Grirolametto, 2011; Martin, Bat-Chava, Lalwani, & Waltzman, 2010; Yuhan, 2013). Children with hearing loss experience greater difficulty than their hearing peers in establishing and maintaining peer interaction, especially in groups. Language level, gender, mode of communication, factors associated with the use of hearing assistive technology, familiarity with hearing loss, and hearing status are often cited variables. There continues to be a need to study and develop the social interaction skills in students with hearing loss. The AR clinician should monitor the social adjustment of the student with hearing loss and make appropriate referrals as needed. The school counselor or other mental health professional can be supportive in addressing the social integration of the student. Refinement of social language skills can also be supportive of this goal area.

Hearing Conservation.   School-age children should be educated regarding the importance of protecting their hearing from damage due to noise exposure. Children exposed to excessively loud sounds can experience noise-induced hearing loss. Specific groups of students, such as band members, students who use firearms, and students who are exposed to loud agricultural or recreational equipment or who participate in shop or automotive classes, may be more at risk to experience noise-induced hearing loss. Healthy People 2020 retains Healthy People 2010 objective 28-17, which advocates reducing the proportion of adolescents who have elevated hearing thresholds, or audiometric notches, related to noise-induced hearing loss. Bennett and English (1999) summarize the literature regarding the need for hearing conservation programs, including an increasing incidence of hearing loss due to noise exposure among the school-age population, and describe the benefits of using a problem-based learning approach compared to a more traditional lecture-based approach for presenting hearing conservation programs. Johnson and Seaton (2012) suggest that developing materials to be integrated into ongoing curriculum rather than single, short opportunities, such as guest lectures regarding hearing loss prevention, will increase the probability that students will integrate and use this information and that hearing loss prevention will occur. The AR clinician can create activities to stimulate the student's thinking regarding the structure and function of the normal ear, pathways of sound, dangerous levels of sound, and ways to protect individual hearing sensitivity.

Self-Advocacy.   The AR clinician should encourage students with hearing loss to develop self-advocacy skills. These skills may include understanding the legal rights associated with the Individuals with Disabilities Education Act and the Americans with Disabilities Act, developing an understanding of individual needs, appropriately expressing communication needs, locating and accessing services within the community, and empowering the individual to take responsibility for meeting his or her unique needs. Students in a school setting might be encouraged to develop a PowerPoint presentation to introduce themselves to the class. English (1997) states that potential employers and college instructors may not know the rights of individuals with hearing loss. It is the responsibility of individuals to know the law and advocate for individual rights once leaving the school environment so that they can be advocates for themselves.

Audibility, Amplification, and Hearing Assistive Technology Issues.   If children obtain their hearing aids during the early intervention period and go through the adjustment and orientation steps described earlier in this chapter, they have a good start on dealing with amplification concerns. However, this area requires a continued focus since hearing assistance technology needs or problems may arise when children enter school. Regular hearing aid and hearing assistance technology reassessment at six-month to one-year intervals and daily monitoring of the aid by school personnel should occur. Unfortunately, such regular monitoring is often neglected (Langdon & Blair, 2000). Therefore, AR clinician personnel need to be vigilant in this area (see Chapter 8). The major deficit for these children is their hearing loss. Therefore, the most obvious management is to restore as much of that hearing through hearing assistive technology and excellent acoustic listening conditions as possible. In this manner, we may lessen or remove the need for some therapy that would otherwise be required.

Daily hearing assistive technology monitoring is an essential but often neglected practice.

Hearing Aids. Some children with hearing loss are not identified until they reach school, and some of them receive their first amplification attention at this time. As indicated in the section on early intervention, when children with hearing losses are identified, they should also be evaluated medically and audiologically. After specific assessment information has been obtained, the way is cleared for carefully evaluating the place of hearing assistance technology in the overall management program. Children with mild or more serious losses in the speech frequencies should proceed with a hearing aid assessment, and additional AR can assist them in hearing aid orientation aspects, as described previously.

Children with slight losses, high-frequency losses, or chronic conductive losses present a more difficult problem in terms of amplification or other hearing assistance technology. It has been suggested that 30 to 40 percent of children with minimal or mild bilateral hearing loss and unilateral losses may experience some type of speech, language, academic, or psychoeducational difficulties (Holstrum, Gaffney, Gravel, Oyler, & Ross, 2008). It is difficult to determine which children will experience difficulties and which children will not. A careful assessment of such children's language and speech status and a report on their ability to function in the classroom will help determine whether they can function successfully without hearing assistance technology (see Case 4 in Chapter 11). The fitting of amplification devices is an option that should be discussed with the family. Preferential seating can provide some help, but this is, at best, an imperfect and perhaps only temporary solution. Careful control of the environment, including the reduction of unwanted background noise, optimizing classroom acoustics, and the provision of good lighting, may help maximize communication opportunities. Surgically implanted devices such, as the bone-anchored hearing apparatus (Baha), may be used for children with unilateral losses. Currently, these devices are approved by the U.S. Food and Drug Administration for use in children over 5 years of age. Another possible solution is temporary use of FM amplification devices until the hearing problems are resolved. Such units may also be used for children with slight sensorineural losses or chronic conductive losses. However, when a family chooses to pursue amplification and a hearing aid can be fitted comfortably, it is generally better to fit children with the aid(s) while they are younger. As they get older, they tend to become more concerned about the unfortunate social stigma associated with amplification devices. In contrast, children who use amplification from an early age know how much it can help them and are less likely to become nonusers as they get older. Nevertheless, encouraging children to use their hearing aid(s) or other hearing assistive technology on a regular basis may be one of the greatest challenges faced by the AR clinician.

Teachers and parents and, later, the child him- or herself can provide information on how regularly the hearing aid is used; however, Munoz, Preston, and Hicken (2014) report that parents often overestimate the amount of time the hearing aids are being used. Many hearing aids have a feature called *data logging*, which tracks various parameters of hearing aid usage. This feature provides an accurate record of hearing aid use time. The AR clinician should seek out this information and try to support the child and family in increasing use time when necessary. Young children will often respond to methods like public charting of their daily hearing aid use. The child can be made responsible for the charting. Older children should understand the purpose for amplification. When they are old enough, therefore, they need to receive the same instruction and information about their hearing loss as their parents were given previously (see the section "Audibility, Amplification, and Assistive Device Issues on page 265 this chapter).

Full-time use of hearing aids is preferable, in part because the child is less likely to forget or lose the instruments. With older children, however, it is sometimes unrealistic. The AR clinician may help the young person identify the situations where the aids should be used.

As the child gets older, he or she can begin to assume the responsibility for the care and management of the hearing aids. At that point, the AR clinician should

Data logging: A feature found in hearing aids that allows for electronic monitoring of use time.

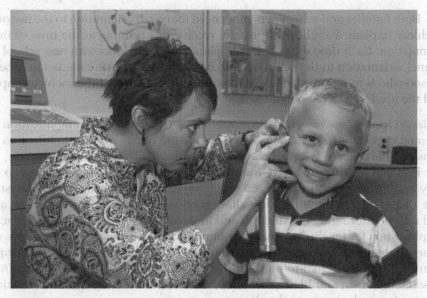

Successful hearing aid fitting requires the making of an accurate ear impression, which can be challenging with a young child.

teach the child about hearing aid function, repair, and use (see Chapter 2 and Chapter 10, including HIO BASICS). Maintenance of children's hearing aids for decades was often neglected, as shown in a series of studies reported by Langdon and Blair (2000). These studies found that approximately half the hearing aids were not in working order, and parents were generally ill informed about the rudiments of aid care. Fortunately, that situation can be improved appreciably by regular maintenance as shown by (Langdon & Blair, 2000). Johnson and Seaton (2012) suggest that incidental reports of hearing technology malfunctions continue to be a frequent concern and recommend frequent monitoring to ensure proper functioning of devices. Teachers should be encouraged to keep daily logs that document device functioning.

In cases where the child's management skills are deficient due to age or length of experience with the aid, help and instruction should be provided (see Chapter 8 for suggestions).

Cochlear Implant Support and Orientation. As the number of children with cochlear implants increases, so does the demand for cochlear implant services. Like hearing aids, cochlear implants must be properly fitted or mapped and their function monitored. The AR clinician should establish communication with the mapping audiologist to develop a relationship. The AR clinician, parent, or other trained person can complete basic monitoring (see Ertmer, 2005). The cochlear implant manufacturers provide excellent troubleshooting guides for educators.

Older children can be taught to take full responsibility for the care and maintenance of their amplification devices, including recognizing times when devices are not functioning properly.

Basic monitoring of a cochlear implant may include the following:

1. Checking battery function
2. Monitoring the child's ongoing ability to detect or discriminate the Ling sounds
3. Use of a signal check device to monitor if a signal is being transmitted
4. Checking all cords for shorts or intermittencies
5. Keeping a supply of extra cords, magnets, and batteries

Both families and school personnel need thorough orientation to the use of the cochlear implant. Families will usually receive this training at the time of initial stimulation. Each time the cochlear implant recipient works with new school personnel, orientation to the device should be provided. The AR clinician may be the person who is most knowledgeable regarding the function of the cochlear implant and the needs of the recipient.

Assistive Listening Devices and Classroom Acoustics. Other aspects of amplification that become important in the school years include use of classroom amplification systems and the concern for quiet classroom environments.

Personal hearing aids have improved appreciably over the past years so that they now provide good fidelity, cosmetic appeal, and often built-in FM systems (see Chapter 2). In addition, they allow good student-to-student communication and self-monitoring by the student, and in small groups they provide satisfactory amplification for teacher-to-student communication purposes. In classrooms with appropriate unoccupied acoustic environments and a proper installation of equipment, a favorable signal-to-noise ratio may be attained for each student in the classroom. Larsen and Blair (2008) documented a +13 dB signal-to-noise ratio on average for students across the classroom.

FM radio-frequency, digital modulation, infrared, and other hearing assistive technology systems are commonly used in classroom settings to control the effects of background noise and distance on understanding of the spoken message.

Chapters 2 and 8 contain a description of the different types of classroom amplification equipment in use. *FM radio-frequency* systems allow teacher and students more freedom and flexibility than other systems. One other device is the *infrared system*, which utilizes light rays for transmission. These classroom amplification systems, or auditory distribution systems, are usable in classes, auditoriums, and public buildings and for personal use and TV watching by some persons with hearing loss. These auditory distribution systems have the advantage that they provide improved listening to students with hearing loss without any stigma, which may be associated with using special equipment that they alone must wear. Personal FM systems may also be integrated within hearing aids or by direct audio hookup and by induction loop transmission.

The AR clinician must be knowledgeable about the various types of equipment and must be able to instruct others in daily operation and monitoring. Occasionally, AR professionals will also be asked to recommend the best arrangement for a particular setting. More frequently, they will simply be responsible for regularly evaluating (or getting someone else to evaluate) the function of existing systems. Several sources (American Academy of Audiology [AAA], 2008; Johnson & Seaton, 2012) contain thorough discussions of factors that should be considered when evaluating amplification equipment. Suffice it to say that attention should be given to (1) electroacoustic considerations, (2) auditory self-monitoring capability of the units, (3) child-to-child communication potential, (4) signal-to-noise ratios, (5) binaural reception, and (6) simplicity and stability of operation.

Other Assistive Devices. It is important that the youngster who is deaf or hard of hearing be introduced to other available accessory devices that can be useful in a variety of situations. Such devices include amplifiers for telephone, television, and radio; decoders for television; signal devices for doorbells and alarm clocks; and so forth. These devices are described in Chapter 2.

Reverberation time is a measure of how long it takes for a sound to be reduced by 60 dB once it is turned off. The signal-to-noise ratio measures the level of the teacher's voice in relation to background noise. Both of these characteristics of a room can influence word recognition.

Sound Treatment. Well-functioning personal and group amplifying systems will be more effective if used in an acoustically treated environment. In this regard, youngsters with sensorineural losses will have more serious difficulties than the child with normal hearing when noise is present. When all sounds are amplified, it is important to avoid excessive reverberation in the amplified environment. Reverberation occurs when reflected sound is present and added to the original sound. In an unbounded space (anechoic chamber), there is no reverberation. A sound occurs, moves through space, and is absorbed. However, in the usual listening environment, such as a classroom, sound hits various hard surfaces as it fans out in all directions, and it is reflected back. Consequently, not only the original unreflected sound but also a variety of reflected versions of the sound are present at once. This results in less distinct signals since signals are "smeared" in the time domain. Management of a student's listening environment is an important factor for educational success.

Reverberation time (RT) is a measure of how long it takes before a sound is reduced by 60 dB once it is turned off. In an anechoic chamber, RT is near 0 seconds. In a typical classroom, it is around 1.2 seconds. However, in a sound-treated classroom, one with carpets, acoustical tile, and solid-core doors, the RT can be on the order of 0.4 second. Finitzo-Heiber and Tillman (1978) showed the effect of RT and environmental signal-to-noise (S/N) ratio. The S/N ratio is a measure of how loud the desired signal (such as a teacher's voice) might be, compared to other random classroom noise. A +12-dB S/N ratio or better is considered acceptable for children with hearing loss, while +6 dB S/N and 0 dB S/N ratios are more typical of ordinary classrooms. As seen in Table 9.8, the speech identification of both children with normal hearing and children with hearing loss is adversely affected when S/N ratios are poorer and RTs are increased. The performance of the child who is hard of hearing is more adversely affected by poor conditions than children with normal hearing.

In the ordinary classroom, noise levels tend to be about 60 dBA, but in an open classroom, they rise to 70 dBA. Gyms and cafeterias have noise levels of 70 to 90 dBA, with high amounts of reverberation. A carpeted classroom with five students and a teacher generates about 40 to 45 dBA of random noise. According to Finitzo-Heiber (1988), since voices at close range average 60 to 65 dBA, the S/N ratio in sound-treated classrooms may be +20 dB if the listener is close to the teacher. If the listener is farther away from the teacher, the signal will get weaker, and the S/N ratio will be poorer. In view of poor performance by youngsters who are hard of hearing in noisy conditions (see Table 9.8), it is recommended that class noise levels be 45 dBA for gym and arts and crafts classes but 30 to 35 dBA in the classrooms where these students spend most of their time. It has also been suggested that noise levels of about 50 dBA may be more feasible. This would allow

TABLE 9.8 Mean Word Recognition Scores of Children with Hearing Loss and Typical Hearing under a High-Fidelity (Loudspeaker) and through an Ear-Level Hearing Aid Condition for Various Combinations of Reverberation and S/N Ratios

Reverberation Time (RT) (sec)	S/N Ratio (dB)	Mean Word Recognition Score (%)		
		Normal Group (PTA = 0 to 10 dB HL) *Loudspeaker*	HH Group (PTA = 35 to 55 dB HL) *Loudspeaker*	*Hearing Aid*
0.4	+12	83	69	60
	+6	71	55	52
	0	48	29	28
1.2	+12	69	50	41
	+6	54	40	27
	0	30	15	11

Source: Adapted from Finitzo-Heiber and Tillman (1978).

minimally acceptable S/N ratios of +15 to +20 dB. Reverberation times are easier to reduce than noise levels. Thus, carpeting, acoustical tile, and even commercially available foam sheets may be placed in classrooms to help absorb noise. A feasible goal may be to reduce the RT to 0.3 to 0.4 second. In addition, provisions should be made to keep the child with hearing loss close to the speaker (teacher). This can be accomplished through use of amplification equipment, when the location of the microphone is, in effect, the position at which listening occurs. Extensive rationale and methods for providing sound treatment are available elsewhere (Berg, 1993; Crandell & Smaldino, 2000).

To summarize, the AR clinician plays a crucial role in providing and encouraging both routine and extensive checks of individual and group amplifying systems and in obtaining adequate sound treatment in the educational setting.

Remediate Communication and Language Stimulation: School-Age Level.
The goal is for all facets of the child's program to be closely integrated, with the focus of the AR program being on building language skills to support academic success. To accomplish this goal, the AR clinician must be in regular communication with the child's educational team and be aware of the communicative demands of the classroom and the academic curriculum.

School-age students are placed in a variety of educational settings. Yet many students who are deaf and hard of hearing spend some time in inclusive educational environments, where the language demands can be complex. Several premises guide quality practices when serving these students:

1. *Intervention goals should be based on a comprehensive evaluation of a student's individual strengths and areas of need in communication and language.* In designing a comprehensive evaluation for an individual school-age student, the AR clinician should consider the language demands of the classroom and curriculum. Questions similar to the following can be helpful in designing a classroom-relevant evaluation process:

- Does the student understand paragraph-length or story-length conversation?
- Can the student recall facts from information presented by the teacher?
- Does the student understand abstract questions related to the curriculum?
- Is the student able to recall past events in well-organized narratives?
- Does the student take the listener's perspective into account when sharing information?
- Is the student able to use complex language functions efficiently (e.g., persuading someone, making comparisons and contrasts, summarizing ideas, justifying an answer, using cause–effect reasoning)?
- Does the student recognize when she or he does not understand? If so, what strategies are used to seek clarification?
- Does the student have strong vocabulary skills, supported by extensive world knowledge? How does the student go about learning new words?
- Can the student shift the manner of conversation for different partners (e.g., peer versus person in authority)? Is the student able to follow multitalker discourse in the classroom in an efficient manner? If not, what supports can be given?
- Is the student able to use complex grammatical forms in spoken and written language (e.g., embedded, subordinate clauses, temporal cohesion devices)?

Although this is not an exhaustive list, it illustrates the process of probing the kinds of language skills that are typically challenged in school environments. Formal tests need to be supplemented with informal procedures and language sampling in order to examine some of these issues (see Case 5 in Chapter 11).

Barriers

Two common barriers to successful education of deaf and hard of hearing students in regular education settings are the following:

1. Classroom educators and administrators often underestimate the student's level of functioning and the impact of language gaps or delays on academic performance. Because the child who is hard of hearing, for example, may speak well on the surface and carry on conversations effectively, the teacher assumes that the child's language is "intact." Teachers may focus on whether the child can "hear" the instruction rather than whether the child can effectively process and understand the language of instruction. Blair, Peterson, and Viehweg (1985) documented significant lags in achievement of students with mild hearing loss by the fourth grade when compared to their grade-mates with normal hearing. Teachers need to become aware of common language weaknesses that will interfere with academic development unless addressed.

2. Too often, support services are provided in a fragmented fashion. Pullout speech services may not be closely aligned with academic challenges the child is facing in the classroom. Collaborative consultation and opportunities to observe the child in the classroom setting can be helpful in identifying priority communicative needs and goals so that they may be addressed.

2. *Intervention should focus on skills that will support the student's functioning in the classroom* (Wallach & Miller, 1988). The AR clinician can support classroom functioning by focusing on skills that lead toward *successful classroom listening behaviors.* Examples include the following:

1. Listening for the main idea in a paragraph
2. Drawing a conclusion from several details
3. Making comments relevant to the remarks of other students in a discussion
4. Recognizing when a critical piece of information has been missed and appropriately seeking clarification

It can be helpful to observe the student in the classroom and/or request input from the teacher on the student's listening habits.

3. *School-age students often need opportunities to expand their world knowledge and link new vocabulary words to existing knowledge.* Delays or gaps in vocabulary and word knowledge are common in some students with hearing loss. Vocabulary delays can interfere with reading comprehension and with understanding of academic discussions. It is not sufficient to teach new words in isolation (e.g., sending home a list of unrelated spelling words to be practiced and memorized). Rather, students need support in building networks of associated meanings. As an example, suppose that you heard the word *barracuda* in a conversation. Immediately, you would consider options for what the word might mean (e.g., a fish, a type of car, a song, an aggressive person). Then you hear your friend say, "Oh, I forgot my barracudas this morning." Right away, you revise your hypothesis. In essence, you do a "best of fit analysis." You draw on your knowledge of grammar to help you. The words "*my* barracudas" tip you off that it cannot be any of the word meanings mentioned before and that it is likely a personal item that can be carried. If you knew that your friend was a swimmer and then the friend added, "I prefer my barracudas because they don't leave rings around my eyes," you would conclude that she was talking about goggles. Vocabulary training needs to help students to use their fund of word knowledge and experience to figure out what words mean and to store new words in relation to associated meanings. Some excellent strategies for implementing such an approach are discussed by Yoshinaga-Itano and Downey (1986).

4. *Many students will benefit from opportunities to work on self-expression at the narrative level.* During a school day, students are asked to express themselves in various modes (e.g., giving an explanation, justifying a response, or writing a theme). If

Narratives involve the telling of stories in various forms. One commonly used narrative form is a personal narrative through which a student shares a past event with another.

a need is identified in this area, the AR clinician can provide practice and support at the narrative level of conversation. Emphasis on the organization of face-to-face narratives may positively influence written language as well. Some narrative functions that are common in school include explaining, describing, debating, negotiating, comparing and contrasting, justifying, summarizing, predicting, and using cause–effect reasoning. AR clinicians can devise activities that address these literate language functions. For example, a student might be encouraged to take an opinion poll related to a recent political event. Functional speech intelligibility can be reinforced while the student asks others for their opinions. He or she can then be asked to draw summary statements and explain them to a peer. Finally, the student could be encouraged to write an article for the school paper about his or her discoveries.

5. *As the school years progress, demands for verbal reasoning increase. Therefore, students may benefit from interventions designed to encourage verbal reasoning skills.* AR clinicians can take advantage of any daily problem to support the student's expansion of problem-solving skills. It is useful to guide the student in analyzing the nature of the problem (e.g., I left my assignment at home, and I will get an F if I fail to turn it in) and alternative solutions (e.g., brainstorming ways to get the assignment finished in time). The student can then be guided in evaluating the various alternatives and needed resources, leading to the selection of the best alternative. The student should evaluate both the outcomes and ways to prevent this problem in the future. These strategies can help the student learn useful problem-solving processes that can be implemented when faced with peer conflicts, social pressures, or other everyday problems. It is also useful to discuss the feelings that result from problems and their consequences. Students may have a limited fund of affective vocabulary. Gaining a

Early cochlear implantation generally will support the development of language skills, but these devices require consistent monitoring to ensure proper function.

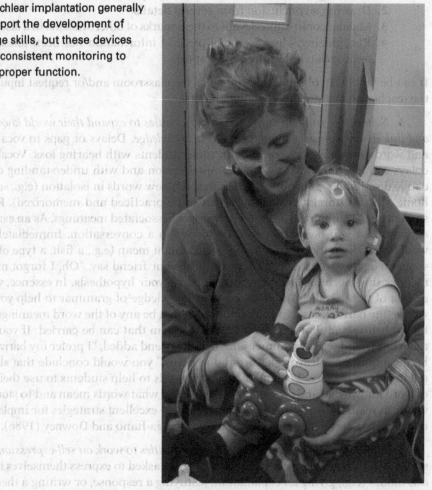

better understanding of affective words and their relation to problem situations can increase students' awareness of themselves and of the perspectives of others.

6. *Some school-age students will profit from emphasis on study skills and other classroom survival skills.* If at all possible, the AR clinician should observe a student in the classroom or interview the teacher about the student's responsiveness in the classroom. Input from these sources is useful in the identification of priority needs. For example, one student had significant difficulty identifying key points for note taking. He tried to write down all the points from a class lecture. This resulted in a lack of organization and many missing elements in his notes. The IEP team decided to provide a note taker to ease the processing demands on the student. The AR clinician used the note taker's transcripts to illustrate some key points about organizing notes and studying from notes. The student learned about what to attend to in the lecture from this process. Through observation and discussions with the teacher, a priority need was effectively addressed.

This list is not meant to be all-inclusive. Rather, it illustrates examples of priority areas for many students who are of school age. It emphasizes the importance of selecting goals that will support the student to function as well as possible in the learning and social environments at school. This can come about only when the AR clinician works closely with the educational team to identify skills that need to be addressed so that the student can communicate more effectively in the classroom. Sensitivity to the language-learning demands of a student's school program will lead to the selection of relevant interventions.

Counseling and Psychosocial Aspects.

Counseling. The AR clinician needs to be a good listener and information/personal adjustment counselor. Students with hearing loss and their families may need a supportive and knowledgeable person to empathize with personal-social concerns associated with hearing loss. The AR clinician should learn to be a good listener and establish a trusting relationship with students so they feel free to communicate needs and feelings. Some school-age children may experience isolation, need help developing a sense of self-confidence (Moeller, 2007), and need someone with whom they can share their feelings freely.

Adjustments for Mild Losses and Auditory Processing Problems. Children with mild hearing problems (i.e., mild sensorineural loss, unilateral or conductive loss) and those with central auditory processing disorders (CAPD or APD) may require communication rehabilitation along with children who demonstrate more pronounced losses. Although the language-related problems may be minimized in the case of milder losses, they are apt to be present and require attention. In cases of auditory processing problems, careful multidisciplinary assessment of the child's difficulties should be conducted consisting of reports from teachers, parents, and the child, in addition to observation and diagnostic testing (see Chapter 8, text website; Schow & Seikel, 2007).

A central auditory processing disorder (CAPD) involves either a delay in development, a disorder in development, or a specific central lesion. CAPD often accompanies other disabilities.

Most authorities agree that CAPD involves one of the following:

1. Delay in development

2. Disordered development

3. A specific central lesion

Such difficulties involve a deficit in neural processing of auditory stimuli not due to higher order language or cognitive function (AAA, 2010; ASHA, 2005.) CAPD may occur in isolation, but CAPD often occurs in conjunction with attention deficit hyperactivity disorder (ADHD) and/or learning disorder (LD), autistic spectrum disorders, reading problems, and/or speech–language deficits.

When intelligence and peripheral hearing are within normal limits and the child seems to be showing deficits mainly in listening tasks, then CAPD rather than a more general problem may be the cause, and this is possible with or without these other conditions (ADHD, LD, etc.). In these cases, a rehabilitation evaluation focused on CAPD is indicated. ASHA (2005) has proposed that seven different related symptoms or assessment areas may be evaluated in CAPD, but current test batteries usually assess only a more limited number of these. This ASHA consensus paper recommended that problems in any one of these areas constitute CAPD. Musiek and Chermak (1994) recommended that the following ASHA areas be assessed: (1) auditory pattern (temporal) recognition, (2) tasks involving dichotic (binaural) separation and integration, and (3) monaural tasks in background competition. Electrophysiologic or electroacoustic tests are also recommended, but only rarely are they a key issue in APD diagnosis.

A Multiple Auditory Processing Assessment (MAPA) battery that follows this three-pronged recommendation has been found to separately measure each of these tasks (Domitz & Schow, 2000; Schow, Seikel, Chermak, & Berent, 2000). MAPA became available in 2007 from Auditec and in 2017 MAPA-2 was further developed through a national normative study and will become available through Academic Therapy Publications, Novato, CA (Schow, Seikel, Brockett, & Whitaker, 2017, in Press). Support for using these three main assessment areas can be found in AAA (2010) and in Bellis (2003). Bellis refers to the three domain areas as Prosodic deficits (temporal), Integration deficits (binaural), and Auditory decoding deficits (monaural). Another assessment method, the SCAN3 tests for children and adolescents (Keith, 2009), also has a focus on temporal, binaural, and monaural test domains. Another APD assessment, the Listening in Spatialized Noise-Sentences (LISN-S; Cameron & Dillon, 2007), is a related and promising approach. This approach relates nicely to classroom listening issues and therefore has good face value. Cameron and Dillon have suggested that deficits on this test show the presence of a spatial processing disorder that they suggest is a form of CAPD. The test is presented binaurally with background competition and uses temporal cues. It is unclear at present which of the three domains is most prominent within LISN-S. Also, various self-report tools, such as S.I.F.T.E.R., are being used with CAPD. The Scale of Auditory Behaviors, also described in Chapter 8, follows the recommendations of the Bruton Conference (Jerger & Musiek, 2000) and has gone through a careful process of development and refinement (Schow et al., 2007, in Press; Schow and Seikel, 2007) including a national normative study. This scale may be used to assist in assessment and to track common behaviors in these youngsters during the rehabilitation process.

Dillon, Cameron, Glyde, Wilson, and Tomlin, (2012) have recommended a simple CAPD screening by using a listening test, such as a speech-in-noise test along with some form of self-report. This would then be followed by more detailed tests in the different domains. Further research will be needed to evaluate how a listening test approach and/or the three-domain approach plus self-report will work together most effectively.

Audiologists do have some remaining questions about defining CAPD. Nevertheless, the advantage of these developments in assessment is that the profession is emerging from the imprecision of an earlier era in CAPD. It is important that ASHA and AAA have defined the areas of concern in APD and assessments have been developed to measure these areas of auditory weakness because this means that focused rehabilitation is possible.

Remediation strategies will include the following:

- Direct therapy for any or all of the three deficit areas. For example, Bellis (2003) has outlined many methods for direct therapy in the three domain areas and the use of commercial products like Fast Forword (see resource website) to remediate problems in one or more of the domain areas. After therapy, these skill areas can then be measured again posttherapy to determine improvement. A new method for remediating difficulties in using temporal cues or directional listening is being tested by the National Acoustic Laboratories of Australia. There, Cameron and Dillon (2013) reported the first of several studies of children between the ages of 6 and 11 getting daily therapy with video games. This approach is designed to work along with their spatialized listening test (LISN-S). Once children are identified, they receive direct therapy to help them improve their processing of cues coming from different directions. In this and subsequent reports, they found significant improvement in self-reported rating of listening ability, attention, and memory.

- Children with CAPD can also be helped with strategies to improve the signal (via improvement of the S/N ratio through noise control and amplification).
- Another major approach is to teach the child cognitive strategies to assist in learning and remembering.

Chermak and Musiek (1992) offered a series of helpful suggestions (see Table 9.9) that address such improved signal and cognitive strategies. As data using these and other remediation methods are gathered to establish evidence-based practice, more will be learned about ways to help children.

In the future, it appears that AR clinicians working with school-age children will be equipped with ever more improved methods for evaluating and remediating CAPD.

TABLE 9.9 Management of Central Auditory Processing Disorders

Functional Deficit	Strategies	Techniques
Distractibility and inattention	Increase Signal-to-Noise Ratio	ALD/FM system; acoustic modifications preferential seating
Poor memory	Metalanguage	Chunking, verbal chaining, mnemonics, rehearsal, paraphrasing, summarizing
	Right hemisphere activation	Imagery, drawing
	External aids	Notebooks, calendars
Restricted vocabulary	Improve closure	Contextual derivation of word meaning
Cognitive inflex: predominantly analytic or predominantly conceptual	Diversify cognitive style	Top-down (deductive) and bottom-up (inductive) processing, inferential reasoning, questioning, critical thinking
Poor listening comprehension	Induce formal schema to aid organization, integration, and prediction	Recognize and explain connectives (additives; causal; adversative; temporal) and patterns of parallelism and correlative pairs (not only/but also; neither/nor)
	Maximize visual and auditory summation	Substitutions for note taking
Reading, spelling, and listening problems	Enhance multisensory integration	Phonemic analysis and segmentation
Maladaptive behaviors (passive, hyperactive, impulsive)	Assertiveness and cognitive behavior modification	Self-control, self-monitoring, self-evaluation, self-instruction, problem solving
Poor motivation	Attribution retraining: internal locus of control	Failure confrontation, attribution to factors under control

Source: Based on Chermak and Musiek (1992).

Concluding Remarks

This chapter has provided an introduction to the process of AR at two distinct levels: the early intervention level and school-age service level. Although services in these settings are provided by a variety of personnel and in various communication modes, one professional—the parent advisor or the AR clinician—often assumes the important roles of coordinating service provision and serving as an advocate for children and families. This chapter has emphasized the critical importance of family-centered practice and the role of the family throughout the child's educational program. After appropriate assessment and selection of intervention priorities, including a communication system, AR services throughout the child's life focus on four major areas (CARE): (1) counseling and psychosocial support for the child and family; (2) audibility, amplification, and assistive device issues; (3) communication activity rehabilitation within a model of language and literacy attainment; and (4) environmental coordination and integration of services, which includes family-centered issues;. At the school-age level, the importance of integrated service delivery that considers the unique communicative demands of the classroom setting has been emphasized. Rehabilitation presents challenges to parents, children, and therapists. Nevertheless, if proper attention is given to all of these aspects, prospects for effective management can be very good. If the problems of the child who is deaf or hard of hearing are underestimated or neglected, the student may experience long-term negative consequences for language, literacy, and social skill attainment. Aggressive and early management of children who are deaf or hard of hearing through AR is therefore critical.

Summary Points

- Rehabilitative management of children who are deaf and hard of hearing begins with comprehensive, transdisciplinary evaluation. During intervention, ongoing assessment is necessary to document outcomes, make appropriate adjustments to therapy routines, and identify additional intervention priorities.

- Universal newborn hearing screening procedures allow for identification of hearing loss in the neonatal period, much earlier than in the past. To gain maximal benefit, early identification needs to be paired with early intervention programs that seek to involve and support families.

- Most early intervention programs seek to offer family-centered practices. In this approach, families are empowered in their roles as decision makers for the child, professionals seek to form balanced partnerships with parents, and family-identified needs are addressed through collaborative teamwork.

- Families in early intervention programs benefit from full access to information on options to guide decision making. Stress is reduced when informal and formal support systems (e.g., support group meetings) are made available. Parent advisors use coaching methods to support families in providing a nurturing language environment for infants with hearing loss. Today, families access a wide range of supports and information sources, including social media, chat rooms, and Internet sources, to expand their knowledge. Professionals need to recognize that families may be accessing a variety of supports and assist families in evaluating advice and information they find and/or serve as a sounding board, as needed.

- Appropriate management of personal amplification, cochlear implants, and FM systems is a primary step in facilitating a child's use of residual hearing. Children benefit from regular monitoring of amplification, encouragement to wear devices their full waking hours, and opportunities to listen throughout daily routines. Auditory learning can be fostered during natural interactions.

- Preschool-age children benefit from language intervention techniques that stimulate thinking, problem solving, and active learning. Children should be encouraged to master question-and-answer routines because this aspect of language supports them in making discoveries about the world.

- Because children who are deaf or hard of hearing may have fewer opportunities to "overhear," they may experience gaps and delays in vocabulary and world knowledge. Both preschool- and school-age children profit from approaches that help them to build networks of word meanings. They need to learn to tie new information to familiar concepts.

- Speech development programs for children with hearing loss should be structured to maximize the child's reliance on residual hearing. When children strengthen their reliance on listening skills, they often learn to self-monitor, which contributes to the generalization of speech training.

- The AR specialist should be involved as a team member in providing input to the child's IFSP (birth to 3 years) or IEP (3 years on). In the school-age years, AR specialists need to communicate regularly with the educational team so that goals will relate to the student's classroom academic needs.

- Family members should be involved in the child's AR program throughout the course of the child's education. Furthermore, children with any type or degree of hearing loss may be candidates for some level of AR service. Team approaches benefit all children but especially those with multiple disabilities.

- School-age children with CAPD should receive assessment and treatment based on recent guidelines and promising new procedures.

Supplementary Learning Activities

See www.isu.edu/csed/audiology/rehab to carry out these activities. We encourage you to use these to supplement your learning. Your instructor may give specific assignments that involve a particular activity.

When this icon appears, visit the companion website for further exploration.

1. The Ling six-sound test discussed in this chapter can be used in a variety of ways to monitor hearing aid or cochlear implant use by children. The text website provides a two-part exercise that you can use to help you become more comfortable in using this procedure.

2. This chapter described the importance of using a partnership approach when working with families. A partnership/coaching approach can apply whether you are in the audiology clinic or working with families on home visits. Go to the text website for a related activity.

3. In this chapter we discuss the MAPA and MAPA-2 which have been developed to measure the three domains of APD assessment. Please review the supplementary supportive material for the MAPA assessment tools and an explanatory video discussing assessment (diagnosis) and management (treatment) based on a three domain approach.

Recommended Reading

Alpiner, J. G., & McCarthy, P. A. (2000). *Rehabilitative audiology: Children and adults* (3rd ed.). Baltimore: Williams & Wilkins.

American Speech-Language-Hearing Association. (2002). *Guidelines for audiology service provision in and for schools.* Rockville, MD: Author.

American Speech-Language-Hearing Association. (2008). *Core knowledge and skills in early intervention speech-language pathology practice* and *Service provision to children who are deaf and hard of hearing, birth to 36 months.* Retrieved from http://www.asha.org/policy

Anderson, K. (2000). *Early listening function.* Retrieved from http://successforkidswith hearingloss.com/uploads/ELF_Questionnaire.pdf

Cole, E. B., & Flexer, C. (2016). *Children with hearing loss: Developing listening and talking—birth to six* (3rd ed.). San Diego, CA: Plural Publishing.

Johnson, C. D., & Seaton, J. B. (2012). *Educational audiology handbook* (2nd ed.). New York: Delmar, Cengage Learning.

Moeller, M. P., Ertmer, D. J, & Stoel-Gammon, C. (Eds.). (2016). *Promoting language and literacy in children who are deaf or hard of hearing.* Baltimore: Paul H. Brookes.

Moeller, M. P., Tomblin, J. B., & the OCHL Collaboration. (2015). Epilogue: Conclusions and implications for research and practice. *Ear and Hearing, 36,* 92S–98S.

Niparko, J. K., Tobey, E. A., Thal, D. J., & the CDaCI Investigative Team. (2010). Spoken language development in children following cochlear implantation. *Journal of the American Medical Association, 303,* 1498–1506.

Roeser, R., & Downs, M. (Eds.). (1995). *Auditory disorders in children* (3rd ed.). New York: Thieme.

Roush, J., & Matkin, N. D. (1994). *Infants and toddlers with hearing loss.* Baltimore: York Press.

Watkins, S. (2004). *SKI*HI curriculum. Family-centered programming for infants and young children with hearing loss.* Logan, UT: Hope, Inc.

Recommended Websites

http://www.agbell.org

National Center for Hearing Assessment and Management:
http://www.infanthearing.org

Hands and Voices: Deaf Awareness and Support:
http://www.handsandvoices.voices.org

Laurent Clerc National Deaf Education Center, Gallaudet University:
http://www3.gallaudet.edu/clerc-center

Boys Town National Research Hospital:
http://www.boystownhospital.org

Outcomes of Children with Hearing Loss
http://ochlstudy.org

Zero to Three National Center for Infants, Toddlers, and Families:
http://www.zerotothree.org

SKI-HI Institute of Communicative Disorders and Deaf Education
http://www.skihi.org

My Baby's Hearing, Boys Town National Research Hospital
http://www.babyhearing.org

References

Alpiner, J. G., & McCarthy, P. A. (2000). *Rehabilitative audiology: Children and adults* (3rd ed.). Baltimore: Williams & Wilkins.

American Academy of Audiology. (2003). *Pediatric amplification protocol.* Retrieved from http://www.audiology.org

American Academy of Audiology. (2008). *Clinical practice guidelines: Remote microphone hearing assistance technologies for children and youth from birth to 21 years.* Retrieved from http://www.audiology.org

American Academy of Audiology. (2010). *Clinical practice guidelines. Diagnosis, treatment and management of children and adults with central auditory processing disorder.* Retrieved from www.audiology.org/resources/documentlibrary/Documents/CAPD%20Guidelines%208-2010.pdf

American Academy of Audiology. (2013). *Clinical practice guidelines: Pediatric amplification.* Retrieved from http://www.audiology.org/publications-resources/document-library/pediatric-rehabilitationhearing-aids

American Academy of Pediatrics. (1999). Newborn and infant hearing loss: Detection and intervention. *Pediatrics, 103*, 527–530.

American Speech-Language-Hearing Association. (1997). *Guidelines for audiologic screening.* Rockville, MD: Author.

American Speech-Language-Hearing Association. (2002). *Guidelines for audiology service provision in and for schools.* Rockville, MD: Author.

American Speech-Language-Hearing Association. (2005). Central auditory processing: Current status of research and implications for clinical practice. *American Journal of Audiology, 5*(2), 41–54.

American Speech-Language Hearing Association. (2008). *Guidelines for audiologists providing informational and adjustment counseling to families of infants and young children with hearing loss birth to 5 years of age.* Retrieved from www.asha.org/docs/html/GL2008-00289.html

American Speech-Language Hearing Association & Council on Education of the Deaf. (2006). *Fact sheet: Natural environments for infants and toddlers who are deaf or hard of hearing and their families.* Retrieved from www.asha.org/advocacy/federal/idea/nat-env-child-facts.htm

Anderson, K. L. (2000). *Early Listening Function* (ELF). Retrieved from http://www.hear2learn.com

Anderson, K. (2004). *Auditory skills checklist: Success for kids with hearing loss.* Retrieved from https://successforkids with hearing loss.com/resources-for-professionals/early-intervention-for-children-with-hearing-loss

Barrera, I., Kramer, L., & Macpherson, T. D. (2012). *Skilled dialogue: Strategies for responding to cultural diversity in early childhood* (2nd ed.). Baltimore: Paul H. Brookes.

Batten, G., Oakes, P. M., & Alexander, T. (2014). Factors associated with social interactions between deaf children and their hearing peers: A systematic literature review. *Journal of Deaf Studies and Deaf Education, 19*(3), 285–302.

Bellis, T. J. (2003). *Assessment and management of central auditory processing disorders in the educational setting: From science to practice* (2nd ed.). Clifton Park, NY: Thomson Learning.

Bennett, J., & English, K. (1999). Teaching hearing conservation to school children: Comparing the outcomes and efficacy of two pedagogical approaches. *Journal of Educational Audiology, 7*, 29–33.

Bentler, R. A. (1993). Amplification for the hearing-impaired child. In J. G. Alpiner & P. A. McCarthy (Eds.), *Rehabilitative audiology: Children and adults.* Baltimore: Williams & Wilkins.

Berg, F. S. (1993). *Acoustics and sound systems in schools.* San Diego, CA: Singular Publishing.

Blair, J., Petersen, M., & Viehweg, S., (1985). The effects of mild sensorineural hearing loss on academic performance of young school-age children. *Volta Review, 87*(2), 87–93.

Blair, J., Wright, K., & Pollard, G. (1981). Parental understanding of their children's hearing aids. *Volta Review, 83*, 375–382.

Blank, M., Rose, S., & Berlin, L. (1978). *The language of learning: The preschool years.* New York: Grune & Stratton.

Boothroyd, A. (1982). *Hearing impairments in young children.* Englewood Cliffs, NJ: Prentice Hall.

Brandwein, M. (2010). *Powerful and practical techniques to train and supervise staff.* Retrieved from http://www.michaelbrandwein.com

Bredekamp, S. (2009). *Developmentally appropriate practice in early childhood programs serving children from birth through age 8* (Expanded ed.). Washington, DC: National Association for the Education of Young Children.

Brinker, R., Frazier, W., & Baxter, A. (1992, Winter). Maintaining involvement of inner city families in EI programs through a program of incentives: Looking beyond family systems to social systems. *OSERS News in Print, 4*(1), 9–19.

Brown, P. M., & Nott, P. (2006). Family-centered practice in early intervention for oral language development: Philosophy, methods, and results. In P.E. Spencer & M. Marschark (Eds.), *Advances in spoken language development of deaf and hard-of-hearing children* (pp. 136–165). New York: Oxford University Press.

Busch, C., & Halpin, K. (1994). Incorporating deaf culture into early intervention. In B. Schick & M. P. Moeller (Eds.), *Proceedings of the Seventh Annual Conference on Issues in Language and Deafness* (pp. 117–125). Omaha, NE: Boys Town National Research Hospital.

Cameron, S., & Dillon, H. (2007). Development of the Listening in Spatialized Noise-Sentences Test (LISN-S). *Ear and Hearing, 28*(2), 196–211.

Cameron, S., & Dillon, H. (2013). Remediation of spatial processing issues in CAPD. In G. D. Chermak & F. E. Musiek (Eds.), *Handbook of central auditory processing disorders. Comprehensive intervention* (Vol. 2, pp. 201–224). San Diego, CA: Plural Publishing.

Carotta, C., Cline, K. M., & Brennan, K. (2014). *Auditory consultant resource network handbook.* Omaha, NE: Boys Town National Research Hospital.

Chermak, G. D., & Musiek, F. E. (1992). Managing central auditory processing disorders in children and youth. *American Journal of Audiology,* 61–65.

Ching, T. Y., Dillon, H., Marnane, V., Hou, S., Day, J., Seeto, M. et al. (2013). Outcomes of early- and late-identified children at 3 years of age: Findings from a prospective population-based study. *Ear and Hearing, 34,* 535–552.

Ching, T. Y. C., & Hill, M. (2007). The Parents' Evaluation of Aural/Oral Performance of Children (PEACH) scale: Normative data. *Journal of American Academy of Audiology, 18*(3), 220–235.

Cole, E., & Flexer, C. (2016). *Children with hearing loss: Developing listening and talking—Birth to six* (3rd ed.). San Diego, CA: Plural Publishing.

Crandell, C., & Smaldino, J. (2000). Classroom acoustics for children with normal hearing and with hearing impairment. *Language, Speech, and Hearing Services in Schools, 31,* 362–370.

Davis, J., Effenbein, J., Schum, R., & Bentler, R. (1986). Effects of mild and moderate hearing impairments on language, educational, and psychosocial behavior of children. *Journal of Speech and Hearing Research, 51*(1), 53–63.

DeBonis, D. (2015). It is time to rethink central auditory processing disorder protocols for school aged children. *American Journal of Audiology, 24,* 124–136.

DeLuzio, J., & Girolametto, L. (2011). Peer interactions of preschool children with and without hearing loss. *Journal of Speech, Language, and Hearing Research, 54*(4), 1197–1210.

DesGeorges, J. (2004a). *Parent wish list for audiologists.* Retrieved from http://www.handsandvoices.org

Des Georges, J. (2004b). Providing emotional support to families. In S. Watkins (Ed.), *SKI*HI curriculum: Family-centered programming for infants and young children with hearing loss* (pp. 202–244). Logan, UT: Hope, Inc.

Dillon, H., Cameron, S., Glyde, H., Wilson, W., & Tomlin, D. (2012). An opinion on the assessment of people who may have an auditory processing disorder. *Journal of the American Academy of Audiology, 23,* 97–105.

Domitz, D., & Schow, R. L. (2000). Central auditory processes and test measures: ASHA revisited. *American Journal of Audiology, 9,* 63–68.

Downs, S. K., Whitaker, M. M., & Schow, R. (2003). *Audiological services in school districts that do and do not have an audiologist.* Paper presented at the Educational Audiology Association Summer Conference, St. Louis, MO.

Dunst, C. J. (2001). *Parent and community assets as sources of young children's learning opportunities.* Asheville, NC: Winterberry Press.

Eisenberg, L. S. (2009b). *Clinical management of children with cochlear implants.* San Diego, CA: Plural Publishing.

English, K. (1997). *Self-advocacy for students who are deaf and hard of hearing*. Austin, TX: PRO-ED.

English, K. (2010). Family informational and support counseling. In R. Seewald & A. Tharpe (Eds.), *Comprehensive handbook of pediatric audiology* (pp. 767–776). San Diego, CA: Plural Publishing.

Erber, N. P. (1982). *Auditory training*. Washington, DC: Alexander Graham Bell Association for the Deaf.

Ertmer, D. J. (2003). *Contrasts for auditory and speech training*. East Moline, IL: Linguisystems.

Ertmer, D. J. (2005). *The source for children with cochlear implants*. East Moline, IL: Linguisystems.

Ertmer, D. J. (2008). The conditioned assessment of speech production (CASP). *Volta Review, 108*(1), 59–80.

Estabrooks, W. (Ed.). (2012). *101 frequently asked questions about auditory verbal practice*. Washington DC: Alexander Bell Association for Deaf and Hard of Hearing.

Estabrooks, W. (1998). Listening skills for kids with cochlear implants, Appendix D, In W. Estabrooks (Ed.), *Cochlear implants for kids*. Washington, DC: Alexander Graham Bell Association for the Deaf.

Eze, N., Ofo, E., Jiang, D., & O'Connor, A. F. (2013). Systematic review of cochlear implantation in children with developmental disability. *Otology and Neurotology, 34*, 1385–1393.

Finitzo-Heiber, T. (1988). Classroom acoustics. In R. Roeser & M. Downs (Eds.), *Auditory disorders in school children* (pp. 221–233). New York: Thieme-Stratton.

Finitzo-Heiber, T., & Tillman, T. (1978). Room acoustics' effects on monosyllabic word discrimination ability for normal and hearing impaired children. *Journal of Speech and Hearing Research, 21*, 440–458.

Fink, N. E., Wang, N. Y., Visaya, J., & CDaCI Investigative Team. (2007). Childhood development after cochlear implantation (CDaCI) study: Design and baseline characteristics. *Cochlear Implants International, 8*, 92–116.

Gallaudet Research Institute. (2011, April). *Regional and national summary report of data from the 2009–2010 annual survey of deaf and hard of hearing children and youth*. Washington, DC: Gallaudet University Press.

Geers, A., Tobey, E., & Moog, J. (2011). Supplement, long-term outcomes of cochlear implantation in early childhood. *Ear and Hearing, 32*, 1S–92S.

Glover, B., Watkins, S., Pittman, P., Johnson, D., & Barringer, D. G. (1994). SKI*HI home intervention for families with infants, toddlers, and preschool children who are deaf or hard of hearing. *Infant–Toddler Intervention: The Transdisciplinary Journal, 4*(4), 319–332.

Hanft, B., Rush, D. D., & Sheldon, M. (2004). *Coaching families and colleagues in early childhood*. Baltimore: Paul H. Brookes.

Harrison, M., Page, T. A., Oleson, J., Spratford, M., Berry, L. U., Peterson, B., et al. (2015). Factors affecting early services for children who are hard of hearing. *Language, Speech, and Hearing Services in Schools*, 47:16–30.

Hatfield, N., & Humes, K. (1994). Developing a bilingual-bicultural parent-infant program: Challenges, compromises and controversies. In B. Schick & M. P. Moeller (Eds.), *Proceedings of the Seventh Annual Conference on Issues in Language and Deafness*. Omaha, NE: Boys Town National Research Hospital.

Hohmann, M., Banet, B., & Weikart, D. (1979). *Young children in action*. Ypsilanti, MI: High/Scope Press.

Holstrum, W. J., Gaffney, M., Gravel, J. S., Oyler, R. F., & Ross, D. S. (2008). Early intervention for children with unilateral and mild bilateral degrees of hearing loss. *Trends in Amplification, 12*(1), 35–41.

Idol, L., Paolucci-Whitcomb, P., & Nevin, A. (1986). *Collaborative consultation*. Rockville, MD: Aspen.

Jerger, J., & Musiek, F. (2000). Report of the consensus conference on the diagnosis of auditory processing disorders in school-age children. *Journal of the American Academy of Audiology, 11*(9), 467–474.

Johnson, C. D., & Seaton, J. B. (2012). *Educational audiology handbook* (2nd ed.). New York: Delmar, Cengage Learning.

Joint Committee on Infant Hearing. (2000). *Position statement.* Retrieved from http://www.asha.org/about/legislation-advocacy/federal.ehdi

Joint Committee on Infant Hearing. (2007). Year 2007 position statement: Principles and guidelines for early hearing detection and intervention programs. *Pediatrics, 120,* 898–921.

Keith, R. W. (2009) SCAN–3:C Tests for Auditory Processing Disorders for Children. San Antonio, TX: Pearson, The Psychological Corporation.

Koch, M. (1999). *Bringing sound to life.* Timonium, MD: York Press.

Langdon, L., & Blair, J. (2000). Can you hear me: A longitudinal study of hearing aid monitoring in the classroom. *Journal of Educational Audiology, 8,* 34–37.

Larsen, J., & Blair, J. (2008). The effect of classroom amplification on the signal to noise ratio in classrooms while class in in session. *Language, Speech and Hearing Services in Schools, 39,* 456–460. doi:10.1044/0161-1461(2008/07-0032)

Ling, D. (1989). *Foundations of spoken language in hearing impaired children.* Washington, DC: Alexander Graham Bell Association for the Deaf.

Luterman, D. (1987). *Deafness in the family.* San Diego, CA: College-Hill Press.

Luterman, D. (2004, November 16). Children with hearing loss: Reflections on the past 40 years. *ASHA Leader,* 6–7, 18–21.

Luterman, D. (2008). *Counseling persons with communication disorders and their families* (5th Edition). Austin, TX: PRO-ED.

Mahoney, G. (2009). Relationship focused intervention (RFI): Enhancing the role of parents in children's developmental intervention. *International Journal of Early Childhood Special Education, 1*(1), 79–94.

Marge, D. K., & Marge, M. (2005). *Beyond newborn hearing screening: Meeting the educational and healthcare needs of infants and young children.* Report of the National Consensus Conference on Effective Educational and Healthcare Interventions for Infants and Young Children with Hearing Loss, September 10–12, 2004. Syracuse, NY: SUNY Upstate Medical Center.

Martin, D., Bat-Chava, Y., Lalwani, A., & Waltzman, S. (2010). Peer relationships of deaf children with cochlear implants: Predictors of peer entry and peer interaction success. *Journal of Deaf Studies and Deaf Education, 16,* 108–120. doi:10.1348/00709908X368848

McClatchie, A., & Therres, M. K. (2009). *Auditory Speech Language (AuSpLan): Summary of a guide to expectations and auditory, speech and language goals for a child with a cochlear implant.* Retrieved from http://www.advancedbionics.com

McWilliam, R. A. (2010). *Routines-based early intervention: Supporting young children and their families.* Baltimore: Brookes Publishing.

Mindel, E. D., & Vernon, M. (1987). *They grow in silence: The deaf child and his family* (2nd ed.). Silver Spring, MD: National Association of the Deaf.

Moeller, M. P. (2007). Current state of the knowledge: Psychosocial development in children with hearing impairment. *Ear and Hearing, 28*(6), 729–739.

Moeller, M. P., & Carney, A. E. (1993). Assessment and intervention with preschool hearing-impaired children. In J. Alpiner & P. McCarthy (Eds.), *Rehabilitative audiology: Children and adults* (2nd ed., pp. 106–136). Baltimore: Williams & Wilkins.

Moeller, M. P., & Condon, M.-C. (1994). D.E.I.P.: A collaborative problem-solving approach to early intervention. In J. Roush & N. D. Matkin (Eds.), *Infants and toddlers with hearing loss* (pp. 163–194). Baltimore: York Press.

Moeller, M. P., Hoover, B., Peterson, B., & Stelmachowicz, P. G. (2009). Consistency of hearing aid use in infants with early-identified hearing loss. *American Journal of Audiology, 18,* 14–23. PMCID: PMC2692469

Moeller, M. P., Tomblin, J. B., & the OCHL Collaboration. (2015). Epilogue: Conclusions and implications for research and practice. *Ear and Hearing, 36,* 92S–98S.

Moeller, M. P., Tomblin, J. B., Yoshinaga-Itano, C., Connor, C. M., & Jerger, S. (2007). Current state of knowledge: Language and literacy of children with hearing impairment. *Ear and Hearing, 28*(6), 740–753.

Moeller, M. P., White, K. R., & Shisler, L. (2006). Primary care physicians' knowledge, attitudes and practices related to newborn hearing screening. *Pediatrics, 118*(4), 1357–1370.

Moog, J. S., Bildenstein, J., & Davidson, L. (1995). *Speech perception instructional curriculum and evaluation (SPICE).* St. Louis, MO: Central Institute for the Deaf.

Moog, J., & Geers, A. (1990). *Early Speech Perception Test*. St. Louis, MO: Central Institute for the Deaf.

Moog-Brooks, B. (2002). *My baby and me: A book about teaching your child to talk*. St. Louis, MO: Moog Center for Deaf Education.

Munoz, K,, Olson, W. A,, Twohig, M. P., Preston, E., Blaiser, K., & White, K. R. (2015). Pediatric hearing aid use: Parent-reported challenges. *Ear and Hearing, 36*(2), 279–287.

Munoz, K., Preston, E., & Hicken, S. (2014). Pediatric hearing aid use: How can audiologists support parents to increase consistency? *Journal of the American Academy of Audiology, 25*, 380–387.

Munoz, K., Shisler, L., Moeller, M. P., & White, K. (2009). Improving quality of early hearing detection and intervention services through physician outreach. *Seminars in Hearing, 30*(3), 184–192.

Musiek, F. E., & Chermak, G. D. (1994). Three commonly asked questions about central auditory processing disorders: Assessment. *American Journal of Audiology, 3*, 23–27.

National Association for the Education of Young Children. (2009). *Developmentally appropriate practice in early childhood programs serving children from birth through age 8*. Washington, DC: Author. Retrieved from http://www.naeyc.org/DAP

National Institute on Deafness and Other Communication Disorders. (2005). *Statistical report: Prevalence of hearing loss in U.S. children, 2005*. Bethesda, MD: Author.

National Institute on Deafness and Other Communication Disorders. (2016). *Cochlear implants*. Bethesda, MD: Author. Retrieved from https://www.nidcd.nih.gov/health/cochlear-implants

National Institutes of Health and National Institute on Deafness and Other Communication Disorders. (1993, March 1–3). *National Institutes of Health Consensus Statement: Early identification of hearing impairment in infants and young children*. Bethesda, MD: Author. Retrieved from http://odp.od.nih.gov/consensus/cons/092/092intro.htm

Niparko, J. K., Tobey, E. A., Thal, D. J., Eisenberg, L. S., Wang, N. Y., Quittner, A. L., et al. (2010). Spoken language development in children following cochlear implantation. *Journal of the American Medical Association, 303*, 1498–1506.

Niskar, A. S., Kieszak, S. M., Holmes, A., Esteban, E., Rubin, C., & Brody, D. (1998). Prevalence of hearing loss among children 6 to 19 years of age: The Third National Health and Nutrition Examination Survey. *Journal of the American Medical Association, 8*, 279(14), 1071–1075.

Nittrouer, S. (2010). *Early development of children with hearing loss*. San Diego, CA: Plural Publishing.

Norton, S. J., Gorga, M. P., Widen, J. E., Folsom, R. C., Sininger, Y., Cone-Wesson, B., et al. (2000). Identification of neonatal hearing impairment: Summary and recommendations. *Ear and Hearing, 21*(5), 529–535.

Palmieri, M., Berrettini, S., Forli, F., Tresvisi, P., Genovese, E., Chilosi, A. M., et al. (2012). Evaluating benefits of cochlear implantation in deaf children with additional disabilities. *Ear and Hearing, 33*, 721–730.

Pepper, J. and Weitzman, E. (2004), *It takes two to talk A practical guide for parents of children with language delays*. 3rd edition, Hanen Centre.

Porter, H., & Bess, F. H. (2011). Children with unilateral hearing loss. In R. Seewald & A. M. Tharpe (Eds.), *Comprehensive handbook of pediatric audiology*. San Diego, CA: Plural Publishing, 175–191.

Pretti-Frontczak, K., & Bricker, D. (2004). *An activity-based approach to early intervention* (4th ed.). Baltimore: Paul H. Brookes Publishing.

Robbins, A. M. (1993). *Mr. Potato Head task*. Indianapolis: Indiana University School of Medicine.

Robbins, A. M., Zimmerman-Phillips, S., & Osberger, M. J. (1998). *Infant-Toddler Meaningful Auditory Integration Scale (IT-MAIS)*. Retrieved from http://www.bionicear.com

Rossi, K. G. (2003). *Learning to talk around the clock*. Washington, DC: Alexander Graham Bell Association for the Deaf.

Rotfleisch, S. F. (2009). Auditory-verbal therapy and babies. In L. S. Eisenberg (Ed.), *Clinical management of children with cochlear implants* (pp. 435–494). San Diego, CA: Plural Publishing.

Roush, J., Harrison, M., & Palsha, S. (1991). Family-centered early intervention: The perceptions of professionals. *America Annals of the Deaf, 136*(4), 360–366.

Saxon, T. F. (1997). A longitudinal study of early mother-infant interaction and later language competence. *First Language, 17,* 271–281.

Schleper, D. (1996). Gallaudet University and Pre-College National Mission programs. *15 principles for reading to deaf children.* Retrieved from http://www.gallaudet .edu/~pcnmplit/literacy/srp/15princ.html

Schow, R. L., & Seikel, J. A. (2007). Screening for (central) auditory processing disorder. In F. Musiek & G. Chermak (Eds.), *Handbook of (central) auditory processing disorder* (Vol. 1). San Diego, CA: Plural Publishing. Chapter 6, 137–161.

Schow, R. L., Seikel, J. A., Brockett, J. E., & Whitaker, M. M. (2007) *Multiple Auditory Processing Assessment.* St. Louis, MO: Auditec.

Schow, R. L., Seikel, J. A., Brockett, J. E., & Whitaker, M. M. (In Press) *Multiple Auditory Processing Assessment-2. Novato, CA* Academic Therapy Publications.

Schow, R. L., Seikel, J. A., Chermak, G. D., & Berent, M. (2000). Central auditory processes and test measures: ASHA 1996 revisited. *American Journal of Audiology, 9,* 65–68.

Schuyler, V., & Sowers, N. (1998). *Parent infant habilitation: A comprehensive approach to working with hearing-impaired infants and toddlers and their families.* Portland, OR: HIR Publications.

Shepard, N., Davis, J., Gorga, M., & Stelmachowicz, P. (1981). Characteristics of hearing impaired children in the public schools: Part I. Demographic data. *Journal of Speech and Hearing Disorders, 46,* 123–129.

Sindrey, D. (1997). *Listening games for littles.* London, ON: Word Play Publications.

Stredler-Brown, A. (2005, January 18). The art and science of home visits. *ASHA Leader,* 6–7, 15.

Stredler-Brown, A., & Johnson, C. (2004). *Functional auditory performance indicators.* Retrieved from http://www.arlenestredlerbrown.com/docs/FAPI.pdf

Stredler-Brown, A., Moeller, M. P., Gallegos, R., Cordwin, J., & Pittman, P. (2004). *The art and science of home visits* [DVD]. Omaha, NE: Boys Town Press.

Tharpe, A. M. (2011). Permanent and mild bilateral hearing loss in children: Implications and outcomes. In R. Seewald & A.M. Tharpe (Eds.), *Comprehensive handbook of pediatric audiology.* San Diego: Plural Publishing, 193–202.

Tsiakpini, L., Weichbold, V., Kuehn-Inacker, H., Coninx, F., D'Haese, P., & Almadin, S. (2004). *LittlEARS Auditory Questionnaire.* Innsbruck: MED-EL.

Vincent, L., Davis, J., Brown, P., Broome, K., Funkhouser, K., Miller, J., et al. (1986). *Parent inventory of child development in nonschool environment.* Madison: University of Wisconsin, Department of Rehabilitation Psychology and Special Education.

Wallach, G., & Miller, L. (1988). *Language intervention and academic success.* Boston: College-Hill Press.

Watkins, S. (2004). *SKI*HI curriculum: Family-centered programming for infants and young children with hearing loss.* Logan, UT: Hope, Inc.

Watkins, S., Pittman, P., & Walden, B. (2004). *Bilingual-bicultural enhancement for infants, toddlers, and preschoolers who are deaf through deaf mentors in family-centered early home-based programming (The Deaf Mentor Project).* Final Report to U.S. Department of Education, Office of Special Education Programs. Logan, UT: SKI*HI Institute.

Watkins, S., Pittman, P., & Walden, B. (1998). The deaf mentor experimental project for young children who are deaf and their families. *American Annals of the Deaf,* 29–34.

Yoshinaga-Itano, C. (2015). *Evolution of a public health revolution: Universal newborn hearing screening.* Paper presented at the American Auditory Society Conference, Phoenix, AZ.

Yoshinaga-Itano, C., & Downey, D. (1986). A hearing-impaired child's acquisition of schemata: Something's missing. *Topics in Language Disorders, 7*(1), 45–57.

Young, A., & Tattersall, H. (2007). Universal newborn hearing screening and early identification of deafness: Parents' responses to knowing early and their expectations of communication development. *Journal of Deaf Studies and Deaf Education, 12*(2), 209–220.

Yuhan, X. (2013). Peer interaction of children with hearing Impairment. *International Journal of Psychological Studies, 5*(4), 17–25. doi:10.5539/ijps.v5n4p17

Audiologic Rehabilitation across the Adult Life Span: Assessment and Management

M. Kathleen Pichora-Fuller, Ronald L. Schow

CONTENTS

Visit the companion website when you see this icon to learn more about the topic nearby in the text.

Learning Outcomes

After reading this chapter, you will be able to

- Define presbycusis
- Define "baby boomers" and explain how they are affecting the age profile of the population
- Describe how estimates of the prevalence of hearing loss based on audiometry and self-report measures differ depending on age
- Explain why nonauditory age-related health conditions (e.g., dementia, falls, vision loss) are relevant to audiologic rehabilitation (AR)
- Explain why family-centered care is important in AR for older adults
- List and provide examples of four strategies for enhancing self-efficacy in AR
- Identify two self-report measures and explain how they would provide information that you could use to plan and/or evaluate AR

- Compare and contrast two speech-in-noise tests and explain how useful they are for assessing a person's ability to listen in everyday life
- Identify one AR program and one tinnitus treatment that have been shown to be effective based on evidence from randomized controlled trials (RCTs)

INTRODUCTION

Some adults lose their hearing suddenly, but most lose it very gradually.

Some individuals who lived with hearing loss as children or teenagers continue to experience hearing loss as adults. Some adults experience sudden hearing loss, and others become late deafened. Adults may undergo medical or surgical treatments, such as middle ear reconstruction, removal of acoustic neuroma, or cochlear implantation. For many, exposure to hazardous levels of recreational or occupational noise over extended periods of time results in permanent sensorineural hearing loss. Recent research even suggests that the audiogram may return to normal following temporary threshold shifts induced by noise, but long-term neural damage can persist and hamper the understanding of speech in noise (Kujawa & Liberman, 2009). Public education about safe listening (World Health Organization [WHO], 2015a; see "Recommended Websites") and hearing conservation programs to prevent hearing loss and identify early signs of hearing loss in industrial workers could be considered as an early type of hearing care along a continuum of care for adults who, sooner or later, will need various forms of audiologic rehabilitation (AR). Overall, the etiology of hearing loss is well known for some adults, but the vast majority of adults experience very gradual age-related declines in hearing for which there may be no obvious cause or explanation.

Today, there is historically unprecedented aging of the population.

Various health conditions (e.g., diabetes or cardiovascular disease related to smoking) are risk factors for hearing loss (Agrawal, Platz, & Niparko, 2009). Conversely, hearing loss is correlated with increased risk of age-related declines in many aspects of health, including falls and dementia. It has never been so important as it is now to consider how hearing health is related to other aspects of aging (Institute of Medicine, 2014) because the population is aging dramatically. In 2011, the baby boomers (people born between 1946 and 1964) started turning 65 years of age, and they will double the numbers of older adults over the next two decades (U.S. Census Bureau, 2014). According to the American Community Survey Reports on *Older Americans with Disability: 2008–2012* (He & Larsen, 2014), there were 40.7 million people aged 65 years and older in the United States (13.2% of the total population), of whom 15.7 million (38.7%) reported having one or more disabilities. The prevalence of disabilities increases with age and is the highest in those who are 85 years of age and older. The segment of the population over 85 years old is increasing in numbers faster than any other age-group. There are also more centenarians in the United States today than there have ever been before, and their numbers are expected to double with each future decade until 2050 (Krach & Velkoff, 1999).

AR will shift more toward a life-course approach to better meet the needs of adults as they age.

As the population continues to age over the coming decades, AR will likely shift more toward a life-course approach that is in line with the WHO's *World Report on Aging and Health* (WHO, 2015b; Davis et al., 2016). A *life-course approach* in AR would focus on starting hearing care earlier to promote healthy aging. New health education programs for younger adults could help to prevent hearing loss. New programs for middle-aged adults could begin when they first notice hearing-related problems, even though they are not yet ready for hearing aids. Such programs could foster adjustment to hearing loss, facilitate readiness for help seeking, and support decision making regarding rehabilitative options. For the oldest adults and their families or caregivers, innovations in hearing care could help to maintain quality of life as these clients struggle to continue to live independently, move into shared living arrangements with family, enter residential care, or receive palliative care at the end of life.

A key to promoting healthy aging and maintaining quality of life is to optimize communication. Most individuals experiencing hearing loss will retain some residual hearing, but what they lose will erode their ability to hear others effectively such that *communication activity* will become compromised. Unaddressed hearing problems will gradually reduce *participation* in many rewarding activities and threaten the individual's ability to preserve positive self-perceptions and to fulfill social roles in the family and in the community. Both *personal* and *environmental factors* will interact to complicate how individuals adjust to these changes. The focus in society today on successful aging brings exciting new opportunities to connect hearing health with many other initiatives to promote physical, mental, and psychosocial health throughout adult development and aging (Pichora-Fuller, 2014). Adopting a life-course perspective on adult development and aging, AR would follow the evolving abilities, needs, and aspirations of clients and their communication partners over many decades of their adult life until their death (see also Stephens & Kramer, 2010; Worrall & Hickson, 2003).

The provision of services for adults who are hard of hearing has always been challenging, but this challenge is larger than ever because of the expanding population of older adults and their increased life expectancy. More needs to be done, and more can be done for adults, whether they are busy middle-aged adults in the workforce or frail older adults in palliative care and whether they have milder or more severe degrees of hearing loss. More than ever before, evidence based on systematic reviews of the literature is being used to evaluate whether AR practices are effective (Wong & Hickson, 2012). In a review of AR practices based on the evidence, Boothroyd (2007) concluded that the best approach in AR is a holistic one that combines technologies, various types of training, and counseling. Current advances in AR combine new technologies, better training, and counseling for clients and their communication partners. Advances are also being made to shape new social policies to improve hearing accessibility.

During the past decade, the improved technology of open-fit hearing aids and other technological improvements likely produced slight increases in the percentage of those with hearing loss who used amplification (Abrams and Kihm, 2015; Kochkin, 2007; Winkler, Latzel, & Holube, 2016). Today, leading manufacturers boast many new hearing aid technologies that converge with assistive technologies and other communication technologies to extend the functionality of conventional hearing aids beyond simply amplifying sound. The Phonak Roger blends a hearing aid with FM assistive technology to offer listeners more options for better listening in complex acoustical environments. The Starkey Halo is a hearing aid made for use with Apple devices, such as iPhones. Oticon has developed BrainHearing products, such as the Opn, which accesses the If This Then That (IFTT) network so that listeners can connect to and control other devices, such as alarms, televisions, and computers (Beck & Le Goff, 2016). Personal sound amplification products have also entered the marketplace as a cheaper alternative to hearing aids (Smith, Wilber, & Cavitt, 2016). In parallel with rapid changes in hearing aid and assistive technologies, there have been ongoing developments in computer-based technologies to provide perceptual, speech understanding, and cognitive training as a component of AR for adults (Pichora-Fuller & Levitt, 2012). Computer-based programs such as Listening and Communication Enhancement (LACE; Sweetow & Henderson-Sabes, 2004, 2006) produced considerable interest, including being adopted by some hearing aid manufacturers, but dispensers and clients sometimes have given such software a cool reception, and a recent randomized control trial did not find evidence of its effectiveness (Saunders et al., 2016). Importantly, new insights have been gained into what motivates successful use of computer-based training programs in AR (Henshaw, McCormack, & Ferguson, 2015). Turning from the technological to the psychosocial aspects of AR, a recent position paper based on a review of the evidence by leading rehabilitative audiologists advocates for more family-centered AR that includes both clients and their significant others (Singh et al., 2016). New educational and counseling approaches based on health psychology (Saunders, Frederick, Silverman, & Papesh, 2013) and social psychology (Pichora-Fuller, Mick, & Reed, 2015) have been advocated for clients and their

Advances in AR combine new technologies, better training, and counseling for clients and their communication partners and changes in social policy to improve hearing accessibility.

families to help them change attitudes toward hearing loss, adopt positive communication behaviors, and make informed decisions about lifestyle choices as they begin to seek help and adjust to living with hearing loss. Finally, social policies to promote healthy aging provide new opportunities to change stigmatizing attitudes toward older people with hearing loss and to improve hearing accessibility in public venues, including health care facilities, such as doctors' offices and hospitals. For example, new acoustical guidelines may greatly benefit older adults in noisy hospital settings where their health is the most vulnerable and when communication may be especially important for their health (Pope, Gallun, & Kampel, 2013). Comprehensive AR that effectively combines technologies, behavioral interventions, and social policies demands that the audiologist thoroughly understand adult clients; thus, these clients are the first major topic in this chapter.

PROFILE OF THE ADULT CLIENT

Hearing Loss across the Life Span

> Hearing loss affects adults of all ages, but it increases dramatically as they grow older; however, the estimated prevalence of hearing loss depends on the methods used to measure it.

The *prevalence of hearing loss* increases with advancing age, as shown in Figure 10.1. Note that hearing loss affects more men than women and it affects men earlier than women. Figure 10.1 gives estimates of hearing loss based on audiometric criteria and on self-report data (Brainbridge & Wallhagen, 2014). The numbers based on self-report are higher than those based on audiometry for younger adults, but the pattern is reversed for older adults. This means that adults can begin to report problems listening in everyday life even if their audiometric thresholds are mostly still in the range of normal hearing. With increasing age, estimates based on audiometric loss may overtake those based on self-reported hearing problems because older adults have slowly adjusted to living with hearing loss. It is interesting that a systematic review of AR research suggests that self-reported disability is more important than audiometric thresholds in explaining why people seek help for hearing loss (Knudsen, Öberg, Nielsen, Naylor, & Kramer, 2010).

> Self-reported problems in everyday functioning can be more important for AR than audiometric thresholds.

> Older adults may notice problems hearing in noisy everyday situations, even though they have normal audiometric thresholds in the speech range and little difficulty hearing in quiet situations.

Inevitably, loss of hearing leads to misunderstandings and stress for individuals, their families, and communication partners. After first realizing that hearing has become difficult, adults often need time to accept that they have a hearing loss and to decide that they should get help. It is common for adults to delay seeking

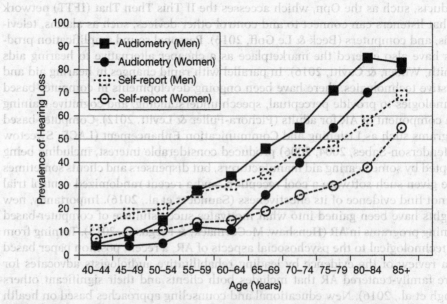

FIGURE 10.1 **Prevalence of hearing loss for males and females estimated based on audiometry and on self-report in the adult population of the United States.**

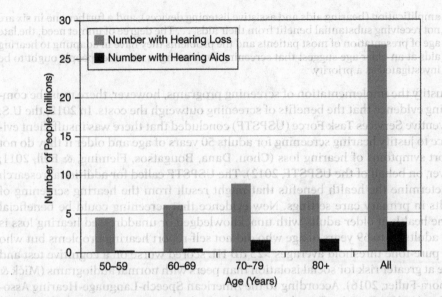

FIGURE 10.2 Prevalence and number of individuals 50 years or older with hearing loss using hearing aids in the United States.

Source: Adapted from Chien and Lin (2012) based on data from the 1999–2006 National Health and Nutrition Examination Survey.

help for hearing problems by years and sometimes even decades. Figure 10.2 shows a portion of those with hearing loss as found in the 1999–2006 National Health and Nutrition Examination Survey (Chien & Lin, 2012). The number of Americans over the age of 50 years with mild or moderate hearing loss (26.7 million) was much greater than the number using hearing aids (3.8 million), although the prevalence of hearing aid use increased from only 4.3 percent in those between 50 and 59 years of age to 22.1 percent in those 80 years of age and older (Chien & Lin, 2012). According to the MarkeTrak IX survey (Abrams & Kihm, 2015), more younger adults are starting to wear hearing aids sooner, and the average age of first-time hearing aid wearers dropped to 63 years in 2015 compared to 69 years in the MarkeTrak VIII survey conducted in 2008.

Help Seeking and Screening

Eventually, it is common for family, friends, or the stress associated with hearing loss to convince the individual to have his or her hearing screened or tested, leading to a confirmation of hearing loss. Rather than dismissing adults in the early stages of hearing loss as poorly motivated or "not yet ready for a hearing aid," innovative audiologists around the world are discovering how to use health education or health promotion approaches to prepare adults and their families for the eventuality of needing AR (Grenness et al., 2016; Singh et al., 2016). By taking the first step to identify hearing loss, the process of acceptance and adjustment can begin.

In the wake of the successful implementation of early newborn hearing screening programs around the world, health care delivery researchers are now tackling the problem of how best to screen adult hearing to reduce the delay in accessing hearing services for those who are most likely to benefit (Davis, Smith, Ferguson, Stephens, & Gianopoulos, 2007). According to the executive summary of the report of these British researchers,

> About one in five adults in the UK has a bilateral hearing problem that affects their hearing and communication. The major problems occur in listening to speech in a background of noise (e.g., in social and family settings, shops, cafés or bars, watching television), which makes communication or enjoyment very difficult. Previous estimates have suggested that at least one in ten people might benefit from amplification, but currently only one in six of those who might benefit have and fully use their

After noticing a hearing problem, it may take years for adults to seek help from an audiologist.

amplification (hearing aids and assistive listening devices), and a further one in six are not receiving substantial benefit from their aids. . . . The degree of unmet need, the late age of presentation of most patients and the problems they have in adapting to hearing aids at an older age suggest that screening for hearing . . . in older people ought to be investigated as a priority.

To justify the implementation of screening programs, however, there must be compelling evidence that the benefits of screening outweigh the costs. In 2012, the U.S. Preventive Services Task Force (USPSTF) concluded that there was insufficient evidence to justify hearing screening for adults 50 years of age and older if they do not report symptoms of hearing loss (Chou, Dana, Bougatsos, Fleming, & Bell, 2011; Moyer, on behalf of the USPSTF, 2012). The USPSTF called for additional research to determine the health benefits that might result from the hearing screening of adults in primary care settings. New evidence that screening could be beneficial to the health of older adults with unacknowledged or unaddressed hearing loss is that adults 60 to 69 years of age who did not self-report hearing problems but who had pure-tone threshold averages >25 dB HL scored worse on a cognitive test and were at greater risk for social isolation than peers with normal audiograms (Mick & Pichora-Fuller, 2016). According to the American Speech-Language-Hearing Association (ASHA) Practice Portal, more evidence that hearing screening is beneficial for healthy aging could justify revisions to the 2012 USPSTF clinical guidelines.

New approaches for reaching adults with unacknowledged or unaddressed hearing loss have been developed using social media and wireless technologies. The exploding use of downloadable applications for mobile phones offers worried individuals a way to test their own hearing and quickly find information about where to get help. One of the earliest apps produced by a manufacturer, Unitron's *uHear*, was released in 2009 and is still available on iTunes (https://itunes.apple.com/ca/app/uhear/id309811822?mt=8). Telephone hearing screening testing using digit triplets was pioneered in the Netherlands (Smits, Govert, & Festen, 2013) and then implemented in other countries. In the United States, the National Hearing Test (Williams-Sanchez et al., 2014) is offered for free by the nonprofit organization AARP (formerly the American Association of Retired Persons) to its almost 38 million members (AARP; https://www.nationalhearingtest.org/wordpress). In addition, validated and relatively inexpensive computer-based pure-tone home hearing tests are now available (Margolis, Killion, Bratt, & Saly, 2016). Innovations in screening and early identification of hearing loss in adults and other research on help seeking and adjustment to hearing loss should help rehabilitative audiologists develop new management approaches to reach adults with hearing problems earlier.

PROFILE OF THE OLDER ADULT CLIENT

In this chapter, we focus special attention on older adults because the prevalence of hearing problems increases with age and most of those who seek hearing rehabilitation are older adults. As a group, older adults are similar in many ways to younger adults, but there are differences, and the complex needs of each person will have to be considered on an individual basis. In addition to considering the effects of auditory aging, audiologists need to consider age-related changes in other health conditions and how hearing loss may interact with other disabilities.

Auditory Aging

Presbycusis.   Willott (1991) defined *presbycusis* as "the decline in hearing associated with various types of auditory system dysfunction (peripheral and/or central) that accompany aging and cannot be accounted for by extraordinary ototraumatic, genetic, or pathological conditions. The term *presbycusis* implies deficits not only in absolute thresholds but in auditory perception, as well." In its most common form, *presbycusis, or age-related hearing loss (ARHL),* is characterized as high-frequency

Presbycusis, or age-related hearing loss (ARHL), includes the decline in hearing thresholds and other declines in auditory processing associated with aging.

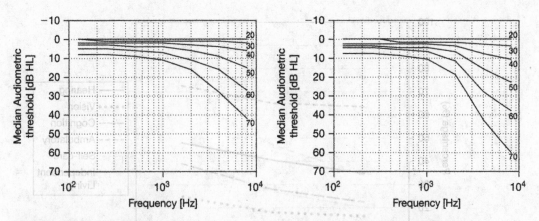

FIGURE 10.3   **Median pure tone audiometric thresholds for women (left panel) and men (right panel) by age decade.**
Source: Adapted from ISO (2000).

sensorineural loss that progresses gradually. Figure 10.3 shows the median thresholds at standard audiometric test frequencies for men and women across decades of age as specified in a standard (7029) of the International Organization for Standardization (ISO, 2000). In addition, median thresholds at higher frequencies have been reported (Stenklev & Laukli, 2004).

Elevated thresholds in the higher frequencies of the audiogram usually result from damage to the cochlea. To the extent that ARHL involves outer hair cell damage (e.g., from noise), the hearing problems of older clients should be very similar to those of younger clients who have similar audiograms. However, a more age-specific cause of high-frequency threshold elevation is reduced endocochlear potentials associated with changes in the blood supply to the stria vascularis in the cochlea (Mills, Schmiedt, Schulte, & Dubno, 2006). Aging adults are also likely to have auditory processing problems that are not predictable from the audiogram (Gates & Mills, 2005). Other characteristics of auditory aging that could be related to neural damage are temporal processing problems and difficulties hearing speech in noise (Kujawa & Liberman, 2009; Pichora-Fuller & Souza, 2003). Knowledge about ARHL has advanced incredibly over the past two decades (for a comprehensive review, see Gordon-Salant, Frisina, Popper, & Fay, 2010).

Suprathreshold Auditory Processing.   In some older individuals, ARHL is characterized by a more severe word recognition problem than would be expected on the basis of the pure tone audiogram. This phenomenon, first referred to as *phonemic regression* (Gaeth, 1948), involves perceptual confusions and distortions of the phonetic elements of speech, resulting in problems that may not be solved by amplification alone. A frequent complaint of older adults with ARHL is that sounds are jumbled or unclear even if they are loud enough. Increasing the intensity of speech is not always helpful because ARHL may involve damage to the auditory neural pathways (Lopez-Poveda, 2014).

Phonemic regression is a term coined almost 70 years ago for a form of hearing loss found in older adults where speech understanding is unexpectedly poor.

Recently, the term *hidden hearing loss* was coined to refer to auditory processing disorders (APD), such as those experienced by older listeners, that are not explained fully by the audiogram; however, others have argued that such auditory processing problems have been recognized for a long time and are really *not-so-hidden hearing loss* (Kraus & White-Schwock, 2016).

Research on the neural aspects of auditory aging offers new insights into the well-established clinical observation that older individuals with auditory processing disorders experience greater hearing difficulties than those without it (Jerger,

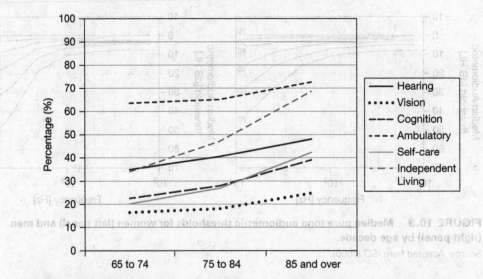

FIGURE 10.4 Percentage of those in each age-group who reported a hearing, vision, cognition, ambulatory, self-care, or independent living disability in the 2008–2012 American Community Survey.
Source: Adapted from He and Larsen (2014).

Oliver, & Pirozzolo, 1990). The report on a review of evidence by the American Academy of Audiology (AAA) Task Force on Central Presbycusis concluded, "Recent evidence has been accumulating in support of the existence of central presbycusis as a multifactorial condition that involves age- and/or disease-related changes in the auditory system and in the brain" (Humes et al., 2012, p. 636). Alternative AR approaches beyond just fitting hearing aids may be needed to address the communication problems of the many older adults who have auditory processing disorders (APD) regardless of whether or not they have significant audiometric threshold elevations (Gates & Mills, 2005).

Physical, Psychological, and Social Aspects of Adult Aging

To further complicate matters, an older listener's peripheral and/or central auditory processing difficulties may interact with age-related strengths and weaknesses in other senses, motor skills, and cognition (Committee on Hearing, Bioacoustics, and Biomechanics, 1988). Figure 10.4, based on data from the American Community Survey for 2008–2012 (He & Larsen, 2014), shows how self-reported disabilities increase with age. Self-reported hearing disability is less common than ambulatory disability (difficulty walking or climbing stairs) and more common than vision disability (serious difficulty seeing, even when wearing glasses), but there is a similar rate of increase for hearing, vision, and ambulatory disabilities across age-groups. In contrast, disabilities in the areas of cognition (difficulty remembering, concentrating, or making decisions), self-care (difficulty bathing or dressing), and independent living (difficulty doing errands alone, such as visiting a doctor's office or shopping) rise more sharply for those in the oldest age-group. Figure 10.5 shows how the number of disabilities affecting a person increases with age, with over 40 percent of those over 85 years of age having two or more disabilities.

The complexities of ARHL and how it interacts with other areas of ability require the audiologist to consider many facets of the client's life as a communicator in everyday life (Kiessling et al., 2003; Kricos, 2006). One obvious example is that about 20 percent of those over the age of 70 years have dual sensory losses in hearing and vision (Brabyn, Schneck, Haegerstrom-Portnoy, & Lott, 2007). Many age-related vision losses are not correctable by lenses, and, depending on the specific age-related pathology (cataracts, macular degeneration, diabetic retinopathy), reduced access to visual environmental information and reduced ability to use

There are many interactions between hearing loss in older adults and other age-related changes in health. Declines in vision, balance, and cognition are especially relevant to AR for older adults.

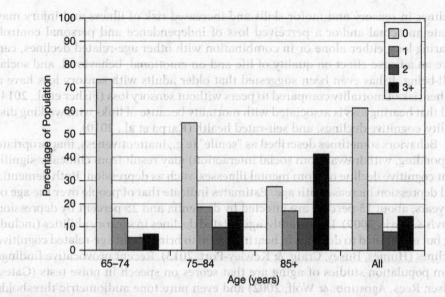

FIGURE 10.5 **Percentage of the population aged 65 or more years old by number of disabilities and age: 2008–2012.**

Source: Adapted from He and Larsen (2014).

visual speech cues during speechreading can seriously hamper communication and social interaction (Echt & Saunders, 2014; Gagné & Wittich, 2009). In trying to understand how adults experience hearing loss, it is important to consider the nonauditory age-related changes they experience (Kricos, 2000), especially changes that alter real or perceived communicative competence and participation in the challenging conditions of everyday life.

Of course, various age-related declines will limit how well older adults communicate and function, but some changes may help to preserve their ability to communicate successfully (Pichora-Fuller & Singh, 2006). In general, studies comparing patterns of brain activation in younger and older adults have found that older adults have more widespread brain activation than younger adults when they perform similarly (e.g., Cabeza, Anderson, Locantore, & McIntosh, 2002; Grady 2012). Research about brain plasticity is very encouraging for rehabilitation professionals because it suggests that older adults can compensate by finding new ways to successfully perform complex tasks, such as listening to speech in noise (e.g., Peelle, Troiani, Wingfield, & Grossman, 2010). In particular, older adults may compensate for sensory declines by using contextual information, which can be advantageous if the context supports the intended meaning of the message (Pichora-Fuller, 2008), although it can sometimes be disadvantageous if the context is misleading (Rogers, Jacoby, & Sommers, 2012). Of course, compensation will be undermined as other disabilities, including cognitive loss, conspire to compromise the level of functioning in everyday life that is needed for independent living.

It is impossible to assess accurately the effect of aging based solely on a person's chronological age. Not all individuals of the same age experience aging in the same way. Some people appear youthful well into their eighties, while others manifest old-age behaviors by their early forties. Importantly, how old a person feels is more related to health and longevity than how old a person is chronologically (Rippon & Steptoe, 2015). To some degree, most older adults adjust to a certain amount of physical disability and reduced activity level, but how well they adjust depends not only on biological factors but also on psychological and social factors. As each new physical problem becomes apparent and deterioration continues, the consequences of aging can significantly affect an individual's attitude toward self-fulfillment. This is why it is difficult to discuss the physical and mental factors contributing to the aging process separately. The interaction between the two can be symbiotic, with changes in one almost certainly influencing the other. Concomitant

Some people appear youthful well into their eighties, whereas others manifest old-age behaviors by their early forties. How old a person feels can be more important than how old they are chronologically.

declines in sensory and motor skills and increased risk of illness and injury may create an actual and/or a perceived loss of independence and personal control. Hearing loss, either alone or in combination with other age-related declines, can have an adverse effect on quality of life and on emotional, behavioral, and social well-being. It has even been suggested that older adults with sensory loss have a higher risk of mortality compared to peers without sensory loss (Fisher et al., 2014) and that hearing loss is associated with mortality because of links with walking disability, cognitive declines, and self-rated health (Karpa et al., 2010).

Behaviors sometimes described as "senile" (e.g., inattentiveness, inappropriate responding, withdrawal from social interaction) may result from clinically significant cognitive decline or from mental illnesses, such as depression. Both dementia and depression increase with age. Estimates indicate that of people over the age of 75 years, about 15 percent are affected by dementia and 25 percent by depression (Davis & Davis, 2009). Importantly, age-related declines in sensory abilities (including but not limited to declines in hearing) seem to bring about age-related cognitive declines (Humes, Busey, Craig, & Kewley-Port, 2013). Recent provocative findings from population studies of aging are that scores on speech in noise tests (Gates, Beiser, Rees, Agostino, & Wolf, 2002) and even pure tone audiometric thresholds (Lin et al., 2011) may predict the onset of dementia 10 years later. Those with dual sensory loss are likely to be at even greater risk (Lin et al., 2004). For first-time hearing aid owners who are 70 years of age, audiologists can expect that more than 1 in 10 may also have clinically significant psychological health issues in addition to the typical psychological stresses related to coping with biological changes (Pichora-Fuller, Dupuis, Reed, & Lemke-Kalis, 2013).

On a positive note, audiologists have become aware of the possibility that by helping older adults maintain active and healthy lifestyles, AR could play a role in helping to stave off or slow down the effects of cognitive decline (Pichora-Fuller, 2009b). Nevertheless, it is premature to make claims that hearing aids or other forms of AR can prevent or cure dementia because there is insufficient high-quality research to provide solid evidence that these interventions are effective in altering the course of cognitive declines! In the broader context of health care, ensuring that older adults can hear as well as possible may make a significant difference to how other health conditions are diagnosed and treated because communication is a necessity in just about every interaction with most health professionals.

Experimental research has shown that when healthy younger and older adults perform cognitive tasks such as remembering and comprehending spoken speech, there seem to be age-related differences in cognitive performance, but these age-related differences are minimized when the test conditions are adjusted so that perceptual difficulty is equal for all listeners (Schneider, Pichora-Fuller, & Daneman, 2010). It follows that if older people have more trouble hearing incoming information, they in turn become disadvantaged when performing cognitive tasks such as comprehending or remembering information that has been heard. For example, Amsel and Weinstein (1986) found that about a third of those assessed for dementia were recategorized to a milder category when they were retested with amplification. It is important for audiologists to provide information about the hearing abilities and needs of older individuals to health professionals (e.g., family doctors, neuropsychologists, and geriatricians) who may be conducting cognitive screening or diagnostic evaluations. Interprofessional collaboration will help to ensure that test stimuli are optimally perceived and results are appropriately interpreted to differentiate the contributions of sensory and cognitive losses on test performance (Dupuis et al., 2015; Jorgensen, Palmer, Pratt, Erickson, & Moncrieff, 2016).

Personal and Environmental Factors

The audiologist must consider the resources or supports that are available to aging clients as they try to adjust to hearing loss. Some older individuals may find it easier than younger adults to adjust to hearing loss because they are able to apply a lifetime of other experiences and generalize lessons they have learned about how

[Margin notes:]

Adjustment to hearing loss can interact with age-related changes in physical, cognitive, emotional, and social function.

Interprofessional collaboration will help to ensure that the effects of hearing loss on cognitive test performance are taken into account.

to cope with other health problems. Nevertheless, others may be less fortunate and face greater challenges, especially if they are adjusting to a number of other changes. According to experts in health promotion, health can be defined as the capacity of people to adapt to, respond to, or control life's challenges and changes (Frankish, Green, Ratner, Chomik, & Larsen, 1996). Leaders in our field have even argued that, rather than focusing on the *rehabilitation* of the individual who has hearing loss, we should shift to a process of *"enablement"* (Stephens & Kramer, 2010). Stephens and Kramer (2010) define "audiologic enablement" to be "a problem-solving process aimed at: enhancing the activities and participation of an individual with hearing difficulties; improving their quality of life; minimizing any effect on significant others; facilitating their acceptance of any residual problems" (p. 3).

With age, the frequency and severity of significant health and lifestyle changes continue to increase, as described by Ronch and Van Zanten (1992) and summarized next. Although most aging persons undergo a certain degree of change in every area listed, their capacity to adapt to these changes is highly individualized, depending on genetic inheritance, life experiences, traditional ways of dealing with life, and past and present environmental factors.

1. *Physical condition:* Loss of youth; changes in physiological and biological aspects of the body cause poor health and its emotional consequences.

2. *Emotional and sexual life:* Loss of significant others through death, separation, and reduction in sexual activity due to societal expectations, health, personal preference, or death of partner.

3. *Members of the family of origin:* Parents, brothers, and sisters become ill or die.

4. *Marital relationship:* Strain due to death or illness of spouse, estrangement due to empty-nest syndrome, pressures due to retirement.

5. *Peer group:* Friends die or become separated by geographical relocation for health, family, or retirement reasons.

6. *Occupation:* Many older people retire; some may feel that their identity has been eroded, and they may have reduced levels of activity and participation outside of work.

7. *Recreation:* Social leisure activities and physical fitness activities become infrequent due to sensory, cognitive and/or mobility limitation, or unavailability of opportunities.

8. *Economics:* Income is reduced by retirement; limited income is tapped by inflation or medical costs not covered by insurance.

Individuals may experience stress if they have difficulty adapting to change. The characteristics of stressful situations are summarized in the acronym NUTS: Novelty, Unpredictability, Threat to self, and Sense of a lack of control (Lupien, Sindi, & Wan, 2012). It seems likely that hearing loss would increase stress reactions as older adults struggle to adapt to significant life changes. It is difficult enough for a person to learn that he or she has been diagnosed with a health condition (e.g., diabetes) and to learn how to manage it, but just imagine the extra stress that a person with hearing loss might have (e.g., if he or she could not hear the instructor or other group members at the diabetes education course). Compounding emotional reactions, stress hormones can alter brain physiology and functioning, resulting in immediate stress-induced reductions in memory performance and in permanent changes to the brain and memory declines in those exposed to chronic stress (Lupien, McEwen, Gunnar, & Heim, 2009). Hearing loss can make attending medical appointments more stressful, but optimizing the physical and social environment of the clinic can improve patient–clinician communication and reduce stress (for practical suggestions, see Lupien et al., 2012). Whereas the causal direction of the link between hearing loss and personal or social adjustment and cognitive performance may be open to debate, the eventual establishment of the link between them for most aging adults is evident. The nature of these links needs to be better understood and incorporated into our approaches to working with adults who have hearing loss (Pichora-Fuller et al., 2015).

Retirement, Leisure, and Economic Status

Staying physically, mentally, and socially active promotes healthy aging.

Retirement is one of the biggest changes in the lives of many older adults. On the one hand, retirement can provide older adults with an opportunity to enjoy many rewarding experiences, such as having more time for leisure activities (e.g., going to the theater or eating in restaurants), engaging in physical activity (e.g., walking or playing golf), working on old hobbies (e.g., playing a musical instrument), or learning new skills (e.g., speaking a foreign language), traveling, or volunteering in community activities. On the other hand, loss of employment may reduce financial security, resulting in reduced social interaction and eroding self-esteem. For some older adults, their identities and social status are bound tightly to their occupation, whereas other older adults look for new ways to find meaning in their lives. In general, staying physically, mentally, and socially active, including participating in leisure activities, seems to promote cognitive health in older adults (Fratiglioni, Paillard-Borg, & Winblad, 2004).

On average, adults with hearing loss have lower rates of employment and lower incomes than peers with normal hearing (Jung & Bhattacharyya, 2012). In general, disability rates are much higher for those with lower education and poorer socioeconomic status, more women than men are disabled, and more people who are black are disabled compared to people who are white (He & Larsen, 2014). Adjustments to lifestyle changes in retirement are easier when people are more educated and economic factors are not a concern. Given that adults with hearing loss and other disabilities may be relatively disadvantaged socioeconomically, it follows that they may have more difficulty adjusting to age-related lifestyle changes than those without disabilities. A higher income allows greater mobility to seek better health care and to continue supportive social contacts. Those with higher incomes may use various options to counteract the effects of hearing loss on their life. For example, they may opt to use technologies, interact with communication partners who are supportive, or select or modify activities and environments according to their communication needs (Wu & Bentler, 2012). An affluent, socially active, and well-educated older person may be inclined to seek information and be willing to purchase medications, eyeglasses, dentures, or hearing aids. Low-income persons with less education may have fewer options. Women are particularly vulnerable to economic stresses, especially if they have not been in the workforce. Of course, the financial disparity between men and women is decreasing because, compared to their mothers, more women in the baby-boom cohort attained higher education and pursued professional careers.

Of the older adult population living in private households in the United States in 2008–2012, 12.6 percent of those with a disability but only 7.2 percent of those without disability were living in poverty, although the poverty rate varied considerably across states (He & Larsen, 2014). Most older individuals are not considered to be poor, but many live on fixed incomes, and the equity in their home is their prime financial asset. The financial benefit of selling the house frequently increases emotional stress produced by the subsequent loss of neighborhood friends and familiar environmental surroundings.

The economic status of older adults who live in long-term extended care facilities is usually lower than that of those who reside in privately owned homes. Where they live and the nature of their prior employment may influence the status of their health care insurance, pensions, and preretirement savings, with some being able to maintain a comfortable lifestyle free of significant financial worries and others experiencing extreme financial stress. In the past decade, recessions and economic worries in the United States and around the world may have magnified these stresses, especially for those at the more disadvantaged end of the social spectrum. Affordable health care, including affordable hearing health care, has become a hotly debated topic, and future changes in social policies may reduce some of the financial barriers to hearing care (Blazer, Domnitz, & Leverman, 2016; see also the National Academies of Sciences, Engineering, and Medicine website at www.nationalacademies.org).

Living Environments

Most older adults live independently in their own residences, and about half live with their spouse. On average, because women live longer than men, it follows that most of the older adults who live on their own are women. About 30 percent of those with disability are married and live with their spouse, but over half are widowed, with equal numbers of widows living either alone or with other family members (He & Larsen, 2014). Many frail older adults are cared for by their spouses or children who live with them. Considerable stress and "caregiver burden" is experienced by those born in the baby-boom cohort who are described as being in the "sandwich" generation because they look after frail parents as well as dependent children who may continue to live at home until they are adults. It is worth noting that changes in the structure of the family over the last half of the twenty-first century, including a trend for families to have fewer children and for more people to remain single, mean that those who enter retirement in the coming decades may have less social support from family.

Of course, a person who spends most of his or her time at home alone may have reduced opportunities for conversation. Nevertheless, hearing may become extremely important from a safety perspective because they must be able to hear fire alarms, doorbells, and the phone ringing and respond appropriately in emergency situations without the help of others or request help when they need it. In the future, with the development of new speech-based information and communication technologies, hearing may become even more important in enabling more older adults to stay at home longer and/or receive health care at home. For example, new *e-health technologies* are being developed to monitor health conditions remotely using the Internet or mobile phones, and new smart home designs will use speech to interact with those living alone who have dementia or who are at risk for adverse events, such as falls or heart attacks (Boger & Mihailidis, 2011).

Older individuals may require professional health care beyond the capabilities of the family environment. Home care services may help to offset the burden that would otherwise fall on family members. Professionally run day programs may provide a much-needed opportunity for social interaction and stimulation in a supportive environment when it is no longer safe for an older adult to remain at home alone during the day while adult children are at work and grandchildren are at school. Almost 10 percent of older adults who have disabilities live in a group residence (He & Larsen, 2014). For some older adults, residential facilities with only limited assisted care may be appropriate. However, the health care facilities most often associated with the aging population are nursing homes that provide long-term care. About half of women and a third of men will use a nursing home before they die. Of women who reach 90 years of age, 70 percent have lived in a nursing home. Those in nursing homes represent an older segment of the geriatric population with generally more advanced physical and mental health problems. Often they are more socially isolated, with about half having no nearby relatives.

In the past, nursing homes often operated following a hospital model, but a rapidly growing number of baby boomers with ample financial resources and higher expectations are seeking high-quality living options with "graduated care" for their parents and for themselves. This demand has fueled the development of the businesses specialized in "retirement living" residences that provide resort-style accommodation and meals, along with in-house recreational, nursing, and other supportive services that can be phased in as the needs of the person change.

Just over 50 percent of the elderly live with a spouse.

Especially for older adults living alone, hearing is important to ensure safety and to enable the use of e-health technologies.

Assistive living options are creating new settings for AR.

For those in the highest level of care, these facilities often feature special "reminiscence" areas specialized for the care of people with dementia, including those who need a living space with secured entry and exit because they are at risk of wandering and becoming lost. These new settings open up new alternative living options with opportunities for audiologists to provide AR on-site in collaboration with other health care providers, volunteers, and family members.

In the future, as recreation-oriented programming in retirement living and assisted living facilities offers more opportunities for social interaction for those living in such residences, the importance of preserving hearing function will only become more important. For nursing home residents and hospitalized older adults, hearing loss is extremely common. In a seminal study, Schow and Nerbonne (1980) evaluated 202 nursing home residents from five facilities and found that 82 percent of their sample demonstrated pure tone threshold averages of 26 dB HL or greater, and 48 percent had averages of at least 40 dB HL. The finding that most residents in long-term care have hearing loss has not changed over the decades. In addition to hearing loss, residents in long-term care often have comorbid conditions that could affect communication, including dementia, depression, and aphasia. Speech-language pathologists providing services in long-term care settings should consider hearing loss when they work with staff and family to develop communication plans for residents, but the communication needs of residents are typically the responsibility of nurses and other on-site workers who usually do not have sufficient knowledge or training regarding hearing care (Lane, 2016; Solheim, Shiryaeva, & Kvaerner, 2016). There are many opportunities for more audiologists to join interprofessional teams working with older adults living in residential settings.

Palliative care occurs when patients are being nursed through the final stages of life. Nurses providing palliative care sometimes make audiology referrals because they want to communicate with people at this stage, even though hearing may have seemed less important at earlier stages of care. We should not underestimate the value of working with very ill people who have little time to live. Maintaining communication with loved ones may become the highest priority for family members and close friends who have gathered to share final days and moments with one another and the person in palliative care. A recent survey found that about one in five audiologists has provided services to clients in palliative care, and most audiologists want to learn more about how to deliver services in this setting (Ricky & English, 2016).

Palliative nursing care occurs in the final stages of a person's life.

The main components of our model are like those in an international model: assessment (or evaluation) and management (or intervention), with feedback from outcome measurement (or surveillance and maintenance).

MODEL FOR REHABILITATION

In Chapter 1 and in Schow (2001), a model and flowchart were presented to provide an overall framework for AR. The flowchart is shown in Figure 10.6 to provide a frame of reference as we describe rehabilitation for adults. As noted there, this work is divided into rehabilitative assessment and management, and it includes an outcome measurement feedback loop. Our model is highly compatible with other models inspired by the WHO's International Classification of Functioning, Disability, and Health (ICF) (WHO, 2001), even though there may be slight differences in terminology. An international consensus paper, including the model shown in Figure 10.7 based on the WHO ICF, was published over a decade ago by a working group, including many of the world's leading rehabilitative audiologists (Kiessling et al., 2003). The WHO ICF model has continued to be a leading model inspiring new approaches to AR (Meyer et al., 2016; Stephens & Kramer, 2010), although more work remains to be done, especially in terms of the participation component of the model (Granberg et al., 2014). The main components of our model—assessment and management with feedback from outcome measurement—parallel the main components of the model proposed by this international consensus group that labels the components, respectively, as evaluation and intervention, with ongoing

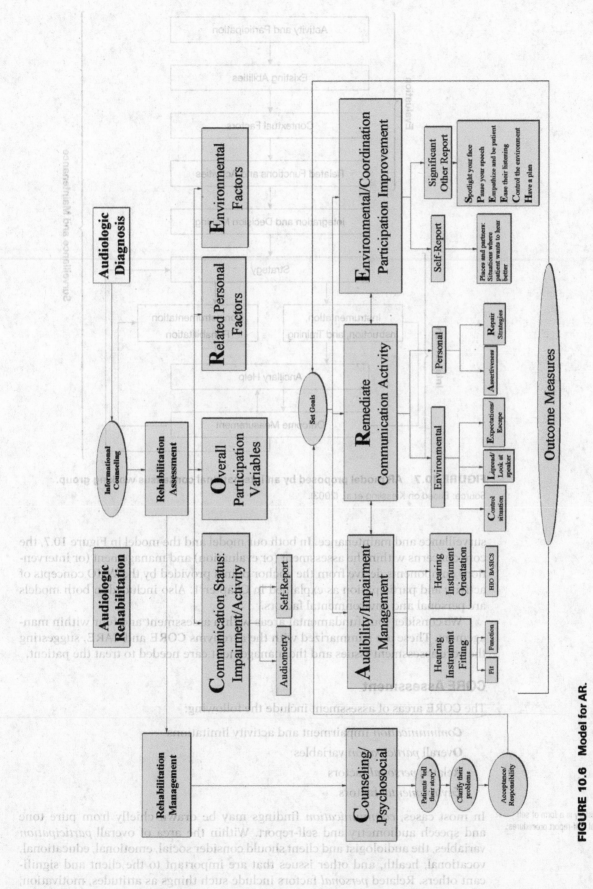

FIGURE 10.6 Model for AR.

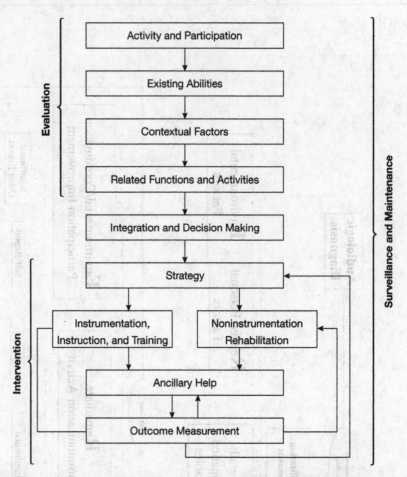

FIGURE 10.7   AR model proposed by an international consensus working group.
Source: Based on Kiessling et al. (2003).

surveillance and maintenance. In both our model and the model in Figure 10.7, the core concerns within the assessment (or evaluation) and management (or intervention) components derive from the anchor points provided by the WHO concepts of activity and participation as explained in Chapter 1. Also included in both models are personal and environmental factors.

We consider four fundamental areas within assessment and four within management. These are summarized with the acronyms CORE and CARE, suggesting the core assessment issues and the management care needed to treat the patient.

CORE Assessment

The CORE areas of assessment include the following:

Communication impairment and activity limitations

Overall *participation* variables

Related *personal* factors

Environmental factors

> The traditional case history is a form of self-report, but more formal self-report procedures are also available.

In most cases, *communication* findings may be drawn chiefly from pure tone and speech audiometry and self-report. Within the area of overall *participation* variables, the audiologist and client should consider social, emotional, educational, vocational, health, and other issues that are important to the client and significant others. Related *personal* factors include such things as attitudes, motivation, and other disabilities or personal conditions that may affect treatment. Finally, the physical and social aspects of the *environment* in which the person lives and must communicate should be considered because treatment options may depend on the auditory ecology of the person (Gatehouse, Naylor, & Elberling, 2006) and the social support available to them from family members and others (Singh et al., 2016). Through this assessment process, the audiologist is invited to consider the fundamental issues that bear on rehabilitation. This need not be an extended process because a good case history and a focused self-report often help us to address these issues. Nevertheless, we need to see these four matters as constituting an assessment battery, and none of these important elements should be neglected.

CARE Management

On the management (treatment) side, we see the four aspects summarized by the acronym CARE:

For many adults, treatment must go beyond amplification alone.

Counseling

Audibility–amplification

Remediation for *communication activities*

Environmental coordination and *participation* issues

Counseling should include information provided to the client and significant others based on the assessment findings. Through an interactive process, counseling should allow the client and significant others to help set goals for treatment. Treatment goals will fall into three areas: *audibility*, *activities*, and *participation*.

The treatment for *audibility* problems usually involves amplification. All too often, however, technology is the only focus of treatment. But through the current model, we propose not only a more precise understanding of the elements within audibility management but also a broader focus on treatment that includes activity and participation issues as proposed by the WHO ICF model. Hearing technologies and audibility treatment involve the fit and function of the device, plus *hearing instrument orientation*. *Fit* has to do with matters such as the style of the aid or the specific assistive device preferred by the client plus issues such as obtaining a suitable earmold impression. *Function* refers to matters such as whether audibility targets are met. These matters of *fit and function* were thoroughly discussed in Chapter 2. Hearing instrument orientation (HIO) should cover some *basic* topics. The typical dispensing audiologist may use a printed handout or other materials (e.g., Internet resources) to cover the basics when this part of the audibility management is performed.

Communication activity issues should be addressed by any professional who fits hearing aids or is involved in AR. One approach involves asking the client to consider at least five important communication concepts captured by the acronym CLEAR: (1) *control* the communication situation, (2) *lipread* and use visual information during communication, (3) *evaluate* the importance of successful communication in the various situations and set realistic *expectations* for or *escape* the situation, (4) *assert* your needs and rights so others know how to modify communication behaviors and environments to *accommodate* your needs, and (5) *repair* miscommunications as needed. As noted in the model, these matters involve both personal and environmental factors. Again, a short handout or other resource material can be used to help reinforce these concepts, which would be explained by the audiologist to the client and significant others and reinforced throughout the entire rehabilitative process. More advanced communication work may be used to follow up and provide more intensive help.

The final area of treatment involves *environmental and participation* issues. We recommend, for most audiologists dispensing hearing aids, that this concern can be most easily addressed through the use of self-report. When clients select a few areas of major concern wherein they have serious communication difficulties, as they do when appropriate self-report approaches are used, these generally translate into goals specifying how the client would like to improve his or her communication activities and participation possibilities. The audiologist helps the client to select goals by identifying at least one high-priority area of concern that the person believes to be important and achievable. Outcome measures can be used to measure improvement for the specific goal(s) of the individual. Moreover, when self-report questionnaires contain standard situations in which persons with hearing difficulties experience problems, standardized data are available that allow comparisons between the client being treated and other clients who have completed the same measures.

Feedback Based on Outcome Measures

Three important outcome measures: benefit, use, and satisfaction.

Outcome measures are used in research to establish the evidence base on which new programs are introduced into practice and/or old ones are changed or phased out. During counseling and when discussing management options with a client, the audiologist should share current research evidence regarding various treatments so that the client can make informed decisions about his or her care (Hickson, 2009; Wong & Hickson, 2012). Following initial assessment and management, it will be essential to use outcome measures to determine if the treatment worked. If the treatment has not addressed the initial goal(s) of the client or if new goals have emerged since the initial assessment, then new rehabilitation plans must be developed and implemented. Follow-up using outcome measures can be thought of as a kind of reassessment. In effect, the process of assessment and treatment cycle repeatedly over time, and changes are introduced based on the results obtained using outcome measures. Three important categories of outcome measures concern how much it helps the person (benefit), how much use he or she makes of the treatment (use), and how satisfied he or she is with it (satisfaction).

Importance of the Conceptual Framework to AR Practice

The WHO ICF model helps to standardize approaches to AR, and it has been used to develop new approaches to AR.

The AR approach described in this textbook is based on the WHO ICF, which has inspired many fresh perspectives on rehabilitative practice (Meyer et al., 2016). We believe that this AR model will be helpful for audiologists doing the most common form of AR: hearing instrument fitting and follow-up for adults. It is also ideal for those providing more comprehensive AR that goes beyond amplification. For most adults, hearing aids and sometimes hearing assistive technology (HAT), along with pre- and postpurchase counseling and orientation tailored to the life circumstances of the individual, will be the key components of AR. However, hearing aid dispensing on its own, with no goal other than making a sale, will be woefully inadequate. Unfortunately, such narrow, sale-focused hearing aid counseling and orientation are often provided in a terribly abbreviated fashion. A current trend to "unbundle" the sale of the device from the provision of services may help to rebalance the focus on technology and rehabilitative services as described on the ASHA Practice Portal (see www.asha.org).

The main challenge facing rehabilitative audiologists is to find approaches based on a deeper understanding of adults with hearing loss and how different forms of rehabilitation can be combined to achieve solutions tailored to meet their specific abilities, needs, and aspirations in a timely and effective fashion (Dillon & So, 2000; Stephens, Jones, & Gianopoulos, 2000). By laying out a recommended protocol for those involved in dispensing and by providing example materials to facilitate the adoption of a more holistic approach based on the WHO ICF concepts, we hope to move toward the acceptance of a more standardized procedure in rehabilitation while at the same time fostering innovative approaches (Schow, 2001).

REHABILITATION SETTINGS

Traditionally, rehabilitative care for adults with hearing loss has been delivered in a variety of settings. These include university speech and hearing clinics, community hearing centers, hospitals, otologic clinics, senior citizen centers, vocational rehabilitation offices, audiology private practices, and hearing aid sales offices.

In keeping with the philosophy of "aging in place," there seems to be a trend for more services to be provided outside of the four walls of traditional clinical settings. To reach older adults who are too frail to attend office visits, programs to deliver hearing rehabilitation as community outreach or home care services have been developed, and such services are likely to increase in the future with the aging of the population. The newest setting to emerge and one that is rapidly expanding is the virtual clinic where tele-audiology is delivered remotely using the Internet or mobile phones (see the ASHA Practice Portal acces via the text website see also Gladden, Beck, & Chandler, 2015; Cleveland Nielsen, Ingo, Grenness, & Laplante-Lévesque, 2016; Saunders & Chisolm, 2015; Singh, Pichora-Fuller, Malkowski, Boretzki, & Launer, 2014). The provision of tele-audiology services may be especially useful for older adults who otherwise would not be able to visit a traditional clinic or office setting.

Research and Teaching Settings: Universities

The earliest adult AR centers in the United States were provided in university training programs that served World War II veterans with hearing loss. The focus of these programs was to improve communication skills through the use of appropriate amplification and communication training, including counseling and education of adults with hearing loss, their families, and significant others. The dual missions of universities to educate new audiologists and to conduct research have also influenced the AR programs developed and delivered in these settings. The approach used in early university-based programs continues to influence many present-day programs. The range of services provided to clients also broadens the educational experience of students.

An example of a university-based AR setting is the Idaho State University Hearing Clinic, where faculty and students have been providing a comprehensive program of hearing care for many years (see Brockett & Schow, 2001; Schow, 2001). After diagnostic audiology, rehabilitation assessment, and counseling, consideration is given to solving audibility deficits through the use of personal amplification systems used alone or in conjunction with assistive devices. After the devices are fitted, the client is given hearing instrument orientation through a process called HIO BASICS, and the client is given a handout (Appendix A) to facilitate this process. Communication activities are routinely treated through the use of a program called CLEAR, and this has a handout also (Appendix B). Self-report information is used to assess aspects of participation that the client is concerned about and chooses to address. In addition, a handout called SPEECH (Appendix C) is provided for family members and for friends to teach them some basic concepts about communication. In this manner, rehabilitation addresses these broad concerns in working to solve hearing problems through improved audibility, communication activity is targeted with common useful remedies, and participation issues are chosen by the client that, when solved, will improve his or her quality of life. Usually, clients are seen on an individual basis, but at times they can attend four two-hour group sessions. Significant others, usually spouses, may be included in AR sessions.

In addition to teaching, another mission of universities is to conduct research. Excellent examples of program development and evaluation research conducted at university audiology clinics are the *Active Communication Education* program (Hickson, Worrall, & Scarinci, 2007b) and the auditory training programs developed at the University of Nottingham to improve working memory, attention,

Systematic reviews are carefully planned and documented searches of reference databases to find all studies meeting criteria set by the researcher to answer a well-formulated key question, often a question about the effectiveness of an intervention.

and communication in adverse conditions (Ferguson & Henshaw, 2015). In both cases, the clinician/researchers used a randomized controlled trial experimental approach to establish an evidence base to show that their respective programs were effective. *Systematic reviews* are an increasingly common type of intervention research whereby the researcher assembles and evaluates the evidence published across multiple studies. This type of research provides an excellent foundation for evidence-based practice, and the number of published systematic reviews of audiology interventions has been growing steadily (Wong & Hickson, 2012). For example, a recent Cochrane review investigated the evidence from 37 studies of over 4,000 hearing aid users regarding the effectiveness of interventions to improve hearing aid use in adult rehabilitation; the authors concluded that at present, there is some evidence of benefit to support the use of self-management support, which includes giving information or practice in listening/communicating or by asking people to practice tasks at home. They made recommendations for future research that could strengthen the evidence (Barker, Mackenzie, Elliott, Jones, & de Lusignan, 2016). Students and clinicians can join online systematic review teams such as the Cochrane Consumer Network (http://consumers.cochrane.org/join-us).

Military and Veterans Administration Medical Centers

Various AR programs are available in military and Veterans Administration (VA) medical centers, with the VA dominating the purchasing of hearing aids in the public sector in the United States (Staab, 2015). Some of the earliest AR programs were developed for those returning after World War II with noise-induced hearing loss. Programs range from one-time, one-hour hearing instrument orientation sessions after hearing aid fitting to comprehensive programs meeting over multiple sessions. Although most military personnel will have a history of significant noise exposure, hearing loss may result from other causes. Ongoing research is aimed at new and more specialized needs; for example, many of the troops returning from Iraq and Afghanistan who sustained traumatic brain injury following blasts from improvised explosive devices complain of difficulties hearing speech in noise and tinnitus despite having audiograms that are mostly normal (Dennis, 2009).

Community Centers, Agencies, and Consumer Groups

Community centers and hearing societies provide rehabilitation and classes where participants are usually highly motivated to manage their hearing problems. Often, consumers have taken the initiative to establish nonprofit agencies to provide professional services to meet consumer needs that were otherwise not being met (e.g., Communication Real-Time Access Translation; see "Recommended Websites"). Vocational rehabilitation provides adults with access to networks of assessment and management services that are often important for optimizing their potential for gainful employment and for helping them function as contributing members of a community. Consumer groups can be described as self-help, social, outreach, and advocacy groups. Consumer groups such as the Hearing Loss Association of America (HLAA; founded as SHHH in 1979) are an important source of help for adults with hearing loss. HLAA maintains a website with a chat room and message board, publishes a magazine, and sponsors an annual convention (see "Recommended Websites"). Local chapters hold monthly social activities and informative meetings. Consumer groups provide a vehicle by which adults with hearing loss can learn from peers about how to improve their ability to self-manage their hearing problems. For example, they promote the installation of group amplification systems in theaters, churches, lecture halls, and other public meeting places. They may also lobby politicians and policymakers regarding standards and laws that affect their lives. But the involvement of informed hearing specialists is important if these groups are to do the most good. There is also an International Federation of Hard of Hearing People (see "Recommended Websites").

Hospitals, Medical Offices, Private Practice Audiologists, and Hearing Instrument Specialists

Services offered in medical and private practice settings vary considerably, but they do not necessarily extend beyond the fitting of a hearing aid, orientation to its use, and counseling regarding management of hearing problems. For most adults with hearing loss, this service appears to satisfy their rehabilitative needs. But in many cases, the hearing aid does not resolve their major communication difficulties. Nor do such limited services begin to meet the needs of clients who have very complex rehabilitation issues. Audiologists dispense about 69 percent of all hearing aids in the United States, with the remainder dispensed by hearing instrument specialists in sales offices (Kochkin et al., 2010). Hearing instrument specialists tend to provide only limited help with hearing aids and associated devices and assist in initial adjustment to hearing aid use. Few of these specialists are trained or inclined to provide extensive rehabilitative services. In the future, given the great advances in hearing aid technology that have taken place over the past decade and given the increasing importance of the connection between the quality of service and customer satisfaction, it is predicted that practice may shift by putting less emphasis on the device and more emphasis on the provision of comprehensive AR services.

AR will become even more important in the future.

Over the decades, the number of dispensing audiologists working in private practice has increased. According to ASHA (2014), fewer than half of the audiologists who responded to their survey worked in a private practice (as owner, full-time salaried employee, part-time salaried employee, or contractor/consultant), while over half worked in health care settings. A recent development in the hearing aid marketplace has been the entry of hearing aid manufacturers into the sales of hearing aids to consumers through their own chains of retail distribution stores. ASHA (2014) reported that about 60 percent of those in private practice were self-employed or worked for other audiologists, whereas about 40 percent worked for nonaudiologists. According to Wayne Staab (2015), "50% of U.S. unit sales are directly to manufacturer-owned outlets/franchises, or to a large company-owned store group (e.g., Costco). . . . It has been reported that only 39% of dispensers in the U.S. are independent, meaning that they are not part of a hearing aid manufacturer company-owned or franchised operation." Some audiologists feel that they will retain autonomy in how they choose to practice if they remain independent but that their choices may be constrained if they work for large companies.

REHABILITATION ASSESSMENT

The overall effect of hearing loss is called *disability* by the WHO (2001). One part of disability (called *impairment* by the WHO) can be measured audiometrically to quantify hearing loss, and another part, communication activity limitation, can be measured most readily by self-report. Hearing loss can be measured easily in terms of decibels on an audiometric grid or percent correct on a word recognition test in quiet or as a threshold for word recognition in noise (expressed as the decibels of the signal-to-noise ratio, or dB SNR, at which 50% of the target words presented in noise are recognized). These behavioral test results yield numerical indicators of the amount of hearing loss. Unfortunately, these numbers are not necessarily indicators of the day-to-day experiences of the person with hearing loss. Two individuals with the same numerical hearing test results may encounter entirely different communication problems in their everyday lives. Although researchers have developed many measures, we still do not have well-established clinical measures of many important aspects of auditory functioning that may help to explain why individuals differ in how they perform as listeners in the real world outside of the sound booth.

Some researchers have been trying to develop tests of listening performance in more realistic conditions (Keidser, 2016). Another active area of research has been the development of new measures of *listening effort* that may one day be used in

In a recent consensus paper, *effort* was defined as the deliberate allocation of mental resources to overcome obstacles in goal pursuit when carrying out a task, with the term *listening effort* applying more specifically when tasks involve listening, including speech understanding, but also listening to other signals, such as music, vocal emotions, and alarms (Pichora-Fuller et al., 2016).

Audiologists can choose from a wide range of self-report measures.

In AR assessment, we look at hearing loss, communication activity, and participation issues (i.e., personal and environmental factors). Loss can be measured with an audiogram, but activity and participation issues require self-report or observational methods.

rehabilitation, including behavioral measures of cognition (e.g., working memory, attention, and speed of processing), physiological measures (e.g., pupil, cardiac, and skin responses), and measures of brain activity (Pichora-Fuller et al., 2016). The auditory, cognitive, and emotional aspects of tinnitus are also being investigated using self-report and measures of brain activity, but there is still no objective behavioral or physiological method to measure tinnitus that is ready for use in the clinic (Baguley, Andersson, & McFerran, 2013).

Assessment of the consequences of hearing loss is important in the AR process. It helps us to understand the individual's hearing loss and its consequences for speech understanding, listening, and communication. In addition, an assessment of the psychosocial consequences of the hearing loss is needed. As explained earlier in the chapter, emotional and psychological problems may magnify or be magnified by hearing loss. Input from the client and significant others is helpful in dealing with this aspect of AR. *Self-report* procedures can be used to evaluate communication function and emotional, social, and vocational well-being. Decades ago, audiologists recognized the value of self-report techniques for measuring the primary and secondary consequences of hearing loss (e.g., Noble, 1998; Schow & Smedley, 1990). There is now a wide range of measures that can be chosen by audiologists for rehabilitative assessment and the evaluation of outcomes (Abrams, 2000; Cox, 2005; Taylor, 2007). In a 2000 survey, 53 percent of audiologists reported using self-report measures for screening or to evaluate outcomes (Millington, 2001) and in 2014, 31 percent of the audiologists surveyed by ASHA reported using self-report questionnaires to validate treatment outcomes.

The final piece of the assessment puzzle is finding out what listening environments are encountered by clients as they engage in activities and participate in everyday life. The specific nature of the individual's listening environments must be known so that the most appropriate technology can be selected and fitted and so that the most appropriate noninstrumental rehabilitation can be designed. Technology to log data about the acoustics of the listening environments of clients can be an important source of information about the acoustical environments that challenge listening in the client's everyday life (Fabry, 2005). A powerful combination of assessment tools, audiometric performance measures, self-report questionnaires, and data logging or other observational methods provides the most complete approach to understanding the abilities and needs of our clients.

Assessing Hearing Loss and Consideration of Comorbid Health Conditions

Audiometric assessment assists in two areas: (1) diagnosis and (2) rehabilitation. The basic diagnostic test battery includes pure tone air- and bone-conduction audiometry, speech threshold tests, word recognition tests in quiet and in noise, immittance, and measures of uncomfortable level. The results of the basic audiometric battery indicate whether a hearing loss exists, the degree and type of loss, and if the loss is likely to be remedied medically or surgically or resolved with amplification. A variety of test procedures may be added to the standard assessment battery to differentiate cochlear from retrocochlear problems, determine vestibular function, assess middle ear function, measure central auditory processing ability, or evaluate tinnitus.

Basic speech audiometry involving the repetition of simple words heard monaurally in quiet is part of the typical audiometric test battery. More ecologically valid tests of ability to understand speech have become increasingly popular among rehabilitative audiologists who are interested in obtaining speech performance measures that are more representative of everyday listening. For example, tests such as the Quick Speech-in-Noise test (Quick SIN; Killion, Niquette, Gudmundsen, Revit, & Nanerjee, 2004), the Words in Noise test (WIN; Wilson, McArdle, & Smith, 2007), or the Multiple Auditory Processing Assessment (MAPA or MAPA-2) (Schow, Seikel, Brockett & Whitaker, 2007, In Press; see Chapter 9) can be used to measure how well a person can hear sentences or words in different amounts of background noise, and the Hearing in Noise Test (HINT; Nilsson, Soli, & Sullivan, 1994) can be used to determine whether the listener is able to take advantage of spatial separation between the target speech and the source(s) of the steady-state, speech-shaped background noise.

It is relatively easy to hear the speech of a talker when the competing masker is a steady-state noise, but it is more difficult to hear speech when there is competing speech. In addition to energetic masking, there is also informational masking if the listener has to attend to one voice but ignore another voice. The Listening in Spatialized Noise—Sentences (LISN-S; Cameron & Dillon, 2007) is a recently developed test in which target speech is masked by competing speech. In some conditions, the target and masking speech are spoken by the same talker, and in other conditions, they are spoken by different talkers. In some conditions, the target speech and the competing speech are co-located, and in other conditions, they are spatially separated. Scores can be used to calculate the advantage that a listener gains when the target and masking speech differ in terms of voice and/or spatial cues. The LISN-S is commercially available, and data have been gathered for listeners of varying ages and with varying degrees of audiometric hearing loss (Besser, Festen, Goverts, Kramer, & Pichora-Fuller, 2015; Cameron, Glyde, & Dillon, 2011).

The hearing assessment can be augmented by tests of nonauditory health conditions, including screening tests for vision, dexterity, balance and fall risk, and cognitive loss. Vision and dexterity problems (Singh, 2009) can make it difficult to handle hearing aids. Age-related changes in balance and mobility are also highly relevant considerations in AR. Older adults with hearing loss walk more slowly (Li, Simosick, Ferrucci, & Lin, 2013) and are three times more likely to fall than peers with normal hearing (Lin & Ferrucci, 2012). Notably, over half of the clients over 60 years old seen in an audiology clinic reported falling in a 12-month period (Criter & Honaker, 2013), and over twice as many clients reported a history of falls compared to a control group (Criter & Honaker, 2016). Audiologists seldom ask older adults about their history of falls or fear of falling, but these issues may be even more important to them than hearing problems. According to a national Canadian survey, individuals with hearing loss identified their most commonly reported limitations to be related to mobility and agility (65%), with these concerns being much more common compared to concerns about communication (12%) or memory (12%) (Statistics Canada, 2006). Hearing loss likely interacts with age-related declines in the sensorimotor systems involved in balance and gait, including the vestibular, visual, kinesthetic, and cognitive systems (Albers et al., 2015). Currently, research is being conducted to examine how age-related declines in multiple sensory systems combine to increase the cognitive demands on older listeners in everyday multitasking situations, such as conversing while walking to cross a busy street and monitoring traffic (Lau, Pichora-Fuller, Li, Singh, & Campos, 2016). This research points to the need for audiologists to consider balance and mobility difficulties that may increase risk of falls and also functioning in everyday multitasking activities that involve listening. For some older clients, AR may become an important part of collaborative work with interprofessional geriatric teams that include experts in fall prevention and rehabilitation, such as physiotherapists, and experts in cognition, such as neuropsychologists. Similarly, audiologists may work on teams with neuropsychologists or geriatricians assessing mild cognitive decline and dementia, and in some settings audiologists may screen for cognitive loss (Phillips, 2016) using tools such as the Montreal Cognitive Assessment (MoCA; Nasreddine et al., 2005). A good start would be to include questions about nonauditory health issues as part of the AR assessment and remain alert to concerns that clients or their significant others have about health issues that may interact with hearing loss in everyday life.

Assessing Activity and Participation and Considerations of Social Factors

The information gathered in the standard diagnostic battery is necessary for hearing aid fitting. However, there is a need to go further in gathering information before

The case history, self-report questionnaires, and data logging or other observational or monitoring techniques provide a powerful combination of tools to complete the activity and participation aspects of an AR assessment. The same pretreatment assessment tools are often used as posttreatment outcome measures.

relevant goals can be set and treatments planned that will improve communication skills and address the implications of the hearing loss for activity and participation by the person in his or her everyday life situations. Audiologists usually work in offices and clinics where they assess the rehabilitative needs of people in highly artificial conditions. Most clinical tests are conducted in a sound-attenuating booth using standardized materials presented under earphones or over one or two loudspeakers. Many of the most challenging social and physical situations that confront listeners in everyday life are difficult if not impossible to assess directly in typical clinical settings. For example, even though the concerns of family members often motivate first visits to the audiologist, the problems plaguing the communicative interactions between the person with hearing loss and family members have been appraised infrequently, either indirectly or directly (Hétu, Jones, & Getty, 1993). Fortunately, the need for family-centered AR has become a hot topic (Singh et al., 2016). The assessment should include identification of those circumstances under which clients experience their greatest communication difficulties and tailor treatment to improve their functioning as they select places where (or persons who) they want to hear better.

Case History. A case history interview can be considered to be a form of self-report and is one way of obtaining information on the day-to-day activity limitations resulting from hearing problems. The history should also be used to gather information about tinnitus and age-related conditions (e.g., vision, dexterity, balance and falls, mobility, cognitive loss, depression) that may need to be considered. The history and the audiogram provide the clinician with an initial impression of the client. The case history usually includes a list of predetermined questions to elicit specific answers (e.g., "Have you ever had ear surgery?"). By including some open-ended questions (e.g., "What brings you here today?"), clients are given an opportunity to tell their own stories and explain their own needs in their own words (Carson, 2005). Stephens and Kramer (2010) recommend sending a simple question with the appointment letter, such as "Please make a list of the effects your hearing problems have on your life. Write down as many as you can think of." When the clinician then interviews the patient, he or she can request clarification of the response as needed. Valuable information may also be found in the referral letter or medical chart or electronic health record.

Speech performance measures, self-reports of benefit and satisfaction, and hearing aid usage provide the essential types of outcome measures.

Outcome Measurement. Behavioral performance measures (e.g., speech tests), self-report instruments, and data logging (and other observational or monitoring methods) provide information that is very useful for initial assessment, and they can also guide reassessment and promote systematic follow-up. In fact, based on an analysis of many measures collected in a large sample of older adults over a period of years (Humes & Wilson, 2003), four different types of measures were determined to be important in assessing the overall outcome of hearing aid fittings. These four types can be measured validly four to six weeks after fitting: (1–2) two of these four involve speech understanding performance using the sorts of speech tests described earlier but with modifications (e.g., presentation over loudspeakers) to enable the measurement of performance when the hearing aid is worn and also comparison to unaided performance (aided and pre/post benefit measures), (3) self-reported satisfaction and benefit (benefaction), and (4) amount of hearing aid usage. A standardized set of outcome measures that cover these important domains should thus be used to determine whether hearing aids are adequate and/or if other rehabilitation efforts have been successful (Schow, Brockett, Bishop, Whitaker, & Horlacki, 2005). Speech performance measures provide information about how much the person can hear with the hearing aid. Data logging or observational methods can provide information about how much and in which acoustical environments the client uses the hearing aid. But self-report measures are essential to understanding how much the person benefits from and is satisfied with treatment. Self-report measures may be the most important measures in the cycle of assessment and treatment and then reassessment based on feedback gathered using outcome measures.

Self-Report Questionnaires. Over the past 50 years, significant efforts have been made to assess the consequences of hearing loss using tools to extend the traditional case history. Most of the instruments involve self-report by questionnaire. Such questionnaires have been used in an abbreviated form for screening purposes to select rehabilitation candidates, in longer versions to explore a number of consequences and needs resulting from a hearing problem, or in pre- and posttreatment versions or simply posttreatment versions to measure the benefits from hearing aid fitting.

A number of reviews have summarized a variety of fundamental concerns related to self-report methods, lists of instruments used in self-report of hearing, specific applications for which self-report may be used, and a variety of psychometric issues that need careful attention (Abrams, 2000; Cox, 2005; Gagné, 2000; Noble, 1998; Schow & Gatehouse, 1990; Taylor, 2007). Self-report instruments are easy and inexpensive to use, but some can be time consuming to complete in the clinic. They can be used for a wide variety of purposes and with different populations and are noninvasive and nonthreatening. These factors account for their wide popularity for hearing and other concerns, such as tinnitus and dizziness. Taylor (2007) has provided an overview of questionnaires in common use to measure outcomes.

In this chapter, because most rehabilitation is being done in hearing aid dispensing settings, we will mention several highly recommended self-report tools that lend themselves to use by those fitting hearing aids. Copies of three questionnaires are provided in the Appendices to facilitate their use, and for others links can be found on the text website and/or at in "Recommended Websites." These tools include the International Outcome Inventory—Hearing Aids (IOI-HA; Cox et al., 2000; Appendix D), the Client Oriented Scale of Improvement (COSI; Dillon, James, & Ginis, 1997; Appendix E), the Glasgow Hearing Aid Benefit Profile (GHABP; Gatehouse, 1999; for proposed norms, see Whitmer, Howell, & Akeroyd, 2014), and the Speech, Spatial and Qualities of Hearing Scale (SSQ; Gatehouse & Noble, 2004). The companion Self-Assessment of Communication/Significant Other Assessment of Communication (SAC/SOAC; Schow & Nerbonne, 1982; Appendix F) is included due to availability of psychometric data (Hodes, Schow, & Brockett, 2009) and easy access to online mean data on the ISU/text website when the client is placed in one of eight common hearing loss groups (see Chapter 1). There is some overlap among these tools since the electronic version of SAC/SOAC contains an open-ended item similar to COSI and GHABP, and it also covers the seven items on the IOI-HA. Some audiologists use more than one tool in order to assess the consistency of responses, to obtain more complete data on a client, and, in the case of IOI-HA, to allow international comparisons using the same wording.

The IOI-HA can be used only posttreatment and was designed to be very simple and generic so that it could be used to compare rehabilitation treatments across programs and countries (Cox et al., 2000; see text website link for the IOI-HA in English and many other languages). The questions can be interpreted by clients in terms of their own life situations, but the IOI-HA does not specifically gather information about the nature of those situations. The IOI has been adapted to evaluate other aspects of AR besides hearing aids (Noble, 2002).

The COSI is also very useful as an assessment and outcome measure and is designed to meet individual needs. It encourages the client to pick up to five situations in which help with hearing is desired or where he or she wants to hear better. After the hearing aid is fitted, the client is asked to rate on a 5-point scale how much improvement or change the hearing aid has provided and how well he or she now hears in those situations when the hearing aid is used. It is a very simple and straightforward scale, but it has been shown to be as valid as much longer scales. The COSI is thus more individualized but does not have a set of standard questions about specific listening situations (e.g., TV listening, one-on-one situations, etc.) as are found in other questionnaires, such as the GHABP (see "Recommended Websites").

The SSQ can be used to evaluate outcomes in different domains of listening relevant to everyday life by comparing pre- and posttreatment scores (see "Recommended Websites"). The SSQ is an excellent self-report questionnaire that provides a window into how people use their hearing in realistic complex environments and how their hearing loss affects ease of listening and abilities such as localizing and attending to sounds. The SSQ has good test–retest reliability, and similar results are obtained whether it is given in person using an interview format or completed as a paper-and-pencil exercise at home and returned by mail (Singh & Pichora-Fuller, 2010). The SSQ may also be an excellent instrument for assessing the everyday listening complaints of older adults who are not candidates for amplification because they have normal or near-normal audiograms (Banh, Singh, & Pichora-Fuller, 2012). Shorter versions more suited to clinical use have also been developed, including a 12-item version (SSQ12; Noble, Jensen, Naylor, Bhullar, & Akeroyd, 2013; see "Recommended Websites"). and a five-item version (SSQ5; Demeester et al., 2012; see "Recommended Websites").

In contrast to the IOI-HA and SSQ, which have only standard questions with a closed set of response options, the open-ended items of the COSI, GHABP, and SAC/SOAC help the audiologist to understand more about the specific situations relevant to the individual client. The SAC/SOAC use some general questions as a framework, but the client also replies with reference to his or her own life situation, so these tools can be adapted nicely for any individual or unique purpose. The SAC/SOAC (10 items each) is a brief, practical tool for hearing aid fitting and is one of the few questionnaires that was designed for both the person with hearing loss and a significant other person. It was picked by the USA HearX company (now known as HearUSA) as its first choice of 20 different self-report outcome measures it tried (Neemes, 2003).

> Self-efficacy is the beliefs in one's capabilities to organize and execute the courses of action required to produce given attainments.

There has been an explosion in the use and development of self-report measures that provide new kinds of information about nonauditory personal and social psychological factors. Cox, Alexander, and Gray (2007) investigated the "Big Five" dimensions of personality (Saucier, 1964). Singh, Lau, and Pichora-Fuller (2015) used another measure from social psychology that was not specific to hearing: the Duke-University of North Carolina Functional Social Support Questionnaire (DUFSS; Broadhead et al., 1988). Another psychological construct in AR that can now be measured by questionnaire is self-efficacy. The famous social psychologist Albert Bandura introduced self-efficacy theory and defined self-efficacy as the "beliefs in one's capabilities to organize and execute the courses of action required to produce given attainments" (Bandura, 1997, p. 3). Self-efficacy has been shown to play an important role in the successful management of a variety of chronic health conditions. The new focus on self-efficacy in AR could reduce delays in seeking help and pursuing treatment recommendations as well as enhancing outcomes and improving adherence over the long term (for a review of self-efficacy enhancing techniques that can be used by clinicians to increase self-efficacy during AR, see Smith & West, 2006). To date, self-report measures have been developed to evaluate hearing aid self-efficacy (West & Smith, 2007), listening self-efficacy (Smith, Pichora-Fuller, Watts, & La More, 2011), and tinnitus-related self-efficacy (Fagelson & Smith, 2016; Smith & Fagelson, 2011). Other recently developed questionnaires can be used to gather information such as the responses of the significant other to the hearing loss of their partner (Preminger & Meeks, 2012; Scarinci, Worrall, & Hickson, 2009a, 2009b), to evaluate the readiness of a client for AR (Laplante-Lévesque, Hickson, & Worrall, 2013), or beliefs about hearing (Saunders et al., 2013).

Acoustic Environment and Hearing Aid Use Data Logging. Data-logging options built into digital hearing aids enable audiologists to gain insights into the acoustic ecologies of their clients by recording information about the sound environments in which the hearing aid is used. Some hearing aid manufacturers have also developed a prefitting data logger that can be worn by a person for a period of time prior to his or her first appointment to discuss hearing aids. Self-report by clients about their experiences in the everyday listening situations that are sampled by the new data-logging technology should enable the audiologist to improve the fitting of devices and to provide more tailored noninstrumental rehabilitation to complement and/or augment the fitting of devices. A new observational research approach that has promise for clinical use is ecological momentary assessment (EMA; Shiffman, Stone, & Hufford, 2008). This approach can be used to observe or monitor clients' listening experiences and environments by using digital assistants or smartphones that may come with a GPS (Global Positioning System) or dosimeters to determine, for example, when, where, and how hearing aids are used (e.g., Galvez et al., 2012; Wu & Bentler, 2012). Importantly, the auditory ecology of the person was found to play a significant role in his or her success with hearing aids (Gatehouse et al., 2006).

To recap, outcome measures provide feedback and continue the cycle of assessment and treatment. Self-report questionnaires are especially useful because they enable the audiologist to look at use, benefit, and satisfaction with interventions, and they can be used to help document the effectiveness of programs (Cox et al., 2000), while goal-specific outcome measures can be helpful in determining the progress of individuals (Gagné, McDuff, & Getty, 1999). Questionnaires to probe nonauditory factors, including social, psychological, and quality-of-life factors, enrich assessment and outcome measurement in AR as well as self-report, there are other tools that can be used to measure the outcomes of rehabilitation, such as daily use of hearing aids (Brooks, 1989). In addition to evaluating treatment focused on hearing aids, outcome measures have also been developed and used to demonstrate the value of hearing assistive technology (HAT) (Lewsen & Cashman, 1997; Pichora-Fuller & Robertson, 1997), communication therapies (Erber, 1988, 1996; Robertson, Pichora-Fuller, Jennings, Kirson, & Roodenburg, 1997), and interventions involving modification of the social and physical environment (Pichora-Fuller & Carson, 2000).

Further development of outcome measures can be expected, especially as the rehabilitative tool kit expands and objectives shift from an emphasis on loss and audibility to a greater emphasis on participation in everyday life, including new tools to assess environmental and personal factors (Granberg et al., 2014; Noble, 2002; Worrall & Hickson, 2003). Audiologists have begun to use psychological measures to evaluate personality, social support, and cognition, and future work in this area is anticipated. Given the increasingly wide range of choices of outcome measures, audiologists need to know which suit their particular purposes in planning individual treatments or group programs and in evaluating the results of rehabilitation. Research strongly suggests that a combination of measures tapping speech/audibility issues, usage, and satisfaction, combined with benefit (benefaction), are the essential outcome measures (Humes & Wilson, 2003). Evidence of the effectiveness of interventions is extremely important if audiologists are to continue to improve service delivery. There are many disbelievers among those who need our services, and favorable outcome findings are increasingly needed to document the evidence base to justify our services to those who pay for them.

CORE Assessment Summary

Audiologic testing and self-report are the fundamental tools for assessment, but a continuing need exists for assessment protocols that present a broader, meaningful profile of the adult with hearing loss. Loss of hearing sensitivity is only one aspect of a complex set of interacting variables, both personal and environmental, that cumulatively affect hearing problems. Therefore, it cannot be stressed enough how the assessment process should focus widely, and all four assessment aspects in the model used throughout this book need to be considered as outlined in CORE.

1. *Communication status* assessment should include both impairment and activity limitations. Once audiologic testing and self-report are completed, there should be reasonably thorough information in these areas.

2. *Overall participation goals* may address social, psychological, educational, and vocational issues. Self-report procedures, such as SAC/SOAC, provide useful information about the social and emotional-psychological dimension of the experience of hearing loss because they ask about four different social/emotional issues (items 6 to 9). Vocational and educational issues may also be identified by the client in specific situations. Open-ended items on self-reports are valuable for teasing out participation concerns, but a follow-up interview may help uncover other areas of concern, and an effort should be made to touch on any aspect of a person's life that may have special relevance.

3. *Related personal factors* that interact with hearing loss include, among others, health status, activity level, and manual dexterity. Self-efficacy may be critical in determining whether the person seeks, adopts, and adheres to treatment. Attitude and motivation also are key issues, but for older persons changes in health status have perhaps the most significant effect on an individual's ability to participate actively in remediation. Difficulties with motor coordination, vision, memory, or general health may prohibit an aging person from initiating or sustaining interest in the intervention process. The older person may not be enthusiastic about involvement in AR when other disabilities, unrelated to the hearing loss, when other disabilities, unrelated to hearing loss, cause greater concern.

4. *Environmental factors/context* includes not only where a person lives and the social circumstances in which he or she chooses to participate but it also includes all aspects of the environment that may facilitate or impede adjustment to and improvement from the effects of the loss. The acoustic environment can be assessed with the help of data logging. Environmental challenges like those depicted in the SSQ questions may underlie difficulties that are not explained fully by the audiogram and may evade measurement in the sound booth. Social environmental assessment includes information about the community and support systems of the client. Environmental factors can often be modified, but first we have to know and understand how they contribute to the problem.

REHABILITATION MANAGEMENT

Following assessment, various forms of AR can be undertaken. A common set of management principles applies to most cases, and a large number of adults have similar auditory abilities and quality-of-life issues. Nevertheless, the specific form of rehabilitation will vary between individuals and over time because of the personal and dynamic nature of adjustment to hearing loss in adulthood. In the management process, the rehabilitative audiologist works together with the individual with hearing loss and his or her communication partners to find a combination of solutions that will enable listening goals to be attained and maintained in a wide range of life circumstances. The audiologic management process coherently integrates specific forms of rehabilitation consistent with CARE.

1. *Counseling*, which focuses on identifying, understanding, and shaping the attitudes and goals that influence help seeking, decision making, and action taking, with an emphasis on the factors that predispose, enable, and reinforce individuals in their adjustment to hearing difficulties and associated stresses. The audiologist gives the client information based on the results of the assessment and the available evidence regarding specific treatment options. Through an interactive process with the client, goals are set to address needs at three levels: audibility, activity, and participation.

2. *Audibility and instrumental interventions*, in which hearing aids, cochlear implants, and/or various types of HAT are discussed, selected, and fitted, with provision of pre- and posttrial education to ensure the effective use of these technologies. This level of intervention addresses amplification issues in terms of the fit and function of devices and orientation to them.

3. *Remediation for communication activities*, which focuses on changing behaviors that will contribute to enhancing the communication performance of listeners with their communication partners in hearing-demanding activities and environments, including when and how to use devices and

other strategies. Building self-efficacy and counteracting stigma may be a prerequisite to changing specific target behaviors.

4. *Environmental coordination and participation improvement*, with an emphasis on the social and physical supports (in the health care system, the community, and occupational, educational, and/or family contexts) are required to ensure that rehabilitation achieves the individual's goals for participation in everyday life, especially in the priority situations that are targeted in the client-specific goals for rehabilitation.

Most rehabilitation programs combine several important components. These components are consistent with the CARE management model used in this text (see Figure 10.6). First, the audiologist counsels the adult who is hard of hearing about hearing loss, explores its significance in the particular life circumstances of the individual, and determines the needs and goals of the person. This step is crucial insofar as it culminates in the statement of prioritized objectives for rehabilitation. Treatment goals fall into three main areas to be improved: audibility, activity, and participation. Depending on the objectives that have been set, a customized combination of interventions can be initiated and continued contingent on ongoing reevaluation. To improve audibility, the client will likely be familiarized with instruments, usually hearing aids and/or HAT. Activity-specific communication skills may be improved through training in areas such as visual attentiveness to speech and communication cues, use of repair strategies or communication tactics, conversational management, and enhancement of goal-directed decision making and assertiveness. Participation can be improved by modifying the physical environment, including the use of HATs in public places, and considering the social environment of the client by effectively involving key communication partners, such as family members, other professionals, or caregivers, in rehabilitation.

Counseling and Psychosocial Considerations with a Health-Promoting Approach

In counseling, the audiologist needs to begin by listening to the client so that the person's attitudes toward hearing loss and his or her goals in seeking help for hearing loss can be identified and understood. Not surprisingly, the way in which the client experiences hearing loss and expresses issues and concerns about these experiences is unlikely to be cast in scientific terms such as decibels and Hertz or hair cell counts. By listening to the client, the audiologist begins to build a bridge between the client's lived experience of hearing loss and his or her own professional understanding of the results of the formal audiologic and self-report assessments. Building the bridge between these kinds of knowledge sets the stage for the important relationship that must develop between the client and clinician if rehabilitation is to succeed (Clark, 1996).

The comments made to audiologists by adults who are hard of hearing provide rich insights into how they experience communication situations in everyday life. The sample of quotes in the following box illuminates various obstacles to communication and how the causes and consequences of hearing problems may be manifested. These words also suggest areas to be addressed in rehabilitation. In counseling, the audiologist must be alert to such comments because of their value in guiding rehabilitation planning and because they provide insight into the problems of the client as well as hints about the resources and supports that are available to the client. Furthermore, as a communication expert, the audiologist is uniquely positioned to provide a positive communication experience for the client and to increase the client's self-efficacy by demonstrating that solutions to the problems that they describe can be achieved. It is especially important that the audiologist rise above ageist stereotypes when interacting with older adults.

Counseling builds the bridge between the client's lived experience of hearing loss and the audiologist's professional and scientific knowledge about hearing.

Hearing Loss

These comments provide insights into some of the psychosocial effects of hearing loss:

Mary: I can appreciate young children being considered inattentive or disruptive in school from this lack of hearing and assimilation and not comprehending why because they don't know that they can't hear. It's not that I don't understand but rather that it is so tiring to listen.

Tom: Jokes aren't funny if you have to ask for a repetition.

Patricia: It's hard to be intimate with my partner when whispers can't be heard and the lights have to be on for lipreading.

Henry: There's no privacy in this home for the aged—no one would hear a knock on the door so people just barge into rooms to find a resident; conversations are never quiet.

These comments about communication breakdowns suggest helpful tactics that could be addressed in conversational therapy:

Marjorie: By completely sounding each word, the speaker goes more slowly and it gives me time to translate the sounds to meaning. Most TV or radio speakers are too fast, and while I am trying to make sense of the first statement, they are away on to the third or fourth sentence, so I soon have to drop out and so lose interest. Asking for repetition seems to be a way of giving the brain cells time to put sounds into meaning.

Mike: In a group, when someone new begins talking, by the time I figure out who it is, I have lost the thread of the conversation. When I know the topic, I have no problem, but when the topic changes I get lost.

Harry: At family parties, when I get discouraged trying to talk and I start thinking about going into the den to be by myself away from the crowd, I remind myself how important it is to stay so that they know I am interested in their lives even if I don't always understand every word. I try to focus on what I do understand instead of dwelling on what I don't understand.

The client will succeed in taking and maintaining rehabilitative action if the factors that predispose, enable, and reinforce change are optimized.

Counseling can then turn to reflection on these experiences, attitudes, and goals as well as to a consideration of possible courses of rehabilitative action. Decision making may be guided by discussing factors specific to the life circumstances of the client that have or will do the following:

- *Predispose or impede*—taking rehabilitative action (e.g., the positive or negative reaction of a middle-aged husband to his wife's new hearing aid)
- *Enable*—taking a rehabilitative step (e.g., providing a college student with written information about FM systems to give to the professors who will be asked to wear a transmitter in class)
- *Reinforce*—the continuation of the rehabilitative action (e.g., joining a peer support group of people with hearing loss who can empathize with and encourage a recently retired individual in the early stages of adjusting to living with hearing loss)

It should be abundantly clear that, although two clients may have the same audiogram and hearing aids, the personal and environmental factors that influence their decision making and action taking may be quite different. It is also important to note that the role of the audiologist is itself one of the factors to be considered (e.g., easy access to a drop-in clinic or fast responses on the Internet may be important in supporting a client in their moment of need, whereas a routine schedule of follow-up appointments may be critical to the success of a client who might otherwise give up rather than asking for help).

Communication goals may emphasize information exchange or social interaction.

Communication Goals and Style. Communication is never perfect; even people with normal hearing experience miscommunication and vary in their communication behaviors and styles (Coupland, Wiemann, & Giles, 1991). Differences between communicators will influence how hearing loss affects communication. Compounding the effects of hearing loss on communication, individual differences and age-related changes in emotional, social, cognitive, perceptual, and linguistic status are likely to influence the process of adjustment and readiness for AR.

Two main functions of communication are *exchange of information* and *social interaction*. Both functions contribute to communication, but their relative importance varies depending on the communicators and their roles in a situation (Pichora-Fuller, Johnson, & Roodenburg, 1998). As people age, emotional aspects of social interaction, especially with close friends and family, tend to become increasingly important, but acquiring new knowledge or exchanging information tends to become relatively less important. Even mild hearing loss can interfere with information exchange (e.g., when a college student listens to the details of instructions in the classroom, phonemes must be perceived with a high degree of accuracy and new vocabulary must be learned). In contrast, social interaction may remain well preserved in the early stages of hearing loss (e.g., when an elderly spouse judges a partner's emotions, prosodic, or visual cues may be adequate) (Villaume, Brown, & Darling, 1994). In setting rehabilitative goals, it is important to understand the kind of communicator that the person has been in the past and determine his or her current and anticipated priorities for communication in the context of specific relationships and roles.

One adult may be a well-educated professional who has always been socially active and a leader in the community. Such a person may be an exceptionally skilled communicator who is motivated to listen carefully and to draw from nonverbal cues during difficult information-intense communicative situations (e.g., at committee meetings). Although participation in such situations may be restricted by a mild hearing loss, the person may be well prepared and motivated to embark on rehabilitation to resolve communication problems. Another adult with the same hearing loss may not have been so socially outgoing or adept at adjusting to new situations and may be concerned primarily about being able to communicate with close family members in the confines of the familiar surroundings of his or her home. The same hearing loss may pose less of a threat to participation for this individual, partly because the spouse is able and willing to manage communication breakdowns and partly because unfamiliar and challenging communication situations are avoided. However, the individual may be far less able to overcome communicative obstacles when it becomes necessary to do so (e.g., when admitted to hospital). It is noteworthy that gender differences in adult adjustment to hearing loss have been recognized to be important, and growing evidence continues to show that hearing loss may take a greater toll on women than men (Mick, Kawachi, & Lin, 2014) and may be a factor in the uptake of hearing aids by older adults (Jenstad & Moon, 2011). Women may be more affected because of the centrality of communication in the roles of wife and mother or because women receive less social support from others in adjusting to hearing loss (Hallberg & Jansson, 1996; Hétu et al., 1993). There is still much more to learn about the functional significance of hearing and hearing loss in everyday communication.

> The hard of hearing adult may hear well enough to participate successfully in many communication situations yet struggle in other communication situations.

Stereotypes and Adjustment. The ageist stereotypes held by family members and professional caregivers can influence an individual's success in adjusting to hearing loss because such stereotypes can have a profound effect on actual behavior over the long term (Ryan, Giles, Bartolucci, & Henwood, 1986). In challenging situations, verbal messages are likely to be misinterpreted and inappropriate responses may result. Many of these difficulties may be caused by hearing problems, but other age-related declines may also result in conversational miscommunications. In addition, age-related stereotypes may aggravate communication problems, and the way in which communication is affected by a combination of stereotypes and various losses can be confusing to the older individual, significant others, and even the audiologist. Clients may also be influenced by media and advertising that suggest negative stereotypes of aging and the use of assistive technologies, including material related to hearing problems and hearing aids (Fraser, Kenyon, Lagacé, Wittich, & Southall, 2016). Whether in spoken or written communication, audiologists should beware of ageism. Eliassen (2016) emphasizes that both the recipients and the providers of health care must be alert to ageism in their communication and interactions and reminds us that "elders have the potential to teach medical personnel through narratives of resilience as well as tribulation" (p. 990). Some leading consumer advocates who are hard of hearing have shared their insights in books about living with hearing loss (e.g., Hannan, 2015).

Age-Related Changes in Health That Interact with Hearing in Older Adults As described earlier, there are increases with age in the prevalence of declines in a range of health conditions (e.g., vision and cognition) that may interact with age-related declines in hearing to affect communication and social interaction. In addition, there are increases in the prevalence of loss in balance, mobility, touch, and dexterity that may increase barriers to communication and constrain rehabilitative options. For example, reduced manual dexterity (e.g., due to arthritis) or reduced tactile sensation (e.g., from neurological diseases) may affect the person's ability to use some communication technologies, such as small hearing aids (Singh, 2009). Multitasking may be too demanding, such as when a person is trying to listen while moving with the assistance of a walker or cane. Opportunities for social interaction may also be constrained; for example, those in wheelchairs may not be able to position themselves to speechread or otherwise optimize communication because seating locations are designated and some venues may not be accessible at all if the only entrance is by stairs. Thus, hearing problems may magnify the activity limitations and participation restrictions of older adults when combined with other health problems. Conversely, by preserving hearing abilities, some functional declines associated with other health problems may be offset. Ultimately, hearing may even be a critical factor in enabling older adults to maintain independent living, with associated cost savings for the health care system if the need for residential care is averted. Information about any relevant nonauditory health issues that could affect communication, everyday functioning, and engagement in rehabilitation should be gathered during the assessment and taken into consideration during management.

Even in healthy older adults, there are declines in some aspects of cognitive processing, including working memory, speed of processing, and divided attention (Phillips, 2016; Pichora-Fuller & Singh, 2006; Pichora-Fuller et al., 2016; Schneider et al., 2010; Wingfield & Tun, 2007). Declines in cognitive processing can interact with hearing loss to affect communication. For example, one of the most commonly reported changes in the conversational patterns of older adults is that they often retell stories and seem not to be aware that they are repeating themselves.

Older adults may also miss or misunderstand or forget information. Some older adults may ask communication partners to repeat information, but others may just pretend to understand. Family and friends may be confused by the inconsistency in the person's apparent communicative ability, and they may attribute the person's moments of seeming inattentiveness and lack of appropriate social interaction to a number of causes, ranging from indifference to senility, any of which may lead to less and less social interaction between the aging individual and various communication partners. When deprived of social interaction, due to either a hearing loss and/or cognitive problems and/or the stereotyped attitudes of those around them, older persons become frustrated and may increasingly avoid situations in which difficulties are encountered (i.e., family gatherings, church, movies, and other social activities that they enjoyed previously). Such a loss in close interpersonal communication can lead to decreased stimulation, resulting in depression and self-stereotyping. The stereotyped expectations become a self-fulfilling prophecy in what has been called the "communication predicament of aging" (Ryan et al. 1986).

In addition to negative stereotypes held by others, self-stereotyping can cause older adults to underperform on many tasks. "Stereotype threat" may occur when the situation poses a risk of confirming a negative stereotype of a group with which a person identifies (Schmader, Johns, & Forbes, 2008). For example, if an older person believes that older people have poor hearing and the situation makes her aware that she is likely to have poor hearing because she is older, then she may perform worse during audiometric testing in the clinic or during conversation at a party than she might under conditions that do not pose a stereotype threat. The ability to use new technologies, including hearing aids, may also be undermined by stereotype threat (Czaja et al., 2006; Gonsalves & Pichora-Fuller, 2008). Indeed, behaviors ranging all the way from walking speed (Bargh, Chen, & Burrows, 1996) to audiometric thresholds (Levy, Slade, & Gill, 2006) can be affected by such age-related stereotype threats. In a recent study, data from about 300 adults over the age of 50 years were modeled to examine the influences among age, negative views of aging, and self-perceived and actual memory and hearing abilities (Chasteen, Pichora-Fuller, Dupuis, Smith, & Singh, 2015). The resulting model confirmed prior findings: Negative views of aging were not associated significantly with chronological age, but self-reported hearing (SSQ scores) influenced self-reported memory, and performance on behavioral tests of hearing (pure tone and word in noise thresholds) influenced performance on memory tests. An interesting new finding was that negative views of aging directly influenced self-reported memory abilities and self-reported hearing abilities (SSQ scores). Furthermore, through self-reported abilities, negative views of aging also influenced actual performance on the behavioral tests of memory and hearing. Stigmatization may result from negative stereotypes. Perceptions of stigmatization fuel the denial of hearing problems, delays in help seeking, and nonadherence to rehabilitative treatments (Gagné, Jennings, & Southall, 2009). Counteracting age-related stigmatization and building self-efficacy for specific behaviors such as using hearing aids or carrying on a conversation in a group situation may be critical prerequisites to successful AR. It won't matter how much speech acoustics are improved if stereotype threats, stigmatization, and low self-efficacy prevent a person from using a hearing aid. These psychosocial factors may also affect the person's experience of effortful listening (Pichora-Fuller, 2016). Fatigue for listening has also become an active topic of research (Hornsby, Naylor, & Bess, 2016). Ultimately, many older persons with hearing loss exhibit what has been described as the "geriapathy syndrome" (Maurer, 1976, p. 72):

> The individual feels disengaged from group interaction and apathy ensues, the product of the fatigue that sets in from the relentless effort of straining to hear. Frustration, kindled by begging too many pardons, gives way to subterfuges that disguise misunderstandings. The head nods in agreement with a conversation only vaguely interpreted. The voice registers approval of words often void of meaning. The ear strives for some redundancy that will make the message clearer. Finally, acquiescing to fatigue and frustration, thoughts stray from the conversation to mental imageries that are unburdened by the defective hearing mechanism.

Ageist stereotypes and geriapathy may make hearing problems more difficult to overcome.

Coping. To deal with obstacles to communication and the fatigue and stress associated with hearing loss, the effort of listening, and frequent miscommunications, adults adopt coping behaviors. Rehabilitation planning requires that the audiologist appreciate how persons experience stress and how they cope with it. Lazarus and Folkman (1984) proposed a model of stress and coping that can be readily applied to the situations of adults who are hard of hearing. In their model, the person and the environment are considered to be in a dynamic, bidirectional relationship. Stress entails the constant appraisal of this person–environment relationship. When the relationship is perceived to pose a threat, challenge, or harm to the person and when the person does not feel that he or she has the capacity to contend with the challenge, then it becomes stressful, and a coping response is required to try to reinstate balance in the person–environment relationship. Problem-focused coping responses are directed at the cause of stress (e.g., gathering information or solving problems). Emotion-focused coping responses are directed at regulating stress (e.g., avoiding problems). Distress continues until coping is successful in restoring balance in the relationship between the person and the environment.

Hard of hearing adults cope by avoiding and/or controlling the situation.

Coping responses can be problem focused or emotion focused.

Geriapathy versus Not Giving Up

The pattern described by clinicians as geriapathy has also been expressed by older adults themselves. The following comment, written by an older woman at a meeting of the Canadian Hard of Hearing Association, demonstrates how she evaded geriapathy: "When you are hard of hearing, you struggle to hear; when you struggle to hear, you get tired; when you get tired, you get frustrated; when you get frustrated, you get bored; when you get bored, you quit.—I didn't quit today."

The relationship between *personal factors* and *environmental factors* and the ensuing stress can lead to coping responses.

Studies of adults who are hard of hearing have found that coping behaviors fall into two general categories: (1) *controlling* the social scene and (2) *avoiding* the social scene (Hallberg & Carlsson, 1991). *Controlling* is similar to problem-focused coping. The person actively manages communication situations assertively by altering the social and physical environment and taking responsibility for the outcomes of these actions. Coping behaviors include giving verbal and/or nonverbal instructions to communication partners, using technology, and/or adjusting seating or lighting in a room. Although these coping behaviors seem laudable, they may create feelings of helplessness and negative feelings when attempts to control the situation fail, and it begins to seem that it is not possible to maintain control. Repeated experiences of helplessness may ultimately result in abandonment of attempts to control the situation.

Avoiding is similar to emotion-focused coping. The person who is hard of hearing minimizes hearing loss by joking about it or making positive comparisons between the self and others. The person may avoid challenging communication situations and choose not to use conspicuous hearing technologies. Rather than disclose the hearing problem or the need for accommodation, strategies such as lipreading, positioning oneself near a talker, pretending to understand, or remaining silent may be used to camouflage hearing problems (Jaworski & Stephens, 1998). Avoiding behaviors seem maladaptive, but they may be essential during some phases of adjustment when the person's self-esteem is vulnerable or the person has too little energy to solve problems. It is intriguing to consider that such avoidance may be a key factor in the limited use of hearing aids by those with hearing loss. However, prolonged avoiding may result in social isolation or redefinition of the self as less competent.

Others may influence how well a person copes and adjusts.

Everyone encountering stress engages in a mixture of coping behaviors, and it is important to reexamine these adjustment methods as they relate to hearing loss in adulthood. What works for one person may not work for another, and what works for a given person at one time may not work at another time, with success necessarily depending on the nature of the person, the environment, and the person–environment relationship at a given time. There is no universally correct form of coping and no stock recipe for managing hearing loss. A number of social psychological factors (self-efficacy, stigma, stress, social support) may interact as individuals evaluate their ability and willingness to muster the cognitive capacity or mental energy required to meet the demands of everyday listening (Pichora-Fuller, 2016).

Coping styles learned in childhood continue to be utilized throughout one's lifetime to deal with the normal stresses of living, but the ways in which aging adults cope with communicative challenges are also influenced and modified by their interactions with others who may or may not support particular coping behaviors. Given the strong influence of family and caregivers on communicative behavior in older adults, it is helpful to the audiologist to consider how the adjustment of the client may be predisposed or reinforced not only by the client's own behaviors but also by the behaviors of significant others. In the model of learned dependency, two main patterns of interactions between older people and their social partners in everyday activities (in private dwellings and in residential care facilities) were described as the *dependence-support script* and the *independence-ignore script* (Baltes & Wahl, 1996).

These scripts highlight how older adults maintain and develop dependent and independent behaviors. In the dependence-support script, the dominant pattern was one in which older people engaging in dependent behaviors were immediately attended to and given positive reinforcement. For example, when a man who is hard of hearing waits for his wife to answer the phone, she reinforces his avoidance of the phone by answering it herself, and, in the ensuing phone conversation with a mutual friend, she makes decisions for her husband without passing the phone to him or even consulting with him. After many such events, he begins to doubt his ability to manage conversations on the phone to the extent that he doesn't answer it at all, even when he is alone, thereby eventually losing independence. The more common independence-ignore script was one in which older people engaging in independent behaviors were ignored or discouraged. For example, if a woman tried to put on her own hearing aid (an independent act), her husband might say, "I told you I would help you with that; you never get it in right" (a dependence-supportive act). Sadly, in the study of Baltes and Wahl, constructively engaged or proactive social behaviors (e.g., talking to another person) were reinforced only 25 percent of the time, and, more frequently, such independent behaviors were discouraged. Ultimately, the older person surrenders independence and complies with the expectations of dependence.

Trade-Offs

An example of the trade-offs between controlling and avoiding are demonstrated in the following example. A middle-aged man, attending a peer support group for the hard of hearing, proudly explained to the group how he and his wife had decided to manage the "going to a restaurant for dinner scene." The couple were united in their conviction that the most important part of going out for dinner was for them to enjoy each other's company. By comparison, the man was clear in his mind that he had no interest in social interaction with the restaurant staff. Furthermore, the man did not feel that his masculinity was threatened in any way if his wife did the talking with the restaurant staff, and his wife did not have any hesitation about taking on the responsibility for the required information exchange with these strangers. Both members of the couple were prepared to use an audio input extension microphone to increase the privacy and reduce the stress of their conversation throughout the dinner. After clearly defining what was important (or not) to them in the situation, they agreed on solutions that accomplished their goals without jeopardizing their roles and relationships. On the one hand, the scenario demonstrates control insofar as action was taken to address important needs (enjoying each other's company); on the other hand, avoiding was a reasonable choice to minimize stress associated with unimportant aspects of the situation (who communicated with the staff). Deciding what is important and what is not is crucial to goal setting and sets the stage for developing an action plan for coping.

On a positive note, the *communication enhancement model* in Figure 10.8 suggests how to counteract the communication predicament of aging (Ryan, 2009; Ryan, Meredith, Maclean, & Orange, 1995). Accordingly, the audiologist should encourage family and caregivers to use independence-supporting behaviors. A daughter can make comments like "It is so great to get your input on this decision" when the hearing aid is worn or a conversational repair strategy is used, thereby encouraging her mother to take an active role in family discussions. Successful communication experiences will predispose, enable, and/or reinforce the behavior changes targeted as goals for the client.

In a similar vein, the principles of self-efficacy can be used in AR to bolster support for the kinds of behavior change that may be necessary as the person adjusts to hearing loss, learns new skills, and faces challenges in maintaining new behaviors, such as wearing a hearing aid. Self-efficacy can be enhanced by using four main strategies: mastery experiences, vicarious experiences, verbal persuasion, and modulation of physiological and emotional states, as outlined in the excellent tutorial by Smith and West (2006) and summarized in Table 10.1.

The communication enhancement model illustrates how to counteract the effects of stereotypes on communication.

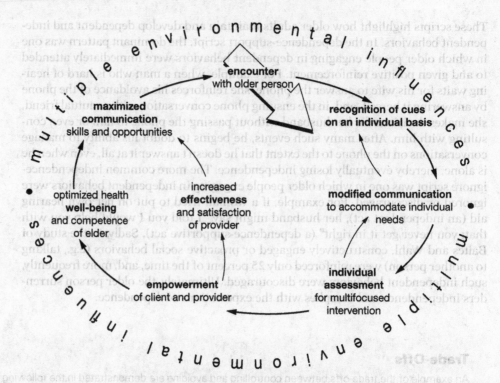

Effective Communication Strategies
Why?
Enhance the interaction
Increase adherence to the rehabilitation plan
Facilitate successful aging

Key Features
Be "inspiring" vs. "dispiriting"
Convey high expectations
Facilitate communication skills of older client
Seek feedback about how communicating
Affirm personhood by listening
Recognize individual life goals and strategies
Assess collaboratively
Assess and build on strengths
Negotiate treatment plan

FIGURE 10.8 Communication enhancement model.
Source: Based on Ryan et al. (1995).

Setting Objectives. In counseling, the audiologist and client explore the complex backdrop against which the rehabilitation plan will be enacted, including the client's attitudes, activity and participation goals, coping and communication styles, and coexisting health issues. It will be important to consider the influence of family and caregivers and the personal and environmental factors that have and will support or impede adjustment to hearing loss. On the one hand, there is mounting evidence that hearing loss can impose burden on significant others, with negative effects on their health and well-being (Wallhagen et al., 2004). On the other hand, there is also mounting evidence that social support from significant others can exert a strong influence on success in all phases of AR (Singh & Launer, 2016; Singh et al., 2015). New approaches to decision making by clients and significant others can help guide this phase of CARE (Laplante-Lévesque, Hickon, & Worrall, 2010; Preminger & Lind, 2012).

Counseling culminates in setting objectives. Objectives should be clearly stated and specify *who* will do *what, how much,* and by *when.* Objectives can target

TABLE 10.1   Strategies to Enhance Self-Efficacy

Strategy to Enhance Self-Efficacy	Examples of How to Use the Strategy in AR
Mastery experience	Practice or role play
	Break complex behaviors into subbehaviors
	Grade difficulty of tasks to progress from easy to hard
Vicarious experience	Teach skills to significant other
	Watch others role play in a group
	Videotape a peer model performing a behavior
Verbal persuasion	Give appropriate feedback
	Recruit social support
	Provide training materials with explanations using pictures
Physiological and emotional states	Allow plenty of time
	Offer frequent breaks
	Use calming, reassuring feedback
	Work in an environment conducive to the behavior

Source: Adapted from Smith and West (2006, p. 49).

behavioral or environmental changes to be adopted by the person who is hard of hearing or by significant others. Examples of a priority rating of objectives developed from an analysis of complaints for a particular client are provided in Table 10.2 (explained in more detail later). Over time, evaluation of whether goals have been achieved will become an important topic of discussion between the audiologist and the client and significant others as they go on to make new decisions and set new rehabilitative goals to meet new or changing needs.

Goals must state who will do what, how much, and by when.

Amplification and Instrumental Interventions to Achieve Audibility

Amplification is the most common form of rehabilitation. In the prefitting stage, the audiologist must determine if the client is ready for hearing aids or HAT. A decision to go ahead with instrumental rehabilitation will depend on the nature and degree of the client's hearing loss, the nature of the client's activity and participation needs, and the client's willingness to trade the potential benefits against the burdens of using an instrument. In the fitting stage, having decided to go ahead with instrumental rehabilitation, the audiologist determines which device is most appropriate, ensures that it functions as expected, and counsels and orients the client to its use and care. In the postfitting stage, follow-up is essential to confirm that a successful fitting has been achieved and that no further rehabilitative issues have emerged and to reinforce adherence to using the device.

Wearing a hearing aid increases the audibility of sound, but it is often stigmatizing.

Is the Client Ready for an Instrument?   Sensorineural hearing loss is generally managed by amplification, but many adults are not eager to wear hearing aids. In addition to age being stigmatizing, hearing loss is stigmatizing (Hétu, 1996; Wallhagen, 2010). By putting on a hearing aid for the first time, the hard of hearing person discloses to the world that he or she has a hearing loss and is not "normal." Hearing aids are considered to be unattractive, unkind associations are made between deafness and intelligence, and uncharitable jokes about deafness and aging are prevalent. In addition to the social costs, wearing a hearing aid also has other costs: the initial high financial costs of hearing aids, ongoing costs for batteries and maintenance, continued lack of knowledge and confusion about the service delivery system, and transportation costs and time needed for visits to clinics and hearing aid offices. Ideally, these costs are balanced by the acoustic benefits of amplification. Nevertheless, sometimes the acoustical benefits may fall short, especially in noisy or reverberant acoustical environments. In a survey of members of the hard of hearing association in the United Kingdom conducted two

TABLE 10.2 Complaints, Objectives, and Recommended Action Steps in Priority Order for an Example Case

Initial Complaint	Objectives for End of the Third Week of the Trial Period	Action
A. Audibility objectives addressed by practicing volume control skills with hearing aid		
1. Turning TV up too loud (daughter's complaint)	Mrs. Carter will find her comfortable TV listening level 100 percent of the time when watching the news by adjusting her hearing aid after the daughter has preset the level.	Practice adjusting TV and hearing aid volume with Mrs. Carter and daughter in a quiet room.
2. Inability to hear whispers, soft sounds	Mrs. Carter will detect car turn indicator sound 100 percent of the time when driving in her neighborhood (to be confirmed by daughter on a trip at the end of the three weeks).	Explain and practice how to adjust hearing aid volume depending on the level of the target signal and degree of background noise.
B. Activity objectives addressed by conversational therapy with client and partner		
3. Daughter tired of repeating conversation	Mrs. Carter's daughter will reduce needed repetitions in a 10-minute sample of daily conversation by 50 percent from the amount needed on samples taken on three days pretrial.	Instruct daughter to turn off background sounds (e.g., radio, TV), make eye contact before talking, state and confirm topic changes, and slow speech rate during conversation.
4. Difficulty understanding conversation with friends in the dining room	Mrs. Carter will understand the gist of 90 percent of conversations with her friend Mrs. Brown during lunch in the dining room at their facility (to be self-assessed by Mrs. Carter).	Explain benefits of visual attention to the talker and how to select a seat away from noise sources and discuss when two preferred repair strategies could help.
C. Participation objectives addressed by use of HAT (FM system)		
5. Confusion at church services	Mrs. Carter will demonstrate to her daughter that she understood 100 percent of the announcements made at the Sunday service of the third week.	Explain and try new hearing aid with existing FM system at her church.
6. Frustration on Senior Adult Center bus outings	Mrs. Carter will increase her understanding of messages from the driver by 75 percent as demonstrated to the recreation staff who accompany the seniors on outings.	FM system and its use with the hearing aid to be explained to the bus driver and the recreation staff and to be used on the bus.

decades ago, the first priority was to improve hearing aids (endorsed by 100%), and the second priority (endorsed by 95%) was to educate the general public about hearing loss (Stephens, 1996). Improving technology and increasing public awareness remain in Hearing Loss Association of America (HLAA's) current top 10 priorities (see "Recommended Websites"). Perhaps not surprisingly, HLAA's top priorities today focus on matters that are feasible for a consumer organization to change: Seven priorities concern public awareness and accessibility, two concern the affordability of technology, but only one is about being "actively involved in the design and development of emerging hearing assistive technology" (see "Recommended Websites"). It is essential for future progress that there be a combination of improved and appropriately fitted technology, but new ways must also be found to reduce stigma by changing societal attitudes toward hearing, hearing loss, and increasing hearing accessibility. Put another way, balancing the benefits and costs of wearing hearing aids can be accomplished by increasing benefit and/or reducing costs.

A client may not be ready to purchase hearing aids for a number of reasons. A recent review of the 39 selected studies published from 1980 to 2009 (Knudsen et al., 2010) identified 31 factors that can influence help seeking, hearing aid uptake, hearing aid use, and satisfaction with hearing aids. These include personal factors (e.g., sources of motivation, expectations, attitudes), demographic factors (age, gender), and external factors (e.g., cost, type of clinic, hearing aid

Factor	Pre-fitting	Fitting	Post-fitting
Counseling	X	X	X
Age	X		X
Gender	X		X
Personality	X		X
Health	X		X
Educational level	X		
Socio-economic status	X		X
Living arrangement	X		X
Married	X		
Amount of social interaction	X		
Source of motivation	X		
Age of onset of hearing loss	X		
Duration of hearing loss	X		
Time/longitudinal change			X
Hearing sensitivity	X		X
Self-reported hearing problems	X		X
Attitude towards own hearing loss	X		X
Attitude towards hearing aid	X		
General health attitude	X		
Expectations	X		
First impression of hearing aid		X	
Lifetime experience with hearing aid			X
Cosmetic appearance of hearing aid			X
Costs	X		
Type of clinic (private vs. public)	X		
Hearing aid professional		X	X
Speech reading	X		
Dexterity	X	X	
Activity of daily living (ADL)			X
Medication			X
Number of major life events			X

FIGURE 10.9 Factors related to the prefitting, fitting, and postfitting stages.

professional, counseling). Figure 10.9 lists the factors related to the prefitting, fitting, and postfitting stages. Notably, only self-reported hearing disability affected outcomes for help seeking, uptake, use, and satisfaction. A systematic review of the literature identified the main barriers and facilitators to the uptake of hearing aids in healthy adults 65 years of age or older who were nonusers of hearing aids despite having been diagnosed with a hearing loss and recommended a hearing aid (Jenstad & Moon, 2011). These factors are shown in Table 10.3. Again, the strongest evidence points to self-reported hearing disability.

Social pressure, especially from family members, can be a major incentive in seeking help for hearing loss. However, family members themselves may experience what is known as *third-party disability* (Scarinci, Worrall, & Hickson, 2009a, 2009b), and by seeking help for the person with hearing loss, they may also gain help for themselves too. Lack of referral from primary care physicians can be a major disincentive to help seeking for hearing problems. Older persons who accept hearing loss as a "normal part of aging," tend to report less disability and tolerate greater loss than younger persons before seeking audiologic assistance for their problems. Of course, it is possible that hearing loss has less effect on many older adults because of their particular life circumstances, including their greater social expertise and less demanding communication goals.

Knowledge has advanced regarding the personality factors that influence rehabilitation outcomes. In a study of 230 older adults who were seeking a hearing aid

TABLE 10.3   Summary of Evidence about the Factors Influencing the Uptake of Hearing Aids by Older Adults

Factors	Main Findings	Number of Studies
Self-reported hearing disability	As self-reported hearing loss increased, participants were more likely or willing to obtain hearing aids.	6
Degree of hearing loss	As degree of loss increased, participants were more likely to adhere to hearing aid use. This effect may be modified by gender differences and contribute more to adherence by females than males.	5
Stigma	The contribution of stigma varied across studies, and it may be gender dependent, being of concern to male nonadherents.	5
Personality or psychological factors	Internal locus of control was strong in hearing aid seekers and may be gender dependent, influencing females acceptance of hearing aids. Those reporting fewer maladaptive coping strategies in communication were more likely to reject hearing aids.	3
Age	Age was found to be a contradictory predictor: two studies found increases and one study found a decrease in hearing aid uptake with increasing age.	3
Cost	Cost of hearing aids was reported to be a barrier in two of the three studies. This factor may conflate affordability and cost–benefit evaluations that hearing aids are not worth the expense.	3

Source: Adapted from Jenstad and Moon (2011).

for the first time, Robyn Cox, Alexander, and Gray (2005) explored how personality characteristics might contribute to help seeking. They found that "compared with the typical adult, hearing aid seekers tended to be more pragmatic and routine-oriented and probably less imaginative in coming up with novel approaches to dealing with a complex problem such as hearing loss. These individuals also were found to feel relatively more personally powerful in dealing with life's challenges. Further, hearing aid seekers reported using social support coping strategies less frequently than their non-hearing-impaired peers" (p. 12). Strikingly, Cox and her colleagues concluded that personality traits were more closely related than measures of audiometric hearing loss to self-reports of hearing problems, sound aversiveness, and hearing aid expectations obtained before hearing aid fitting. Recent research exploring the role of social support found that those with more social support had greater satisfaction with hearing aids (Singh et al., 2015). More generally, the social context of the person with hearing loss has been identified as a significant but relatively understudied factor affecting the adoption of hearing aids that warrants further research (Singh & Launer, 2016). In keeping with the communication enhancement model, the audiologist will need to explore the participation goals of each person as an individual in his or her own person–environment relationships.

For older adults, acknowledging the need for amplification follows acknowledging disabling hearing problems, often linked to an acknowledgment of aging. As one woman emphatically stated during a hearing aid counseling session, "Well, I suppose this thing will go along with my dentures, glasses, and support brace. It's

Prefitting readiness and postfitting follow-up can be as or more important than the fitting itself.

getting so it takes me half the morning to make myself *whole!*" Fortunately, most older persons can benefit from appropriately fitted hearing aids and/or HAT if the predisposing, enabling, and reinforcing conditions are optimized.

Fit and Function of the Instrument.   Although amplification is worn by individuals of all ages, most people who wear hearing aids are beyond the sixth decade of life. The number of older adult using hearing aids is only likely to increase as the population ages, especially as the number of people over 85 years of age reaches unprecedented proportions. Overall, it seems that progress has been made, with more adults (81%) being satisfied with their hearing aids today than ever before (Abrams & Kihm, 2015). Some of this welcomed increase in satisfaction is no doubt due to improvements in technology, but evolution in AR practice has also helped to optimize satisfaction with the fitting of technologies. Over the past few decades, hearing aids have become increasingly miniaturized, and there have been innovations to provide many more options, such as open fit, extended-wear technologies, and convergence with Bluetooth and even cell phone apps. Hearing aid selection and fitting techniques have become more sophisticated. For example, practice has evolved by the widespread adoption of standard hearing aid fitting algorithms and the use of real-ear measurement. Audiologists have also become more systematic in applying solutions when fine-tuning hearing aids in response to how clients describe their problems (for an excellent overview, see Jenstad, Van Tasell, & Ewert, 2003). Even self-fitting and self-training devices that adapt to users' listening preferences and environments are moving from research to practice (Wong, 2011). Cochlear implants, hybrid hearing aid (acoustic) and cochlear implant (electric) modality devices, bone-anchored hearing aids, and other specialized technologies continue to advance and can be important solutions for some people for whom conventional hearing aids do not provide an adequate solution. Along with these technological advances, there has

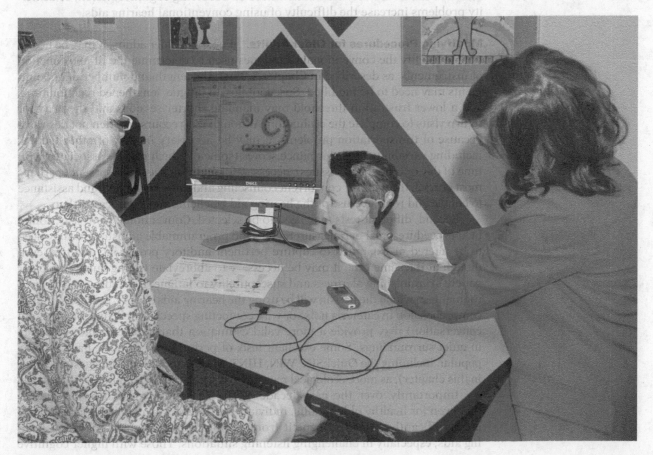

Cochlear implants are being fitted on a growing number of adults worldwide.

been a rise in consumer advocacy, better consumer protection through U.S. Food and Drug Administration regulations, and the recognition that policy changes are needed to ensure affordability and access to hearing care. Professionals have become more aware of the importance of patient-centered and family-centered approaches in which providers, clients, and their significant others collaborate in decision making to optimize both prefitting readiness and postfitting follow-up.

The hearing aid may be looked on as a general-purpose device to be used in almost any situation, while HAT serves a variety of special listening needs, such as telephone listening, TV listening, or listening in large meeting rooms where the listener is some distance from the talker. A number of other listening and speaking devices are available, ranging from simple hardwire amplification systems for use in automobiles to infrared and FM systems for use in nursing homes, churches, and auditoriums (see Chapter 2 for a complete listing of devices; for an overview of issues concerning HAT and older adults, see Jennings, 2009). Some HATs are used instead of conventional hearing aids, while others are used in conjunction with them. Recently, there has also been convergence between hearing aids and HATS to facilitate the use of hearing aids with other communication technologies, such as cell phones (Lesner & Klingler, 2011). Aligned with the principles of universal design, a new trend is to strive for the convergence of specialized and ordinary technologies; for example, innovations in communication technologies, such as the use of texting or Internet services such as Skype, now offer people with hearing loss "normal" ways to use visual communication as an alternative to auditory communication. New international standards may help ensure that hearing (and vision) problems are overcome to a greater extent by improved design (ISO, 2011). HATs, cell phone apps, or Internet services may be preferred over conventional hearing aids by those in the early stages of hearing loss who have very specific needs (e.g., hearing on the telephone or in an auditorium). They may also be the device of choice for very old adults whose co-occurring cognitive, vision, or dexterity problems increase the difficulty of using conventional hearing aids.

Modifying Procedures for Older Adults.   For some older adults, it may be necessary to modify the conventional techniques used to determine the fit and function of instruments, as described in Chapter 2. First, the length and number of appointments may need to be modified. Susceptibility to fatigue, lengthened reaction time, and a lower frustration threshold may mandate shorter sessions and the need for return visits to complete the evaluation. Although this recourse is often not desirable because of transportation problems, it may be necessary in view of other factors, including variability in performance scores (some of which may be associated with time of day or other health issues), necessity for additional assessment, and, perhaps most crucial, the need for concurrent counseling and ongoing support and assistance to enable and reinforce use of the hearing aid by clients and significant others.

Second, different tests may need to be selected. Conventional word lists, sound field procedures, real-ear measurements, and programmable adjustments may need to be altered or expanded to capture pertinent auditory processing abilities, even though at the same time it may be necessary to abbreviate testing due to the older patient's diminishing alertness and susceptibility to fatigue. Depending on the environments in which the person will be using the hearing aids or HAT, tests for sentence comprehension in cafeteria noise or with competing speech (intelligible background conversation) may provide a more valid estimation than monosyllabic word lists in quiet surroundings. Some excellent tests of performance in noise have become popular, including the QuickSIN, WIN, HINT, MAPA, and LISN-S (suggested earlier in this chapter), as more ecological measures of speech understanding performance.

Importantly, over the past decade, groundbreaking research has suggested that even for healthy older adults, individual differences in cognitive performance are significantly related to benefit from complex digital signal processing hearing aids, especially in challenging listening situations. Those with higher cognitive

Conventional techniques used to determine the fit and function of instruments may need to be modified for older adults.

performance are able to take advantage of faster processing schemes, especially in noise with speechlike temporal fluctuations, whereas those with lower cognitive performance are less able to do so (e.g., Gatehouse et al., 2006; Lunner, Rönnberg, & Rudner, 2009). At the present time, there are no standardized audiologic clinical tests of cognition, but it has been recognized that there is the need to develop and incorporate such tests in the hearing aid fitting test battery (Pichora-Fuller, 2003, 2007, 2009a). A promising new test that is being standardized for clinical use in AR is the Word Auditory Recognition and Recall Measure (WARRM; Smith, Pichora-Fuller, & Alexander, 2016). Real-time physiological responses (pupil dilation, skin, cardiac, and brain responses) during listening are also garnering increasing interest as new ways to understand better and to quantify listening effort, and one day some of these experimental methods may mature to the point where they can be applied in practice (Pichora-Fuller et al., 2016). More research is needed to determine how early hearing aid experience relates to brain reorganization and how brain plasticity may be affected by training in individuals with different cognitive processing abilities (Arlinger, Lunner, Lyxell, & Pichora-Fuller, 2009; Pichora-Fuller & Singh, 2006). Care should be taken to assess use, benefit, and satisfaction from a hearing aid after a period of acclimatization following 6 to 12 weeks of hearing aid use because the degree of improvement in listening performance over time may vary from person to person as they become more adept and comfortable using amplification in their everyday lives and improve in handling the device. Older listeners may require more time to acclimatize.

Third, hearing aid selection may be highly influenced by nonauditory considerations. The number of hearing aid choices may be restricted by the individual's lack of management skills, especially if they have vision, dexterity, or cognitive problems. Those with cognitive issues may require more support from others, including frequent prompting or assistance in order to handle and care for hearing technologies. Choices may also be governed by low self-efficacy, stigma, and firmly entrenched attitudes as to what type of instrument will or will not be tolerated.

Fourth, additional types of appointments may need to be planned. The aging segment of the population often requires more extensive follow-up for a variety of possible reasons, including counseling, supervised orientation, hearing aid earmold modifications, and consultation with caregivers, communication partners, and/or other health care professionals. It may be necessary to discuss expected and actual benefit from the hearing aid in different situations once the person has been able to use it in his or her everyday life.

Adjustment to amplification needs to be reviewed over time.

Binaural Fitting. The question of whether aging persons should wear one hearing aid or binaural amplification is an individual one. This decision will depend on the degree of central processing deficit in binaural hearing. It will also depend to a great extent on prosthesis management and financial capabilities, which should be weighed against perceived gains in communication and social participation. An added variable is the attitudinal difference between wearing one instrument as opposed to two. It is not uncommon to hear an older person comment, "I don't need two of these, do I? I'm not deaf!" Apparently, if one hearing aid represents a milestone in adjustment to sensorineural aging, two become a millstone! Nevertheless, everyday functioning is generally greater for those who can adjust to appropriately fitted binaural amplification, and these benefits are likely to increase as more sophisticated binaural signal processing schemes are implemented in newer technologies that may offset some kinds of central auditory processing deficits. As long as 40 years ago, when technology was much simpler, Birk-Nielsen (1974) noted in comparing monaural versus binaural amplification that two aids reduced the amount of social hearing handicap among older persons. This two-ear advantage includes better speech perception in noise, reduced localized autophony (voice resonance), improved spatial balance and localization, and improved sound quality. Research using the SSQ suggests that binaural hearing aids and binaural cochlear

Benefits of binaural fitting must be considered for each individual.

implants are beneficial and that the segregation of sounds in complex environments is perhaps the most important possible benefit of wearing two hearing aids (Noble, 2010). An emerging innovation in digital signal processing that promises to make binaural fittings even more beneficial is the coordination of signal processing by the left-ear and right-ear hearing aids such that interaural difference cues (e.g., the interaural intensity difference cues resulting from head shadow) are preserved and not destroyed when compression is applied. Spatial hearing could be greatly improved by preserving or even augmenting interaural cues, especially in complex auditory ecologies in which different sounds originate at different locations. For adults who have physical, financial, or cosmetic issues or whose quiescent lifestyles fail to justify the need for two instruments, the choice of which ear to fit becomes an issue. Considerations that enter into this decision among older adults include (1) if one ear is better for communication in quiet or in noise, (2) severity of arthritic or other physical involvement in the arms and hands as related to prosthesis manipulation, (3) handedness, (4) ear used for telephone, and (5) lifestyle factors affecting sidedness, such as driving a car or location of bed in a convalescent home.

> Rehabilitation can be successful even for the most challenging situations if the appropriate supports are in place.

> Dexterity and memory may be important factors in selecting a device.

Special Device Features. On the one hand, signal processing hearing aids with built-in automatic controls have provided relief for some whose dexterity problems would make manipulations such as adjusting the volume control difficult. On the other hand, some advanced hearing aid features may be inappropriate for the frail older adult who has co-occurring *cognitive (memory)* vision, and *dexterity* problems. In particular, success with hearing aids depends to a great extent on the individual's ability to handle and maintain the device. Some hearing aid companies have developed special features to accommodate the physical limitations of older persons by offering oversize or touch-type volume controls, modified battery compartments to make it easier for those with dexterity problems to change batteries or to make it harder for those with dementia to remove batteries to prevent them from being lost or even swallowed, attachments to reduce risk of loss of the aid, and fingernail slots or removal handles for easier removal of in-the-ear hearing aids. Choices such as open fit may eliminate problems inserting earmolds, but they may also introduce other handling problems. A few hearing aid manufacturers have become aware about the special needs of older persons in nursing homes and rehabilitation hospitals, including persons whose dexterity and visual, tactile, neuromuscular, and memory difficulties contraindicate conventional forms of amplification. The visibility of a body aid may benefit nursing home residents with poor management skills and visual limitations. There is also less risk that a large device will become lost. Similarly, when earmold insertion becomes prohibitively challenging, headset-style HATs are often preferred because they are easier to put on but also because they can be removed without assistance, thereby supporting independence. A set of helpful tips concerning hearing aid and earmold choices for the specific challenges posed by frail elderly clients with co-occurring cognitive, vision, and dexterity has been prepared (D. Fairholm, Vancouver/Richmond Health Board Community Audiology Centre Outreach to Hard of Hearing Seniors Program, personal communication, 2001).

Extra Adjustment Time: Outcome Measures. Older adults with physical and cognitive limitations require special accommodations, and it is often even more important to include family and/or professional caregivers in the rehabilitation plan for such individuals. Furthermore, those with central auditory processing problems may derive less benefit from hearing aids because increased audibility of the amplified signal does not overcome their need for better signal-to-noise conditions. Such central auditory processing deficits, usually involving declines in temporal and binaural processing, may not be apparent from the results of conventional hearing testing but may be revealed during a comprehensive audiologic assessment including speech-in-noise tests. Hearing aids may not produce significantly improved word recognition scores but may allow persons with central auditory involvement to maintain awareness of their environment (e.g., hearing people approaching). HATs may provide some help for these cases of central auditory processing deficit because they are designed specifically to overcome adverse signal-to-noise conditions. When the rehabilitation program incorporates appropriate supports, it has been shown that even those living in residential care are able to benefit from HATs (Jorgensen & Messersmith, 2015; Lesner, 2003; Lewsen & Cashman, 1997; Pichora-Fuller & Robertson, 1997). Certainly, the recommendation for amplification should not be ignored or contraindicated because of central processing or cognitive problems without a quantitative assessment of potential benefits during a reasonable trial period with different devices and with the involvement of significant others who can support the person as needed in handling devices. A consideration of contextual factors will guide decision making.

For *frail* clients, it may be easier to assess benefits in the actual real-world context than relying only on clinic-based assessment. In particular, assessing the person in his or her usual surroundings may provide crucial information about the nature of the social and physical environment and the supports that are available to the person. This information will guide the choice of technology best suited to the participation needs of the individual. Greater opportunity for communication will provide motivation for using a hearing aid. Peer support may boost self-efficacy and inspire a new hearing aid user to try to continue the use of a hearing aid (Carson, 1997; Dahl, 1997). If caregivers or volunteers are willing to assist with the hearing aid and their involvement becomes part of the rehabilitation plan, a hearing aid may be an option for a person with cognitive issues who would not be able to manage the device independently (Hoek, Pichora-Fuller, Paccioretti, MacDonald, & Shyng, 1997). If a participation priority of the person is attending group activities (e.g., bingo in the cafeteria), an FM system may provide a vital improvement in signal-to-noise ratio that would not be achieved with a personal hearing aid. If telephone conversations with family in another city are a participation priority, a telephone amplifier may be sufficient, cheaper, and easier to manage than a hearing aid with a T-switch. The hearing aid evaluation process for older adults may encompass the entire 30- to 60-day trial period offered by the dispenser, often taxing the patience of those whose primary interest is sale closure. However, the clinical audiologist must remain steadfast in terms of ethical responsibilities toward even the slowest clients and must remain open to alternative or complementary solutions.

Several methods are available for measuring the perceived benefit of amplification and, indeed, self-report has been shown to be useful in dealing with acclimatization issues. Diligent follow-up is perhaps even more important for the frail elderly because their needs and abilities may change unexpectedly. When appropriate supports are in place for this special population, regular use and benefit from amplification can be maintained by experienced hearing aid wearers, even though a first-time user of a hearing aid would be unlikely to succeed (Hoek et al., 1997; Parving & Phillip, 1991; Pichora-Fuller & Robertson, 1997). Use or benefit or satisfaction may be useful measures for those who are still participating in activities; for those who have stopped participating in activities and have already become more socially isolated, increases in the number of activities in which the individual participates may provide a telling outcome measure (Pichora-Fuller & Robertson, 1994). For those with a significant *cognitive problem*, questionnaires are too difficult, but benefit from amplification has been demonstrated by other kinds of outcome measures, such as staff observations of reductions in behavioral problems (Palmer, Adams, Bourgeois, Durrant, & Rossi, 1999). Clearly, counseling and ongoing support and follow-up are necessary for success in many cases.

Orientation to Instruments. Initial experiences with hearing aids or HAT, especially in the first few weeks, are critical. The audiologist should be ready for any problem that might occur concerning the client, the instrument, and/or the

Benefits from rehabilitation for frail older adults can be improved by considering the social and physical environment.

Observation of behavior may be used to evaluate benefit for those who have cognitive problems.

Improvement may be reported by the person with the new hearing aid or by a significant other.

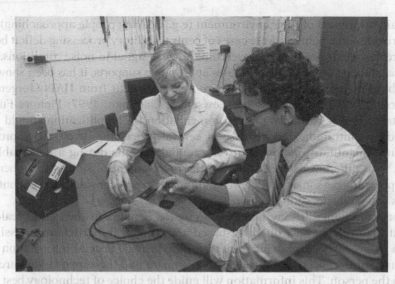

A client being familiarized with HAT.

environment. Counseling, whether face-to-face, by telephone, or on the Internet, is a continuing commitment that is based on the adjustment needs of the individuals and their communication partners. As pointed out earlier, the reasons for rejection of devices are numerous, ranging from fine-tuning solutions to address the client's description of problems hearing with the device to simple difficulties handing the device to complex attitude adjustment problems. The clinician must allow these reasons to surface early in the trial period before rejection becomes ingrained. An important concept to be aware of during counseling is that rejection often works in tandem with other age-related deficits that undermine appropriate use of the device. For example, rejection and reduced short-term memory may combine to become counterproductive, as summed up in the statement of an 89-year-old woman who, during a moment of exasperation, announced, "I can never remember which way the battery goes in, and I hear better without this thing, anyway!" Needless to say, she had the battery inserted backward. Other problems may be less obvious.

Even if the person wearing the hearing aids does not notice much benefit from amplification, it is possible that his or her communication partner does notice improvement in terms of not finding talking so stressful: "Harry doesn't think my voice is any easier to hear, but now I don't have to shout at him so it really makes my life a lot easier!" The primary complaints of the client, family members, and friends during the prefitting phase can be readdressed during the trial period. Information from the example case of Mrs. Carter in Table 10.2 illustrates the utility of this approach. The prefitting counseling session included the list of complaints and associated objectives to be reviewed at follow-up. Consequently, audiologic surveillance in the first two weeks was aimed not only at use of the hearing aid but also at taking appropriate measures to reduce or eliminate each complaint. Two additional strategies for addressing the complaints were an introduction to conversational therapy for the client and her daughter and familiarization with the use of an FM system in challenging acoustical conditions. The conversational therapy targeted the frustration of the daughter during conversation with her mother, and it also targeted communication with a close friend in the dining hall at the residence of the client. An FM system was already available in the client's church, and its use in conjunction with the hearing aid was practiced with both client and daughter. Furthermore, the use of an FM system would enable listening to the bus driver on group outings, and the driver and recreational staff were involved in implementing this solution. Considered separately from the environment, the hearing aids would have been doomed to failure given the person's usual seating choices, the high level of reverberation in the church, and the high level of noise on the bus. Similarly, the overloud TV volume control was corrected by allowing the daughter to adjust the loudness to a "comfortable" level while the client was seated in her customary chair with her aids turned to half-gain. This listening level was subsequently marked on the TV volume control with an easily visible fingernail polish. Had this solution failed to meet the objectives, the next step would have been to consider using a device providing FM transmission of the TV signal directly to the hearing aid wearer. Setting clear and measurable objectives helped to clarify that the rehabilitation plan was on track during the follow-up appointment during the trial period.

Individual Orientation. Based on survey data, the majority of hearing aid and HAT users receive help within an individual rather than a group orientation structure (Millington, 2001; Schow, Balsara, Smedley, & Whitcomb, 1993). Although group sessions have certain advantages that will be discussed later, many people are unable to meet regularly in the group environment. Individual sessions permit rehabilitation to focus more on accomplishing the specific goals of the individual. Whenever possible, it is important to have significant others in attendance during therapy sessions or even to conduct sessions on-site in locations where the target activities take place (e.g., at the chapel or in the dining hall of a care facility), one reason being to facilitate carryover to the person's everyday participation in real-world environments.

> The necessary skills in operating and caring for hearing aids and assistive devices should be checked to be sure that no further training is needed.

Frequently, individual device orientation focuses on developing competence in using the device. A prerequisite to achieving audibility is for the clients and/or their caregivers to become skilled at handling, operating, and caring for the hearing aid or HAT. These skills are difficult for older adults to acquire, and even middle-aged adults may need more help than is routinely provided. Hearing aid handling skills can be evaluated using a structured test (Doherty & Desjardins, 2012). Common problems for users of all ages are improper placement of the aid, insertion of the mold, operation of the controls, and battery insertion. Even if the new wearer has mastered the skills necessary to operate the hearing aid, it may take more time to become proficient in taking full advantage of the advanced features of a hearing aid. All clients should be given instruction in both the essential and the advanced skills needed to take full advantage of the hearing aids as well as being given written information that they can continue to refer to over time. To personalize take-home materials, some clinicians are even using common recording technologies on phones and computers to make photographs or videos during sessions so that the client can replay the images themselves operating their own devices. An example handout for clients is HIO BASICS (Appendix A). Handouts may need to be translated into foreign languages for some clients or produced in large print for those with vision problems.

For those requiring more intensive instruction, it will help to focus on specific skills and to use step-by-step training to improve each skill (Maurer, 1979). In such training, the skill to be acquired (e.g., inserting the earmold) is broken down into discrete steps that are repeated until each is mastered. At each step, encouraging comments are provided by the audiologist as successes are achieved. It is also crucial for the client to learn how to judge if he or she has been successful, often on the basis of tactile and visual cues regarding how the earmold looks and "feels in the ear" when it is properly seated, how it "feels to the fingers" when it is properly seated, and how it "feels to the fingers" when it is grasped properly. Such programs may be completed in a single session or over multiple sessions. Caregivers may be trained to prompt, assist, and/or check that the person is using the skills on an ongoing basis. Skills should always be reevaluated at follow-up to ensure that they have been maintained and to further reinforce and refine them. An example of this is as follows.

> Mrs. Andrew's chief complaint about her new hearing aid was lack of battery life.
>
> "Are you opening the battery case at night when you're not using the instrument?" the audiologist inquired.
>
> "Heavens, no. You didn't tell me to do that!"

"Yes, she did, mother," the daughter chimed in. "Don't you remember? It's even stated in that booklet in your purse."

"Well, this is the first time I've *heard* about it," the older woman retorted.

Orientation in Groups. Some persons may fit into a group training structure rather than or in addition to individual sessions. This will not be feasible for everyone, however, because some do not have attitudes or cultural beliefs that favor group interaction with strangers, some may prefer meeting times that do not coincide with the group meeting time, and some may simply prefer or need the individual attention created by a one-on-one situation. But when group sessions are feasible, they can be very helpful. Aging individuals may become socially isolated and group AR may be one of the few opportunities for socialization in these cases. As noted earlier, their network of peers is smaller than in previous years, and the opportunity to participate in a group experience is often welcomed. The Hard of Hearing Club at Baycrest Hospital in Toronto has continued for many years to meet the needs of older adults with severe hearing loss for whom social isolation poses a risk to mental health (Reed, 2010). An important aspect of a small AR group is the opportunity to share information. In addition to the benefits to those receiving information, sharing information is often a positive experience for the information giver. In such meetings, the audiologist takes the position of group leader and facilitates discussions by (1) bringing out those persons who are reluctant to share their experiences, (2) inhibiting those few who might dominate the group, (3) permitting the discussion topics to surface from the group rather than from the clinician, (4) acting as a resource person when expertise is needed, and, most important, (5) acting as a *good listener* and establishing a safe and positive situation for communication. A very well documented and successful group AR program for older adults is Active Communication Education (Hickson, Worrall, & Scarinci, 2007a, 2007b; Oberg, Bohn, & Larsson, 2014). Achieving homogeneous grouping (i.e., bringing together persons who have similar perceived communication problems, as revealed in self-assessment profiles), when feasible, may be desirable. It may also be advantageous to mix more expert, experienced hearing aid users with beginners so that peer teaching and modeling can be incorporated into group sessions.

It is important for the audiologist to be a good listener.

Like individual orientation sessions, traditional group sessions have tended to focus mostly on the use of hearing aids, with lesser amounts of attention on communication strategies, auditory training, HATs, and speechreading (Schow et al.,

Group AR activities can help clients learn about hearing aids.

1993). In addition to the ideas on hearing aid orientation listed in Chapter 2 and in the HIO BASICS (Appendix A), a good group meeting is one that (1) is oriented primarily to building successes rather than problems, (2) is engaging and provides an element of entertainment, (3) focuses on no more than three learning objectives, (4) incorporates sharing of ideas in a counseling medium, and (5) culminates with a clear understanding of how each member can take charge of his or her newly acquired learning through carryover activities. The clinician may improve group cohesiveness by asking members to contact each other by telephone between sessions; for example, the objective of a homework assignment might be for the person called to guess who the "mystery caller" is and report on the experience at the next group meeting. Additional help in planning group meetings can be found by consulting the references cited in this section.

The Significant Other.   The significant other should understand the device, its main components, and the conditions under which it should be worn; should possess information regarding basic troubleshooting, warranty, and repair; and should be proficient at inserting and removing the instrument. It is helpful to provide a written description of this information and resources for obtaining further information on particular topics. Resource information always includes the audiologist's contact information as well as information such as the following: the location and contact information for an accessible source of low-cost batteries; suppliers of special alerting, wake-up, or other communication devices; information on captioned films for television; lists of local facilities with hearing accessibility options (e.g., loops or FM systems); a schedule for planned hearing aid checks; notices of AR meetings; and call-back for annual audiologic assessment. Furthermore, in addition to learning new information and communication skills so that they can help the person with the hearing loss, because significant others themselves must adjust to living with a person with hearing loss, they may benefit as much as the client from group discussions with peers in which information and common experiences may be shared (see SPEECH handout, Appendix C). (See also Chapter 12, Case 3.)

Advocacy in Restrictive Environments or Residential Care.   Just as it is important to set objectives that address the goals of individuals, at the institutional level, the best method for securing the participation of the *administration and staff* of convalescent hospitals, nursing homes, high-rise facilities for the aging, senior adult centers, or assistive living facilities is to find out what client and staff needs that the organization leaders perceive can be addressed by the AR program. Unfortunately, they may perceive the hearing problems of their clientele to rank low in priority when compared to the sleeping, eating, bathing, recreation programs, and other health needs within the facility. Most staff lack knowledge of hearing loss and hearing aids, and they may not perceive hearing help to fall within their job descriptions. Sometimes it is difficult to gain entry into a restrictive environment on the basis of one client who has a hearing loss and needs on-site follow-up. A workable strategy for overcoming staff resistance is to seek out the staff member who is most likely to appreciate the communication and listening needs of the person (e.g., the activities director) and explain that you are working with the client and his or her family. Improvements in the person's communication functioning can make the work of staff easier and more satisfying. Sometimes housekeeping or nutrition staff spend more time communicating with residents than do nurses. Offer to provide services that will help all staff involved in the case to work more easily with the client. Another possibility is to offer a more general information session on hearing and aging as an in-service activity aimed at helping the staff understand and manage all clientele with hearing difficulties. A stimulating, solution-oriented in-service presentation nearly always produces advocates among residents, family, volunteers, and staff members, individuals who later may become allies in the rehabilitation plan. Once allies are

It is important to find out what staff and administrators perceive to be the AR needs of older adults residing in their facility.

TABLE 10.4   Multistep Program for Those in Residential Care

1. Screening of hearing, as required by federal law, with pure tones, visual inspection (including determination of need for removal of cerumen), and self-assessment and staff members' assessment of hearing (e.g., Nursing Home Hearing Handicap Index; Schow & Nerbonne, 1977).
2. Cerumen management as indicated, followed by thorough diagnostic testing for those who fail screening, along with charting and informing staff of results and arranging for referrals as needed.
3. Consultation with communication partners if appropriate to identify objectives of staff, family, or significant others.
4. Identification of objectives for rehabilitation for individuals and subgroups of residents who share particular interests or activities (e.g., attending services in chapel, going on bus outings).
5. Selection of candidates for devices, trials with hearing aids or HAT in context, and thorough orientation for those who are reestablishing use or becoming new users of devices.
6. In-services, consultations, or team meetings with staff, including explanation of the causes and effects of hearing loss in older adults, discussion of the role of the audiologist and facility staff in hearing health care for individuals or groups of older adults in the facility, development of skills in using and caring for amplification devices, and guidance on how to encourage independent communication behaviors and an environment that facilitates positive interpersonal relationships among residents and staff.
7. Recommend changes to routines and physical environment that will enable best communication and use of amplification and assistive technology.
8. Implement method for ongoing monitoring of and help for all amplification users and key communication partners, including family, staff, peers, and volunteers.

made, interest is maintained through a recognized need for further education as well as an open communication line to the audiologist's office. Leaving a designated staff member with this public service gesture and a copy of your professional credentials removes much of the suspicion frequently associated with the doorstep intervention tactics of some commercial vendors.

Elsewhere, we have reported a variety of experiences in providing hearing services for nursing homes (Hoek et al., 1997; Pichora-Fuller & Robertson, 1997; Schow, 1992). In a number of such homes where hearing was tested, we found that only about 10 percent of potential hearing aid candidates were using amplification, whereas another 20 percent responded that they had hearing aids but were not using them. Importantly, rehabilitation has been shown to be valuable in maintaining the use of devices by those in residential care. Therefore, the need for rehabilitation is apparent, and residents will be at a disadvantage if it is not provided. A multistep program is proposed as an effective plan for ensuring that hearing services are available in these facilities (see Table 10.4).

Alternative Media.   Face-to-face interactions between the rehabilitative audiologist and those in residential facilities will be crucial, but in some situations other media, ranging from posters and videotapes to the Internet, may augment face-to-face interactions. Use of the Internet by older adults in our society is rapidly increasing. About 1 in 10 older adults had Internet access at home in 1999, but by 2014 more than half did (Smith, 2014). Health information on the Internet has growing appeal to many adults who want to find or review information on health topics at a time and place of their own choosing. In the future, Internet connection will no doubt be used to facilitate more immediate communication between the audiologist and staff, family, or residents at locations that are geographically distributed.

Rehabilitative training is being rejuvenated in new programs that emphasize listening.

Remediation for Communication Activities

Traditionally, communication rehabilitation has focused on auditory and visual communication training, with an emphasis on speechreading and auditory training. Typically, it was provided when counseling and instrumental interventions proved insufficient. In light of the growing understanding of the lengthy but important process of adjusting to hearing loss, many rehabilitative audiologists today offer communication rehabilitation to a broader segment of the population and in more varied forms that target more specific activity goals. All clients should be familiarized with the principles of communication rehabilitation in discussion with the audiologist, and written materials should be provided for the client to refer to later or share with significant others. An example of such a handout is CLEAR (Appendix B). In addition to introducing these general principles to clients, their specific activity goals can also be addressed by individual or group communication remediation tailored to their needs.

In addition to communication remediation for those using amplification, communication training is now being provided to assist individuals in the process of adjusting to hearing loss who may not yet be ready to try a hearing aid. Other programs have been developed that use a health promotion approach in programs for older adults with no known clinically significant hearing loss so that they will be better prepared for taking action when they do begin to experience hearing problems (Worrall, Hickson, Barnett, & Yiu, 1998).

"Bridge" Therapy

Individual speechreading instruction was deemed appropriate for a 62-year-old woman who had suffered loss of hearing in one ear due to Ménière's disease. Socially active in the community and reluctant to disclose her loss to others, the woman preferred the privacy of individual therapy. She was an avid bridge player, and participation in her bridge club was of utmost importance to her. To address her single goal of retaining excellent ability to participate in bridge games, individual therapy activities were chosen that satisfied the same five ingredients described earlier for a good group meeting. One such therapy activity consisted of "playing" bridge through a two-way mirror with only visual cues for statements, such as "I bid three spades," "I pass," and so forth. The woman improved her ability to speechread the language of her favorite game. This proved fortuitous since the signs of Ménière's syndrome (roaring tinnitus, vertigo, and nausea) signaled the eventual loss of hearing in her good ear. As her hearing loss continued to deteriorate, additional goals were formulated and therapy activities undertaken.

Conversational Therapy and Tactics. The critical implication of hearing loss for an aging individual is that it affects the lenses through which the client views reality. Thus, when the speech signal and content of messages are altered, the older person comes to distrust what others say as well as his or her own interpretation of communicative events. Restoring control and trust in communication may become an objective for communication rehabilitation that is accomplished in conversational therapy. When communication needs become apparent in a wider range of everyday life situations and when reduced communicative competence comes to have far-reaching effects on the person's well-being, a broader approach to communication training becomes essential. Conversation-based communication training has been promoted for over two decades by Erber (1988, 1996), and it has been extended by Lind (2009), who refers to "interaction as intervention." It is explained in Chapters 4 and 5. Just as in face-to-face communication, conversation-based therapy necessarily engages the person in auditory and visual perception of speech. However, the therapy stresses how the person can take advantage of and manipulate many of the redundant sources of information available in the communicative interaction, including many aspects of the person–environment relationship. Whereas some sources of information come from the external world (e.g., seeing the waitress approach a table in a restaurant), others come from internally stored knowledge of the world (e.g., knowledge that the restaurant script for ordering food often begins by the waitress asking the customers if they are ready to order). During therapy, clients learn how they can optimize the usefulness of available information, especially by using conversational strategies. For example, miscommunication resulting from misperceived speech sounds can be overcome if conversational strategies are used to establish the topic. A peripheral high-frequency hearing loss alters coding of the speech signal, thereby affecting comprehension of the content of the message and even influencing the ongoing response to the message:

> Mr. Jacobson was helping his grandson paint the family shed. "Gramps," the younger person said, "let's quit for a while and go get some thinner."
>
> The older man stared in amazement at his grandson, "Go get some dinner? Son, we just had lunch!"

The confusion arising from the *thinner–dinner* misperception would have been repaired more gracefully if the grandfather had been more cautious and asked, "What do you want to get?" before jumping to a conclusion that he actually recognized to be inconsistent with the situation. For AR to be successful for the older person, positive change must be brought about in the entire social-communicative milieu.

Conversation-based therapy cultivates the communication skills pertaining to the four elements in any communication situation: listener, talker, message, and environment. The client develops skills in each area: (1) listening (and watching) to comprehend, (2) coaching talkers to produce more easily understood speech and language (e.g., by suggesting helpful accommodations such as "Could you keep your hand away from your face and speak slower?"), (3) using linguistic and world knowledge to interpret the meaning of the message, and (4) altering the acoustical and lighting properties of the situation to improve the signal and reduce interference from extraneous sources. The *communication partner* also develops corresponding skills pertaining to each of the skill areas. Both the client and the communication partner develop methods that are effective for them in their relationship with each other. These methods may be different for spouses who have lived together for 50 years than for a college student and his new professor or for a 90-year-old with dementia and the nurse providing her with care in a hospice. The audiologist/ counselor, acting in the multiple roles of diagnostician, hearing aid specialist, AR specialist, and gerontologist, becomes an integral part of the client's milieu.

The communication issues of the partner may need to be addressed, too.

Partner Communication.   It is worth noting that hearing loss in one communication partner may coexist with hearing loss in the other partner. It is also common for one or both partners to have another communication disorder (Orange, 2009). A spouse or daughter may develop vocal pathology as a result of chronically raising her voice to be heard by a husband or parent with hearing loss. Family members may have trouble hearing the poorly intelligible or soft voices of partners with Parkinson's disease. Most individuals who have had total laryngectomy surgery are within the older adult age-group and have hearing difficulties. Furthermore, since esophageal speech generally has reduced intensity and less well defined vowel formants, persons with laryngectomies are less intelligible to peers, who are also likely to be older and hard of hearing. Withdrawal from social situations may result from the combination of hearing and speaking difficulties and may affect the relationship between spouses, family, and friends. Communicative rehabilitation often entails using visual cues to improve speech perception; however, this may not be an option for the many older adults with vision loss. In one home for the aged, the audiologist was surprised when a woman who was blind asked to join the lipreading class until the woman explained that she wanted to learn how to talk more clearly so that her roommate who was hard of hearing would be able to lipread her better. It may become necessary to address the other communication issues of the client or even the communication issues of the spouse in order to achieve a solution in communication rehabilitation.

Simulations and Role Playing.   The counselor/audiologist is positioned between the older client and reality because the counselor's own communication skills and knowledge are called into play to assist the older person in making lifestyle changes to ameliorate or compensate for the hearing loss to achieve participation. The audiologist may even play the role of the client when the communication partner is receiving conversational training or the role of the communication partner when the client is being trained. The ability to re-create these roles is enhanced by the use of hearing loss simulators (e.g., Erber's HELOS) that can be used to introduce the effects of hearing loss into the signal heard by a person with normal hearing (Erber, 1988), but the therapy can also be done without HELOS. Importantly, role playing enables the audiologist to model effective communication strategies, and it also promotes empathy, self-efficacy, mutual respect and consideration, and sharing of experiences with and between the client and his or her communication partner(s).

Empathy and Listening.   During communication rehabilitation, as in all stages of AR, the empathy achieved through listening will have great effect on the outcome of the rehabilitation program. More professional time may be needed for the feelings of older adults to surface insofar as they can be slower in adapting to change and more fixed in their attitudes. In some instances, the audiologist can bring about positive changes by simply *permitting the client to register complaints*, thereby achieving a more favorable outlook in decision making. Listening helps the audiologist appreciate the delicate balance between the client's enjoyment of hearing and the perceived nuisances of the new device. Listening also helps the audiologist learn from the ingenuity of clients who find their own novel solutions to problems. The many personal preferences, attitudes, and beliefs of clients will guide the setting of objectives and the selection of an action plan for rehabilitation that can be reevaluated over time.

A profile of the client focuses on the person's lifestyle and listening needs.

Environmental Interventions to Improve Participation

As demonstrated so far in this chapter, a well-coordinated rehabilitation program for adults requires an organized body of knowledge about the clientele. This includes clinical sensitivity toward persons who are at various life span stages, a thorough understanding of the individual in question, and prioritization of this information into a meaningful rehabilitative plan. Directive, informational counseling that includes "laundry lists" of questions, often constructed on the basis of stereotypes, is not well advised. Although such an approach may be useful for some purposes, the salience of the information sampled in this generic and narrow manner may be lost in the undertow of real needs and feelings that surface when the clinician simply listens to the individual client. In too many instances, failure or rejection of hearing amplification or other treatment during the intervention process is due either to lack of clinical sensitivity toward the individual client's needs, feelings, and goals or to insensitivity toward the subpopulation of adults to which the individual belongs. Adults are heterogeneous, and their particular needs must be determined by the audiologist. The older segment of the world population of persons with hearing loss has a wealth of life experiences that may influence their course of rehabilitation both positively and negatively. There is also variability among younger adults, including young adults completing their education and vocational training, adults raising young families, adults caring for aging parents, working adults in stressful senior positions, and adults with unusual health or occupational challenges. For older and younger adults alike, their need for audiologic services may range from minimal to extensive. Each case must be appreciated in a dynamic context.

The pervading question is whether the rehabilitation program will make a significant, positive impact on the life satisfaction of the person. A well-developed client profile, based on both formal assessment measures and informal information gathering during counseling, substantially increases the probability of successful AR. Such a workup serves to determine client needs rather than those of the clinic or the practitioner. It delineates whether the individual is a candidate for intervention, the particular plan that should be tailored to meet the person's needs, the hypothetical objectives and terminal goals that might be accomplished, significant other persons who should be involved, environmental modifications that will be needed to achieve a solution for the person, and where, when, and under whose auspices the program should be carried out. The individual's adjustment to hearing loss and readiness for taking rehabilitative action is foremost in the rehabilitative agenda, but rehabilitation may fall short of meeting the individual's goals if the importance of social and physical environmental supports is overlooked.

Client Profile

Areas of intake information that provide context for the overall coordination of the program:

- Hearing status, including history, duration, and potential site(s) of lesion, as well as self-assessment of the hearing problems and assessments by significant other persons.
- What problems are the most important to this person and his or her partners?
- What are the past, present, and desired activities of this person?
- Previous help seeking and medical or prosthetic intervention.
- What factors contributed to the success or failure of previous rehabilitative action?
- Associated health issues, such as tinnitus, vision loss, cognitive declines (e.g., memory), risk of or fear of falling, arthritis, neuromuscular limitations, speech or language problems, and mobility difficulties.
- To what extent do physical, mental, social, or economic conditions make this individual dependent on others?
- Personal and environmental factors that will predispose, enable, and reinforce decision making and action taking.
- What kinds of social or environmental supports are needed by the individual in his or her activities, and what are possible negative effects of hearing loss on significant other persons?
- What costs and benefits might influence rehabilitative choices?

Relatives, friends, and professionals can be important partners in AR.

Participation in Situations and Relationships. Most of the complaints of adults about their hearing difficulties, for example, are about participation in a specific situation or role: "I can't hear in church," "I can't understand the lecturer when my classmates are talking," "I don't watch the news on television because the announcer talks too fast," "I feel like I'm letting my teenage son down because I can't have conversation with him without making him repeat all the time." Knowledge about such concerns provides for a practical, operational baseline from which positive rehabilitative changes can be measured. Self-assessment measures such as the SAC and COSI are useful for identifying the needs of the individual and documenting changes with respect to these needs. New tools, such as data logging, can be used to discover more about the communication environments encountered by the client in everyday life. More informal information gathering during counseling, however, is still necessary if the audiologist is to fully appreciate how personal, social, and physical environmental factors should best be tackled to achieve a successful rehabilitative solution.

Social Environmental Supports. The key to whether significant other persons should be included in the plan and subsequent coordination of the rehabilitation program is the extent of their present and potential contribution toward the older individual's life satisfaction and the achievement of his or her top-priority goals. Observing interactions between the client and others may reveal the kind of support that they will provide and whether they will be allies during intervention. Perhaps the paramount questions that the clinician should consider is whether significant others' support seems to be based on a valid concern for the individual or whether it is irregular or counterproductive and whether the support would reinforce independence or dependence. Relatives, friends, and staff in a geriatric setting can be important links in the rehabilitative chain and can be helped by review of a communication handout like the one shown in Appendix C. Others who may act in concert with the audiologist to facilitate adjustment to hearing loss include members of the professional community who have knowledge about the client and his or her family support system, culture, and lifestyle. Relevant parties may include members of the clergy, physicians, welfare workers, home care workers, volunteers, and administrators or leaders of organizations and clubs in which the client holds membership.

When a department head in a large company moved into her new office, she was horrified to discover that she was unable to use her T-switch for the telephone or with HAT in the conference room. To the embarrassment of the architect, the acoustical consultant who was hired to assess the problem determined that the problem was caused by the high level of electromagnetic interference produced in a machine room located directly below the new offices. A large insulating panel was installed to eliminate the problem. The nature of the client's problem and the method for solving it eluded the audiologist, whose clinical measures showed that there was no change in the client's hearing and that her devices were working properly. The cooperation of the employer and the expertise of the architect and acoustical consultant were vital to achieving the environmental piece of the solution.

Physical Environmental Supports.   The physical environment may also be crucial to the client's ability to participate fully. Supports can be optimized by selecting favorable environments or modifying unfavorable environments. For example, a client may need to investigate which restaurants are quiet and well lit and learn how to pick the best table and seat. Where choices are not possible, modifications may be required. Noise and reverberation may be reduced by interior decorating (e.g., carpeting, upholstery, drapes) or by architectural changes to increase sound absorption by room surfaces. Electromagnetic interference can also interfere with participation by people who are hard of hearing. Greater involvement of professionals and policymakers responsible for the built environment will likely be seen as AR catches up with other rehabilitative fields in which accessibility adaptations (e.g., ramps for wheelchairs) have long been accepted as societal obligations, especially in workplaces or public educational, health, and law facilities. It is encouraging that in 2014, the Facility Guidelines Institute (2014a, 2014b) recommended a maximum level of 45 dBA in hospital patient areas and that in the same year that these recommendations were published, they were incorporated into the building codes of 42 states (Swallow & Wesolowsky, 2014; Van Wyk & Murphy, 2014a, 2014b).

> Acoustical consultants may help with architectural solutions.

OTHER IMPORTANT ISSUES IN THE SCOPE OF AR PRACTICE

Vestibular/balance disorders and tinnitus are disturbances frequently associated with hearing loss that sometimes require assessment and rehabilitation efforts by audiologists and other professionals. Since they are not as common as communication disorders but affect mainly adults and elderly adults, we have chosen to place brief pertinent information on them at the end of this chapter. Some prevalence and assessment information is followed by management (treatment) options for each.

Vestibular Assessment and Management

The evaluation and treatment of vestibular disorders often requires an interdisciplinary approach involving physicians, physical therapists, and audiologists. Vestibular assessment and rehabilitation is a growing area of specialization for audiologists, and expanded training is needed to increase knowledge and skills in this area because new techniques and procedures have been developed recently to better assess the vestibular system (Nelson, Akin, Riska, Andresen, & Mondelli, 2016).

About half the people in the United States will experience some form of balance or dizziness problem in their lifetimes (AAA, 2005). Between 5 million and 8 million physician consults per year are due to dizziness (Desmond, 2000). These disorders increase with age, with one study finding that 65 percent of individuals over age 60 experience dizziness or loss of balance (Hobeika, 1999). Falls are a major health concern in older adults, and those with hearing loss have an increased risk of falling.

Often balance and dizziness disorders are thought to be related to inner ear problems, but there are complex interactions between several systems required to maintain our stability. The somatosensory (our sense of body location) and visual

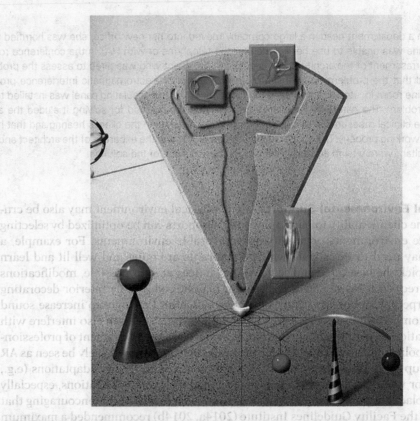

FIGURE 10.10 **Sensory input contributing to balance are the visual, somatosensory, and vestibular systems.**
Source: Courtesy of Natus Medical, Inc.

systems work with the vestibular portion of the inner ear to perceive our environment and position in space. This complex sensory input is analyzed by the brain stem, cerebellum, and cortex to trigger reflexive and voluntary motor responses (Figure 10.10). Normally, somatosensory input from the legs, hips, ankles, and feet plays a major role in balance maintenance. The visual system becomes dominant in the sensory integration hierarchy when somatosensory input is compromised. If both visual and somatosensory inputs are compromised, we rely more heavily on inner ear function. Sensory conflicts within the central nervous system impair our ability to maintain equilibrium. For example, it is easy to stand on a ladder to change an overhead light bulb, but it is more difficult if the light bulb is over a bed and we need to stand on the mattress. The mattress moves when we reach up, and input from the lower half of our body is compromised such that it takes more concentration and time and is fatiguing because we need more resources, both mental and physical, to replace the bulb.

The inner ear is a dual sensory organ: the cochlea, which is responsible for hearing, and the vestibular portion for interpreting and reporting head and body position information to the brain. The vestibular portion of the inner ear is made up of three semicircular canals and two otolith organs. The three semicircular canals in each ear are fluid-filled structures that respond to angular acceleration of the head, allowing us to monitor head changes in various planes of motion. The otolith organs provide an interpretation of motion in a straight line, such as going up in an elevator or accelerating in a car. The vestibular system is connected with the visual system in the brain stem and helps maintain a stable visual image of the world around us. This sensory integration is important for keeping our eyes focused on targets of interest when we are in motion. This is accomplished by a very important neurological relationship called the vestibular-ocular reflex (VOR). This reflex has the responsibility of stabilizing an item of interest in our visual system by means of a series of adjustments of the eye muscles. These adjustments are coordinated through a set of complex neural networks in the brain stem and cerebellum. Vestibular testing involves measuring the magnitude and direction of the *nystagmus* produced by the VOR in order to monitor the function of peripheral and central vestibular systems.

Nystagmus involves rapid, involuntary movements of the eye.

Causes of Balance Problems Damage to visual, vestibular, and proprioception systems (the ability to sense position and motion) are often the main sources of balance problems. However, medication that has unwanted side effects or interactions with other prescriptions may also impair one's abilities to process this complex sensory integration. Consequently, we depend on a multidisciplinary approach to balance assessment that typically begins with a physician.

Assessment An otolaryngologist can complete a thorough exam of the head, neck, and functional balance. Since disease processes may affect both the hearing and the vestibular portions of the inner ear, a thorough audiologic evaluation is conducted. If abnormal results (e.g., asymmetric hearing loss) are obtained on standard audiologic tests, then advanced testing, such as Auditory Brainstem Responses (ABR), may be conducted. A battery of vestibular tests can be conducted, including the analysis of the VOR. This involves a complex observation of the patient's eyes by capturing eye movement with infrared video recording systems. This testing is called *videonystagmography (VNG)*. The eye movements are subsequently analyzed by computer to evaluate the vestibular portion of the inner ear structures, sensory and motor function of ocular muscles, and brain stem processing. Caloric testing involves using warm or cool air or water in the ear canal to stimulate the vestibular system. This creates a predictable eye response called nystagmus. The nystagmus can then be quantified and compared to the performance of the other ear vestibular system, much like a hearing test.

VNG is a sensitive process for testing inner ear function that involves recording eye movements via cameras.

Caloric testing involves using warm or cool air or water in the ear canal.

Another way to initiate a response of nystagmus from the patient is to rotate the head or body either passively (e.g., rotary chair testing) or actively (e.g., the Vestibular Autorotation Test [VAT]). If the etiology of chronic balance disturbances is unknown, as is often the case for older adults, other tests, such as computerized dynamic posturography (CDP), can be particularly useful and provides a more functional evaluation.

One subtest of CDP, called Sensory Organization Testing (SOT), is useful for assessing a patient's static balance. The patient is asked to maintain balance under a variety of conditions. These findings help document patients' balance problems, assist in development of a rehabilitation plan, and confirm progress gained from individualized therapies.

A self-report tool called the Dizziness Handicap Inventory (Jacobsen & Newman, 1990) can be administered to explore the effects that dizziness has in the lives of patients. It was designed to investigate the physical, emotional, and functional problems related to dizziness. It is very useful to document patient improvement before and after treatment.

Vestibular Rehabilitation Therapy The goal of Vestibular Rehabilitation Therapy (VRT) is to improve balance and gait by retraining the sensory/motor systems described above. Those who respond well to VRT usually have chronic conditions of motion-provoked dizziness or generalized disequilibrium. Individuals with *benign paroxysmal positional vertigo (BPPV)*, asymmetrical vestibular disorders, or abnormal postural control or gait problems are typically good candidates. In addition, people who have demonstrated difficulties integrating visual, vestibular, or somatosensory input as verified by CDP or during clinical evaluations can benefit from VRT. In contrast, people experiencing progressive medical pathologies that involve balance or severe disability may not realize the same level of improvement (see Chapter 12, Case 7).

BPPV is a form of vertigo caused by loose crystals from the vestibule relocating in the semicircular canals.

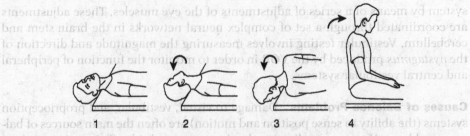

FIGURE 10.11 Canalith repositioning maneuver. Right CRT. (1) right head hanging position; (2) leftward roll; (3) further leftward roll; (4) sitting up.

Canalith repositioning, which involves simple head movements is successful in treating about 80 percent of cases with BPPV.

The Epley Maneuver is a type of canalith repositioning therapy.

Vestibular therapy works due to the ability of the central nervous system to change depending on need or condition. Treatment of BPPV is done through a series of precise head and body movements, termed *canalith repositioning*, that are utilized to move displaced carbonate crystals from the semicircular canal back into the vestibule of the inner ear. As shown in Figure 10.11, the patient is laid back on the side where the dizziness occurs with his or her head hanging over the edge of the table and slightly to the right. A series of movements are then carried out to gradually move the crystals back into their original position, like moving sand through a hula hoop. The success rate of this procedure is very high and often can result in an immediate return to all activities, with the number of sessions depending on the severity of the case.

Common individualized VRT therapy programs encourage patients to do the opposite of what may come naturally. Inactivity is substituted with safe activity. They may be asked to withdraw from "dizziness medication" that affects the brain and delays recovery. Exercises are demonstrated in the clinic, and the client is given written instructions with specific details, thereby building self-efficacy and preparing the individual to continue therapy at home safely. Counseling, education, and compliance with at-home exercises are crucial to success. Retrospective studies found that 85 percent of those enrolled in a customized VRT program improved and that about 30 percent reported complete recovery (Smith-Wheelock, Shepard, & Telian, 1991). Improvements can be seen in several weeks, with the typical program lasting about two months. These protocols normally are appropriate regardless of age or gender. Older individuals often require longer programs and closer monitoring but experience similar gains in function as younger patients.

Tinnitus Assessment and Management

Tinnitus: A ringing or buzzing sound in the ear that is not caused by external sound stimulation.

Tinnitus is a perception of sound without the presence of an external stimulus. Patients frequently describe tinnitus as a ringing, hissing, or buzzing sound in their ears or head. These sounds can be intermittent or continuous and are frequently high pitched in nature, although they can manifest as a vast array of auditory experiences. Tinnitus can range from a minor annoyance to a debilitating condition. While hearing loss and age have been linked with the experience of tinnitus (Newell et al., 2001; Shargorodsky, Curhan, & Farwell, 2010), not all older people with hearing loss encounter this problem, and not all people with tinnitus have hearing loss. According to ASHA (2015), about 10 to 15 percent of adults have prolonged tinnitus requiring medical evaluation and, consistent with that, the AAA (2001) reported that 40 million to 50 million people in the United States have some presence of tinnitus, with as many as 2.5 million reporting feeling debilitated by the symptom.

There are many causes of tinnitus. Noise exposure, aging, acoustic trauma, head injury, and even excess cerumen have been associated with tinnitus. Ménière's disease, multiple sclerosis, and acoustic neuromas can result in long-term tinnitus. Ototoxic effects from aspirin, certain antibiotics, and chemotherapy can cause deleterious effects on the peripheral and central auditory system that may also result in tinnitus. The brain may be involved in the generation of neural activity that contributes to the perception of tinnitus. There are also many consequences of tinnitus. Tinnitus can be associated with sleep disorders, depression, anxiety, and other medical problems.

Assessment A team approach, including an audiologist, otolaryngologist, and psychologist or psychiatrist, is helpful, especially for severe cases of tinnitus. A thorough medical examination by an otolaryngologist is advised to rule out any significant medical or pharmacologic issues that could cause tinnitus. A psychologist or psychiatrist can be a valuable team member because many patients experience emotional and psychological problems (e.g., depression, anxiety, sleep disorders) as a result of or in addition to tinnitus. Medications can be prescribed for mood or sleep disorders, and therapies, such as biofeedback and cognitive behavioral therapy (CBT), can be provided. The audiologist conducts a comprehensive audiologic assessment and offers sound-based therapy and training. Quantification of the tinnitus is often completed using methods to match the pitch or frequency of the tinnitus, its loudness, and at what levels it can be "masked" by another sound. Loudness discomfort levels are obtained for a variety of stimuli. The tinnitus work-up also includes otoacoustic emission testing. An important facet of the tinnitus evaluation includes exploring how tinnitus affects the person's life. Currently, there are a variety of questionnaires that are used to help assess symptoms and evaluate treatment outcomes. The Tinnitus Functional Index (Meikle et al., 2012) is a comprehensive questionnaire developed by a team of tinnitus experts.

Management A systematic review comparing the effectiveness of various treatments for tinnitus (Pichora-Fuller, M. K., Santaguida, P., Hammill, A., Oremus, M., Westerberg, B., Usman, A., et al..., 2013) concluded that there was insufficient evidence that medical or surgical treatments were effective, weak evidence for the effectiveness of some pharmacological treatments, but stronger evidence for the effectiveness of psychological behavioral treatments, such as CBT. Until recently, there have not been randomized control trials to evaluate the effectiveness of sound-based treatments, although these are in widespread use.

One of the key principles of sound-based tinnitus treatment is to avoid total quiet and develop a rich auditory environment. Sound-based treatment uses technology. For those with hearing loss, amplification of external sounds by a hearing aid can make tinnitus less noticeable. If amplification does not reduce the perception of tinnitus, noise generators or ear-level masking devices may help. Noise generators can be as simple as a radio station or audio recording that diverts attention from the tinnitus to soothing music or the sound of waves breaking on a beach. They can be specifically tuned devices that cover up, or "mask," the tinnitus. Combination devices can generate a specifically tuned sound to mask the tinnitus and also provide amplification. By using these devices, habituation to tinnitus can occur slowly. *Habituation* can be defined as a disappearance in reactions induced by a stimulus. This phenomenon allows for adaptive changes in the central nervous system.

Habituation can be defined as a disappearance in reactions induced by a stimulus.

Most sound-based treatments involve listening retraining. One person can experience a very loud level of tinnitus and find it only mildly annoying, while another finds even the slightest sounds in the head extremely disturbing. Frequently, individuals suffering from clinically significant tinnitus engage in thinking patterns that are counterproductive. Jastreboff coined the term "Tinnitus Habituation Therapy," which has received widespread acceptance as *Tinnitus Retraining Therapy (TRT)*. The objective of TRT is to condition the patient not to respond emotionally to tinnitus. Protocols are designed to make the tinnitus an unimportant sound that is in the background of consciousness (Jastreboff & Jastreboff, 2006). TRT is carried out through directive counseling and sound therapy. Directive counseling is used to educate the patient not to view the tinnitus in a threatening manner. Information

Tinnitus Retraining Therapy (TRT) conditions the patient not to respond emotionally to tinnitus.

is delivered and coping strategies are developed to help make this transition occur. TRT may take months to produce noticeable improvement and up to two years for habituation to be complete.

Cognitive behavioral therapy (CBT) is another psychological approach that has been used successfully to treat tinnitus. It is based on the assumption that the thoughts we have learned over time have a great deal to do with our feelings and subsequent behaviors. By directing individuals away from maladaptive thinking regarding their tinnitus, new cognitive processes and new behaviors can be incorporated into daily living. Therefore, it is not the tinnitus that dictates how you feel but rather the way you think about your tinnitus that influences your response to this condition. For example, some people may feel that because they have tinnitus, they will never be able to enjoy life. Dysfunctional thought patterns can be ingrained in their lives and include minimizing positive information and all-or-nothing thinking patterns that can make dealing with their tinnitus difficult. By challenging these thoughts and learning new ways of thinking, changes can occur in current belief systems. In combination with other psychotherapy techniques and guidance by a skilled therapist, many can find significant relief from tinnitus (Sweetow, 2000).

Some technologies have advanced the research investigating the mechanisms involved in tinnitus. For example, one treatment of tinnitus is transcranial magnetic stimulation (TMS) (Dornhoffer & Mennemeier, 2010). A series of magnetic pulses is delivered over the surface of the cortex to achieve neural reorganization in tinnitus-producing areas of the brain. TMS has been found to alter tinnitus perception in some people; however, tinnitus relief is not always long lasting.

The American Tinnitus Association funds research and provides information to tinnitus sufferers and the professionals who treat patients (American Tinnitus Association, 2005). It also publishes *Tinnitus Today*, a quarterly journal, and maintains an up-to-date website on tinnitus.

Conclusion Tinnitus remains one of the most challenging conditions to treat, but progress continues to be made. The key elements in most therapy plans are to (1) provide counseling so that the patient is not afraid of his or her tinnitus, (2) expose the patient to low levels of background noise, and (3) add some elements of cognitive behavior modification.

Summary

The AR specialist has a unique opportunity to provide services to the adult population over many decades of their life, although the majority of services will be provided to older adults, with the average first-time hearing aid user being in their sixties. Even if AR does not start until an older adult reaches 65 years of age, AR services would span over two decades for those with a typical life expectancy of 85 years and over four decades for those who become centenarians. The complexity of changes occurring in advanced age, together with the difficulties encountered due to auditory deficits, requires that the audiologist become resourceful and willing to tailor established techniques and protocols for the individual and his or her communication partners. The audiologist can contribute to a positive future for aging persons who are hard of hearing—a future that is of higher quality, more productive, and/or less isolated. Better communication skills may promote healthy aging and help lessen the stress caused by other disabilities as well as facilitating ongoing social interaction between older adults and their environments.

The need for specialized training in adult life span changes and gerontology among graduate students specializing in speech and hearing sciences is becoming increasingly apparent as longevity increases and the population ages. The past two decades have seen a substantial growth in our knowledge of aging in general and auditory aging in particular. Following on these advances in research, it is now time for a greater commitment to training in gerontology among graduate programs so that audiologists can take on a leadership role in the care of aging persons who are hard of hearing. Many future innovations will no doubt involve the use of tele-audiology and increasing use of the Internet and wireless communication to build new ways for professionals and clients to interact outside of the four walls of the clinic. Addressing the problems of adults who are hard of hearing is a professional challenge that we must all face together. It is an exciting time to form interprofessional collaborations and work in geriatrics teams united by a common goal to promote active, healthy, and successful aging.

Summary Points

- Adults acquire hearing loss due to illness, accident, noise exposure, and aging, but most lose their hearing through the aging process.

- The population is aging, and many older people with hearing loss also have other health-related health issues that are relevant to AR, including vision, dexterity, balance, and cognition.

- Hearing loss leads to misunderstandings and stress for the individual, family, and friends.

- A number of personal and environmental factors may complicate the situation for older persons with hearing loss.

- Presbycusis is the name for age-related hearing loss (ARHL), but it does not have a single cause.

- Phonemic regression is a common presbycusic problem wherein there is a more severe word recognition problem than would be expected on the basis of hearing thresholds.

- Speech in noise tests such as the WIN, HINT, QuickSIN, MAPA, or LISN-S are more representative of listening ability in the conditions encountered in everyday life.

- It is not uncommon for the majority of a nursing home population to have hearing loss.

- The CORE and CARE models of rehabilitation employed throughout this text provide the framework for rehabilitation assessment and management.

- Rehabilitation settings include university speech and hearing clinics, military facilities, community centers, medical clinics, private practice offices of dispensers, and new tele-audiology services.

- Assessment begins with audiometry and self-report and progresses using a patient-centered or family-centered approach to address concerns about participation, personal, and environmental factors.

- Three self-report measures, the IOI-HA, COSI, and SAC/SOAC (see appendices), are used in assessment and are also extremely valuable later as outcome measures.

- Data logging can be used by the audiologist to track how much and in what kinds of acoustical environments the hearing aid has been used. The SSQ can also be used to appraise the kinds of environments that challenge the client, including the need for binaural or spatial hearing.

- Cell phone or computer-based observational ecological momentary assessment (EMA) methods can be used to gather information about a person's experiences and responses in the moment rather than relying on later recall.

- Rehabilitative goals must be set by considering the current audibility, activity, and participation needs of the individual.

- The personal, social, and physical environmental factors supporting or impeding decision making and action taking must be considered when goals are set.

- Goals should clearly state and specify *who* will do *what*, *how much*, and by *when*.

- Goals must be reevaluated and reset as needed at the time of follow-up, a crucial step in the rehabilitative cycle.

- An essential list of outcome measures should include tests of speech understanding, hearing aid usage, and self-reported benefit and satisfaction.

- Rehabilitation involves change on the part of the individual who is deaf or hard of hearing but may also involve the participation of his or her communication partners or necessitate changes in the physical environment.

- More people will seek and benefit from rehabilitation as technology improves, but it will also be crucial for stigma to be reduced by social change.

- Stereotype threats and low self-efficacy can be counteracted in AR to overcome delays in help-seeking, barriers to action taking, and lapses in the maintenance of target behaviors.

- Even individuals who do not or cannot use amplification might benefit from other forms of AR, such as HATS or cochlear implants.

- Adjustment to hearing loss is a dynamic process that we do not yet fully understand.

- Patients with balance problems or complaining of tinnitus no longer must be told that there are no successful treatment plans available.

- Research in vestibular and tinnitus rehabilitation promises hope to the many individuals suffering from vertigo and tinnitus. New advances in these areas have helped many patients resume active and productive lives.

Supplementary Learning Activities

See www.isu.edu/csed/audiology/rehab to carry out these activities. We encourage you to use these to supplement your learning. Your instructor may give specific assignments that involve a particular activity.

1. Sound environment is an important concept discussed in this chapter. It plays a role in setting AR goals and fitting hearing aids. On the text website, you will find a series of activities that will help you understand your sound environment much better and give you experience in activities that could be helpful to the person who is being fitted with hearing aids or having hearing difficulties.

2. The 2016 Phonak position paper advocates for audiologists to embrace family-centered care. What do you think would be the advantages or disadvantages to this approach? Can you think of a case you have seen where the involvement of the client's family member was important?

3. Look up the WHO guide to age-friendly communities (see "Recommended Websites"). Find out if your community has an age-friendly strategy. Propose three ways that hearing accessibility strategies could help older adults in your community.

4. Evidence-based practice in AR is flourishing with more randomized control trials (RCT) and systematic reviews being published. Find such a study or a systematic review of an AR intervention and explain how you could incorporate the findings of the study into counseling.

5. Look up the WHO ICF Comprehensive Core Set for Hearing (see "Recommended Websites"). Which aspects of hearing problems have been covered best by existing AR measures: impairment, activity, or participation? Do you

think that the coverage has changed with the development of new AR measures over the past 10 years?

6. Interview an older adult with a history of falls or balance problems. Go to the text website to find directions on this activity.

7. Over several days or a week, observe if you perceive occasional or persistent tinnitus. If you do, record the timing and features of the tinnitus (how often, duration of each episode, intensity and pitch) and what may have been linked with its onset.

8. This chapter discusses a number of hearing related self report tools. Study the helpful supplementary materials on self report on the text website under this item 8. For SAC and SOAC you can find mean and standard deviation summaries based on different pure tone configurations. Also, find comparisons with other self reports, and electronic versions of SAC and SOAC.

Recommended Reading

Baguley, D., Andersson, G., & McFerran, D. (2013). *Tinnitus: A multidisciplinary approach* (2nd ed.). Hoboken, NJ: Wiley-Blackwell.

Gordon-Salant, S., Frisina, R. D., Popper, A., & Fay, D. (Eds.). (2009). *The aging auditory system: Perceptual characterization and neural bases of presbycusis*. Berlin: Springer.

Katz, J. (2014). *Handbook of clinical audiology* (7th ed.). Philadelphia: Lippincott Williams & Wilkins.

Kiessling, J., Pichora-Fuller, M. K., Gatehouse, S., Stephens, D., Arlinger, S., Chisolm, T., et al. (2003). Candidature for and delivery of audiological services: Special needs of older people. *International Journal of Audiology*, 42(Suppl. 2), 2S92–2S101.

Pichora-Fuller, M. K., Kramer, S. E., Eckert, M., Edwards, B., Hornsby, B., Humes, L., et al. (2016). Hearing impairment and cognitive energy: The framework for understanding effortful listening (FUEL) [Special Issue]. *Ear and Hearing*, 37(Suppl.), 5S–S27.

Spitzer, J., & Montano, J. (Eds.).(2013) *Adult audiologic rehabilitation: Advanced practices* (2nd ed.). San Diego, CA: Plural Publishing.

Tye-Murray, N. (2015). *Foundations of aural rehabilitation: Children, adults and their family members* (4th ed.). Stamford, CT: Cengage Learning.

Tyler, R. S. (2005). *Tinnitus treatment: Clinical protocols*. New York: Thieme.

Valente, M., & Valente, L. M. (2014). *Adult audiology casebook*. New York: Thieme.

Weinstein, B. (2012). *Geriatric audiology* (2nd ed.). New York: Thieme.

Wong, L., & Hickson, L. (Eds.). (2012). *Evidence-based practice in audiology: Evaluating interventions for children and adults with hearing impairment*. San Diego, CA: Plural Publishing.

Worrall, L., & Hickson, L. (2003). *Communication disability in aging: Prevention and intervention*. San Diego, CA: Singular Publishing.

Recommended Websites

World Health Organization (WHO) Resources

World Health Organization *Comprehensive ICF Core Set for Hearing Loss*:

http://www.icf-research-branch.org/search?searchword=Hearing&searchphrase=all

World Health Organization *International Classification of Functioning, Disability, and Health*:

http://www.who.int/classifications/icf/en

World Health Organization *Global Age-Friendly Cities: A Guide*:

http://www.who.int/ageing/publications/Global_age_friendly_cities_Guide_English .pdf?ua=1

World Health Organization *Make Listening Safe*:

http://www.who.int/pbd/deafness/activities/MLS/en

http://www.who.int/pbd/deafness/activities/MLS_Brochure_English_lowres_for_web.pdf

World Health Organization *World Report on Ageing and Health*:

http://www.who.int/ageing/publications/world-report-2015/en

Consumer Associations and Resources for the Public

AARP *Consumer Guide to Hearing Aids*:

https://assets.aarp.org/www.aarp.org_/articles/health/docs/hearing_guide.pdf

International Federation of Hard of Hearing People:

http://www.internationaldisabilityalliance.org/IFHOH

http://www.IFHOH.org

Hearing Loss Association of America (HLAA) Policy Statements, Advocacy Agenda and CART:

http://www.hearingloss.org/content/policy-statements

http://www.hearingloss.org/content/advocacy-people-hearing-loss

http://www.hearingloss.org/content/captioning-and-cart

American Tinnitus Association:

https://www.ata.org

Tinnitus Research Initiative:

http://www.tinnitusresearch.net

NIDCD on Tinnitus:

https://www.nidcd.nih.gov/health/tinnitus

McMaster University Optimal Aging Portal:

https://www.mcmasteroptimalaging.org

Gael Hannan: Hearing Loss Advocate, Writer, Speaker, Humorist:

http://www.gaelhannan.com/bio

Websites about AR Tools

Outcome measurement from ISU site:

http://www2.isu.edu/csed/audiology/profile

Perry Hanavan's site that defines AR and includes about 30 links:

http://www.augie.edu/perry/ear/ardefine.htm

International Collegium of Rehabilitative Audiology (SSQ; IOI in English and other languages):

https://icra-audiology.org/Repository/self-report-repository/IOI-HA%20list-of-questionnaires

Glasgow Hearing Aid Benefit Profile (GHABP):

http://studentacademyofaudiology.com/sites/default/files/journal/JAAA_10_02_03.pdf

National Acoustics Laboratory Australia (COSI and LISN-S):

https://www.nal.gov.au/outcome-measures_tab_peach.shtml

https://capd.nal.gov.au/lisn-s-about.shtml

"Apps with Amps" by S. Lesner and M. Klingler:

http://leader.pubs.asha.org/article.aspx?articleid=2280067

Listening and Communication Enhancement (LACE):
https://www.neurotone.com/lace-interactive-listening-program

Montreal Cognitive Assessment (MoCA):
http://www.mocatest.org

References

Abrams, H. B., (2000). Outcome measures in audiology: Knowing we've made a difference. *Audiology Online*. http://www.audiologyonline.com/articles/outcome-measures-in-audiology-knowing-1277

Abrams, H. B., Kihm, J. (2015). An introduction to MarkeTrak IX: A new baseline for the hearing aid market. *Hearing Review*, 22(6), 16. http://www.hearingreview.com/2015/05/introduction-marketrak-ix-new-baseline-hearing-aid-market

Agrawal, Y., Platz, E. A., & Niparko, J. K. (2009). Risk factors for hearing loss in US adults: data from the National Health and Nutrition Examination Survey, 1999 to 2002. *Otology and Neurotology*, 30(2), 139–145.

Albers, M. W., Gilmore, G. C., Kaye, J., Murphy, C., Wingfield, A., Bennett, D. A.,et al. (2015). At the interface of sensory and motor dysfunctions and Alzheimer's disease. *Alzheimer's and Dementia*, 11(1), 70–98.

American Academy of Audiology. (2001, March/April). American Academy of Audiology position statement on audiologic guidelines for the diagnosis and management of tinnitus patients. *Audiology Today*, 13, 2.

American Academy of Audiology. (2005). Position statement on the audiologist's role in the diagnosis and treatment of vestibular disorders. *Audiology Today*, 17.

American Speech-Language-Hearing Association. (2014). 2014 audiology survey: Clinical focus patterns. http://www.asha.org/uploadedFiles/2014-Audiology-Survey-Clinical-Focus-Patterns.pdf

American Speech-Language-Hearing Association. (2015). Tinnitus. http://www.asha.org/public/hearing/Tinnitus

American Tinnitus Association. (2005). About ATA. http://www.ata.org/about_ata

Amsel, B. E., & Weinstein, B. E. (1986). Hearing loss and senile dementia in the institutionalized elderly. *Clinical Gerontologist*, 4, 3–15.

Arlinger, S., Lunner, T., Lyxell, B., & Pichora-Fuller, M. K. (2009). The emergence of cognitive hearing science. *Scandinavian Journal of Psychology*, 50, 371–384.

Baguley, D., Andersson, G., & McFerran, D. (2013). *Tinnitus: A multidisciplinary approach* (2nd ed.). Hoboken, NJ: Wiley-Blackwell.

Bainbridge, K. E., & Wallhagen, M. I. (2014). Hearing loss in an aging American population: Extent, impact, and management. *Annual Review of Public Health*, 35, 139–152.

Baltes, M. M., & Wahl, H-W. (1996). Patterns of communication in old age: The dependence-support and independence-ignore script. *Health Communication*, 8(3), 217–231.

Bandura, A. (1997). *Self efficacy: The exercise of control*. New York: Freeman.

Banh, J., Singh, G., & Pichora-Fuller, M. K. (2012). Age affects responses on the Speech, Spatial, and Qualities of Hearing Scale (SSQ) for adults with minimal audiometric loss. *Journal of the American Academy of Audiology*, 23, 81–91.

Bargh, J. A., Chen, M., & Burrows, L. (1996). The automaticity of social behaviour: Direct effects of trait concept and stereotype activation on action. *Journal of Personality and Social Psychology*, 71, 230–244.

Barker, F., Mackenzie, E., Elliott, L., Jones, S., & de Lusignan, S. (2016). Interventions to improve hearing aid use in adult auditory rehabilitation. *Cochrane Database of Systematic Reviews*, 8.

Beck, D. L., & Le Goff, N. (2016). A paradigm shift in hearing aid technology. *Hearing Review*, 23(6),18. http://www.hearingreview.com/2016/05/paradigm-shift-hearing-aid-technology

Besser, J., Festen, J. M., Goverts, S. T., Kramer, S. E., & Pichora-Fuller, M. K. (2015). Speech-in-speech listening on the LiSN-S test by older adults with good audiograms depends on cognition and hearing acuity at high frequencies. *Ear and Hearing*, 36, 24–41.

Birk-Nielsen, H. (1974). Effect of monaural versus binaural hearing and treatment. *Scandinavian Audiology, 3,* 183–187.

Blazer, D. G., Domnitz, S., & Liverman, C. T. (Eds.). (2016). *Hearing health care for adults: Priorities for improving access and affordability.* Washington, DC: National Academy Press. http://www.nap.edu/23446

Boger, J., & Mihailidis, A. (2011). The future of intelligent assistive technologies for cognition: Devices under development to support independent living and aging-with-choice. *NeuroRehabilitation, 28,* 271–280.

Boothroyd, A. (2007). Adult aural rehabilitation: What is it and does it work? *Trends in Amplification, 11*(2), 63–71.

Brabyn, J. A., Schneck, M. E., Haegerstrom-Portnoy, G., & Lott, L. A. (2007). Dual sensory loss: Overview of problems, visual assessment, and rehabilitation. *Trends in Amplification, 11*(4), 219–226.

Broadhead, W., Gehlbach, S., de Gruy, F., Kaplan, B. H. (1988). The Duke-UNC Functional Social Support Questionnaire: Measurement of social support in family medicine patients. *Medical Care, 26,* 709–723.

Brockett, J., & Schow, R. L. (2001). Web site profiles common hearing loss patterns. *Hearing Journal, 54*(8), 20.

Brooks, D. (1989). The effect of attitude on benefit obtained from hearing aids. *British Journal of Audiology, 23,* 3–11.

Cabeza, R., Anderson, N., Locantore, J. K., & McIntosh, A. R. (2002). Aging gracefully: Compensatory brain activity in high-performing older adults. *NeuroImage, 17,* 1394–1402.

Cameron, S., & Dillon, H. (2007). Development of the Listening in Spatialized Noise-Sentences Test (LISN-S). *Ear and Hearing, 28,* 196–211.

Cameron, S., Glyde, H., & Dillon, H. (2011). Listening in Spatialized Noise-Sentences Test (LiSN-S): Normative and retest reliability data for adolescents and adults up to 60 years of age. *Journal of the American Academy of Audiology, 22,* 697–709.

Carson, A. J. (1997). Evaluation of the "To Hear Again" program. *Journal of Speech–Language Pathology and Audiology, 21,* 160–166.

Carson, A. J., (2005). "What brings you here today?" The role of self-assessment in help-seeking for age-related hearing loss. *Journal of Aging Studies, 19,* 185–200.

Chasteen, A., Pichora-Fuller, M. K., Dupuis, K., Smith, S., & Singh, G. (2015). Do negative views of aging influence memory and auditory performance through self-perceived abilities? *Psychology and Aging, 30*(4), 881–893.

Chien, W., & Lin, F. R. (2012). Prevalence of hearing aid use among older adults in the United States. *Archives of Internal Medicine, 172,* 292–293.

Chou, R., Dana, T., Bougatsos, C., Fleming, C., & Bell, T. (2011). Screening adults aged 50 years or older for hearing loss: A review of the evidence for the US Preventive Services Task Force. *Annals of International Medicine, 154*(5), 347–355.

Clark, P. G. (1996). Communication between provider and patient: Values, biography, and empowerment in clinical practice. *Aging and Society, 16,* 747–774.

Cleveland-Nielsen, A., Ingo, E., Grenness, C., & Laplante-Lévesque, A.,. (2016). eHealth Activities and Hearing Aids-A Systematic Review. Presented at the British Society of Audiology Annual Conference 2016, April 25–27. Downloaded on March 31, 2017 from http://www.eriksholm.com/publications.aspx

Committee on Hearing, Bioacoustics, and Biomechanics. (1988). Speech understanding and aging. *Journal of the Acoustical Association of America, 83,* 859–895.

Coupland, N., Wiemann, J. M., & Giles, H. (1991). Talk as "Problem" and communication as "Miscommunication": An integrative analysis. In N. Coupland, H. Giles, & J. M. Wiemann (Eds.), *"Miscommunication" and problematic talk* (pp. 1–17). Newbury Park, CA: Sage.

Cox, R. M. (2005). Choosing a self-report measure for hearing aid fitting outcomes. *Seminars in Hearing, 26*(3), 149–156.

Cox, R. M., Alexander, G. C., & Gray, G. A. (2005). Who wants a hearing aid? Personality profiles of hearing aid seekers. *Ear and Hearing, 26,* 12–26.

Cox, R. M., Alexander, G. C., & Gray, G. A. (2007). Personality, hearing problems, and amplification characteristics: Contributions to self-report hearing aid outcomes. *Ear and Hearing, 28,* 141–162.

Cox, R., Hyde, M., Gatehouse, S., Noble, W., Dillon, H., Bentler, R., et al. (2000). Optimal outcome measures, research priorities, and international cooperation. *Ear and Hearing, 21*(4, Suppl.), 106S–115S.

Criter, R. E., & Honaker, J. A., (2013). Falls in the audiology clinic: A pilot study. *Journal of the American Academy of Audiology, 24*(10), 1001–1005.

Criter, R. E., & Honaker, J. A. (2016). Audiology patient fall statistics and risk factors compared to non-audiology patients. *International Journal of Audiology, 55*(10), 564–570.

Czaja, S. J., Charness, N., Fisk, A. D., Hertzog, C., Nair, S. N., Rogers, W. A., et al. (2006). Factors predicting the use of technology: Findings from the Center for Research and Education on Aging and Technology Enhancement (CREATE). *Psychology and Aging, 21*, 333–352.

Dahl, M. (1997). To Hear Again: A volunteer program in hearing health care for hard-of-hearing seniors. *Journal of Speech–Language Pathology and Audiology, 21*, 153–159.

Davis, A., & Davis, K. (2009). Epidemiology of aging and hearing loss related to other chronic illnesses. In L. Hickson (Ed.), *Hearing care for adults* (pp. 23–32). Stäfa: Phonak.

Davis, A., McMahon, C., Pichora-Fuller, M. K., Russ, S., Lin, F., Olusanya, B.O. et al. (2016). Ageing and hearing health: The life-course approach. *The Gerontologist, 56*(Suppl. 2), S256–S267.

Davis, A., Smith, P., Ferguson, M., Stephens, D., & Gianopoulos, I. (2007). Acceptability, benefit and costs of early screening for hearing disability: A study of potential screening tests and models. *Health Technology Assessment, 11*(42). http://www.hta.ac.uk/project/1025.asp

Demeester, K., Topsakal, V., Hendrickx, J. J., Fransen, E., van Laer, L., Van Camp, G., et al. (2012). Hearing disability measured by the speech, spatial, and qualities of hearing scale in clinically normal-hearing and hearing-impaired middle-aged persons, and disability screening by means of a reduced SSQ (the SSQ5). *Ear and Hearing, 33*(5), 615–626.

Dennis, K. C. (2009). Current perspectives on traumatic brain injury. http://www.asha.org/aud/articles/CurrentTBI.htm

Desmond, A. L. (2000). Vestibular rehabilitation. In M. Valente, H. Hosford-Dunn, & R. J. Roser (Eds.), *Audiology treatment*, 639–667, New York: Thieme.

Dillon, H., James, A., & Ginis, J. (1997). Client Oriented Scale of Improvement (COSI) and its relationship to several other measures of benefit and satisfaction provided by hearing aids. *Journal of the American Academy of Audiology, 8*(1), 27–43.

Dillon, H., & So, M. (2000). Incentives and obstacles to the routine use of outcome measures by clinicians. *Ear and Hearing, 21*(4, Suppl.), 2S–6S.

Doherty, K. A., & Desjardins, J. L. (2012). The Practical Hearing Aid Skills Test—Revised. *American Journal of Audiology, 21*, 100–105.

Dornhoffer, J., & Mennemeier, M. 2010 Using repetitive magnetic stimulation for the treatment of tinnitus. *Hearing Journal, 63*(11), 16–18, 20.

Dupuis, K., Pichora-Fuller, M. K., Marchuk, V., Chasteen, A., Singh, G., & Smith, S.L. (2015). Effects of hearing and vision impairments on performance on the Montreal Cognitive Assessment. *Aging, Neuropsychology, and Cognition, 22*(4), 413–427.

Echt, K. E., & Saunders, G. H. (2014). Accommodating dual sensory loss in everyday practice. *American Speech-Language-Hearing Association Sig 15 Perspectives on Gerontology, 19*, 4–16.

Eliassen, A. H. (2016). Power relations and health care communication in older adulthood: Educating recipients and providers. *The Gerontologist, 56*, 990–996.

Erber, N. P. (1988). *Communication therapy for hearing-impaired adults.* Victoria: Clavis Publishing.

Erber, N. P. (1996). *Communication therapy for adults with sensory loss* (2nd ed.). Melbourne: Clavis Publishing.

Fabry, D. (2005). DataLogging: A clinical tool for meeting individual patient needs. *Hearing Review.* http://www.hearingreview.com/issues/articles/2005-01_05.asp

Facility Guidelines Institute. (2014a). *Guidelines for design and construction of hospitals and outpatient facilities.* Chicago: American Society for Healthcare Engineering of the American Hospital Association.

Facility Guidelines Institute. (2014b). *Guidelines for design and construction of residential health, care, and support facilities.* Chicago: American Society for Healthcare Engineering of the American Hospital Association.

Fagelson, M. A., & Smith, S. L. (2016). Tinnitus self-efficacy and other tinnitus self-report variables in patients with and without post-traumatic stress disorder. *Ear and Hearing, 37*(5), 541–546.

Ferguson, M. A., & Henshaw, H. (2015). Auditory training can improve working memory, attention, and communication in adverse conditions for adults with hearing loss. *Frontiers in Psychology, 6,* 556.

Fisher, D., Li, C.-M., Chiu, M. S., Themann, C. L., Petersen, H., Jonasson, F., et al. (2014). Impairments in hearing and vision impact on mortality in older people: The AGES-Reykjavik Study. *Age and Ageing, 43*(1), 69–76.

Frankish, C. J., Green, L. W., Ratner, P.A., Chomik, T., & Larsen, C. (1996). Health impact assessment as a tool for population health promotion and public policy: A report submitted to the health promotion development division of Health Canada. http://catalogue.iugm.qc.ca/GEIDEFile/healthimpact.PDF?Archive=192469191064

Fraser, S. A., Kenyon, V., Lagacé, M., Wittich, W., & Southall, K. E. (2016). Stereotypes associated with age-related conditions and assistive device use in Canadian media. *The Gerontologist, 56,* 1023–1032.

Fratiglioni, L., Paillard-Borg, S., & Winblad, B. (2004). An active and socially integrated lifestyle in late life might protect against dementia. *The Lancet Neurology, 3*(6), 343–353.

Gaeth, J. (1948). *A study of phonemic regression associated with hearing loss.* Unpublished doctoral dissertation, Northwestern University, Evanston, IL.

Gagné, J.-P. (2000). What is treatment evaluation research? What is its relationship to the goals of audiologic rehabilitation? Who are the stakeholders of this type of research? *Ear and Hearing, 21*(4, Suppl.), 60S–73S.

Gagné, J.-P., Jennings, M. B., & Southall, K. (2009). Understanding stigma associated with hearing loss in older adults. In L. Hickson (Ed.), *Hearing care for adults* (pp. 203–212). Stäfa: Phonak.

Gagné J.-P., McDuff, S., & Getty, L. (1999). Some limitations of evaluative investigations based solely on normed outcome measures. *Journal of the American Academy of Audiology, 10,* 46–62.

Gagné, J.-P., & Wittich, W. (2009). Visual impairment and audiovisual speech perception in older adults with acquired hearing loss. In L. Hickson (Ed.), *Hearing care for adults* (pp. 165–178). Stäfa: Phonak.

Galvez, G., Turbin, M. B., Thielman, E. J., Istvan, J. A., Andrews, J. A., & Henry, J. A. (2012). Feasibility of ecological momentary assessment of hearing difficulties encountered by hearing aid users. *Ear and Hearing, 3,* 497–507.

Gatehouse, S. (1999). Glasgow Hearing Aid Benefit Profile: Derivation and validation of a client-centered outcome measure for hearing-aid services. *Journal of the American Academy of Audiology, 10,* 80–103.

Gatehouse, S., Naylor, G., & Elberling, C. (2006). Linear and nonlinear hearing and fittings. 1. Patterns of benefit. *International Journal of Audiology, 45,* 130–152.

Gatehouse, S., & Noble, W. (2004). The Speech, Spatial and Qualities of Hearing Scale (SSQ). *International Journal of Audiology, 43*(2), 85–89.

Gates, G. A., Beiser, A., Rees, T. S., Agostino, R. B., & Wolf, P. A. (2002). Central auditory dysfunction may precede the onset of clinical dementia in people with probably Alzheimer's disease. *Journal of the American Geriatric Society, 50,* 482–488.

Gates, G. A., & Mills, J. H. (2005). Presbycusis. *The Lancet, 366,* 1111–1120.

Gladden, C., Beck, L., & Chandler, D. (2015). Tele-audiology: Expanding access to hearing care and enhancing patient connectivity. *Journal of the American Academy of Audiology, 26*(9), 792–799.

Gonsalves, C., & Pichora-Fuller, M. K. (2008). Effect of hearing ability on use of communication technology by older adults. *Canadian Journal on Aging, 27,* 145–157.

Gordon-Salant, S., Frisina, R. D., Popper, A., & Fay, D. (Eds.). (2010). *The aging auditory system: Perceptual characterization and neural bases of presbycusis.* Berlin: Springer.

Grady, C. (2012). The cognitive neuroscience of ageing. *Nature Reviews Neuroscience, 13,* 491–505.

Granberg, S., Swanepoel de W, Englund U, Möller C, Danermark B., (2014). The ICF Core Sets for Hearing Loss Project: International expert survey on functioning and disability of adults with hearing loss using the International Classification of Functioning, Disability, and Health (ICF). *International Journal of Audiology, 53*(8), 497–506.

Grenness, C, Meyer C[2], Scarinci N[2], Ekberg K[2], Hickson L[2]. (2016). The International Classification of Functioning, Disability and Health as a framework for providing patient- and family-centered audiological care for older adults and their significant others. *Seminars in Hearing, 37*(3), 187–199.

Hallberg, L., & Carlsson, S. (1991). A qualitative study of strategies for managing a hearing impairment. *British Journal of Audiology, 25,* 201–211.

Hallberg, L. R., & Jansson, G. (1996). Women with noise-induced hearing loss: An invisible group? *British Journal of Audiology, 30*(5), 340–345.

Hannan, G. (2015). *The way I hear it: A life with hearing loss.*: Victoria: Friesen Press.

He, W., & Larsen, L. J. (2014). *Older Americans with a disability: 2008–2012.* Washington, DC: U.S. Government Printing Office, https://www.census.gov/content/dam/Census/library/publications/2014/acs/acs-29.pdf

Henshaw, H., McCormack, A., & Ferguson, M. A. (2015). Intrinsic and extrinsic motivation is associated with computer-based auditory training uptake, engagement, and adherence for people with hearing loss. *Frontiers in Psychology, 6,* 1067.

Hétu, R. (1996). The stigma attached to hearing impairment. *Scandinavian Audiology, 25*(Suppl. 43), 12–24.

Hétu, R., Jones, L., & Getty, L. (1993). The impact of acquired hearing impairment on intimate relationships: Implications for rehabilitation. *Audiology, 32,* 363–381.

Hickson, L. (Ed.). (2009). *Hearing care for adults.* Stäfa: Phonak.

Hickson, L., Worrall, L , & Scarinci, N. (2007a). *Active Communication Education (ACE): A program for older people with hearing impairment.* Bradwell Abbey: Speechmark Publishing.

Hickson, L., Worrall, L., & Scarinci, N. (2007b). A randomized controlled trial evaluating the Active Communication Education program for older people with hearing impairment. *Ear and Hearing, 28,* 212–230.

Hobeika, C. P. (1999). Equilibrium and balance in the elderly. *Ear, Nose and Throat Journal, 78*(8), 558–562.

Hodes, M., Schow, R. L., & Brockett, J. (2009) New support for hearing aid outcome measures: The computerized SAC and SOAC. *Hearing Review, 16*(12), 26–36.

Hoek, D., Pichora-Fuller, M. K., Paccioretti, D., MacDonald, M. A., & Shyng, G. (1997). Community outreach to hard-of-hearing seniors. *Journal of Speech–Language Pathology and Audiology, 21,* 199–208.

Hornsby, B. Y., Naylor, G., & Bess, F. H. (2016). A taxonomy of fatigue concepts and their relation to hearing loss. *Ear and Hearing, 37*(Suppl. 1), 136S–144S.

Humes, L. E., Busey, T. A., Craig, J. & Kewley-Port, D. (2013). Are age-related changes in cognitive function driven by age-related changes in sensory processing? *Attention, Perception and Psychophysics, 75,* 508–524.

Humes, L. E., Dubno, J. R., Gordon-Salant, S., Lister, J. J., Cacace, A. T., Cruickshanks KJ, et al. (2012). Central presbycusis: A review and evaluation of the evidence. *Journal of the American Academy of Audiology, 23,* 635–666.

Humes, L. E., & Wilson, D. L. (2003). An examination of changes in hearing-aid performance and benefit in the elderly over a 3-year period of hearing-aid use. *Journal of Speech, Language, and Hearing Research, 46,* 137–145.

Institute of Medicine. (2014). *Hearing loss and healthy aging: Workshop summary.* Washington, DC: National Academies Press. https://www.ncbi.nlm.nih.gov/books/NBK202191

International Organization for Standardization. (2000). *Acoustics: Statistical distribution of hearing thresholds as a function of age* (SIO 7029). Geneva: Author.

International Organization for Standardization. (2011). No more squinting at small print or leaning forward to hear properly—Thanks to new ISO standards. http://www.iso.org/iso/pressrelease.htm?refid=Ref1397

Jacobson, G. P., & Newman, C. W. (1990). The development of the Dizziness Handicap Inventory (DHI). *Archives of Otolaryngology–Head and Neck Surgery, 116,* 424–427.

Jastreboff, P. J. & Jastreboff, M. M. (2006). Tinnitus Retraining Therapy: A different view of tinnitus. *Journal of Oto-Rhino-Laryngology, 68,* 23–30.

Jaworski, A., & Stephens, D. (1998). Self-reports on silence as a face-saving strategy by people with hearing impairment. *International Journal of Applied Linguistics, 8,* 61–80.

Jennings, M. B. (2009). Hearing accessibility and assistive technology use by older adults: Application of universal design principles to hearing. In L. Hickson (Ed.), *Hearing care for adults* (pp. 249–254). Stäfa: Phonak.

Jenstad, L., & Moon, J. (2011). Systematic review of barriers and facilitators to hearing aid uptake in older adults. *Audiology Research*, *1*, e25. https://www.ncbi.nlm.nih .gov/pmc/articles/PMC4627148/pdf/audio-2011-1-e25.pdf

Jenstad, L. M., Van Tasell, D. J., & Ewert, C. (2003). Hearing aid troubleshooting based on patients' descriptions. *Journal of the American Academy of Audiology*, *14*(7), 347–360.

Jerger, J., Oliver, T., & Pirozzolo, F. (1990). Speech understanding in the elderly. *Journal of the American Academy of Audiology*, *1*, 17–81.

Jorgensen, L. E., & Messersmith, J. J. (2015). Impact of aging and cognition on hearing assistive technology use. *Seminars in Hearing*, *36*, 162–174.

Jorgensen, L. E., Palmer, C. V., Pratt, S., Erickson, K. I., & Moncrieff, D. (2016). The effect of decreased audibility on MMSE performance: A measure commonly used for diagnosing dementia. *Journal of the American Academy of Audiology*, *27*, 311–323.

Jung, D., & Bhattacharyya, N. (2012). Association of hearing loss with decreased employment and income among adults in the United States. *Annals of Otology, Rhinology and Laryngology*, *121*(12), 771–775.

Karpa, M. J., Gopinath, B., Beath, K., Rochtchina, E., Cumming, R. G., Wang J. J., et. al. (2010). Associations between hearing impairment and mortality risk in older persons: The Bluce Mountains Study. *Annals of Epidemiology*, *20(6)*, 452-9.

Keidser, G. (2016). Introduction to special issue: Toward ecologically valid protocols for the assessment of hearing and hearing devices. *Journal of the American Academy of Audiology*, *27*(7), 502–503.

Kiessling, J., Pichora-Fuller, M. K., Gatehouse, S., Stephens, D., Arlinger, S., Chisolm, T., et al. (2003). Candidature for and delivery of audiological services: Special needs of older people. *International Journal of Audiology*, *42*(Suppl. 2), S292–2S101.

Killion, M. C., Niquette, P. A., Gudmundsen, G. I., Revit, L. J., & Nanerjee, S. (2004). Development of a quick speech-in-noise test for measuring signal-to-noise ratio loss in normal-hearing and hearing-impaired listeners. *Journal of the Acoustical Society of America*, *116*, 2395–2405.

Knudsen, L. V., Öberg, M., Nielsen, C., Naylor, G., & Kramer, S. (2010). Factors influencing help seeking, hearing aid uptake, hearing aid use and satisfaction with hearing aids: A review of the literature. *Trends in Amplification*, *14*(3), 127–154.

Kochkin, S. (2007). MarkeTrak VII: Obstacles to adult non-user adoption of hearing aids. *The Hearing Journal*, *60*(4), 24–51.

Kochkin, S., Beck, D. L., Christensen, L. A., Compton-Conley, C., Fligor, B. J., Kricos, P. B., et al. (2010). MarkeTrak VIII: The impact of the hearing healthcare professional on hearing aid user success: Correlations between dispensing protocols and successful patient outcomes *Hearing Review*, *17*(4), 12–34.

Krach, C. A., & Velkoff, V. V. (1999). *Centenarians in the United States*. Washington, DC: U.S. Government Printing Office. http://www.census.gov/prod/99pubs/p23-199.pdf

Kraus, N., & White-Schwoch, T. (2016). Not-so-hidden hearing loss. *Hearing Journal*, *69*(5), 38, 40.

Kricos, P. (2000). Influence nonaudiological variables on audiological rehabilitation outcomes. *Ear and Hearing*, *21*(4), 7S–15S.

Kricos, P. (2006). Audiologic management of older adults with hearing loss and compromised cognitive/psychoacoustic auditory processing capabilities. *Trends in Amplification*, *10*, 1–28.

Kujawa, S. G., & Liberman, M. C. (2009). Adding insult to injury: Cochlear nerve degeneration after "temporary" noise-induced hearing loss. *Journal of Neuroscience*, *29*(45), 14077–14085.

Lane, K. R. (2015). Improving policies hearing loss in long term care environments. *The Gerontologist*, *55*(Suppl. 2), 275.

Laplante-Lévesque, A., Hickson, L., & Worrall, L. (2010). A qualitative study on shared decision making in rehabilitative audiology. *Journal of the Academy of Rehabilitative Audiology*, *43*, 27–43.

Laplante-Lévesque, A., Hickson, L., & Worrall, L. (2013). Stages of change in adults with acquired hearing impairment seeking help for the first time: Application of the transtheoretical model in audiologic rehabilitation. *Ear and Hearing*, *34*(4), 447–457.

Lau, S.-T., Pichora-Fuller, M. K., Li, K., Singh, G., & Campos, J. (2016). Effects of hearing loss on dual-task performance in an audiovisual virtual reality simulation of listening while walking. *Journal of the American Academy of Audiology*, *27*, 567–587.

Lazarus, R. S., & Folkman, S. (1984). *Stress, appraisal and coping.* New York: Springer.

Lesner, S. A. (2003). Candidacy and management of assistive listening devices: Special needs of the elderly. *International Journal of Audiology, 42*(2), S68–S76.

Lesner, S. A., & Klingler, M. (2011). Apps with amps: Mobile devices, hearing assistive technology, and older adults. *The ASHA Leader, 16*, 14–17. http://leader.pubs.asha .org/article.aspx?articleid=2280067

Levy, B. R., Slade, M. D., & Gill, T. (2006). Hearing decline predicted by elders' age stereotypes. *Journal of Gerontology. Series B, Psychological Sciences, 61*, 82–87.

Lewsen, B. J., & Cashman, M. (1997). Hearing aids and assistive listening devices in long-term care. *Journal of Speech–Language Pathology and Audiology, 21*(3), 149–152.

Li, F., Simosick, E. M., Ferrucci, L., & Lin, F. R. (2013). Hearing loss and gait speed among older adults in the United States. *Gait Posture, 38*, 25–29.

Lin, F. R., & Ferrucci, L. (2012). Hearing loss and falls among older adults in the United States. *Archives of Internal Medicine, 172*, 292–293.

Lin, F. R., Metter, E. J., O'Brien, R. J., Resnick, S. M., Zonderman, A. B., & Ferrucci, L. (2011). Hearing loss and incident dementia. *Archives Neurology, 68*(2), 214–220.

Lin, M. Y., Gutierrez, P. R., Stone, K. L., Yaffe, K., Ensrud, K. E., Fink, H. A., et al. (2004). Vision impairment and combined vision and hearing impairment predict cognitive and functional decline in older women. *Journal of the American Geriatrics Society, 52*, 1996–2002.

Lind, C. (2009). Conversation therapy: Interaction as intervention. In L. Hickson (Ed.), *Hearing care for adults* (pp. 103–110). Stäfa: Phonak.

Lopez-Poveda, E. A. (2014). Why do I hear but not understand? Stochastic undersampling as a model of degraded neural encoding of speech. *Frontiers in Neuroscience, 8*, 348.

Lunner, T., Rönnberg, J., & Rudner, M. (2009). Cognition and hearing aids. *Scandinavian Journal of Psychology, 50*, 395–403.

Lupien, S. J., McEwen, B. S., Gunnar, M. R., & Heim, C. (2009). Effects of stress throughout the lifespan on the brain, behavior and cognition. *Nature Reviews Neuroscience, 10*, 434–445.

Lupien, S., Sindi, S., & Wan, N. (2012). *When we test, do we stress? Guidelines for health professionals and scientists working with older adults.* Montreal: Centre for Studies on Human Stress. http://www.humanstress.ca/documents/pdf/KT/KT_document_EN.pdf

Margolis, R. H., Killion, M. C., Bratt, G. W., & Saly, G. L. (2016). Validation of the Home Hearing Test™. *Journal of the American Academy of Audiology, 27*(5), 416–420.

Maurer, J. E. (1976). Auditory impairment and aging. In B. Jacobs (Ed.), *Working with the impaired elderly* (p. 72). Washington, DC: National Council on the Aging.

Maurer, J. E. (1979). Aural rehabilitation for the aging. In L. J. Bradford & W. G. Hardy (Eds.), *Hearing and hearing impairment* (pp. 319–338). New York: Grune & Stratton.

Meikle, M. B., Henry, J. A., Griest, S. E., Stewart, B. J., Abrams, H. B., McArdle, R., et al. (2012). The Tinnitus Functional Index: Development of a new clinical measure for chronic, intrusive tinnitus. *Ear and Hearing, 33*(2), 153–176.

Meyer, C, Grenness C[2], Scarinci N[1], Hickson L[1]. (2016). What is the International Classification of Functioning, Disability and Health and why is it relevant to audiology? *Seminars in Hearing, 37*(3), 163–186.

Mick, P. T., Kawachi, I., & Lin, F. R. (2014). The association between hearing loss and social isolation in older adults. *Otolaryngology—Head and Neck Surgery, 150*(3), 378–384.

Mick, P. T., & Pichora-Fuller, M. K. (2016). Is hearing loss associated with poorer health in older adults who might benefit from hearing screening? *Ear and Hearing, 37*(3), e194–e201.

Millington, D. (2001). *Audiologic rehabilitation practices of ASHA audiologists: Survey 2000.* Unpublished master's thesis, Idaho State University, Pocatello.

Mills, J. H., Schmiedt, R. A., Schulte, B. A., & Dubno, J. R. (2006). Age-related hearing loss: A loss of voltage, not hair cells. *Seminars in Hearing, 27*(4), 228–236.

Moyer, V. A., on behalf of the U.S. Preventive Services Task Force. (2012). Screening for hearing loss in older adults: U.S. Preventive Services Task Force Recommendation Statement. *Annals of Internal Medicine, 157*, 655–661.

Nasreddine, Z. S., Phillips, N. A., Bédirian, V., Charbonneau S, Whitehead V, Collin I, et al. (2005). The Montreal Cognitive Assessment, MoCA: A brief screening tool for mild cognitive impairment. *Journal of the American Geriatrics Society, 53*, 695–699.

Neemes, J. (2003). Despite benefits of outcomes measures, advocates say they're underused. *Hearing Journal, 8,* 19–25.

Nelson, M. D., Akin, F. Q., Riska, K. M., Andresen, K., & Mondelli, S. S. (2016). Vestibular assessment and rehabilitation: Ten-year survey trends of audiologists' opinions and practice. *Journal of the American Academy of Audiology, 27,* 126–140.

Newell, P., Mitchell, P., Sindhussake, D., Golding, M., Wigney, D. Hartley, D., et al. (2001). Tinnitus in older people: It is a widespread problem. *Hearing Journal, 54*(11), 14–18.

Nilsson, M., Soli, S. D., & Sullivan, J. A. (1994). Development of the Hearing in Noise Test for the measurement of speech reception thresholds in quiet and in noise. *Journal of the Acoustical Society of America, 95,* 1085–1099.

Noble, W. (1998). *Self-assessment of hearing and related functions.* London: Whurr.

Noble, W. (2002). Extending the IOI to significant others and to non-hearing-aid based interventions. *International Journal of Audiology, 41,* 27–29.

Noble, W. (2010). Assessing binaural hearing: Results using the Speech, Spatial and Qualities of Hearing Scale. *Journal of the American Academy of Audiology, 21,* 568–574.

Noble, W., Jensen, N. S., Naylor, G., Bhullar, N., & Akeroyd, M. A. (2013). A short form of the Speech, Spatial and Qualities of Hearing scale suitable for clinical use: The SSQ12. *International Journal of Audiology, 53*(6), 409–412.

Oberg M[1], Bohn T[2], Larsson U[2], Hickson L[3]. (2014) A preliminary evaluation of the active communication education program in a sample of 87-year-old hearing impaired individuals. *J Am Acad Audiol.* Feb;25(2):219–28.

Orange, J.B. (2009). Language and communication disorders in older adults: Selected considerations for clinical audiology. In L. Hickson (Ed.), *Hearing care for adults* (pp. 87–102), Stäfa: Phonak.

Palmer, C. V., Adams, S. W., Bourgeois, M., Durrant, J., & Rossi, M. (1999). Reduction in caregiver-identified problem behaviors in patients with Alzheimer disease post-hearing-aid fitting. *Journal of Speech and Hearing Research, 42,* 312–328.

Parving, A., & Phillip, B. (1991). Use and benefit of hearing aids in the tenth decade—And beyond. *Audiology, 30,* 61–69.

Peelle, J. E., Troiani, V., Wingfield, A., & Grossman, M. (2010). Neural processing during older adults' comprehension of spoken sentences: Age differences in resource allocation and connectivity. *Cerebral Cortex, 20,* 773–782.

Phillips, N. A. (2016). The implications of cognitive aging for listening and the Framework for Understanding Effortful Listening (FUEL). *Ear and Hearing, 37*(Suppl. 1), 44S–51S.

Pichora-Fuller, M. K. (2003). Cognitive aging and auditory information processing. *International Journal of Audiology, 42*(Suppl. 2), S26–S32.

Pichora-Fuller, M. K. (2007). Audition and cognition: What audiologists need to know about listening. In C. Palmer & R. Seewald (Eds.), *Hearing care for adults* (pp. 71–85). Stäfa: Phonak.

Pichora-Fuller, M. K. (2008). Use of supportive context by younger and older adult listeners: Balancing bottom-up and top-down information processing. *International Journal of Audiology, 47*(Suppl. 2), S144–S154.

Pichora-Fuller, M. K. (2009a). How cognition might influence hearing aid design, fitting, and outcomes. *Hearing Journal, 62*(11), 32, 34, 36.

Pichora-Fuller, M. K. (2009b). Using the brain when the ears are challenged helps healthy older listeners compensate and preserve communication function. In L. Hickson (Ed.), *Hearing care for adults* (pp. 53–65). Stäfa: Phonak.

Pichora-Fuller, M. K. (2014). A successful aging perspective on the links between hearing and cognition. *SIG 6 Perspectives on Hearing and Hearing Disorders: Research and Diagnostics, 18,* 53–59.

Pichora-Fuller, M. K. (2016). How social factors may modulate auditory and cognitive functioning during listening. *Ear and Hearing, 37*(Suppl.), 92S–100S.

Pichora-Fuller, M. K., & Carson, A. J. (2000). Hearing health and the listening experiences of older communicators. In M. L. Hummert & J. Nussbaum (Eds.), *Communication, aging, and health: Linking research and practice for successful aging* (pp. 43–74). New York: Lawrence Erlbaum Associates.

Pichora-Fuller, M. K., Dupuis, K., Reed, M., & Lemke-Kalis, U. (2013). Helping older people with cognitive decline communicate: Hearing aids as part of a broader rehabilitation approach. *Seminars in Hearing, 34*(4), 307–329.

Pichora-Fuller, M. K., Johnson, C., & Roodenburg, K. (1998). The discrepancy between hearing impairment and handicap in the elderly: Balancing transaction and interaction in conversation, *Journal of Applied Communication Research, 25,* 99–119.

Pichora-Fuller, M. K., Kramer, S. E., Eckert, M., Edwards, B., Hornsby, B., Humes, L., et al. (2016). Hearing impairment and cognitive energy: The Framework for Understanding Effortful Listening (FUEL) [Special issue]. *Ear and Hearing, 37*(Suppl.), S5–S27.

Pichora-Fuller, M. K., & Levitt, H. (2012). Speech comprehension training and auditory and cognitive processing in older adults. *American Journal of Audiology, 21,* 351–357.

Pichora-Fuller, M. K., Mick, P. T., & Reed, M. (2015). Hearing, cognition, and healthy aging: Social and public health implications of the links between age-related declines in hearing and cognition. *Seminars in Hearing, 36,* 122–139.

Pichora-Fuller, M. K., & Robertson, L. F. (1994). Hard of hearing residents in a home for the aged. *Journal of Speech–Language Pathology and Audiology, 18,* 278–288.

Pichora-Fuller, M. K., & Robertson, L. (1997). Planning and evaluation of a hearing rehabilitation program in a home-for-the-aged: Use of hearing aids and assistive listening devices. *Journal of Speech–Language Pathology and Audiology, 21,* 174–186.

Pichora-Fuller, M. K., Santaguida, P., Hammill, A., Oremus, M., Westerberg, B., Usman, A., et al. (2013). *Evaluation and treatment of tinnitus: A comparative effectiveness review.* https://effectivehealthcare.ahrq.gov/ehc/products/371/1649/TInnitus-report-130821.pdf

Pichora-Fuller, M. K., & Singh, G. (2006). Effects of age on auditory and cognitive processing: Implications for hearing aid fitting and audiological rehabilitation. *Trends in Amplification, 10,* 29–59.

Pichora-Fuller, M. K., & Souza, P. (2003). Effects of aging on auditory processing of speech. *International Journal of Audiology, 42*(Suppl. 2), S11–S16.

Pope, D. S., Gallun, F. J., & Kampel, S. (2013). Effect of hospital noise on patients' ability to hear, understand, and recall speech. *Research in Nursing and Health, 36,* 228–241.

Preminger, J. E., & Lind, C. (2012). Assisting communication partners in the setting of treatment goals: The development of the goal sharing for partners strategy. *Seminars in Hearing, 33,* 53–64.

Preminger, J. E., & Meeks S. (2012). The Hearing Impairment Impact—Significant Other Profile (HII-SOP): A tool to measure hearing loss-related quality of life in spouses of people with hearing loss. *Journal of the American Academy of Audiology, 23,* 807–823.

Reed, M. (2010). The Hard of Hearing Club: A social framework for audiologic rehabilitation for seniors with severe hearing difficulties. In L. Hickson (Ed.), *Hearing care for adults* (pp. 147–156).: Stäfa: Phonak.

Rickey, L., & English, K. (2016). Audiology care at the end of life. *Audiology Today, 28*(4), 14–20.

Rippon, I., & Steptoe, A. (2015). Feeling old vs. being old: Associations between self-perceived age and mortality. *JAMA Internal Medicine, 175*(2), 307–309.

Robertson, L., Pichora-Fuller, M. K., Jennings, M. B., Kirson, R., & Roodenburg, K. (1997). The effect of an aural rehabilitation program on responses to scenarios depicting communication breakdown. *Journal of Speech–Language Pathology and Audiology, 21,* 187–198.

Rogers, C. S., Jacoby, L. L., & Sommers, M. S. (2012). Frequent false hearing by older adults: The role of age differences in metacognition. *Psychology and Aging, 27*(2), 33–45.

Ronch, J. L., & Van Zanten, L. (1992). Who are these aging persons? In R. Hull (Ed.), *Rehabilitative audiology* (pp. 185–213). New York: Grune & Stratton.

Ryan, E. B. (2009). Overcoming communication predicaments in later life. In L. Hickson (Ed.), *Hearing care for adults* (pp. 77–86). Stäfa: Phonak.

Ryan, E. B., Giles, H., Bartolucci, G., & Henwood, K. (1986). Psycholinguistic and social psychological components of communication by and with the elderly. *Language and Communication, 6,* 1–24.

Ryan, E. B., Meredith, S. D., Maclean, M. J., & Orange, J. B. (1995). Changing the way we talk with elders: Promoting health using the Communication Enhancement Model. *International Journal of Aging and Human Development, 41,* 89–107.

Saucier, G. (1964). Mini-markers: A brief version of Goldberg's unipolar big-five markers. *Journal of Personality Assessment, 63*(3), 506–516.

Saunders, G. H., & Chisolm, T. H. (2015). Connected audiological rehabilitation: 21st century innovations. *Journal of the American Academy of Audiology, 26*(9), 768–776.

Saunders, G. H., Frederick, M. T., Silverman, S., & Papesh, M. (2013). Application of the health belief model: Development of the hearing beliefs questionnaire (HBQ) and its associations with hearing health behaviors. *International Journal of Audiology*, *52*(8), 558–567.

Saunders, G. H., Smith, S. L., Chisolm, T. H., Frederick, M. T. McArdle, R. A., & Wilson, R. H. (2016). Randomized control trial: Supplementing hearing aid use with Listening and Communication Enhancement (LACE) auditory training. *Ear and Hearing*, *37*(4), 381–396.

Scarinci, N., Worrall, L., & Hickson, L. (2009a). The effect of hearing impairment in older people on the spouse: Development and psychometric testing of the significant other scale for hearing disability (SOS-HEAR). *International Journal of Audiology*, *48*(10), 671–683.

Scarinci, N., Worrall, L., & Hickson, L. (2009b). The ICF and third-party disability: Its application to spouses of older people with hearing impairment. *Disability and Rehabilitation*, *25*(31), 2088–2100.

Schmader, T., Johns, M., & Forbes, C. (2008). An integrated process model of stereotype threat effects on performance. *Psychological Review*, *115*, 336–356.

Schneider, B. A., Pichora-Fuller, M. K., & Daneman, M. (2010). The effects of senescent changes in audition and cognition on spoken language comprehension. In S. Gordon-Salant, R. D. Frisina, A. Popper, & D. Fay (Eds.), *The aging auditory system: Perceptual characterization and neural bases of presbycusis* (pp. 167–210). Berlin: Springer.

Schow, R. L. (1992). Hearing assessment and treatment in nursing homes. *Hearing Instruments*, *43*(7), 7–11.

Schow, R. L. (2001). A standardized AR battery for dispensers. *Hearing Journal*, *54*(8), 10–20.

Schow, R. L., Balsara, N., Smedley, T. C., & Whitcomb, C. J. (1993). Aural rehabilitation by ASHA audiologists, 1980–1990. *American Journal of Audiology*, *2*(3), 28–37.

Schow, R. L., Seikel, J. A., Brockett, J. E., & Whitaker, M. M. (2007) *Multiple Auditory Processing Assessment*. St Louis, Auditec.

Schow, R. L., Seikel, J. A., Brockett, J. E., & Whitaker, M. M. (In Press) *Multiple Auditory Processing Assessment-2*. Novato, CA, Academic Therapy Publications.

Schow, R., Brockett, J., Bishop, R., Whitaker, M., & Horlacki, G. (2005). *Standardization of outcome measures in hearing aid fitting*. Paper presented at the International Collegium of Rehabilitative Audiology Conference, Gainesville, FL.

Schow, R. L., & Gatehouse, S. (1990). Fundamental issues to self-assessment of hearing. *Ear and Hearing*, *11*(5, Suppl.), 6–16.

Schow, R. L., & Nerbonne, M. A. (1980). Hearing levels among elderly nursing home residents. *Journal of Speech and Hearing Disorders*, *45*(I), 124–132.

Schow, R., & Nerbonne, M. (1982). Communication Screening Profile: Use with elderly clients. *Ear and Hearing*, *3*, 135–147.

Schow, R. L., & Smedley, T. C. (1990). Self-assessment of hearing [Special issue]. *Ear and Hearing*, *11*(5, Suppl.), 1S–65S.

Shargorodsky, J., Curhan, G. C., & Farwell, W. R. (2010). Prevalence and characteristics of tinnitus among US adults. *American Journal of Medicine*, *123*(8), 711–718.

Shiffman, S., Stone, A. A., & Hufford, M. R. (2008). Ecological momentary assessment. *Annual Review of Clinical Psychology*, *4*, 1–32.

Singh, G. (2009). The aging hand and handling of hearing aids: A review. In L. Hickson (Ed.), *Hearing care for adults* (pp. 255–276). Stäfa: Phonak.

Singh, G., Hickson, L., English, K., Scherpiet, S., Lemke U. Timmer, B., et al. (2016). Family-centered adult audiologic care: A Phonak position statement. *Hearing Review*, *23*(4), 16. http://www.hearingreview.com/2016/03/family-centered-adult-audiologic-care-phonak-position-statement/

Singh, G., Lau, S.-T., & Pichora-Fuller, M. K. (2015). Social support predicts hearing aid satisfaction. *Ear and Hearing*, *36*(6), 664–676.

Singh, G., & Launer, S. (2016). Social context and hearing aid adoption. *Trends in Hearing*, *20*, 1–10.

Singh, G., & Pichora-Fuller, M. K. (2010). Older adults performance on the Speech, Spatial, and Qualities of Hearing Scale (SSQ): Test-retest reliability and a comparison of interview and self-administration methods. *International Journal of Audiology*, *49*, 733–740.

Singh, G., Pichora-Fuller, M. K., Malkowski, M., Boretzki, M., & Launer, S. (2014). A survey of the attitudes of practitioners toward teleaudiology. *International Journal of Audiology*, *53*(12), 850–860.

Smith, A., (2014). *Older adults and technology use*. Washington, DC: Pew Research Center. http://www.pewinternet.org/2014/04/03/older-adults-and-technology-use

Smith, C., Wilber, L. A., & Cavitt, K. (2016). PSAPs vs hearing aids: An electroacoustic analysis of performance and fitting capabilities. *Hearing Review*, *23*(7), 18. http://www.hearingreview.com/2016/06/psaps-vs-hearing-aids-electroacoustic-analysis-performance-fitting-capabilities

Smith, S. L., & Fagelson, M. (2011). Development of the self-efficacy for tinnitus management questionnaire. *Journal of the American Academy of Audiology*, *22*(7), 424–440.

Smith, S. L., Pichora-Fuller, M. K., & Alexander, G. (2016). Development of the Word Auditory Recognition and Recall Measure (WARRM): A working memory test for use in rehabilitative audiology. *Ear and Hearing*, *37*(6), e360–e376.

Smith, S. L., Pichora-Fuller, M. K., Watts, K. L., & La More, C. (2011). Development of the Listening Self-Efficacy Questionnaire (LSEQ). *International Journal of Audiology*, *50*, 417–425.

Smith, S. L., & West, R. L. (2006). The application of self-efficacy principles to audiologic rehabilitation: A tutorial. *American Journal of Audiology*, *15*, 46–56.

Smith-Wheelock, M., Shepard, N. T., & Telian, S. A. (1991). Physical therapy program for vestibular rehabilitation. *American Journal of Otology*, *13*(3), 224–225.

Smits, C., Goverts, S. T., & Festen, J. M. (2013). The digits-in-noise test: assessing auditory speech recognition abilities in noise. *Journal of the Acoustical Society of America*, *133*(3), 1693–1706.

Solheim, J., Shiryaeva, O., & Kvaerner, K. J. (2016). Lack of ear care knowledge in nursing homes. *Journal of Multidisciplinary Homecare*, *9*, 481–488.

Staab, W. (2015). U.S. hearing aid market. http://hearinghealthmatters.org/waynesworld/2015/u-s-hearing-aid-market

Statistics Canada. (2006) Participation and activity limitation survey: Facts on hearing limitations. http://www.statcan.gc.ca/pub/89-628-x/2009012/fs-fi/fs-fi-eng.htm

Stenklev, N. C., & Laukli, E. (2004). Presbyacusis—Hearing thresholds and the ISO 7029. *International Journal of Audiology*, *43*, 295–306.

Stephens, D., & Kramer, S. E. (2010). *Living with hearing difficulties: The process of enablement*. Chichester: Wiley-Blackwell.

Stephens, S. D. G. (1996). Evaluating the problems of the hearing impaired. *Audiology*, *19*, 105–220.

Stephens, S. D. G., Jones, G., & Gianopoulos, I. (2000). The use of outcome measures to formulate intervention strategies. *Ear and Hearing*, *21*(4, Suppl.), 15S–23S.

Swallow, J. C., & Wesolowsky, M. J. (2014). Acoustic design considerations in modern health care facility design. *Canadian Acoustics*, *42*(3), 108–109.

Sweetow, R. W. (2000). Cognitive-behavior modification. In R. S. Tyler (Ed.), *Tinnitus handbook* (297–311). San Diego, CA: Singular Publishing.

Sweetow, R. W., & Henderson-Sabes, J. (2004). The case for LACE (Listening and Communication Enhancement). *Hearing Journal*, *57*(3), 32–40.

Sweetow, R. W., & Henderson-Sabes, J. H. (2006). The need for and development of an adaptive Listening and Communication Enhancement (LACE) Program. *Journal of the American Academy of Audiology*, *17*, 538–558.

Taylor, B. (2007). Self-Report Assessment of Hearing Aid Outcome—An overview. *Audiology Online*. http://www.audiologyonline.com/articles/self-report-assessment-hearing-aid-931

U.S. Census Bureau. (1990). *The need for personal assistance with everyday activities: Recipients and caregivers, current population reports* (Series P-70, No. 19, Table B). Washington, DC: U.S. Government Printing Office.

Van Wyk, K., & Murphy, K. (2014a). FGI guidelines for healthcare acoustic design. *Canadian Acoustics*, *42*(3), 112–113.

Van Wyk, K., & Murphy, K. (2014b). Hospital noise methodology and survey results. *Canadian Acoustics*, *42*(3), 114–115.

Villaume, W. A., Brown, M. H., & Darling, R. (1994). Presbycusis, communication, and older adults. In M. L. Hummert, J. M. Wiemann, & J. F. Nussbaum (Eds.), *Interpersonal communication in older adulthood: Interdisciplinary theory and research* (pp. 83–106). Thousand Oaks, CA: Sage.

Wallhagen, M. I. (2010). The stigma of hearing loss. *Gerontologist, 50*, 66–75.

Wallhagen, M., Strawbridge, W., Shema, S., Kaplan, G.A.(2004). Impact of self-assessed hearing loss on a spouse: A longitudinal analysis of couples et al. (2004). Impact of self-assessed hearing loss on a spouse: A longitudinal analysis of couples. *Journal of Gerontology. Series B, Psychological Sciences and Social Sciences, 59*, S190–S196.

West, R. L., & Smith, S. L. (2007). Development of a hearing aid self-efficacy questionnaire. *International Journal of Audiology, 46*, 759–771.

Whitmer, W. M., Howell, P., & Akeroyd, M. A. (2014). Proposed norms for the Glasgow Hearing Aid Benefit Profiles (GHABP) questionnaire. *International Journal of Audiology, 53*(5), 345–351.

Williams-Sanchez, V., McArdle, R. A., Wilson, R. H., Kidd, G. R., Watson, C. S., & Bourne, A. L. (2014). Validation of a screening test of auditory function using the telephone. *Journal of the American Academy of Audiology, 25*(10), 937–951.

Willott, J. F. (1991). *Aging and the auditory system: Anatomy, physiology, and psychophysics*. San Diego, CA: Singular Publishing.

Wilson, R. H., McArdle, R. A., & Smith, S. L. (2007). An evaluation of the BKB-SIN, HINT, QuickSIN, and WIN materials on listeners with normal hearing and listeners with hearing loss. *Journal of Speech Language and Hearing Research, 50*, 844–856.

Wingfield, A., & Tun, P. A. (2007). Cognitive supports and cognitive constraints on comprehension of spoken language. *Journal of the American Academy of Audiology, 18*, 567–577.

Winkler, A., Latzel, M., & Holube, I. (2016). Open versus closed hearing-aid fittings: A literature review of both fitting approaches. *Trends in Hearing, 20*, 1–13. http://tia.sagepub.com/content/20/2331216516631741.abstract

Wong, L. L. N. (2011). Evidence on self-fitting hearing aids. *Trends in Amplification, 15*(4), 215–225.

Wong, L., & Hickson, L. (Eds.). (2012). Evidence-based practice in audiology: Evaluating interventions for children and adults with hearing impairment. San Diego, CA: Plural Publishing.

World Health Organization. (2001). *International Classification of Functioning, Disability and Health (ICF)*. Geneva: Author. http://www.who.int/classifications/icf/en

World Health Organization. (2015a). *Make listening safe*. Geneva: Author. http://apps.who.int/iris/bitstream/10665/177884/1/WHO_NMH_NVI_15.2_eng.pdf?ua=1&ua=1

World Health Organization. (2015b). *World report on ageing and health*. Geneva: Author. http://www.who.int/ageing/publications/world-report-2015/en

Worrall, L. E., & Hickson, L. M. (2003). *Communication disability in aging: From prevention to intervention*. Clifton Park, NY: Thomson Delmar Learning.

Worrall, L., Hickson, L., Barnett, H., & Yiu, E. (1998). An evaluation of the *Keep on Talking* program for maintaining communication skills into old age. *Educational Gerontology, 24*, 129–140.

Wu, Y.-H., & Bentler, R. A. (2012). Do older adults have social lifestyles that place fewer demands on hearing? *Journal of the American Academy of Audiology, 23*, 697–711.

APPENDIX A

Hearing Instrument Orientation (HIO) BASICS

Hearing expectations.

- Even the most advanced hearing aid technology will not give you normal hearing.
- Properly fitted hearing aids help you hear soft sounds better and loud sounds appropriately loud.
- Continued use and adjustment to the hearing aids will allow you to be comfortable in your environment.
- Be sure you are using effective communication strategies.

Instrument operation.

- Be sure that you understand the controls on your hearing aid and remotes.
- Your hearing aid may have a program button and/or remotes.
- Review each control and be sure that you can adjust it.
- Be familiar with controls on your assistive devices (telephone/television).

Occlusion effect.

- The occlusion effect is an echo that you may hear that can make your voice sound hollow.
- If you notice this for a period longer than three months with consistent hearing aid use, bring it to the attention of your hearing care professional.

Batteries.

- Your battery size is _____ The color is _____.
- Batteries usually last 1 to 2 weeks depending on how often you wear your hearing aids.
- The battery should be inserted with the flat side facing up and the color tab removed.
- Keep batteries away from children and pets because they can cause choking or danger if swallowed.
- Batteries can be purchased at pharmacies and grocery stores.

Acoustic feedback.

- Feedback is the squealing sound that your hearing aids sometimes make.
- If you get feedback make sure your earmold is fitting snugly.
- Feedback may also occur if there is excess cerumen (wax) in the ear.
- If this may apply to you, call our clinic for an appointment to have it removed.

System troubleshooting.

- If your hearing aid(s) are not working, first check the battery. Then check your filters and wax guard.
- Check for wax in the microphone or receiver opening. Remove the wax using the simple tools that come with your hearing aids.
- If you still have problems, ask your hearing care professional for help.

Insertion and removal.

- It is very important to learn how to insert and remove your hearing aids properly because, if you find it difficult or uncomfortable to do this, you won't want to use the aid(s).

Cleaning and maintenance.

- Wax or other debris can block the opening on the microphone or receiver causing the hearing aid not to function properly.
- Learn how to use tissues, brushes, and wax loops to keep your hearing aids clean. Clean your hearing aids every day and not just when there is a problem.

Service.

- If you have problems or concerns contact our clinic _____
- Take advantage of the regular follow-up appointments that are scheduled for you.
- The usual life of hearing aids is four to five years

Adapted from Brockett and Schow (2001); Schow (2001).

APPENDIX B

CLEAR (for the listener)

Control your communication situations

- Maximize what you are trying to listen to and minimize anything that gets in the way of it.
- Position yourself so that you can see the talker well and hear the person most clearly and with the *least interference* from others.
- Turn on some lights or *move your conversation* to an area that is better lit.
- Move conversations away from noisy areas.
- If the talker is too far away or the interference from others is too bothersome, you can mic that person with an assistive device.
- In short, whenever you can, be sure to control the lighting and your position in the room and favor your better ear if you have one.

Look at/ lipread the talker to ease the strain of listening.

- Watch the person so you can *"read" body language, facial expressions, and lip movements* to clarify information that is hard to hear.
- Remember that much of the information that is hard to hear is easy to see.
- Lipreading is easier if you face the person directly, but you can also get useful visual information from the side.
- In general, the *closer the better*, but 5 to 10 feet away is ideal.

Expectations need to be realistic and when the situation is just too difficult you can *use communication escape strategies to help you reduce frustration.*

- If you are realistic about how well you can hear, you may decide some situations are unreasonably difficult.
- Anticipate the fact that you will likely have difficulty and *plan options* for dealing with a breakdown in communication.
- For example, if a restaurant is a difficult listening situation, rather than staying at home, agree to have another person in your party explain the specials to you or do the ordering.

Assertiveness can help others understand your hearing difficulties.

- Let others in your conversation know that you have difficulty hearing and encourage them to get your attention before talking and to look at you when they speak.
- Let them know that short, uncomplicated sentences are easier to understand than longer, complicated ones.
- *Being timid will not help you* since you must speak up and be assertive in order to move the conversation away from a noisy area or ask the talker to slow down or talk louder.
- Be pleasantly assertive and *let your needs be known*.
- Most people will want to be helpful in these circumstances.

Repair strategies for communication breakdown can help you and the talker.

- If you miss important information and you don't understand enough of what is being said, repeat back what you did hear and ask the person to *clarify what you missed*.
- You can ask others to speak more loudly or slowly or distinctly. You can ask the people to spell a word or even write it down. Counting on your fingers may help with numbers.
- Develop different ways to repair a conversation and do it in an interesting way or with a *sense of humor* if possible.
- Saying "I'm going to listen the best I can now, so please say that once more" as you face and watch the person is a more pleasant way to ask for repetition than simply saying "What?"
- You can also reduce the need for repairs by being the one who begins a conversation or by being sure you know what the topic is before you enter into a conversation.

Adapted from Brockett and Schow (2001); Schow (2001).

APPENDIX C

SPEECH (for the speaker)

Spotlight your face and keep it visible.

- Keep your hands away from your mouth so that the hard of hearing person can get all the visual cues possible.
- Be sure to face the speaker when you are talking and be at a good distance (5 to 10 feet).
- *Avoid chewing gum, cigarettes, and other facial distractions* when possible.
- And *be sure not to talk from another room* and expect to be heard.

Pause *slightly* between the content portions of sentences.

- Slow, exaggerated speech is as difficult to understand as fast speech.
- However, speech at a *moderate pace* with slight pauses between phrases and sentences can allow the hard of hearing person to process the *information in chunks*.
- This procedure is sometimes called CLEAR SPEECH.

Empathize and *be patient* with the person who has hearing loss.

- Try plugging both ears and listen for a short while to something soft that you want to hear in an environment that is distracting and noisy.
- This may help you appreciate the challenge of being hard of hearing and it should help you be patient if the responses seem slow.
- *Re-phrase* if necessary to clarify a point and remember, empathy, patience, empathy!

Ease listening.

- *Get the listener's attention* before you speak and make sure you are being helpful in the way you speak.
- *Ask how you can facilitate communication*. The listener may want you to speak more loudly or more softly, more slowly or faster, or announce the subject of discussion, or signal when the topic of conversation shifts.
- Be compliant and helpful and encourage the listener to give you feedback so you can make it as easy as possible for him or her.

Control the situations and the listening conditions in the environment.

- Maximize communication by getting closer to the person.
- If you can be *5 to 10 feet away*, that is ideal.
- Also, move away from *background noise* and maintain good lighting.
- Avoid dark restaurants or windows behind you that blind someone watching you.

Have a plan.

- When *anticipating difficult listening situations, set strategies* for communication in advance and implement them as necessary.
- This might mean that at a restaurant you communicate with a waitress/waiter instead of having your hard-of-hearing family member or friend do so.

Adapted from Brockett and Schow (2001); Schow (2001).

APPENDIX D

IOI-HA

International Outcome Inventory for Hearing Aids (IOI-HA)

1. Think about how much you used your present hearing aid(s) over the past two weeks. On an average day, how many hours did you use the hearing aid(s)?

none	less than 1 hour a day	1 to 4 hours a day	4 to 8 hours a day	more than 8 hours a day
☐	☐	☐	☐	☐

2. Think about the situation where you most wanted to hear better, before you got your present hearing aid(s). Over the past two weeks, how much has the hearing aid helped in that situation?

helped not at all	helped slightly	helped moderately	helped quite a lot	helped very much
☐	☐	☐	☐	☐

3. Think again about the situation where you most wanted to hear better. When you use your present hearing aid(s), how much difficulty do you STILL have in that situation?

very much difficulty	quite a lot of difficulty	moderate difficulty	slight difficulty	no difficulty
☐	☐	☐	☐	☐

4. Considering everything, do you think your present hearing aid(s) is worth the trouble?

not at all worth it	slightly worth it	moderately worth it	quite a lot worth it	very much worth it
☐	☐	☐	☐	☐

5. Over the past two weeks, with your present hearing aid(s), how much have your hearing difficulties affected the things you can do?

affected very much	affected quite a lot	affected moderately	affected slightly	affected not at all
☐	☐	☐	☐	☐

6. Over the past two weeks, with your present hearing aid(s), how much do you think other people were bothered by your hearing difficulties?

bothered very much	bothered quite a lot	bothered moderately	bothered slightly	bothered not at all
☐	☐	☐	☐	☐

7. Considering everything, how much has your present hearing aid(s) changed your enjoyment of life?

worse	no change	slightly better	quite a lot better	very much better
☐	☐	☐	☐	☐

APPENDIX E

The Client-Oriented Scale of Improvement (COSI)

https://www.nal.gov.au/wp-content/uploads/sites/3/2016/11/COSI-Questionnaire.pdf

Client Oriented Scale of Improvement (COSI)

Name: _____   Category: New _____

Audiologist: _____   Return _____

Date: 1. Needs Established _____

       2. Outcome Assessed _____

Final Ability
(with hearing aid)

Person can hear

10% 25% 50% 75% 95%

SPECIFIC NEEDS

Indicate Order of Significance

	Degree of Change					Category	Person can hear				
	Worse	No Difference	Slightly Better	Better	Much Better		Hardly Ever	Occasionally	Half the Time	Most of Time	Almost Always

Categories

1. Conversation with 1 or 2 in quiet	9. Hear front door bell or knock
2. Conversation with 1 or 2 in noise	10. Hear traffic
3. Conversation with group in quiet	11. Increased social contact
4. Conversation with group in noise	12. Feel embarrassed or stupid
5. Television or Radio @ normal volume	13. Feeling left out
6. Familiar speaker on phone	14. Feeling upset or angry
7. Unfamiliar speaker on phone	15. Church or meeting
8. Hearing phone ring from another room	16. Other

NATIONAL ACOUSTIC LABORATORIES

Reproduced with permission from the National Acoustic Laboratories.

APPENDIX F

Self-Assessment of Communication (SAC)

HEARX VERSION adapted from Schow and Nerbonne (1982).

Self-Assessment of Communication (SAC)

Name: _____   Date:_____

Instructions: The purpose of this form is to identify the problems your hearing loss may be causing you. If you wear hearing aids, answer the questions according to how you communicate *when the hearing aids are NOT in use.*

One of the five descriptions on the right should be assigned to each of the statements below.

(1) Almost never (or never)
(2) Occasionally (about ¼ of the time)
(3) About ½ of the time
(4) Frequently (about ¾ of the time)
(5) Practically always (or always)

Select a number from 1 to 5 next to each statement (please *do not* answer with yes or no, and pick only one answer for each question.)

(1) Do you experience communication difficulties in situations when speaking with one other person? (at home, at work, in a social situation, with a waitress, a store clerk, with a spouse, boss, etc.)

1	2	3	4	5

(2) Do you experience communication difficulties while watching TV and in various types of entertainment? (movies, radio, plays, night clubs, musical entertainment, etc.)

1	2	3	4	5

(3) Do you experience communication difficulties in situations when conversing with a small group of several persons? (with friends or families, co-workers, in meetings or casual conversations, over dinner or while playing cards, etc.)

1	2	3	4	5

(4) Do you experience communication difficulties when you are in an unfavorable listening environment? (at a noisy party, where there is background music, when riding in an auto or bus, when someone whispers or talks from across the room, etc.)

1	2	3	4	5

(5) How often do you experience communication difficulties in the situation where you most want to hear better?
Situation _____

1	2	3	4	5

(6) Do you feel that any difficulty with your hearing negatively affects or hampers your personal or social life?

1	2	3	4	5

(7) How often do others seem to be concerned or annoyed or suggest that you have a hearing problem?

1	2	3	4	5

(8) Does any problem or difficulty with your hearing worry, annoy or upset you?

1	2	3	4	5

(9) How often does your hearing negatively affect your enjoyment of life?

1	2	3	4	5

(10) If you are using a hearing aid: On an average day, how many hours did you use your hearing aids?

hours_____ /16=_____%

Please rate your overall satisfaction with your hearing aids.

1 ☐ *not at all satisfied (0%)*   2 ☐ *slightly satisfied (25%)*   3 ☐ *moderately satisfied (50%)* _____ %

4 ☐ *mostly satisfied (75%)*   5 ☐ *very satisfied (100%)*

FOR OFFICE USE ONLY

☐ Pre-Assessment
☐ Post-Assessment
☐ Not currently using Hearing Aid
☐ Current Hearing Aid User

FOR OFFICE USE ONLY

Score: (Q1-9) _____ (/9) _____ -1 _____ × 25 = _____ %

Score (Q1-5)/5 = _____ (Q6-9)/4 = _____ Q9 _____

−1×25 = _____   D _____ % H _____ % Q _____ %

Significant Other Assessment of Communication (SOAC)

HEARX VERSION adapted from Schow and Nerbonne (1982).

Significant Other Assessment of Communication (SOAC)

Name:_____

Name or Person Completing Assignment:_____

Date:_____

Relationship:_____

Instructions: The purpose of this form is to identify the problems a hearing loss may be causing your significant other. If the patient has a hearing aid, please fill out the form according to how he/she communicates *when the hearing aids are NOT in use.*

(1) Almost never (or never)
(2) Occasionally (about ¼ of the time)
(3) About ½ of the time
(4) Frequently (about ¾ of the time)
(5) Practically always (or always)

One of the five descriptions on the right should be assigned to each of the statements below.

Select a number from 1 to 5 next to each statement (please _do not_ answer with yes or no, and pick only one answer for each question.)

(1) Does he/she experience communication difficulties in situations when speaking with one other person? (at home, at work, in a social situation, with a waitress, a store clerk, with a spouse, boss, etc.)

1	2	3	4	5

(2) Does he/she experience communication difficulties while watching TV and in various types of entertainment? (movies, radio, plays, night clubs, musical entertainment, etc.)

1	2	3	4	5

(3) Does he/she experience communication difficulties in situations when conversing with a small group of several persons? (with friends or families, co-workers, in meetings or casual conversations, over dinner or while playing cards, etc.)

1	2	3	4	5

(4) Does he/she experience communication difficulties when you are in an unfavorable listening environment? (at a noisy party, where there is background music, when riding in an auto or bus, when someone whispers or talks from across the room, etc.)

1	2	3	4	5

(5) How often does he/she experience communication difficulties in the situation where he/she most wants to hear better?
Situation_____

1	2	3	4	5

(6) Do you feel that any difficulty with hearing negatively affects or hampers his/her personal or social life?

1	2	3	4	5

(7) Do you or others seem to be concerned or annoyed that he/she has a hearing problem?

1	2	3	4	5

(8) Do you feel that any problem or difficulty with his/her hearing worries, annoys, or upsets him/her?

1	2	3	4	5

(9) How often does hearing loss negatively affect his/her enjoyment of life?

1	2	3	4	5

(10) If he/she is using a hearing aid: On an average day, how many hours will he/she use the hearing aids?

hours_____/16=_____%

Please rate what you feel is his/her overall satisfaction with the hearing aids.

1 ☐ *not at all satisfied (0%)*   2 ☐ *slightly satisfied (25%)*   3 ☐ *moderately satisfied (50%)*_____%

4 ☐ *mostly satisfied (75%)*   5 ☐ *very satisfied (100%)*

FOR OFFICE USE ONLY

☐ Pre-Assessment
☐ Post-Assessment
☐ Not currently using Hearing Aid
☐ Current Hearing Aid User

FOR OFFICE USE ONLY

Score: (Q1-9) _____ (/9) _____ 1 _____ × 25 = _____ %

Score (Q1-5)/5 = _____ (Q6-9)/4 = _____ Q9 = _____

-1×25 = D _____% H _____% Q _____%

APPENDIX G

Further Illustration of CORE and CARE

The approach recommended in this chapter suggests that the rehabilitation of hearing loss should be based on the strategy suggested by CORE and CARE (see Figure 10.6). We further noted that most of the rehabilitation done by audiologists is in connection with hearing aid fitting. We know that in a certain number of special cases, such as with a cochlear implant client, rehabilitation may be much more involved, but these special cases are the exception. Therefore, we want to provide a clear emphasis on hearing aid fitting. Before concluding this chapter, we would like to describe a hearing aid client seen in our clinic to illustrate how this rehabilitation procedure plays out in real life. This individual, John, was a male, age 54, who had been experiencing hearing problems for the past few years that finally prompted him to have his hearing tested with the idea he might need hearing aids. In the *C (communication) assessment* phase, we tested hearing by audiometry and self-report. The audiogram revealed equal results in both ears, with thresholds of 35 dB HL at 1 kHz, 40 dB HL at 2 kHz, and 45 dB HL at 4 kHz (Figure 10.12). The loss was sensorineural, and, based on better ear thresholds and the system used in this text for sorting hearing loss into exclusive groups, the loss was in the category F1 (see Chapter 1 and text website).

We also had John complete a Glasgow Hearing Aid Benefit Profile (GHABP). At an initial interview and before any decision was made about hearing aids, the GHABP allowed us to measure John's initial disability or communication activity limitation. This score is based on four standard listening situations and up to four situations of concern supplied by the client. John provided two areas of hearing concern beyond the four standard ones, and his GHABP results for the relevant six items are shown in Figure 10.13. The percentage disability score (*activity limitation*) obtained on the GHABP for John was 60 percent.

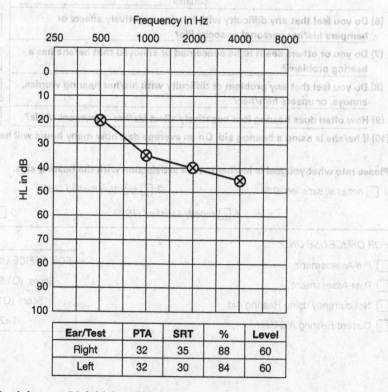

Ear/Test	PTA	SRT	%	Level
Right	32	35	88	60
Left	32	30	84	60

FIGURE 10.12 John, age 54, initial audiogram.

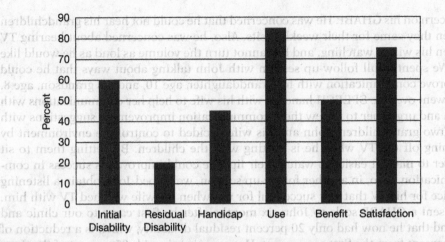

FIGURE 10.13 Glasgow (GHABP) findings for John. Prehearing aid results are initial disability and handicap. Postfitting results are residual disability, use, benefit, and satisfaction.

In terms of *O (overall) participation*, we considered vocational, social, and emotional issues. John said his work as a janitor was not affected by his hearing, but his major concerns were in social activities and some emotional problems related to these social activities. Again, the **GHABP** was helpful in measuring this handicap or *participation restriction* because it measured how much his hearing problems cause him to be worried, annoyed, or upset in the six situations. This score was 45 percent.

We have gathered and published scores on over 800 clients sorted into exclusive hearing categories, and when we compared John's two scores (60% and 45%) with others who have hearing losses in the same category as his, we found that he was within one standard deviation of the mean for all clients with such a hearing loss (see data in Chapter 1 and on the text website). However, his scores were located toward the upper end of that midrange, showing that he has more than average *activity limitation* and *participation restrictions*. We also explored *R (related personal)* and *E (environmental)* factors that had a bearing on John's experience of hearing loss. We found that his attitude about improving his hearing was excellent (a type I) and that he was an extrovert who would like to get out more if his hearing were better. In terms of environmental issues, his wife also wanted him to socialize more and encouraged him to obtain hearing aids. She filled out a **GHABP** also, modified for use by a significant other person. Thus, we considered all four of the **CORE** issues.

As John told us his story during the *C (counseling)* phase of the treatment, goals were determined based on input from him and his wife. These goals were set in the areas of *A (audibility)*, *R (remediation of communication activities)*, and *E (environmental or participation)* goals. By counseling and setting goals in these three areas, we recommended a reasonably standardized procedure in rehabilitation (**CARE**), much as audiologists do in diagnostic audiology (Schow, 2001). After John decided to obtain hearing aids, the necessary decisions were made about fit and function of the aid, and ear impressions were made. When he came back to pick up his hearing aids, we used the **HIO BASICS** handout in a 45-minute session for hearing instrument orientation. A week later in a second 45-minute follow-up session, the remediation of communication issues was addressed with the **CLEAR** handout. This provided John with some help in fundamental areas of concern surrounding communication. Had John been interested in getting more help in these areas, we would have recommended our four sessions of group therapy. These sessions are provided from time to time in our clinic. John did not elect to enroll for these sessions.

John did elect to focus his efforts in the next two 45-minute follow-up sessions on the two environmental participation issues that he had identified as a major concern on his GHABP. He was concerned that he could not hear his grandchildren when they came for their weekly visits. Also, he was concerned about hearing TV when his wife is watching, and he cannot turn the volume as loud as he would like it. We spent a full follow-up session with John talking about ways that he could improve communication with his granddaughter, age 10, and his grandson, age 8. We went over the SPEECH handout with his wife to help her communications with him and urged her to review these communication improvement suggestions with the two grandchildren. John and his wife decided to control the environment by turning off the TV when he is visiting with the children. By getting them to sit closer to make it easier to watch their lips, he could improve his success in communication. Also, in another follow-up session, we helped John obtain a listening device for his TV that was successful for use when his wife watched TV with him. We sent a GHABP scale to John six months after he first came to our clinic and found that he now had only 20 percent residual disability, which is a reduction of 40 percent from the first assessment. He was using the aids 85 percent of the time, was receiving good reported benefit (50%), and was satisfied at a 75 percent level of satisfaction.

Certainly, all rehabilitation outcomes will not be this straightforward and successful. But new goals may be set based on outcome measures when the initial plans do not yield good success. When the entire CORE–CARE package is used with clients, we believe that good outcomes can occur on a consistent basis.

part 3

Implementing Audiologic Rehabilitation: Case Studies

part

Implementing Audiologic Rehabilitation: Case Studies

Case Studies: Children

Mary Pat Moeller, Catherine Cronin Carotta

CONTENTS

Visit the companion website when you see this icon to learn more about the topic nearby in the text.

Learning Outcomes

After reading this chapter, you will be able to

- List three areas that may be considered red flags for autism spectrum disorder
- List five areas that are assessed in developmental evaluations
- List three assessment instruments that can be used to assess speech and language skills in children who are deaf or hard of hearing
- Explain the auditory–visual continuum
- Describe the purpose of the new–review–routine intervention strategy

INTRODUCTION

Children with hearing loss represent a heterogeneous group, with highly individual characteristics and needs. Differences in degree of hearing loss, family constellation and resources, medical history, language abilities, school support, and styles of learning contribute to each child's unique profile. The five case examples that follow describe individualized approaches to case management, with process-oriented strategies for problem solution. In each of the cases that follow, two concepts are central to the intervention: (1) clinicians must ascertain intervention priorities through differential assessment and careful determination of a child and family's

Each child with hearing loss presents with a unique constellation of abilities and needs. An individualized approach to assessment and case management is essential.

Parents should have access to information about all communication options and guidance based on thoughtful evaluation of the child and the family's needs.

primary needs, and (2) individualized management requires a process of clinical decision making and objective monitoring of the efficacy of intervention (see Chapter 9).

The process of pediatric audiologic rehabilitation (AR) is complex and challenging. Parents and clinicians face numerous management decisions early in the course of AR. What will be the best approach(es) to optimize the child's language development? What type of amplification will best meet this child's needs? Should a cochlear implant be considered? Will the child's needs be met in an inclusive educational setting, or will a specialized setting better serve this child? Answers to these and other management questions are rarely simple and rarely without controversy. Parents face many of these questions at a time when they are trying to cope with parenting a newborn and the diagnosis of hearing loss. They deserve objective guidance that is based on thoughtful examination of the child's needs and abilities in light of the options available.

AR service delivery for children is further complicated by the increasing incidence of children with hearing loss who have significant secondary disabilities. These children require sophisticated assessment and management through a team approach. Federal mandates require that early intervention be provided in a family-centered manner (Roush & Matkin, 1994). This has brought about a reconceptualization of the professional's role in the decision-making and management process. The goal of empowering family members in the management of the child's needs also requires a diverse and individualized approach given the wide range of family systems represented in the clinician's caseload. Each of these factors dictates the need for objective, individually tailored approaches and flexible, innovative service delivery models.

The case studies that follow represent five unique concerns that influenced the course of rehabilitative management:

1. Early intervention for a child with multiple disabilities
2. Routes to spoken language after cochlear implantation
3. Issues affecting educational placement decisions
4. Late identification in a child who was hard of hearing: auditory-linguistic considerations
5. Differential diagnosis through professional teamwork: a tool for solving complex intervention problems

In each of the following cases, multidisciplinary service delivery was necessary and advantageous, and it capitalizes on interprofessional practices (see http://www.asha.org/Practice/Interprofessional-Education-Practice). No one discipline has all the skills and expertise to address the complex nature of the problems that often present themselves. The AR specialist needs to cultivate the skills of working as a team member, joining in collaborative consultation with allied professionals and parents. Multidisciplinary perspectives contribute to a holistic understanding of the child's and family's needs.

Although the cases described are based on real persons, names and other biographical facts have been changed to maintain patient confidentiality.

CASE 1: MATTHEW—EARLY INTERVENTION, MULTIPLE DISABILITIES

It has been estimated that between 30 to 40% of children with hearing loss have educationally significant secondary disabilities.

AR specialists working at the parent/infant level are meeting new professional challenges, including the opportunity to work with very young infants in the context of the family system (see Chapter 8). It has been estimated that 30 to 40 percent of children who are deaf or hard of hearing have secondary disabilities (Gallaudet

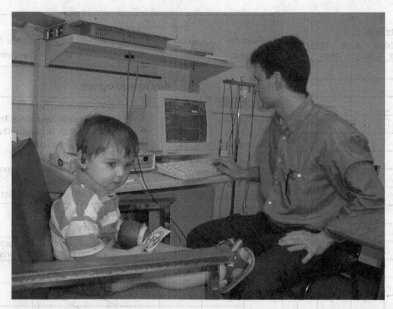

ABR and OAE testing are valuable in identifying hearing loss in a young child like Matthew.

Research Institute, 2008; Moeller, Coufal, & Hixson, 1990). This case illustrates the importance of transdisciplinary approaches to case management. Overall coordination among various professionals and families is essential in meeting the needs of deaf infants with additional disabilities.

Background Information

Matthew was born at 38 weeks' gestation without complication. He did not pass his newborn hearing screening. He was referred for further testing and was diagnosed with a profound bilateral sensorineural hearing loss through auditory brain stem response testing when he was 3 months of age. He was fit with hearing aids at 4 months of age. Matthew achieved his motor milestones at typical ages as noted by his sitting at 5 months and walking at 12 months. Speech and language milestones were significantly delayed. First words did not appear until 2 years of age.

> Significant regression in language behaviors or delays in language development may be associated with autism.

Intervention Plan

Matthew was enrolled in weekly home-based intervention services at 6 months of age. The family attended these sessions consistently. The parent–infant specialist worked with the family to establish hearing aid use, to explore the benefits of the hearing aids, to consider communication options, and to establish a supportive language environment. The family decided they would like to focus on listening and spoken language. Hearing aid use could not be established due to recurrent ear infections and limited benefit from the hearing aid technology. As a result, Matthew was referred for a cochlear implant candidacy evaluation.

Matthew qualified as a cochlear implant candidate and underwent cochlear implant surgery at 16 months for his right side and at 20 months for his left side. After implantation, Matthew was enrolled in weekly listening and spoken language sessions in addition to his home-based early intervention sessions. Matthew demonstrated slow but steady growth in terms of his auditory skills. At six months postimplantation, he was reported to respond to his name inconsistently and attend to such environmental sounds as the blender and television, and he was beginning to show recognition of familiar sounds. For example, when he heard music, he started dancing, and when he heard a knock, he walked toward the door. Although Matthew was responding to sound, he was not able to engage in functional listening assessment due to inability to maintain responsiveness to the tasks.

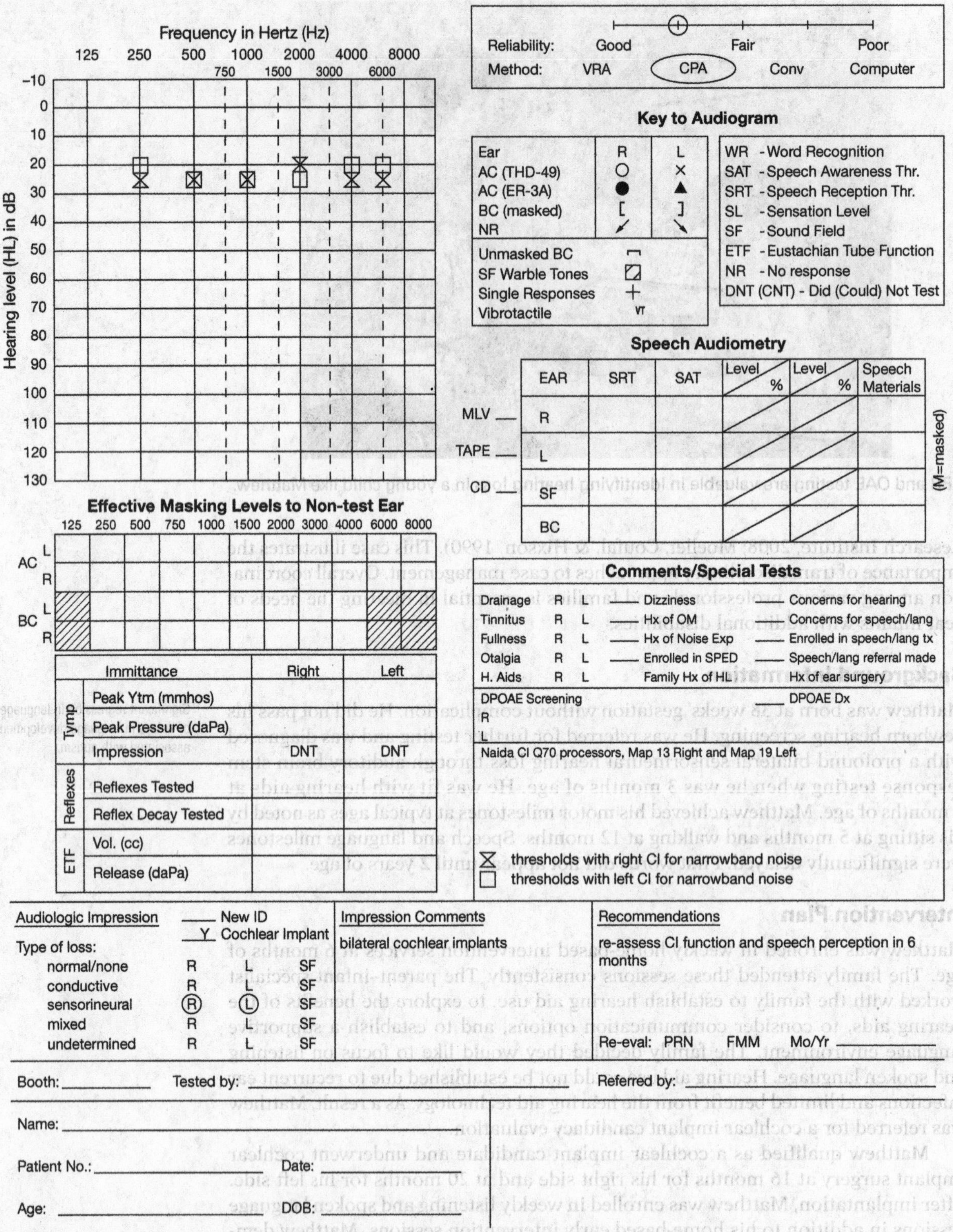

FIGURE 11.1   Case 1: Matthew's cochlear implant audiogram.

Reliability: Good — Fair — Poor
Method: VRA — (CPA) — Conv — Computer

Frequency in Hertz (Hz)

Key to Audiogram

Ear	R	L
AC (THD-49)	○	×
AC (ER-3A)	●	▲
BC (masked)	[	]
NR	↙	↘

Unmasked BC	⌐
SF Warble Tones	▨
Single Responses	+
Vibrotactile	VT

WR - Word Recognition
SAT - Speech Awareness Thr.
SRT - Speech Reception Thr.
SL - Sensation Level
SF - Sound Field
ETF - Eustachian Tube Function
NR - No response
DNT (CNT) - Did (Could) Not Test

Speech Audiometry

	EAR	SRT	SAT	Level %	Level %	Speech Materials
MLV —	R					
TAPE —	L					
CD —	SF					
	BC					

(M=masked) (*=halflist)

Effective Masking Levels to Non-test Ear

125 250 500 750 1000 1500 2000 3000 4000 6000 8000

AC	L	
	R	
BC	L	
	R	

	Immittance	Right	Left
Tymp	Peak Ytm (mmhos)		
	Peak Pressure (daPa)		
	Impression	DNT	DNT
Reflexes	Reflexes Tested		
	Reflex Decay Tested		
ETF	Vol. (cc)		
	Release (daPa)		

Comments/Special Tests

Drainage	R L	— Dizziness	— Concerns for hearing
Tinnitus	R L	— Hx of OM	— Concerns for speech/lang
Fullness	R L	— Hx of Noise Exp	— Enrolled in speech/lang tx
Otalgia	R L	— Enrolled in SPED	— Speech/lang referral made
H. Aids	R L	— Family Hx of HL	— Hx of ear surgery

DPOAE Screening   DPOAE Dx
R
L
Naida CI Q70 processors, Map 13 Right and Map 19 Left

⊠ thresholds with right CI for narrowband noise
☐ thresholds with left CI for narrowband noise

Audiologic Impression	New ID
	Y Cochlear Implant

Type of loss:			
normal/none	R	L	SF
conductive	R	L	SF
sensorineural	(R)	(L)	SF
mixed	R	L	SF
undetermined	R	L	SF

Impression Comments
bilateral cochlear implants

Recommendations
re-assess CI function and speech perception in 6 months

Re-eval: PRN   FMM   Mo/Yr _____

Booth: _____   Tested by: _____   Referred by: _____

Name: _____

Patient No.: _____   Date: _____

Age: _____   DOB: _____

Environmental Coordination and Participation

At age 2 years, 3 months, Matthew's early intervention team had increasing concerns regarding Matthew's slow auditory, speech, and language development. The early intervention team wanted to know if Matthew's progress was typical or if his slow progress could be related to other factors. The team contacted Matthew's cochlear implant team with concerns of (1) inconsistent responsiveness to sound, (2) slow progress with vocalizations and word production, and (3) limited engagement in social exchanges. A meeting was scheduled with the family, early intervention team, and the cochlear implant team. The team members worked together to create an assessment plan that included the cochlear implant team administering a developmental evaluation and speech assessment and the early intervention team obtaining sound, word, and communication function inventories while Matthew was engaged in daily routines in the home environment.

Limited engagement in social exchanges may be associated with autism.

Assessment: Postimplantation

Matthew was administered a developmental evaluation by the cochlear implant team's speech-language pathologist. The Developmental Profile—3 (Alpern, 2007) was used to assess Matthew's development across five key areas: physical, adaptive behavior, social-emotional, cognitive, and communication. All developmental areas were determined to be below age-level expectations with the exception of adaptive skills, which were found to be in the average range. A significantly below-average general development score of 54 was obtained on this measure. The speech-language pathologist also assessed Matthew's speech skills using the Conditioned Assessment of Speech Production (CASP; Ertmer & Stoel-Gammon, 2008). The CASP is an elicited imitation task in which familiar adults provide spoken models of 10 utterances that are presented in three levels of the assessment. Because increased vowel diversity is an early indicator of auditory-guided speech development, three different vowel types serve as stimuli for Level 1, five consonant–vowel syllable forms are stimuli for Level 2, and a consonant + diphthong and a consonant–vowel–consonant syllables form the stimuli for Level 3. Matthew was able to participate in Level 1 of the test, but he did not have the skills to participate in Levels 2 or 3. He obtained 1 out of 6 possible points for Level 1. He was able to imitate "duh" for "uh," "uh" for "ee ee," and "m" for "ae ae ae."

A sound production inventory was collected at age 2 years, 11 months, by Matthew's early interventionist while Matthew was engaged in routine-based home activities. Frequent simple consonant–vowel babbling was observed with limited word or sign production noted. The following consonant sound inventory was obtained: /m, n, b, w, l, z/. The vowel inventory was limited to /i, ae, a/. In addition, the MacArthur-Bates Communicative Development Inventories (Fenson et al., 2007), which is a parent report scale, provided valuable information on Matthew's use of vocabulary and communication functions. Matthew was observed and reported to use gestures (e.g., hands reached out) to request, vocalizations to reject, and physical movements (e.g., pushed people) to demand and call attention. Labeling, commenting, and recurrent communication functions were not observed or reported. Once all the assessments were completed, the cochlear implant and the early intervention teams met to discuss Matthew's test results. The teams agreed that Matthew's progress was more delayed than expected. The parents questioned if Matthew was possibly autistic. The team indicated that Matthew's inattentiveness, lack of social responsiveness, and limited functional communication could be indicators of autism spectrum disorder. The team offered the family a referral to the team psychologist, but the family declined, stating that they would prefer to wait to see if enrollment in preschool supported Matthew's further development.

Fleeting visual attention, reduced functionality of communication, and lack of social responsiveness are not typical of a child who has hearing loss alone.

At 3 years of age, Matthew was enrolled in an early childhood special education classroom for children who are deaf or hard of hearing five mornings a week, and he attended a neighborhood preschool in the afternoons. On enrollment in preschool, he was communicating primarily using gestures, vocalizations, and a few signs. While enrolled in the early childhood special education program, Matthew received weekly individual speech-language therapy and occupational therapy. Matthew was described by his mother as a relatively shy child. His teacher reported that he was curious about what others are doing, but engaged in limited partnered play. Further, Matthew had significant difficulty in transitioning from one preschool activity to another, often engaging in disruptive behavior. Progress in speech, language, and auditory skills was slow, with significant concerns about Matthew's social relatedness skills. Given the slow progress, Matthew's school team and family decided to begin use of a picture communication system. Matthew demonstrated some progress with the picture communication system, but progress was limited and very inconsistent.

At age 3 years, 4 months, Matthew's parents requested an evaluation to determine if Matthew was autistic. According to the multidisciplinary team report, Matthew was communicating using 7 to 10 single words, signs, or pictures. School reports indicated that Matthew had difficulty making friends. He sometimes was noted to get overexcited and scare the other children in the classroom. Inconsistent eye contact was reported, with Matthew maintaining eye contact only when he was requesting a food item or toy. Matthew's favorite activities included puzzles and cars. He reportedly carried around a small pillow as a comfort item everywhere he went. No sensory sensitivities were noted. However, when Matthew did not get what he wanted, he engaged in disruptive behaviors that interfered with daily functioning across settings. Social relatedness, limited responsiveness, and a reduced range of play interests are considered "red flags" for autism spectrum disorder (see http://firstwords.fsu.edu/asd.html). The comprehensive multidisciplinary assessment revealed delays in social/communication, peer socialization, adult socialization, and social/emotional reciprocity. A diagnosis of autism spectrum disorder was provided to the family when Matthew was age 3 years, 6 months.

Psychosocial and Counseling Aspects

It is critical for educational and cochlear implant teams to consider the serial adjustments that families may be experiencing as they are caring for their children who are deaf or hard of hearing. For families of newly identified children who are deaf, there may be an emotional adjustment that the family makes immediately after the child's birth. Very shortly after learning about the diagnosis, many families begin a path of trying to address the hearing loss with hearing technology. When the hearing aid technology option does not provide the child with enough audibility, families adjust again to the fact that medical intervention may be needed, which requires cochlear implant surgery. In this family's case, yet another adjustment needed to be made when they learned about their child's diagnosis of autism. It is important for providers to understand the depth and rate of adjustments families are making so that they can determine how to best support the family through all of the changes they are experiencing.

Assessment and Intervention Postdiagnosis of Autism Spectrum Disorder

Formal administration of Matthew's speech, language, and auditory skills was conducted when Matthew was age 4 years, 4 months. Vocabulary testing was conducted and discontinued, as Matthew was unable to demonstrate a consistent point response. Results of the Preschool Language Scale–5 (Zimmerman, Steiner, & Pond, 2011) revealed a language standard score of 53 and a percentile rank of 1. Matthew was noted to inconsistently follow simple one-step commands when prompting and visual supports were used. He was observed to answer a few yes-or-no questions related to food (e.g., "Do you want a cracker"). He had difficulty labeling and identifying simple pictures. Assessment of Matthew's articulation skills was conducted using an articulation screener. On this measure, he was able to imitate only 1 of the 23 items presented (e.g., "b" in "bird"). Language sample analysis revealed that Matthew used one or two words, signs, or pictures to communicate. Examination of oral motor production was attempted, but Matthew would not cooperate with the tasks. Analysis of Matthew's communication indicated the following communication patterns: (1) 26 percent use of spoken language, (2) 17 percent use of simultaneous communication (voice and sign), (3) 17 percent use of sign only, and (4) 40 percent use of a picture communication system.

Communication Rehabilitation Adjustment

Matthew's individualized education team designed an intervention plan to meet Matthew's complex needs. The following goals were identified to address Matthew's speech, language, auditory, attention, and social relatedness needs:

Children with autism frequently need specific intervention focused on developing their daily communication skills.

1. Given an unstructured setting, Matthew will use his voice four times for each of the following communication functions in a preschool morning: greetings/salutations, requesting, commenting, and protesting.
2. Given a structured setting, Matthew will approximate modeled vocal production of words with the following types of word structures without sign support in four out of five opportunities: CV (consonant–vowel, e.g., "me"), VC (e.g., "on"), CVCV (e.g., "mama"), and CVC (e.g., "mom").
3. Using listening only, in a classroom or therapy setting, Matthew will respond to his name by looking up or turning in four out of five opportunities.
4. Given a listening situation in a classroom or therapy setting, Matthew will participate in listening sound checks by dropping a block in a bucket when he hears the sound presented.
5. Given a classroom setting, Matthew will use 15 different signs, words, or pictures in a preschool morning on three consecutive days.
6. Given an unstructured setting, Matthew will follow simple directions in four out of five opportunities.
7. Given a classroom setting and a set of four choices, Matthew will point to a named object in four out of five opportunities.
8. Given a visual schedule, Matthew will independently transition between five classroom activities on three consecutive days.
9. Given a highly motivating item or activity and wait time, Matthew will demonstrate joint attention while commenting by shifting his gaze from an item to a person and then back to the item four times in a preschool morning.

Given the complexity of this case, ongoing assessment of the intervention plan will be needed. It is hoped with time that Matthew will increase his auditory responsiveness, functional language usage, and social relatedness. The family and school team are currently exploring use of Pivotal Response Treatment (PRT). PRT is a naturalistic intervention based on the principles and practices of applied behavior analysis and developmental approaches. PRT targets pivotal areas of a child's development, including motivation, responsivity to multiple cues, self-management, and social initiations (see https://www.autismspeaks.org/what-autism/treatment/pivotal-response-therapy-prt).

Summary

This case illustrates the importance of careful monitoring of a child's progress across developmental domains. It also demonstrates the amount of time that must be taken when partnering with families as they are receiving and processing information that their child has multiple factors impacting development. Collaboration between the family, educational team, and cochlear implant team ensured that all partners were obtaining a comprehensive view of the child so that a unified intervention approach could be implemented. Finally, this case demonstrates the importance of examining the effectiveness of intervention and the exploration of multiple approaches that may support that child's development.

CASE 2: ANNIE—ROUTES TO SPOKEN LANGUAGE FOLLOWING COCHLEAR IMPLANTATION

Many families electing a cochlear implant have a goal that their child will learn to communicate using spoken language. However, families vary in the routes they may take to this goal.

As a result of newborn hearing screening programs, infants who are deaf or hard of hearing and their families have earlier access to interventions than ever before. Many families whose infants have severe to profound hearing loss elect to pursue cochlear implantation to provide the infant access to sound during sensitive periods for language development. Cochlear implant surgery typically occurs around 12 months of age, with programming of the device occurring a few weeks later. Many families electing this option have a goal that their child will learn to communicate using spoken language. However, families vary in the routes they may take to this goal. This case study describes a family who elected to use total communication (sign + spoken language) with their daughter prior to cochlear implantation. Following cochlear implant mapping, they were strategic in reducing reliance on visual communication in order to promote auditory development and spoken language. This case illustrates some concepts and strategies that can be helpful in determining if such an approach is working to meet the stated goals.

Background Information

Annie was the third child born to a midwestern family. She did not pass newborn hearing screening, and subsequent Auditory Brainstem Response (ABR) testing at 11 weeks of age confirmed the presence of a severe to profound bilateral sensorineural hearing loss. Annie's older brother also had severe to profound hearing loss. He received a cochlear implant at 14 months of age and was performing in the average to above-average range in all areas of spoken language development by 3 years of age. The family planned for Annie to receive a cochlear implant shortly after her first birthday. Annie was fit with powerful hearing aids at 3.9 months of age. She then underwent cochlear implantation on the right side at 13 months of age. She uses an Advanced Bionics device with HiRes processing strategy.

As families explore their options for communicating with their infant, some consider whether to use sign language prior to cochlear implants. They often encounter varied opinions from professionals or other parents. In some cases, the concern is expressed that use of sign-based approaches will interfere with the development of auditory skills and spoken language. Others express the view that signing will not interfere but will support the development of spoken language. What is a family to believe? More important, how can they ensure their child's success and achieve the goals set for their family?

Professionals and parents use the Auditory–Visual Continuum to characterize the child's current "zone of development" in order to provide optimal access to language.

One approach to guiding families is to help them adapt to their own child's learning abilities and needs, which are likely to shift with development. Robbins (2001) suggested that professionals consider children's current performance levels and learning needs on a continuum from fully auditory to fully visual. This concept has been adapted by others to guide decision making and curricular planning (Nussbaum, Scott, Waddy-Smith, & Koch, 2004). The continuum has also been adapted by a program called the Auditory Consultant Resource Network (ACRN; Carotta, Koch, & Brennan, 2014) at Boys Town National Research Hospital. The ACRN project was designed to assist school programs/professionals in creating auditory/spoken language opportunities for children with new technologies who had historically been instructed using visual methods. An Auditory–Visual Continuum is illustrated in Figure 11.2A. Professionals and parents use this tool to characterize the child's current "zone of development" in terms of providing optimal access to language. For example, one child might access familiar information through audition alone (auditory) but require some visual supports (pictures, context support, speechreading, or sign) when encountering new concepts. That child's zone of development would include the A and A$_V$ end of the continuum (see Figure 11.2A). Another child may be reliant on visual supports for most language

	Auditory (A)————A$_V$————AV————V$_A$————Visual (V)	Time 1	Time 2
A	Able to understand through listening alone		
A$_V$	Able to understand primarily through listening but needs some visual support		
AV	Equal need for visual/sign and auditory input		
V$_A$	Mostly a visual/sign user; understands speech for some words/phrases		
V	Visual/sign user; spoken language challenging to understand		

FIGURE 11.2A   Auditory–Visual (A–V) Continuum for receptive communication.

Source: Adapted from Spoken language and sign: Optimizing learning for children with cochlear implants. Paper presented at Laurent Clerc National Deaf Education Center. Washington, DC., © 2004.

learning but could be developing new auditory skills after receiving a cochlear implant. That child's zone of development would include the V to V$_A$ end of the continuum. The scale helps parents and professionals identify the current zone of development for individual children in relation to the goals for the child. The zone of development is a flexible construct; the educational team may be setting goals to shift the child's skills along the continuum.

In Figure 11.2A, the two columns on the right allow the team to capture how the child's abilities may be changing over time in relation to language access. Annie's family elected to use signs and other visual supports before the cochlear implant surgery, so they began at the visual end of the continuum. However, their goals and expectations were for Annie to move toward the auditory end of the continuum as she gained auditory experience following implantation.

Aural Rehabilitation Plan: Preimplantation

Annie's family had signed with their first child, who had normal hearing, and with Annie's older brother, who was born deaf. When asked about their decision to use sign with Annie, the mother replied, "We were signing advocates from the beginning of our parenting. . . . We did begin signing much earlier with Annie than the other two because she was diagnosed with hearing loss at 11 weeks of age. We wanted all of our infants and toddlers to begin communicating with us as soon as possible, and we could only assume that signing would aid in language development prior to the children receiving a cochlear implant. For us it was the concept of filling their 'language tool bucket' with whatever might be useful in their development."

Annie's family began providing visual supports (signing, gestures, visual cues) along with spoken language. They consistently called her attention to sounds in the environment and called her name at close distance before using visual methods to get her attention. Annie's progress in auditory development was limited. However, the AR specialist/family educator stressed the importance of continuing with auditory development activities in preparation for the cochlear implant. Studies have demonstrated that use of residual hearing prior to cochlear implantation is related to improved cochlear implant outcomes (Geers, 2006). Once she received her cochlear implant, the family helped her adjust to full-time use, and they began providing rich auditory stimulation.

Aural Rehabilitation Plan: Postimplantation

The family goal was for Annie to develop the use of spoken language following cochlear implantation. They were aware of the need to gradually reduce their use of visual supports and increase focus on auditory learning opportunities. Once her cochlear implant was programmed, the goals on the Individualized Family Service Plan (IFSP) were modified to include this shift toward increased auditory emphasis.

To reach their goals, the family was aware of the need to gradually reduce their use of visual supports and increase focus on auditory learning opportunities. They made strategic decisions about when to provide visual supports.

	A	Av	AV	Comments/Observations
New			X	New words presented with sign or other visual supports + spoken
Review		X		Spoken → sign/visual supports + spoken → spoken
Routine	X			Auditory input; clarify with sign only if needed

FIGURE 11.2B **Strategies for supporting comprehension during the first year of cochlear implant use.**
Source: Carotta et al. (2014).

Family members were supported to use the following strategies in everyday contexts to build Annie's reliance on auditory skills (for additional auditory strategies with infants, see Rotfleisch, 2009):

1. Consistently giving her opportunities to alert to her name; using their voices to get her attention before using visual means.
2. Optimizing her auditory environment (reducing background noise; ensuring consistent cochlear implant use; limiting overtalk among multiple speakers).
3. Directing her attention to sounds around her ("I hear that. That's the phone." "You heard my voice; it was Mommy!")
4. Encouraging Annie to vocalize and use her voice to get family members' attention and to engage in vocal imitation.
5. Making strategic decisions about when to provide sign supports. The family goal was to build a bridge between Annie's language knowledge in sign and her ability to represent the same ideas in spoken language. Their strategy was guided by three considerations:
   a. The child's level of familiarity with the language. The parents considered whether the concept/phrase was familiar (routine), emerging (review), or new. This is illustrated in Figure 11.2B. Routine language (understood in sign) was the first to be presented in spoken form; sign support was provided for a while to introduce new concepts. When sign was used, it was often incorporated in an "auditory sandwich" format (Koch, 2004). This means that the information was presented first through audition, then signed + spoken, and then audition again. This was used to tie familiar concepts in sign to their spoken forms and to increase Annie's reliance on auditory skills for learning spoken language.
   b. The need to clarify Annie's spoken language attempts. When Annie's speech was unintelligible, her parents would ask, "Can you tell me again?" then, as needed, "Can you sign it?" (so that her message could be understood). They would then repeat the spoken form of the word to her and encourage her to express the idea again in spoken language.
   c. The need to repair communication breakdowns. If Annie misunderstood something the family presented in spoken language, they would make a second attempt in spoken language, and then clarify with sign + spoken language as needed.
6. Establishing links from spoken messages to their meaning. This involved sharing an idea (spoken input) and then showing the idea.
7. Emphasizing important words using acoustic highlighting (added emphasis) and modeling language using infant-directed speech characteristics.
8. Implementing systematic auditory development strategies during natural routines, based on guidance from the AR specialist.
9. Providing auditory imprinting using natural repetition of phrases (Koch, 2004).

Annie made rapid progress in alerting to her name, attaching meaning to sounds and spoken words, and increasing her vocalizations. However, the parents noticed that their little girl was slower to progress in expressive skills than her older brother had been. They realized that it was important to have high expectations for her but to avoid comparisons with her brother's early learning rates. The mother noted that Annie's brother was more of a risk taker when communicating with others: "I think signing 'fits' Annie's expressive personality even today," she added. They continued using the strategies outlined above to increase Annie's reliance on auditory skills and spoken language while using visual supports (signs, speechreading, context) to "bridge" new spoken language development for both of the children. "But I remember Annie transitioning slower, so we continued to use sign whenever needed for language support," her mother added.

The AR team observed that this mother appeared to make wise intuitive judgments about when to sign to Annie. When asked how she did that, the mother stated, "I think I would watch for that 'blank look' that told me she had missed something and then fill in the gap with repetition and visual clarifiers, like sign. Sometimes she just wouldn't respond (or obey an instruction). We made it a practice to use the 'auditory sandwiching' technique taught to us by our team. This took some practice, but became more natural with practice. There was a time when I think Annie would have preferred to watch and not work so hard at listening. We had to try to balance effectively communicating without frustrating her yet encouraging her to be a good 'listener.'"

> "There was a time when I think Annie would have preferred to watch and not work so hard at listening. We had to try to balance effectively communicating without frustrating her yet encouraging her to be a good 'listener.'"

Intervention Outcomes

After one year of cochlear implant use, the family made progress in their reliance on spoken language. As Annie increasingly relied on her auditory skills, visual supports were not needed as often. As shown in Figure 11.3, after one year of cochlear implant experience, new information could be presented in spoken language. Signs were used to support her understanding as needed, but Annie rarely required these clarifications. At this point, sign was used more often to help Annie clarify her language expression when she attempted complex words. That too was changing, as she increasingly expressed herself orally and speech became clearer.

Annie's progress in sign and spoken vocabulary was monitored using the MacArthur Bates Communication Development Inventory (Fenson et al., 2007), a parent report measure. Through 21 months of age, the mother was asked to complete duplicate forms, capturing the words Annie expressed in sign and those expressed in spoken language. What is evident from Figure 11.4 is that Annie's spoken vocabulary developed more slowly than sign vocabulary until about 22 months of age (9 months postimplantation). Her number of spoken words then began to accelerate, and she relied on spoken language more than sign in most situations.

Initially, sign vocabulary greatly exceeded spoken. Sign and spoken vocabulary scores were reported through 21 months; around that time, it was observed that Annie's rate of spoken vocabulary learning was accelerated.

Annie's progress also was monitored with standardized measures of language and speech, administered in spoken language. The results supported the view that Annie was making appropriate progress. She achieved Standard Scores of 93 and 111 on the Goldman Fristoe Test of Articulation (Goldman Fristoe-2, 2000) at 3 and 4 years of age, respectively. A spontaneous language sample collected at 4 years age revealed

	A	Av	AV	Comments/observations
New		X		Spoken; clarify key words with sign, only if needed
Review			X	Spoken; clarify key words with sign, only if needed
Routine		X		Auditory presentation; spoken language

FIGURE 11.3 Strategies for supporting comprehension after one year of cochlear implant use.

Source: Carotta et al., (2014).

FIGURE 11.4 Changes in Annie's expressive vocabulary as a function of age from 12 to 34 months.

It is critical to partner with families to evaluate if the chosen approaches are moving them toward stated goals.

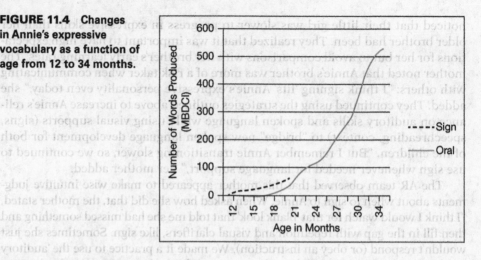

that 89 percent of her utterances were completely intelligible. At this same age, she achieved a Standard Score of 93 on the Peabody Picture Vocabulary Test (Dunn & Dunn, 1997) and a total language standard score of 101 on the Preschool Language Scale 5 (Zimmerman et al., 2011). Figure 11.5 illustrates how Annie's zone of development was shifting in terms of both receiving information and expressing herself.

Summary

The point of this case study was not to advocate for the use of any particular method. Rather, it illustrates a process professionals can use in supporting a family whose stated goal is to transition from visual approaches to spoken language development. Today, Annie is a highly successful student thanks to the strong support from her family. When asked about Annie's current communication preferences,

	Auditory——A_V——AV——V_A——Visual	Time 1	Time 2
A	Able to understand through listening alone		✓
A_V	Able to understand primarily through listening but needs some visual support	✓	✓
AV	Equal need for visual/sign and auditory input	✓	
V_A	Mostly a visual/sign user; understand speech for some words/phrases		
V	Visual/sign user; spoken language challenging to understand		
	Oral——OS——OS——SO——Sign		
O	Oral/spoken language		
O_S	Mostly oral, with some visual/sign use		✓
OS	Equal use of oral/spoken, plus sign		
S_O	Mostly sign/visual communicator, with some spoken words	✓	
S	Uses sign only		

FIGURE 11.5 Changes in Annie's zone of development. Receptive at top; expressive at bottom at 1 and 2 years postimplantation.

Source: Developed for use in the ACRN and adapted from Nussbaum et al. (2004) and Robbins (2001). The expressive continuum was developed by Bettie Waddy-Smith at the Clerc Center at Gallaudet University in 2004.

her mother reported, "Annie does rely primarily on spoken language, but she still enjoys signing. We do use sign in several settings . . . anytime her cochlear implant is off—swimming or bathing, at bedtime when she is asking for yet another drink, at church during the 'quiet times,' and occasionally in a noisy setting or if she is across the room from us. You can find any member of our family using sign in these situations." In summary, this family used sign to support spoken language development, and they did so in a balanced manner. They recognized the importance of promoting Annie's development of auditory skills to achieve their goals. Annie currently performs in the Auditory to A_V zone of development on the continuum. Yet the family recognizes sign as a helpful communication tool that can be employed in situations where Annie needs additional support. For this family, it was helpful to flexibly adapt the tools they used as Annie's abilities changed.

CASE 3: AMBER—ISSUES AFFECTING EDUCATIONAL PLACEMENT

AR management frequently includes provision of input to a child's Individualized Education Plan (IEP) team related to educational placement. This case illustrates the importance of considering audiologic, language, academic, and social factors in such decisions.

Background Information

Amber was referred for a multidisciplinary evaluation by the AR team when she was age 6 years, 7 months. She was born in Korea and spent the first year of her life with a Korean foster family. Birth records indicated a normal, full-term delivery. An American family adopted Amber when she was 14 months of age. Amber walked at 14 months, was toilet trained at 4 to 5 years of age, and had few words at 3 years of age.

At 30 months of age, a bilateral, sensorineural hearing loss was identified. Audiologic records indicated that the loss was progressive in nature, as shown in the serial audiogram in Figure 11.6. At the time of her first evaluation, Amber's

> A serial audiogram is used when progression is suspected. It logs the thresholds over time for ease of comparison.

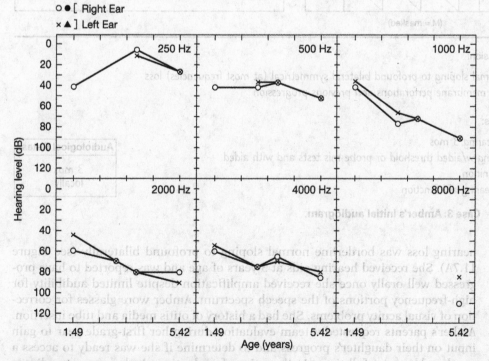

FIGURE 11.6 Case 3: Amber's serial audiogram.

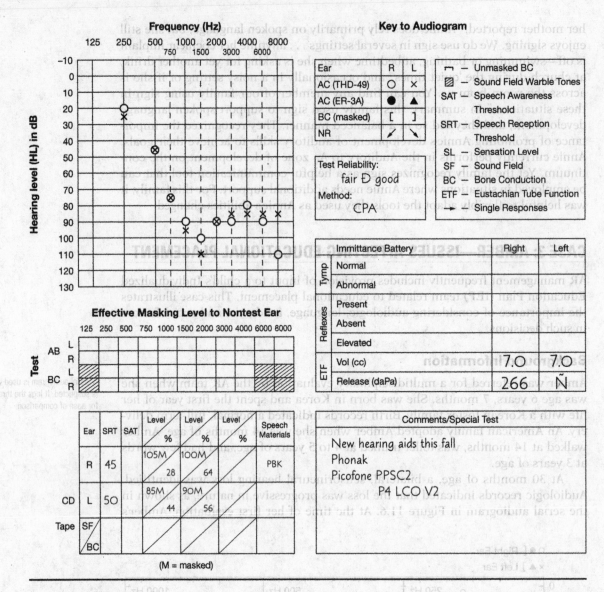

Key to Audiogram

Ear	R	L
AC (THD-49)	O	×
AC (ER-3A)	●	▲
BC (masked)	[	]
NR	↙	↘

⌐ — Unmasked BC
▨ — Sound Field Warble Tones
SAT — Speech Awareness Threshold
SRT — Speech Reception Threshold
SL — Sensation Level
SF — Sound Field
BC — Bone Conduction
ETF — Eustachian Tube Function
→ — Single Responses

Test Reliability: fair Đ good
Method: CPA

Immittance Battery		Right	Left
Tymp	Normal		
	Abnormal		
Reflexes	Present		
	Absent		
	Elevated		
ETF	Vol (cc)	7.0	7.0
	Release (daPa)	266	Ñ

Effective Masking Level to Nontest Ear

125 250 500 750 1000 1500 2000 3000 4000 6000 8000

Test
AB L / R
BC L / R

Ear	SRT	SAT	Level %	Level %	Level %	Speech Materials
R	45		105M / 28	100M / 64		PBK
CD L	50		85M / 44	90M / 56		
Tape SF / BC						

(M = masked)

Comments/Special Test

New hearing aids this fall
Phonak
Picofone PPSC2
P4 LCO V2

Audiologic Impression:

Borderline normal sloping to profound bilateral symmetrical (at most frequencies) loss with tympanic membrane perforations and previous progression

Recommendations:

1. Monitor hearing 3 mos
2. Aided testing w/aided threshold or probe mis tests and with aided word recognition
3. Monitor hearing aid function

Audiological Retest
3 mos locally

FIGURE 11.7A Case 3: Amber's initial audiogram.

hearing loss was borderline normal sloping to profound bilaterally (see Figure 11.7A). She received hearing aids at 3 years of age and was reported to have progressed well orally once she received amplification despite limited audibility for high-frequency portions of the speech spectrum. Amber wore glasses for correction of visual acuity problems. She had a history of otitis media and tube insertion. Amber's parents requested a team evaluation during her first-grade year to gain input on their daughter's progress and to determine if she was ready to access a regular classroom full-time. At the point of evaluation, Amber was attending a

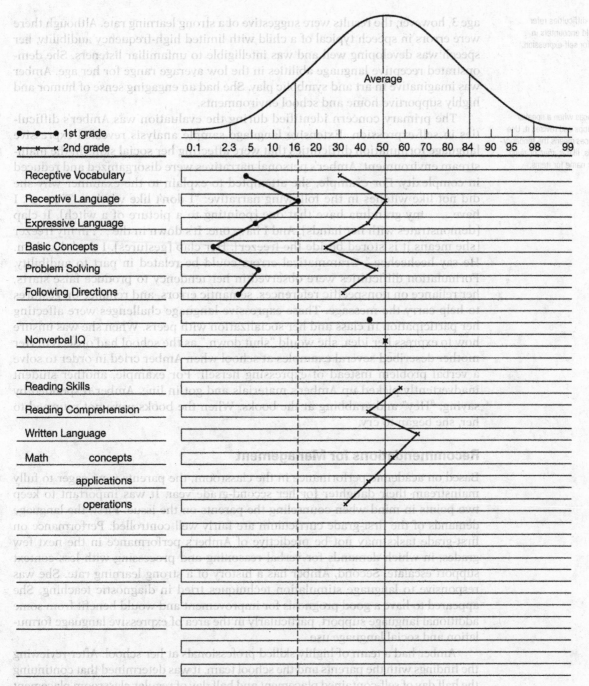

FIGURE 11.7B   Amber's profile of multidisciplinary findings.

self-contained classroom for children who are hard of hearing in the mornings and a mainstream first grade in the afternoons. The only concern raised by the school was Amber's tendency to "shut down" and avoid responding following some adult requests at school.

Assessment Findings

The profile in Figure 11.7B summarizes the result of multidisciplinary findings in the areas of psychology, language, and communication. Filled circles represent the first evaluation; the x's represent a one-year follow-up evaluation. In the first evaluation, Amber's language and academic skills were very delayed in comparison to the hearing peers who were in her class. Considering that she had limited language at

A profile can be a useful way to integrate results across disciplines in order to get a "total child" view.

Language formulation difficulties refer to problems that a child encounters in organization of ideas for self-expression.

age 3, however, the results were suggestive of a strong learning rate. Although there were errors in speech typical of a child with limited high-frequency audibility, her speech was developing well and was intelligible to unfamiliar listeners. She demonstrated receptive language abilities in the low average range for her age. Amber was imaginative in art and symbolic play. She had an engaging sense of humor and highly supportive home and school environments.

False starts are instances when a speaker begins a phrase but stops and revises it. Use of *nonspecific references* means the tendency to use indefinite words, like *it*, *that*, or *thing*, instead of the specific name for items.

The primary concern identified during the evaluation was Amber's difficulties in self-expression. Extensive language sample analysis revealed expressive language formulation difficulties that were affecting her social skills in the mainstream environment. Amber's personal narratives were disorganized and reduced in complexity. For example, she attempted to explain to the examiner why she did not like witches in the following narrative: "I don't like witches. That . . . I have . . . my grandma have that one [pointing to a picture of a witch]. It clap [demonstrates with her hands]. And I have one. It's down in the . . . in my freezer [she means it is stored beside the freezer]. Her clap [gestures]. I don't like him. He say heeheehee." Grammatical errors could be related in part to audibility. Formulation difficulties were observed in her tendency to produce false starts, her reliance on nonspecific references, semantic errors, and reliance on gestures to help carry the message. These expressive language challenges were affecting her participation in class and her socialization with peers. When she was unsure how to express her idea, she would "shut down," as the school had observed. Her mother described several examples at school when Amber cried in order to solve a verbal problem instead of expressing herself. For example, another student inadvertently picked up Amber's materials and got in line. Amber responded by saying, "Hey" and grabbing at the books. When the books were not returned to her, she began to cry.

Recommendations for Management

Based on academic performance in the classroom, the parents were eager to fully mainstream their daughter for her second-grade year. It was important to keep two points in mind when counseling the parents on the issue. First, the language demands of the first-grade curriculum are fairly well controlled. Performance on first-grade tasks may not be predictive of Amber's performance in the next few grades, in which demands for verbal reasoning and processing with less context support escalate. Second, Amber has a history of a strong learning rate. She was responsive to language stimulation techniques tried in diagnostic teaching. She appeared to have a good prognosis for improvement and would benefit from some additional language support, particularly in the area of expressive language formulation and social language use.

Amber had a team of highly skilled professionals at her school. After reviewing the findings with the parents and the school team, it was determined that continuing the half day of self-contained placement and half day of regular classroom placement was advisable. The teaching team selected the following priorities for her support program: (1) strengthen expressive language formulation through daily opportunities to narrate with support from the team, with particular emphasis being placed on school language functions (e.g., problem solving, reasoning, describing, explaining, sharing personal stories); (2) building vocabulary and using specific references; (3) reducing semantic errors, particularly those based in limited audibility (e.g., pronouns and prepositions); (4) strengthening emotive vocabulary; and (5) role-playing, using social scripts to practice verbal social interactions with peers.

Communication and social findings should be considered along with academic performance when making decisions about mainstreaming and support needs.

Follow-Up Assessment

The parent and school team requested a follow-up assessment one year later as a way of monitoring their progress toward the established goals and reconsidering the parental goal of increasing mainstreaming opportunities. Audiologic testing revealed that Amber's hearing thresholds had remained stable over the past year and that she was receiving good benefit from her amplification and FM systems. Language and academic retesting demonstrated significant progress in all areas of language and literacy. As illustrated by the x's on the profile in Figure 11.7B, Amber's language and academic scores were within the average range for her age and grade placement. Although Amber was still working through some formulation struggles at times, her personal narratives were better organized and contained few errors. She was able to express her ideas fluently much of the time. The school reported that Amber was getting along better with her peers and solving problems using verbal means. As a result of the positive findings, the parents and educators made a decision to mainstream Amber in the third grade with support services. This case illustrates that social-emotional and communication factors needed to be considered in the decision-making process. Academic test results, especially in the earliest grades, can be misleading in determining readiness for mainstreaming. Amber benefited greatly from an additional year of support, which resulted in stronger linguistic and social preparation for full inclusion in the mainstream setting.

CASE 4: GREG—LATE IDENTIFICATION OF A CHILD WHO IS HARD OF HEARING

Prior to newborn screening, the average age of identification of hearing loss in the United States was 18 months for deaf children and even older for hard of hearing children (Carney & Moeller, 1998). Since the advent of newborn hearing screening, many hard of hearing infants and families have the combined advantage of early and consistent amplification and early intervention services. Many of these children are able to achieve language skills close to their peers with normal hearing (Moeller, 2000; Yoshinaga-Itano, Sedey, Coulter, & Mehl, 1998) and are able to be successfully educated in mainstream settings. This proactive approach to management is ideal. Some children still slip through system cracks; others develop later-onset hearing loss. This means that professionals and parents must continue to be vigilant and refer for audiologic evaluation if there are concerns for speech, language, or hearing. The following case describes a child who was late-identified prior to the implementation of newborn hearing screening. Inconsistency in his responses to sound led to delays in referral for hearing evaluation. This case illustrates the importance of audibility in the formation of language rules by a child who is hard of hearing. In this case, the child needed to learn new ways of gaining meaning from messages around him. His aural habilitation program needed to focus on helping him develop productive listening and comprehension behaviors.

Background Information

Greg's parents first began to express concerns about his hearing to their pediatrician when he was 2 years old. He was demonstrating inconsistent responses to sound and delayed speech and language development at that time. Results of audiologic testing at a community hospital suggested borderline normal hearing sensitivity in response to speech and narrowband stimuli. One and a half years later, the parents continued to express concern for Greg's hearing, and testing revealed at least a mild to moderate sensorineural hearing loss in the better ear. However, the audiologist reported questionable test reliability, and Greg was referred for auditory brain stem response testing. Results suggested the probability of a moderate to severe sensorineural hearing loss in at least the higher frequencies, with the right ear more involved than the left. Greg was then referred to a pediatric audiologic team. A severe rising to mild hearing loss in the right ear was confirmed through behavioral testing. Left ear testing revealed responses in the mild hearing

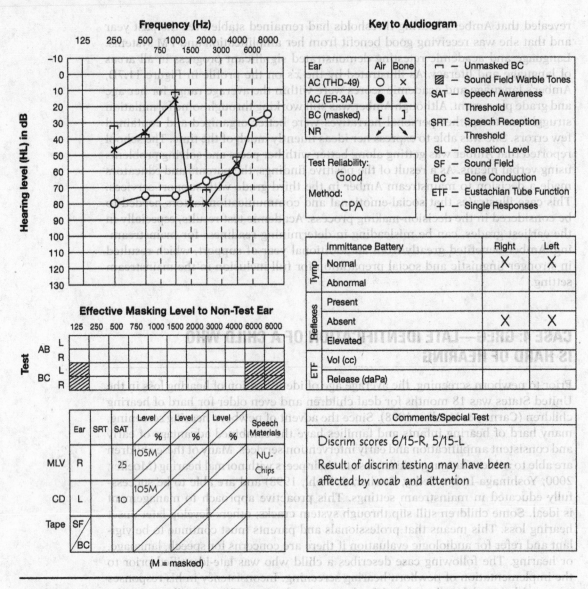

FIGURE 11.8A Case 4: Greg's initial audiogram.

loss range, rising to within normal limits at 1 kHz, steeply sloping to the severe hearing loss range at 2 kHz, and then rising to the mild hearing loss range in the higher frequencies. Given the unusual configuration of Greg's hearing loss (see Figure 11.8A), it was not surprising that he passed a screening evaluation that used speech and narrow bands of noise in the sound field. Unfortunately, the referral for more definitive testing was delayed by the findings of the screening assessment. Medical-genetic evaluation revealed a family history of hearing loss, but etiology could not be confirmed.

Hearing aid fitting was complex given the unusual audiometric configuration in the left ear. However, a binaural fitting was selected, with capability for direct audio input for FM amplification. Greg was immediately referred to an **AR** program for the purposes of evaluating his individual communication needs and determining considerations for educational placement.

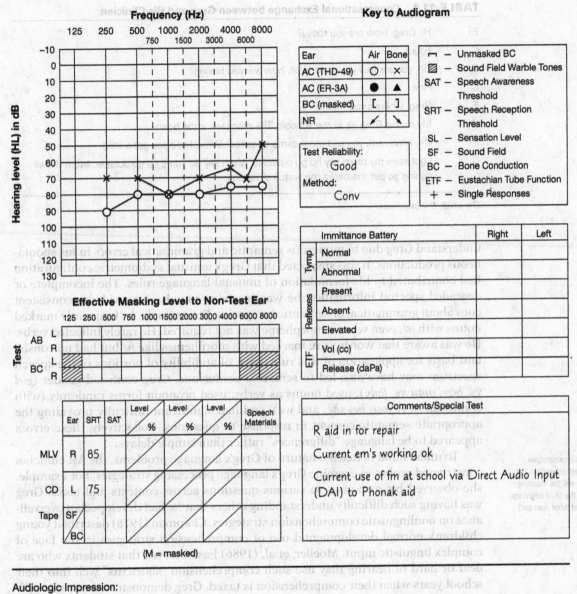

FIGURE 11.8B   Case 4: Greg's recent audiogram (following progression).

Communication Assessment

Greg demonstrated an unusual communication profile at 4 years of age. On standardized tests of language, his receptive language skills were more severely delayed (>2 standard deviations) than his expressive language skills. Analysis of conversational interactions was useful in understanding the complexity of his receptive and expressive language problems. It was evident from the outset that Greg was having serious difficulty understanding those around him. Table 11.1 contains a segment from an interactive language sample where Greg was conversing with an AR clinician.

A number of interesting patterns were reflected in Greg's spontaneous speech. Although most of his words were intelligible to the listener, it was difficult to

Greg's comprehension difficulties were evident in the finding that expressive language was stronger than receptive.

Semantic errors refer to errors in the meaning of the message. For example, referring to a *girl* as a *boy* is an error of meaning.

TABLE 11.1 **Conversational Exchange between Greg and His Clinician**

E	Hi, Greg. How are you today?
C	Fours.
E	Oh, you are four years old. Well, how are you feeling?
C	Fine.
E	Greg, where's your mom?
C	My moms Greg go to the schools. The mom talk it the boats.
E	Oh. Hmmmm, you and mom came to school. Wow, I see you got a star!
C	I got stars my mom say no go outsides. Mom say do sums no go outside. Mom the all raining go put the backs the watch all raining.

C = child; *E* = examiner.

understand Greg due to numerous semantic and grammatical errors in his spontaneous productions. It was suspected that Greg's unusual audiometric configuration had contributed to his formulation of unusual language rules. The incomplete or degraded spectral information he was receiving may have provided inconsistent cues about grammatical or semantic categories. For example, he frequently marked nouns with /s/, even when a morpheme was not required. He rarely inflected verbs. He was aware that words were marked with morphemes like /s/ but had no consistent basis for application of this rule. Lack of audibility of portions of the speech spectrum may have also led to semantic confusions. Greg confused gender (*girl* vs. *boy*; *man* vs. *lady*), used nouns as verbs, used pronoun forms randomly (with confusion of *I*, *you*, *be*, *she*, and *we*), and had significant difficulty providing the appropriate semantic content in response to questions. Collectively, these errors appeared to be language "differences" rather than simple delays.

To understand better the nature of Greg's language problems, the AR clinician constructed probes to examine Greg's language processing strategies. For example, she observed his responses to various questions across contexts and tasks. Greg was having such difficulty understanding others that he had developed an overreliance on nonlinguistic comprehension strategies. Chapman (1978) described young children's normal developmental use of comprehension strategies in the face of complex linguistic input. Moeller, et al, (1986) has observed that students who are deaf or hard of hearing may use such comprehension "shortcuts" well into their school years when their comprehension is taxed. Greg demonstrated extreme reliance on these behaviors due to pervasive comprehension difficulties. Greg used the following strategies in his attempts to make sense of input around him:

Nonlinguistic comprehension strategies refer to a child's use of cues other than the spoken message to figure out the meaning of a phrase. For example, the child might use content cues to understand what was said.

1. Attended to key words in the message to the exclusion of other information
2. Predicted message intention based on situational context cues
3. Nodded his head as if he understood
4. Selected a key, recognizable word and made comments related to that topic (without respect for the current topic of conversation)
5. Controlled the conversational topic to avoid comprehension demands
6. Said everything known about the topic in hopes that the answer was included in the content somewhere (global response strategy)

Greg was not able to answer any types of questions with consistency. Tracking of his responses revealed correct responses in fewer than 25 percent of the instances. In response to commands, he failed to recognize the need for action and would instead imitate the command or nod his head. Greg's reliance on nonlinguistic strategies is evident in the discourse example provided in Table 11.2.

In this example, Greg showed his overdependence on context for determining what questions mean. He also demonstrated his tendency to use a global response strategy and his assumption that "if she asks me the question again, my first

TABLE 11.2   Greg's Replies to Questions about Simple Objects

E	(holding a boy doll) Who is this?
C	Boy.
E	(puts boy in helicopter) Who is this?
C	Boy the helicopter.
E	(holds up a mom doll) Who is this?
C	Mom boy the helicopter

C = child; E = examiner.

response must have been wrong." The clinician observed similar behaviors from Greg in his preschool class setting. He had a "panicked" expression on his face much of the time. Greg did not appear to expect to understand. Rather, he expected to have to guess. In the classroom, he frequently produced long, confused narratives. His teacher, in an effort to be supportive, would abandon her communication agenda and follow Greg's topic to any degree possible. This was problematic, however, in that Greg needed to learn to understand and respond with semantic accuracy to classroom discourse.

Management

Remediation of Communication Activity: Auditory and Linguistic Training.
Once amplification was fitted, Greg was enrolled in a multifaceted AR program. Individual listening and language therapy focused on development of productive comprehension strategies and reduction of semantic confusion through attention to appropriate auditory linguistic cues. A parent program was included, with focus on teaching the family to use routine-based interventions to support Greg's comprehension. Greg had a tendency to imitate each message he heard, which interfered with processing and responding. The parents and therapist agreed to reduce emphasis on imitation and expression until success in comprehension could be increased. Further, the AR specialist provided collaborative consultation to Greg's classroom teacher. The school district provided Greg a diagnostic placement in a language intervention preschool. His teacher was a speech-language pathologist. The teacher and AR specialist developed a scheme for helping Greg repair comprehension breakdowns and for helping him respond accurately in the classroom. Table 11.3 illustrates the type of teaching interaction that was implemented to scaffold or support Greg's emerging comprehension.

Because imitation interfered with processing, clinicians needed to reduce the emphasis on requests for speech imitation. Focus was placed on listening and comprehending.

TABLE 11.3   Classroom Interaction Designed to Support Greg's Emerging Discourse Skills

E	Good morning, Greg. Where's your mommy?
C	Mom Greg go go the school. My moms says Greg no go the school the rain. . . .
E	Just a minute, Greg. Listen to the question (focusing prompt).
E	Where is mom? (highlighting prompt) At home? In the car? Here at school? (multiple-choice prompt).
C	Mom right there. At school! (points to his mother in the hall—on her way in to be room mother today)
E	Good, Greg! You answered my question! I asked, "Where's mom?" You told me . . . right there! There she is!

C = child; E = examiner.

Source: Based on Moeller, Osberger, and Eccarius (1986).

These classroom adaptations were successful in helping Greg begin to focus on the content of what he was hearing. As his auditory-linguistic behaviors strengthened, he began to revise language and discourse rules. His auditory language program focused specifically on helping him discriminate among linguistic elements that marked important semantic or syntactic distinctions. For example, he worked with the AR clinician in learning to distinguish pronoun forms (e.g., *I* vs. *you*), various morphological structures, and the meaning of various question forms. All intervention was incorporated in communicatively based activities to ensure the development of pragmatically appropriate conversational skills.

The AR clinician and teacher worked collaboratively to gradually shape in Greg productive listening and comprehension strategies. This was an essential step in helping Greg revise his expressive language behaviors. He needed to develop the confidence that he could understand and that his responses needed to be related to the conversational topic. Adjustment of Greg's approach to comprehension was necessary to prepare him for learning in a classroom environment.

Once his comprehension of basic questions improved, the clinician worked with the teacher on implementing a classroom discourse model (Blank, Marquis, & Klimovitch, 1995). This model involves a systematic approach to increasing the student's ability to respond to questions at varied levels of abstraction, from simple (close to the present context) to abstract (reasoning about concepts).

Intervention Outcomes

Greg was responsive to the auditory-linguistic training program and to the supportive techniques used in the classroom to strengthen language processing. Greg continued to receive a team approach to his rehabilitation and education into his early elementary years. Although the ultimate objective was to enable him to profit from education in a regular classroom, the initial approach was conservative with emphasis on specialty services to help him develop the language foundation necessary for academic success. In this case, the conservative approach was especially fortuitous because Greg experienced progression in his sensorineural hearing loss during his early elementary years. The audiograms in Figures 11.8A and 11.8B illustrate the progression in thresholds that occurred, with the initial audiogram in Figure 11.8A and the final audiogram in Figure 11.8B. Hearing thresholds finally stabilized at a severe hearing loss level, with bilaterally symmetrical configuration. Although audibility was achieved for some portions of the speech spectrum, portions of the spectrum were not optimally amplified, especially for the lowest and highest frequencies. Fortunately, optimal hearing aid fittings have been achieved (see Figure 11.9). Real-ear measures indicate that much of the speech spectrum is audible to Greg with properly fitted personal and FM amplification. Consideration for cochlear implants could be considered in the future, depending on multiple factors, including progression of the loss.

A language assessment was completed when Greg was 10 years of age. All language test scores were solidly within the average range for his age in comparison to hearing peers. Previous comprehension and discourse problems were no longer present. In the context of a storytelling task, Greg produced complex utterances like "The boy says that the frog should stay on the land while the rest of them sail off on a raft." Greg's expressive language was semantically and grammatically appropriate for his age. Provision of support services will continue to be important for Greg in spite of his strong language performance. When asked if he was having any problems in school, Greg reported, "Well, it is hard sometimes because you have to be quiet to hear the teacher, but the hearing kids keep talking. Then I always have to watch what everybody's doing and then I'll know what I'm supposed to be doing."

Summary

This case has illustrated the critical importance that audibility plays in a child's language. It also underscores the importance of a framework for identifying learning

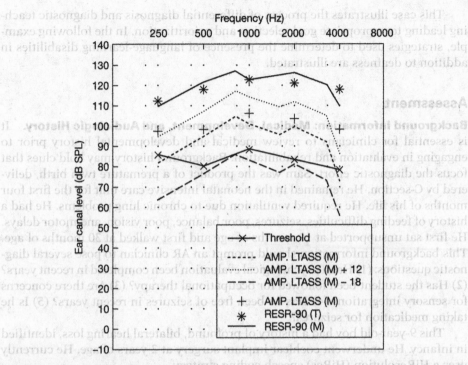

FIGURE 11.9   Results of real-ear measures illustrating audibility in relation to the long-term average speech spectrum (LTASS).

behaviors (e.g., nonlinguistic comprehension strategies) that were interfering with his language development. Teaching staff needed to hold Greg accountable for responding to the language addressed to him rather than to nonlinguistic and/or contextual cues. With aggressive and continuous AR support, this late-identified child who is hard of hearing has an opportunity to continue to make progress. Appropriate management of amplification and auditory learning opportunities play a key role in this process. Given the limitation in audibility of the amplified speech spectrum, this child may be a candidate for cochlear implantation in the future.

CASE 5: SAM—DIFFERENTIAL DIAGNOSIS THROUGH PROFESSIONAL TEAMWORK: A TOOL FOR SOLVING COMPLEX INTERVENTION PROBLEMS

Fundamental to the process of AR is the need to obtain a comprehensive understanding of a child's strengths and areas of need. This requires accurate and thorough differential diagnosis, best accomplished within the context of a transdisciplinary team. Some children present with a complex array of developmental needs. Unless these are well understood, barriers to progress may not be identified, strengths may not be utilized to the child's advantage, and intervention priorities may be misaligned. Children with language processing difficulties in addition to hearing loss may present with a host of communicative needs. One of the "arts" to AR is the ability to prioritize treatment goals so that the impact of intervention on the child as a communicator may be maximized. The selection of intervention priorities following thorough problem analysis is like a craft, requiring skill, theoretical preparation, and insight. It is useful for the clinician to ask the following: (1) If I select this goal, what difference will it make in the child's overall communicative functioning? (2) Will emphasis on this goal lead to generalization or impact on other communicative behaviors? (3) Will work on this goal better prepare the student to handle classroom language demands?

It is important for the clinician to consider the impact that work on a certain goal will have on the student's overall communicative function.

This case illustrates the process of differential diagnosis and diagnostic teaching leading to appropriate goal selection and prioritization. In the following example, strategies used to determine the presence of language-learning disabilities in addition to deafness are illustrated.

Assessment

Background Information: Medical, Development, and Audiologic History.   It is essential for clinicians to review medical and developmental history prior to engaging in evaluation and rehabilitation. Background history may hold clues that focus the diagnostic effort. Sam was the product of a premature twin birth, delivered by C-section. He remained in the neonatal intensive care unit for the first four months of his life. He required ventilation due to chronic lung problems. He had a history of feeding difficulties, seizures, poor balance, poor vision, and motor delays. He first sat unsupported at 18 months of age and first walked at 30 months of age. This background information should prompt an AR clinician to pose several diagnostic questions: (1) Has a psychological evaluation been completed in recent years? (2) Has the student been followed for occupational therapy? (3) Are there concerns for sensory integration? (4) Has he been free of seizures in recent years? (5) Is he taking medication for seizures?

This 9-year-old boy had a history of profound, bilateral hearing loss, identified in infancy. He underwent cochlear implant surgery at 2 years of age. He currently uses a HiResolution (HiRes) speech coding strategy.

Educational/Rehabilitative History and Concerns.   Sam and his family participated in regular early intervention services in the birth-to-age-3 period. At age 3, he attended a public school preschool program for children with special needs and then entered a mainstream educational setting. Due to persistent problems with speech and language skills, Sam repeated his kindergarten year. At the time of referral, he was mainstreamed in a first-grade class with support services from an itinerant teacher of the deaf, a speech-language pathologist, a physical therapist, and an educational interpreter. He relied on both speech and signs for communication. The parents and the school sought support from an AR team due to concerns for (1) behavioral difficulties and limited motivation in the academic setting, (2) lack of clear benefit from the cochlear implant, (3) poor retention of information, (4) limited generalization of concepts taught, (5) limited use of his interpreter, (6) concerns for integration of sensory information, (7) slow progress, and (8) difficulties socializing with peers.

Psychosocial and Communication Findings.   Psychological evaluation revealed that Sam's nonverbal abilities were in the low average range. Observations of verbal cognitive abilities revealed significant difficulty with categorization, making connections between words, and reasoning. He struggled with tasks that required him to use multiple skills simultaneously or to manipulate information in his head without visual cues (i.e., "How are an apple and bread alike?"). These results have important implications for educational and rehabilitative planning and need to be considered as the diagnostic story unfolds.

On formal language measures, Sam performed well below age expectations receptively and showed marked delays in expressive language. Observations of him in language-learning lessons and in the classroom provided important insights about language processing skills. It is challenging to determine if a student has language-learning difficulties beyond what can be explained by the hearing loss. Comparison of behaviors to typically developing children who are deaf can be useful in making this judgment. Table 11.4 summarizes language-learning behaviors exhibited by Sam that are not usual for children and deafness.

Developmental and medical history information helps the AR clinician form diagnostic questions that guide evaluation and further referrals.

The psychologist identified low average nonverbal cognitive skills. Combined with other disabilities, cognition must be considered as a possible limiting factor in Sam's learning.

It is important to consider if the presenting behaviors are "typical" for students who are deaf or hard of hearing.

TABLE 11.4 Atypical Language Behaviors Demonstrated by Sam

Receptive Language Concerns	Expressive Language Concerns
■ Recognizes concepts but cannot manipulate them (i.e., can identify a knife and scissors but cannot answer how they are "alike"). ■ Relies on contextual cues (e.g., pictures, other student responses) for understanding, instead of processing the language, resulting in misunderstanding and confusion. ■ Difficulty redirecting his focus after he misunderstood something. ■ Easily overwhelmed by multiple sources of information (e.g., teacher talking, objects presented, interpreter signing, children answering). Tended to "shut down." ■ Sometimes distracted by visual support materials. ■ Difficulties with visual-spatial organization. ■ Able to answer only basic questions; inordinate difficulty with abstraction.	■ Qualitative concerns with vocabulary development; poor skills in word associations and classification, resulting in disorganized word storage. This contributes to problems recalling words. ■ Word retrieval difficulties seen in misnaming of common words, frustration when naming, misnaming role concepts (i.e., confusing boy/girl). ■ Difficulty planning, sequencing, and executing fine motor movements. ■ Imprecise signed movements, related to poor trunk stability, difficulties with bilateral coordination of movements, and sequencing problems. ■ Significant difficulty responding to nonconcrete questions. ■ Language formulation, planning, and organization difficulties (start, stop, revise, try again)

Analysis of Sam's spontaneous conversational language supported the impression of language formulation (planning/organization) difficulties. Table 11.5 contains an excerpt from his language sample, along with diagnostic impressions of the language behaviors.

Functional Auditory and Speech Production Skills. Sam relied primarily on oral communication for self-expression but at times used both speech and sign. His speech intelligibility was reduced, which led the school to question the

TABLE 11.5 Conversational Sample Showing Language Processing Difficulties

	Impressions
Clinician: Does dad drive a truck? *Sam:* drive a truck . . . truck. a brown truck. Yeah it have a trailer . . . white trailer. *Sam:* a box. Dad put on trailer many many all.	Sam imitates a phrase from the question asked, perhaps to give him time to process the meaning or organize his response. He then answers and adds a relevant comment, which includes pauses and revisions. He attempts to continue his turn on the topic but does not give enough information for his partner to understand.
Clinician: Does dad have a tractor? *Sam:* tractor and wagon and combine.	Appropriate response.
Clinician: What do you do with a combine? *Sam:* a corn. The corn have wagon in. In the wagon . . . corn in the wagon.	Takes three tries to produce the phrase he intends.
Clinician: How do you get up in the combine? *Sam:* It tall very wheel like that. Climb wheel. I climb in that.	Language organizational issues apparent as he tries to answer.

benefit he was receiving from his cochlear implant device. Given their concerns, formal and informal measures of functional auditory skills were administered. He demonstrated a high degree of accuracy in closed-set word and phrase recognition, and his scores had steadily improved over a two-year period. Word lists were created and tested to ensure that they were within his vocabulary. These were then presented auditory-only in an open-set context, and he was asked to repeat the words. Sam recognized 88 percent of those words, with most errors accounted for by place of articulation (e.g., *cat* vs. *hat*). Further, Sam was able to follow basic commands and to correct speech production errors when given auditory-only input. It was the impression of the AR team that Sam was making good progress with his cochlear implant. It did not appear that auditory skills were creating a barrier for speech production. This led to the next diagnostic question, "Are other issues affecting spoken word production?" Given that fine motor sequencing issues were observed, it is possible that oral motor execution and planning may be challenging for Sam.

Sam was seen by a speech-language pathologist, who determined that motor difficulties were complicating speech production. An oral motor evaluation revealed that Sam had problems separating head and tongue movements and demonstrated a restricted range of lingual movements. The speech evaluation revealed a number of behaviors that were consistent with childhood apraxia of speech. These included vowel errors and distortions, inconsistency (variability in error patterns) in production of known words, timing errors, and reduced rate and accuracy when attempting to repeat a string of syllables. This information is essential for interpreting the cochlear implant results. His benefit from the implant simply could not be judged by his spoken language performance because it was affected by language processing and motor planning difficulties. Functional auditory evaluation revealed strength and helped the teaching team recognize a key area in which they had facilitated Sam's learning. Interestingly, Sam's teaching team had experienced only two children with cochlear implants. The other child had outstanding outcomes, leading teachers to conclude that Sam's outcomes were less than satisfactory. Clearly, findings must be interpreted with reference to the child's entire constellation of abilities. For Sam, with his multiple language and learning challenges, the cochlear implant was leading to positive outcomes.

> Motor sequencing or planning difficulties (e.g., praxis) are not typical in deaf and hard of hearing students. Speech training approaches need to be modified in light of the diagnosis.

Management

Diagnostic Teaching: Finding Strengths and Effective Strategies. Several sessions were conducted to identify Sam's learning strengths as well as strategies to address his priority needs. Diagnostic teaching is a process whereby the clinician creates learning tasks and objectively analyzes their effectiveness with the child, modifying the approach as necessary to bring about success. The cyclical nature of this process is illustrated in Figure 11.10.

FIGURE 11.10 Model of cycles of diagnostic teaching in AR.

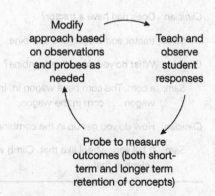

Modify approach based on observations and probes as needed

Teach and observe student responses

Probe to measure outcomes (both short-term and longer term retention of concepts)

An obvious priority for Sam was to build stronger classification and vocabulary skills so that words could be retained and generalized. Six new words were introduced to Sam during diagnostic teaching activities (e.g., Tinkertoy construction barrier game; drawing and creating stories) to identify methods that support word learning. Receptively, he learned all six target words introduced to him. He also learned to express these words, but he retained primarily the signed symbol, suggesting that he needed more trials/opportunities to learn the spoken form. In general, Sam showed enhanced retention of novel words when the learning activity contained the following:

- Experiential components (i.e., hands-on materials, active engagement, problems to solve). Drill and practice in isolation was not effective.
- Contrasts in the purposes of tool used (e.g., knowing the purpose of the Tinkertoy parts made it easier to retain distinctive words for those parts). Pictures alone were ineffective in exploring characteristics of words (such as functions of their parts).
- Recognition to recall opportunities (e.g., place all the word cards out in front of him and give several trials of "find the X" before asking him to "name X.")
- Functional expression (i.e., provide opportunities for him to use the target words in pragmatically appropriate ways).
- Chaining of inputs. Instead of working on all modalities at once, he needed trials where he can: hear it, then say it, then sign it, then read it, then fingerspell it. It was found that simultaneous use of multiple modes was overwhelming. Chaining separate modes was effective. Inclusion of signs aided longer-term recall.
- Extra learning opportunities that focus on oral skills (practice in saying and recalling the target words).

As another illustration of this process, the AR clinicians teamed with an academic specialist to conduct a diagnostic teaching activity related to classification, a priority goal for Sam. To explore ways to blend language and academic objectives, they chose the content area of money, an area in mathematics that was causing Sam some difficulties. The goal of the activity was to help Sam attend to characteristics of money that would help him to compare, contrast, and group bills and coins and eventually help him to problem solve which bill or coin(s) he would need in a given functional situation. Listing characteristics took place in a parallel comparison chart. Two paper bills (a $5 bill and a $20 bill) were placed each at the head of a column on a small whiteboard. A clinician elicited anything that Sam knew about the first bill and wrote the characteristics in a column under the bill:

Five-Dollar Bill	Twenty-Dollar Bill
$5	$20
money	money

Then the clinician used guided questions to elicit additional information:

Five-Dollar Bill	Twenty-Dollar Bill
$5	$20
money	money
made of paper	made of paper
green	green

Finally, the clinician placed new items, one at a time, encouraging Sam to look at the previous examples to help him describe the new items. The contrastive example of the nickel allowed Sam to begin to recognize how things could be similar in one characteristic while different in others.

Five-Dollar Bill	Twenty-Dollar Bill	Ten-Dollar Bill	One-Dollar Bill	Nickel
$5	$20	$10	$1	5 cents
money	money	money	money	money
made of paper	made of paper	made of paper	made of paper	made of metal
green	green	green	green	silver

Sam did not automatically make use of the columns and rows to cue himself about important characteristics. With visual structuring, however, he became more independent as the activity progressed. The resulting matrix could be used in the future to build language elements, such as "They are all . . . ," "These are made of paper, but this one is made of metal," or "The dollar and the nickel are different colors." The amount of complexity of the language would depend on Sam's response. Eventually, this same matrix could be used for problem solving about how much would be necessary to make a purchase, what the money was worth, and so on. His teachers indicated that he had just learned the names of coins and was having difficulty retaining previously learned information about their value. A similar matrix would help him to differentiate between the questions: "What is the name of this coin?" and "What is this coin worth?"

A Quarter	A Dime	A Nickel	A Penny
quarter	dime	nickel	penny
25 cents	10 cents	5 cents	1 cent

At the end of the activity, Sam successful[ly] . . . . money into one group and the coins into another group, start . . . . placing one additional item at a time into the . . . . dation for using language to answer "Why do . . . . . . or to summarize, "They are all . . ." Sam bene . . . . . with appropriate (but not overwhelming) vis . . . .

Sam also demonstrated strengths in epis . . . . . able to remember a paragraph-length story b . . . . . dialogue. The AR clinicians were able to pro . . . . Sam in role-play scenarios and story-retell a . . . .

Putting It All Together: Adapting the Ed . . . . cated teachers had been experiencing frustra . . . . tion difficulties. Many of the findings fron . . . . understand Sam's progress in a new light . . . . the lens when interpreting progress. Sam . . . . in addition to deafness. Therefore, the bes . . . . time. Another key point was that Sam was . . . . *the language of the task was manageable for him.* Sam was inhere . . . he was simply unable to process the multiple inputs in the classroom (explaining why he was not watching the interpreter). This led to behavioral responses, such as shutting out all input. The evaluation process clarified the strengths in auditory learning with the cochlear implant and ability to profit from script-based learning and selected visual tools. These results were used to make adjustment in the classroom curriculum to accommodate Sam's individual language and learning needs. Motor planning issues needed to be considered in speech therapy, in interpreting cochlear implant outcomes, and in working on written language (e.g., keyboarding was recommended). Increased support in the classroom was recommended along with ongoing task analysis during learning activities (e.g., What is Sam doing right now to attempt to complete this task? Is that helping or interfering? Does this activity begin with one of Sam's strengths? How much information is new and is at least part of the activity familiar? Is the task meaningful for Sam, and is he functionally involved?) These "online" strategies help teachers identify paths to success with a student like Sam.

Chapter Summary

the importance of professional collaboration zzles. This is true for all the cases in this chape value in implementing a diagnostic teaching ng priorities and useful solutions to address e continually modified to bring about positive

nd ongoing monitoring of all developmental tional, cognitive, auditory, language, and speech child understanding and programming.

nily, educational team, and clinical teams en-f the child and supports a unified intervention

- Audibility plays a critical role in child language, but may not be the only factor impacting language development. Other factors which may contribute to language delays include inconsistent use of hearing technology, reduced cognition, sound production disorders, limited social relatedness, reduced joint attention, language processing disorders, and other learning disabilities.

- When designing listening intervention programs it is important to identify the family's views on the type and amount of visual supports they wish to be used to enhance their child's spoken language skills. AR interventionists working with children who use sign language should assess how much visual support is needed to understand the spoken message. Strategically reducing visual supports depending on if the content is new, routine, or review is a strategy that can be used for developing auditory skills in increasingly complex contexts. Ongoing assessment of the child's level of comprehension and need for visual supports is essential as the cognitive linguistic demands of the academic environment increase.

- Use of the diagnostic teaching approach enables the clinician's ability to examine how a child approaches academic tasks, identify areas of strength and particular difficulty, and determine strategies that can be used to support learning.

Supplementary Learning Activities

See www.isu.edu/csed/audiology/rehab to carry out these activities. We encourage you to use these to supplement your learning. Your instructor may give specific assignments that involve a particular activity.

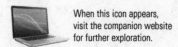

When this icon appears, visit the companion website for further exploration.

1. Dr. Amy Wetherby's research has focused on the early identification of children with autism. As shown in Case 1, this can be a difficult diagnosis when a child has combined challenges of deafness and autism. Review the characteristics in

Dr. Wetherby's table as found on the text website. Determine how many of these characteristics were observed in Matthew.

2. Several of the case studies in this chapter demonstrate the key role of a trans-disciplinary process when children present with complex and/or multiple challenges. It is helpful to understand what perspectives and areas of specialization these professionals can bring to the team. Look at the list of professionals on the text website. You may look up their professional organizations to aid your understanding of their potential roles.

3. Review the special needs section on the following website: www.raisingdeafkids .org/special. These are conditions that may coexist in a child with hearing loss.

Recommended Website

For information on working with deaf and hard of hearing children who have additional disabilities:
http://www.raisingdeafkids.org

References and Recommended Reading

Alpern, G.D. (2007). Developmental Profile—Third Edition. Los Angeles, CA: Western Psychological Services.

Blank, M., Marquis, M. A., & Klimovitch, M. (1995). *Directing early discourse.* Tucson, AZ: Communication Skill Builders.

Carney, A. E., & Moeller, M. P. (1998). Treatment efficacy: Hearing loss in children. *Journal of Speech, Language, and Hearing Research, 41,* S61–S84.

Carotta, C. C., Koch, M. E., & Brennan, K. (2014). *Auditory consultant resource network handbook.* Omaha, NE: Boys Town National Research Hospital.

Chapman, R. (1978). Comprehension strategies in children. In J. Kavanagh & P. Strange (Eds.), *Language and speech in the laboratory, school and clinic.* Cambridge, MA: MIT Press, 308–327.

Dunn, L. M., & Dunn, L. M. (1997). *Peabody Picture Vocabulary Test–III.* Circle Pines, MN: American Guidance Service.

Ertmer, D. J., & Stoel-Gammon, C. (2008). The Conditioned Assessment of Speech Production (CASP): A tool for evaluating auditory-guided speech development in young children with hearing loss. *Volta Review, 108*(1), 59–80.

Fenson, L., Marchman, V. A., Thal, D., Dale, P. S., Reznick, J. S., & Bates, E. (2007). *MacArthur-Bates Communicative Development Inventories: User guide and technical manual, second edition.* Baltimore, Maryland: Paul H. Brookes Publishing Co.

Gallaudet Research Institute. (2008, November). *Regional and national summary report of data from the 2007–2008 annual survey of deaf and hard of hearing children and youth.* Washington, DC: Author.

Geers, A. E. (2006). Factors influencing spoken language outcomes in children following early cochlear implantation. *Advances in Otorhinolaryngology, 64,* 50–65.

Goldman, R. (2000). *Goldman-Fristoe Test of Articulation–2.* Circle Pines, MN: American Guidance Service.

Koch, M. E. (2004). *Bringing sound to life: Principles and practices of cochlear implant rehabilitation.* Valencia, CA: Advanced Bionics Corp.

Moeller, M. P. (2000). Early intervention and language development in children who are deaf and hard of hearing. *Pediatrics, 106*(3), 1–9.

Moeller, M.P., Osberger, M.J., & Eccarius, M. (1986). Cognitively based strategies for use with hearing-impaired students with comprehension deficits. Topics in Language Disorders, *6*(4), 37–50.

Moeller, M. P., Coufal, K., & Hixson, P. (1990). The efficacy of speech-language intervention: Hearing impaired children. *Seminars in Speech and Language, 11*(4), 227–241.

Moeller, M. P., Osberger, M. J., & Eccarius, M. (1986). Cognitively based strategies for use with hearing-impaired students with comprehension deficits. *Topics in Learning Disabilities*, *6*(4), 37–50.

Nussbaum, D., Scott, S. Waddy-Smith, B., & Koch, M. (2004). *Spoken language and sign: Optimizing learning for children with cochlear implants.* Paper presented at the Laurent Clerc National Deaf Education Center, Washington, DC.

Robbins, A. M. (2001). A sign of the times: Cochlear implants and total communication. *Loud and Clear*, *4*(2), 1–8. http://www.advancedbionics.com/userfiles/File/Vol4Issue2-Nov2001.pdf

Rotfleisch, S. F. (2009). Auditory-verbal therapy and babies. In L. S. Eisenberg (Ed.), *Clinical management of children with cochlear implants* (pp. 435–493). San Diego, CA: Plural Publishing.

Roush, J., & Matkin, N. D. (1994). *Infants and toddlers with hearing loss.* Baltimore: York Press.

Wetherby, A., & Prizant, B. (1993). *Communication and symbolic behavior scales.* Chicago: Special Press.

Yoshinaga-Itano, C., Sedey, A. L., Coulter, B. A., & Mehl, A. L. (1998). Language of early- and later-identified children with hearing loss. *Pediatrics*, *102*(5), 1168–1171.

Zimmerman, L., Steiner, V., & Pond, R. (2011). *Preschool-Language Scales 5.* Boston: Pearson.

Case Studies: Adults and Elderly Adults

Michael A. Nerbonne, Jeff E. Brockett, Alice E. Holmes

CONTENTS

Visit the companion website when you see this icon to learn more about the topic nearby in the text.

Learning Outcomes

After reading this chapter, you will be able to

- Identify four topics that are commonly included in group communication training sessions
- Identify what HIO BASICS is and list its main components
- Describe how an individual's significant other (e.g., a spouse) can be a key element in successful rehabilitation for an adult with hearing loss
- Explain how motivation can influence the degree of success experienced from audiologic rehabilitation
- Define and explain the symptoms of BPPV.

INTRODUCTION

The seven adult and elderly cases focusing on audiologic rehabilitation (AR) described in this chapter involve a wide range of clients with hearing loss in terms of both age and communication-related difficulties. While special adjustments must be considered with some elderly patients, such as those found in nursing homes, in general both adult and elderly persons will most often demonstrate the same kinds of communication problems and therefore be candidates for similar rehabilitation strategies. Thus, we have grouped these younger and older cases together and presented them in the same chapter. Although references are made to group therapy (as in Case 1), the major emphasis with each case is on addressing the specific, unique problems that each of these individuals is experiencing. Some of these problems relate as much to psychosocial influences as to auditory effects. Such influences need to be acknowledged in AR approaches.

Although a major goal for each case was to reduce communication-related difficulties, the specific audiologic strategies varied for each client, depending on individual needs and motivation. The sampling of cases presented here ranges from involvement in hearing aid selection and orientation and counseling to traditional and more recently developed forms of individual and group communication rehabilitation. In addition, the pre- and postimplantation AR process for a challenging cochlear implant recipient is presented, and a case of BPPV is included as well.

In the course of performing AR, the audiologist may encounter the wide range of cases described here. We hope that these cases will give some insights into the challenges and possibilities of this work. In general, the model followed here is the one detailed in the introductory chapter of this text (see Figure 1.4), which was inspired by the World Health Organization (WHO) (2001) classification scheme associated with rehabilitation. The model involves both assessment and management phases as part of the total AR process.

A variety of pre- and post-AR tests were used in an attempt to objectify the status of the clients during the assessment and management phases of therapy. Self-assessment tools are receiving increased emphasis in AR, and several different communication assessment instruments have been used here, including both screening and diagnostic tools. Also, real-ear (probe tube microphone) measures are used with some cases, demonstrating the utility of this tool in the rehabilitation process. No single test battery is recommended, nor is it implied that one is best for all purposes. Instead, clinicians must select the tests that will be useful for determining the exact needs of the client, assisting in specific therapy strategies, and providing relevant outcome measures to assess the results of management. In addition to the tests and procedures used in this chapter, the reader may refer to numerous other chapters throughout the book for other relevant test and resource materials that may be useful in AR.

Even though all cases included here are based directly on real persons, minor adjustments have been made in the names used and the material presented in order to maintain the anonymity of the clients.

CASE 1: DR. M.—PROGRESSIVE HEARING LOSS

Case History

Dr. M. was a 69-year-old man who had retired four years earlier after a 40-year career as a college professor. He reported experiencing frequent difficulties in hearing, particularly at church, social functions, and plays that he and his spouse attended at the university's theater. Dr. M. had noted being aware of hearing difficulties for some time, including the last several years of his teaching career. The onset of his hearing loss was reportedly gradual and seemed to affect both ears equally.

AR Assessment

Figure 12.1 contains the audiometric results obtained with Dr. M. In general, he was found to possess a mild to moderate sensorineural hearing loss bilaterally. The results of speech audiometry were consistent with the pure tone findings and indicated that Dr. M. was experiencing significant difficulty in speech perception, especially if speech stimuli were presented at a typical conversational level (50 dB HL).

The Self-Assessment of Communication (SAC) and Significant Other Assessment of Communication (SOAC) (Schow & Nerbonne, 1982) screening inventories were administered to Dr. M. and his spouse to gather further information concerning the degree of perceived hearing difficulty resulting from Dr. M.'s hearing loss. Using both of these measures provides valuable information about how persons with hearing loss view their hearing problems as well as potentially valuable insights from the person who is communicating with the individual on a regular basis. Scores of 50 and 60 percent (raw scores of 30 and 34) on the SAC and SOAC tests, respectively, presented a consistent pattern that, when evaluated according to research (see Table 12.1), provided further evidence that Dr. M. was experiencing considerable hearing-related difficulties (Schow, 1989; see also text website).

Interestingly, some people with hearing loss similar to Dr. M.'s will report much different (less or more) hearing difficulty. This important dimension obviously is quite individualized.

On the basis of these test results and the patient's comments, a hearing aid evaluation was recommended and scheduled.

Management

Hearing Aid Evaluation and Adjustment. Prior to any testing associated with hearing aids, Dr. M. was advised about the option of utilizing a behind-the-ear (BTE) or one of the in-the-ear (ITE) styles of hearing aid. Like some individuals facing this

Obtaining information from the person with hearing loss (SAC) and a significant other (SOAC) regarding perceived hearing difficulties for the client can be valuable in determining AR needs.

Audiological Record

Name Dr. M.   Age 69

Frequency (Hz)							

	PTA	SRT	SAT	HL / PB
R	37	40		80 / 82
L	45	50		90 / 78
SF		35		50 / 52
Aided (Quiet)		20		50 / 80
Aided (Noise)				

Ear	Air	Bone
Right	O	<
Left	×	>
Aided	A	

NR — No Response
DNT — Did Not Test
CNT — Could Not Test
SAT — Speech Awareness Threshold

FIGURE 12.1   Case 1: Audiometric results for Dr. M.

TABLE 12.1 Categories and Associated Scores for Classifying Primary and Secondary Effects of Hearing Loss (Hearing Disability or Handicap) When Using the SAC and SOAC

Category	Raw Scores	Percentage Scores
No disability or handicap	10–18	0–20
Slight hearing disability or handicap	19–26	21–40
Mild to moderate hearing disability or handicap	27–38	41–70
Severe hearing disability or handicap	39–50	71–100

Source: Adapted from Schow (1989), Schow and Tannahill (1977), and Sturmak (1987).

Care must be taken to get accurate and complete ear impressions. No matter how state of the art the circuitry of a hearing aid may be, if it doesn't fit well and feel comfortable, the patient probably will not use it.

choice, Dr. M. expressed a clear preference for the ITE style. Dr. M. was also advised that because of the slope of his hearing loss and open-fit considerations, binaural BTE hearing aids might be advisable. However, Dr. M. chose two ITE hearing aids with moderate gain and high-frequency response.

The hearing aid evaluation consisted of a series of probe-tube microphone real-ear measures with each ear as well as sound field speech audiometry. Audiometric data were applied to an existing prescription approach to determine the desired gain, frequency response, and OSPL-90 values for the hearing aids to be fitted in the right and left ears. This resulted in two ITE hearing aids being recommended with moderate gain and high-frequency emphasis. Venting of each unit was also deemed appropriate. Earmold impressions were taken, and an appointment was scheduled for Dr. M. to be fitted with his new aids once they were received from the manufacturer.

Dr. M. was fitted with his hearing aids at the next session, and real-ear measures were taken to confirm the appropriateness of the insertion gain and OSPL-90 values for each unit. Sound field speech audiometry was also used to evaluate further the degree of improvement provided by the binaural system. As seen in Figure 12.1, Dr. M.'s speech reception threshold and speech recognition score improved significantly with the ITE hearing aids. His comments concerning the aids were favorable, and no further adjustments were made with either hearing aid. Following a thorough orientation to the operation and care of his new aids, Dr. M. was advised to return for subsequent follow-up appointments.

Dr. M.'s experience with his new hearing aids was, for the most part, positive. While still noting some problems hearing in group situations and at the theater, he definitely felt that the hearing aids were assisting him. Further discussion with Dr. M. regarding his hearing difficulties at the theater revealed that he had not yet tried the facility's infrared listening system. Encouraging him to do so, the audiologist explained the manner in which the system functions as well as how Dr. M. could use the infrared receiver either with his hearing aids or as a stand-alone unit. Subsequent contact with Dr. M. revealed that he found the assistive listening device to be remarkably helpful.

While Dr. M. had adjusted well to his hearing aids and received substantial improvement as a result of their use, he did note some persistent communication difficulties. Because of this and his motivation for improvement, Dr. M. agreed to enroll in a short-term group AR program for adults.

Communication Training. Dr. M. was one of eight adults with hearing loss who participated in the weekly group sessions. Although the activities and areas of emphasis varied somewhat as a result of the interests and needs of each group of participants, the main components of the program generally followed those outlined in the section "Recent Trends in Speechreading Instruction" in Chapter 5. The individuals participating with Dr. M. were new hearing aid users with mild to moderate hearing losses. Consequently, emphasis was placed on 1) describing different types and degrees of hearing loss (implications of their loss), 2) the effective use of hearing aids, care and maintenance of the systems, and 3) the way hearing aids can be supplemented by one or more types of assistive devices. Attention was also given to 4) developing more effective listening skills and capitalizing on the visual information available in most communication situations. Interaction among the group participants was encouraged, and valuable information on a variety of topics, including the use of conversation strategies and clear speech, was shared at each session.

Successful AR done with groups of adults will involve both structured content and informal information sharing among the participants. They can learn as much from each other as from the group facilitator.

Following the final session, Dr. M. stated that the sessions had been helpful to him. In addition to the practical information provided, such as where to buy batteries for his hearing aids and the use of hearing aids with the telephone, Dr. M. felt that a number of the communication strategies covered had been of benefit to him. The net result was that he felt much more confident when communicating with others.

Summary

It was clear from the start that Dr. M. had accepted his hearing problem and was motivated to seek out whatever assistance was available to him. His positive and cooperative behaviors, which would be categorized by Stephens and Kramer (2010) as an example of a Type I attitude (see Chapter 10), facilitated the AR process and positively affected Dr. M.'s overall communication abilities. Motivation should be recognized as a key ingredient in successful AR with any individual with hearing loss.

CASE 2: MR. B.—HEARING LOSS, DEPRESSION, AND SUCCESSFUL HEARING AID USE

Mr. B. is a 70-year-old male who was brought in by his neighbor. Mr. B's wife of nearly 50 years passed away one year prior to this visit. His neighbor was concerned that Mr. B. was becoming depressed and a shut-in because of his difficulty in hearing. Mr. B. reported having had hearing problems for a very long time and that he had tried at least three different sets of hearing aids over the past 20 years. His newest set was approximately seven years old and was not working. Even when these instruments were new, they reportedly "did him no good." When asked what he didn't like about his current hearing aids (when they were working), he said that "everything was too noisy and loud" and that he "was constantly fiddling with the hearing aids to try and hear better."

Depression and hearing loss difficulties can be related.

Informational Counseling

Following a complete evaluation, the test findings were explained to Mr. B. in such a way that he could understand why he had so many communication difficulties. The AR process was described to him, but he seemed somewhat reluctant to proceed.

Rehabilitation Assessment

Communication Status: Hearing Loss/Activity Limitations

Audiometry and Communication Assessment. The results of a complete audiologic evaluation (see Figure 12.2) showed a moderate, symmetrical sensorineural hearing loss with a gradually sloping configuration. This is a flat 2 (F2) category (see www.isu.edu/csed/audiology/rehab). His word recognition scores at a comfortable presentation level were 76 percent correct in the left ear and 84 percent correct in the right ear, using the CID W-22 word lists.

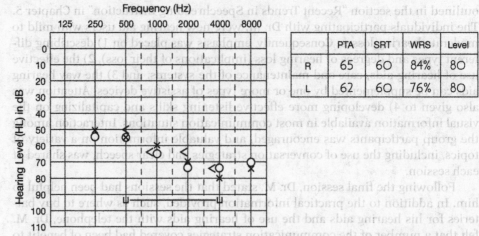

FIGURE 12.2 **Case 2: Audiogram for Mr. B., plus loudness discomfort levels at 500 and 4000 Hz.**

	PTA	SRT	WRS	Level
R	65	60	84%	80
L	62	60	76%	80

Mr. B.'s dynamic range was mapped at 500 and 4000 Hz. Results showed a dynamic range of 40 dB at 500 Hz and a significantly reduced dynamic range of 20 dB at 4000 Hz.

Mr. B.'s perception of his communication difficulty was assessed using the *Self-Assessment of Communication* (SAC) (Schow & Nerbonne, 1982). A raw score of 22 indicated only a mild degree of perceived difficulty. His neighbor was given the *Significant Other Assessment of Communication* (SOAC) to get an estimate of how others perceived Mr. B.'s communication difficulty. A raw score of 30 was computed, indicating a higher perception of communication difficulty.

The Glasgow Hearing Aid Benefit Profile (Gatehouse, 1999) was used to provide additional information about Mr. B.'s perceived disability and handicap. Scoring the unaided portion resulted in an initial disability of 72 percent and an initial handicap of 59 percent.

Overall Participation Variables. Based on his report, Mr. B. had little demand on his hearing. He lived alone and did not participate in any social activities. His family was distant and did not keep in touch with him very much. He avoided using the phone unless absolutely necessary. His neighbor thought that if Mr. B. could hear better, he would start to become more active and enjoy life more.

Related Personal Factors. Mr. B. seemed very quiet, and, although he did not resist being at the evaluation, he did not appear motivated to do anything about his hearing loss. His neighbor mentioned the word "depressed" several times in describing Mr. B.'s behavior.

Environmental Factors. Because Mr. B. lived alone, his communication environment was very restricted. In other words, aside from his neighbor and an occasional trip to the grocery store, he had little communication demand. When he was at home, he watched TV and was able to turn the TV up loud enough to hear.

Rehabilitation Management

Counseling and Psychosocial Issues. Mr. B. did not have any problem believing and admitting that he had a hearing problem. It was difficult, however, for him to manage his communication environment at home. By avoiding the telephone and turning up the TV, his perception of "difficulty" was somewhat distorted.

After some discussion, Mr. B. was asked if there were any situations that he would participate more in if he could hear better. He reported that he would like to

Persons routinely engaging in only a limited amount of communication on a day-to-day basis sometimes tend not to report as much hearing disability as another person who does more communicating.

hear on the telephone so that he could visit with his family and he wanted to hear well in a "group" situation.

It was clear that Mr. B. had some reservations about proceeding, probably due to a combination of three unsuccessful hearing aid fittings in the past and low communication demands. However, getting him to hear better on the telephone and in group environments seemed like appropriate goals.

Audibility Management

Amplification (Modifying Audibility). New technology in amplification was discussed, particularly the ability of hearing aids to address how he needs to hear different levels of sound in the environment. When it was explained that hearing aids could be adjusted so that he could receive more gain for soft sounds, less gain for average sounds, and even less for loud sounds, he seemed very interested in pursuing a trial period. He was comfortable with the BTE style, and, because his dynamic range across frequencies was different, multichannel, programmable instruments were considered in the design. Because the circuitry could manage the gain for different input levels, the hearing aids were ordered without a user-operated volume control.

When the hearing aids arrived, Mr. B.'s threshold and suprathreshold information was entered, and the Desired Sensation Level (DSL) I/O fitting formula (Seewald, 1992, 2000) was followed to preset the initial program for the hearing aids. Predicted insertion gain response curves matched the target gain curves for soft, average, and loud inputs reasonably well.

When Mr. B. arrived for his hearing aid fitting and orientation, he seemed excited and anxious to hear the new sound. The hearing aids were placed in his ears, and the actual fit of the hearing aids was inspected. The aids/molds slipped in easily and seemed stable once in place. Mr. B. said that the hearing aids felt comfortable. The program was activated, and he had an immediate positive reaction.

An informal, functional assessment was performed using a CD containing different types of speech and environmental sounds presented in a sound field. Using this method, gain levels for soft (<45 dB), average (45 to 65 dB), and strong (>65 dB) inputs were adjusted slightly. The compression ratio in the channel assigned to the high frequencies, where Mr. B. had a narrower dynamic range, was adjusted further to reduce loud sound amplification. Mr. B. reported that soft sounds seemed "distant," but he could still identify the sound. Average sounds were reported to be comfortable, and higher level inputs seemed loud but were not uncomfortable.

> Hearing aids with multiple channels allow for greater flexibility in meeting the specific needs that a given individual may have.

As an objective measure, probe microphone measurements using modified DSL targets were used to evaluate insertion gain. Results showed good approximation of target in the low and mid-frequencies, but the insertion response for soft, high-frequency sounds did not meet target gain values in the range of 3000 to 4000 Hz. Gain in the channels assigned to the higher frequencies was increased to better address soft, high-frequency sounds; however, Mr. B. then reported that speech was too "lispy." The hearing aids were returned to the previous setting.

Finally, a formal functional assessment was performed under unaided and aided listening conditions using CID W-22 word lists presented in a sound field at 50 dB HL. Mr. B. was unable to correctly identify any of the words in the unaided condition but scored 88 percent in the aided condition.

Hearing Aid Orientation. Even though Mr. B. was an experienced user, basic hearing instrument orientation, *HIO BASICS* (see Chapters 2 and 10), was discussed in detail. These topics included the following:

Hearing expectations: Realistic ones

Instrument operation: On/off, telecoil, telephone use

Occlusion effect: User's voice with hearing aids in place

Batteries: Tabs, how long they will last, removal, replacement, dangers

Acoustic feedback: What causes it; when is it OK, not OK?

System troubleshooting: What to do when there are problems?

Insertion and removal: Identifying left, right, insertion, and removal

Cleaning and maintenance: Wax and debris cleaning, hair spray, excessive heat, etc.

Service, warranty, repairs, follow-up process, etc.

Mr. B.'s overall speech perception was improved dramatically when listening to speech presented at a normal conversational level.

Mr. B. was encouraged to maintain a journal of his experiences, both good and bad, so that appropriate adjustments to his hearing aids could be made.

Mr. B. returned for his two-week follow-up, and it was apparent from his attitude that his experience had been favorable. Mr. B. reported that he was so pleased about how he was hearing that the night following his fitting he decided to go to a fiftieth wedding anniversary gathering. As expected, it was "too much, too soon," and he had to remove the hearing aids before the end of the evening.

Mr. B.'s journal included positive comments about how much "clearer" the TV sounded and that one-on-one conversations were much easier for him to hear. On the negative side, he felt that in situations where there was "a lot going on" (background noise), he could actually hear better with the hearing aids removed. He also commented that using the telephone was difficult because it sounded too soft. A combination of reducing gain and increasing the compression kneepoint for both channels was used to address his concerns about background noise. However, when he tried the telephone in our clinic, the volume still seemed too soft. Gain for the telephone coil circuit was increased, and he reported that it was much better. He was scheduled for a one-month follow-up appointment.

His one-month follow-up visit was very positive. Competing noise situations were much better, and he also reported doing much better on the telephone.

Remediate Communication Activity. At each of his follow-up visits, Mr. B. was given additional information about how to maximize his communication ability. The information included the following items from our CLEAR handout (see Chapter 10):

Control communication situations by avoiding noisy areas, poorly lit areas, and the like.

Look at the speaker: Visual cues from speakers are important and help make up for lost information.

Escape and expectations: Be realistic about situations where it will be easy or difficult to hear; plan strategies for dealing with unfavorable listening situations.

Assertiveness: Let others know that you have difficulty hearing and encourage them to gain your attention before speaking and to look at you when they are talking.

Repair strategies: If a breakdown occurs in communication, repeat back to the speaker what you *did* hear and then ask him or her to clarify what you *did not* hear.

Environment and Coordination: Participation Improvement. On Mr. B.'s three-month follow-up, his neighbor (who initially referred him to our clinic) accompanied him. Both were extremely appreciative of what the hearing aids had done to improve his quality of life. Mr. B. reported that he is attending more group functions (group communication goal), has kept in better touch with his family through the telephone (telephone goal), and is less intimidated by difficult communication situations. His neighbor reported that Mr. B. seemed much more outgoing and positive about himself and had been praising the effects of his new instruments to others.

Scoring of the aided portion of the Glasgow profile resulted in scores that supported Mr. B. and his neighbor's comments. In the Hearing Aid Use category, he scored 80 percent, indicating a high level of hearing aid use. In the Hearing Aid Benefit category, he scored 39 percent, indicating only a moderate amount of perceived benefit. For the Residual Disability category, he scored 52 percent, indicating a reduced perception of disability (unaided initial disability was 72 percent). Finally, in the Satisfaction category, his mean score was 91 percent, indicating a very high level of satisfaction with his hearing aids.

Summary

This is a classic case because it contains two very common issues in AR. The first issue relates to the amplification (modifying audibility) component of AR. Mr. B. had a dynamic range problem, and his previous three sets of hearing aids did not manage differing input levels appropriately. He would turn the hearing aids up to hear soft sounds, and then loud sounds would be too loud. When he was exposed to loud sounds, he would have to turn the hearing aids down. After a few weeks of use, he would just set the hearing aids to where loud sounds were comfortable, and the result was inadequate gain for soft and average inputs. Current multichannel technology has the ability to address differences in dynamic range associated with hearing loss more effectively. Mr. B.'s new hearing aids were programmed to help him manage his problems related to loudness. This capability contributed much toward enabling Mr. B. to be a successful hearing aid user this time around.

The second issue is that hearing loss often results in communication problems that can be perceived as depression-like symptoms and can ultimately affect one's emotional well-being. Providing amplification can go a long way to relieving some of these problems, but effective rehabilitation should also address other appropriate aspects of communication. For example, effective use of communication strategies, establishing patient-based goals, the inclusion of the communication partner in rehabilitative efforts, and consideration of environmental situations all help to increase communication competence.

Synergy is a process in which the whole is greater than the sum of the parts. As with Mr. B., a definite synergy often occurs when the AR process for adults is managed multidimensionally and includes more than just targeting amplification.

Successful AR often can have a positive impact on an individual that goes beyond simply facilitating communication.

CASE 3: J.D.—AR FEATURING A SIGNIFICANT OTHER

Introduction

J.D. is a 28-year-old male college student who, at his wife's insistence, made an appointment at a local audiology center for a complete evaluation. J.D. and his wife were married six months ago, and the stress of being newlyweds has been amplified considerably by communication difficulties on his part. J.D. had always felt that he had *some* difficulty hearing but not as much as his wife seemed to describe. His wife felt that J.D. "just doesn't listen" and reported that "he tunes me out!"

J.D. was unaware of any history of hearing loss in his family but believed that he first noticed some difficulty hearing after working with a construction firm after graduation from high school. His wife admittedly hadn't had the opportunity to interact with too many people who had difficulty hearing and said that "my grandma and grandpa don't even wear hearing aids."

Hearing problems can result in increased stress for relationships.

Informational Counseling

The policy for the audiology center is to invite the patient's significant other, if possible, to the evaluation. Having the significant other present during the evaluation and informational counseling session helps supplement case history and rehabilitative goal setting. The results of the evaluation and the communication implications were discussed in detail with both J.D. and his wife. It seemed to make perfect sense to J.D., but his wife was concerned that it was more of an "attention" problem than a "hearing" problem and that it seemed like a big expense to proceed with rehabilitation when all he would have to do is "listen."

Rehabilitation Assessment

Communication Status: Impairment and Activity Limitations

Audiometry.   The evaluation revealed a moderate, precipitous, high-frequency sensorineural hearing loss in both ears (see Figure 12.3). The loss was slightly greater at 4000 Hz in the right ear. His word recognition scores using phonetically balanced words (PB) were 88 percent in the right ear and 92 percent in the left ear. However, when high-frequency word lists were used (Gardner's High Frequency Words), his scores dropped dramatically to 68 percent in the right ear and 72 percent in the left ear.

A dynamic range (DR) assessment by frequency showed near-normal DR for the low frequencies (80 dB), reduced dynamic range for the mid-frequencies (50 dB), and a very shallow DR (30 dB) for the frequencies above 2000 Hz.

Communication Assessment.   The SAC and the SOAC (Schow & Nerbonne, 1982) tools were used to help quantify J.D. and his wife's perception of the communication difficulty. Both of these assessment tools use the same 10 questions to sample self-assessed difficulty in a variety of communication situations. The first five questions evaluate Activity Limitation (Disability) and include an open-ended communication situation item for the patient to identify a specific communication concern. Questions 6 through 9 evaluate Participation Restriction (Handicap), and question 10 applies to patients wearing amplification and asks them to estimate their hearing aid use in hours. The SAC and the SOAC are identical; however, the *patient* fills out the SAC, and a "significant other" fills out the SOAC. Patients can be asked to complete the instrument prior to treatment (AR) and following treatment.

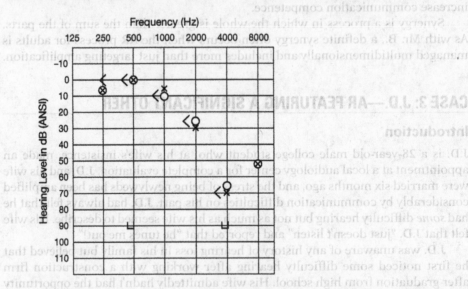

	PTA	SRT	WRS PB Words	Level	WRS HF Words	Level
Right	12	15	88%	50 dB HL	68%	50 dB HL
Left	12	15	92%	50 dB HL	72%	50 dB HL

FIGURE 12.3   Case 3: Audiometric results for J.D.

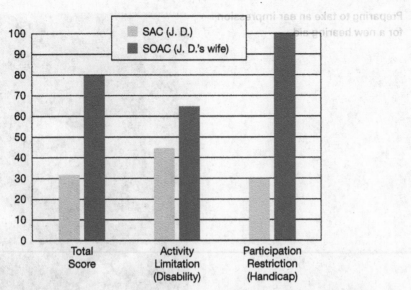

FIGURE 12.4   Summary of results for the initial administration of SAC and SOAC.

J.D.'s assessment of his communication difficulty revealed a total score of 33 percent, but his wife's assessment yielded a score of 80 percent, indicating that *her* perception of *his* communication difficulty was much greater (see Figure 12.4). When the individual items on the SAC and SOAC were compared, both J.D. and his wife indicated similar patterns for the "Various Communication Situations" section. For example, quiet one-to-one situations showed the least difficulty, while group situations or difficult listening environments showed the most difficulty. However, in the "Social and Emotional" section, J.D. felt like his hearing loss "limited or hampered his personal or social life" only "occasionally," while his wife rated this item as "practically always." Similarly, the question asking "Do problems or difficulty with your hearing upset you?" also showed a large difference, with J.D. reporting a 1 (Almost Never) and his wife reporting a 5 (Practically Always).

As shown in Figure 12.4, when the categories of Activity Limitation (Disability) and Participation Restriction (Handicap) were summarized, J.D.'s Activity Limitation (Disability) was computed at 45 percent, and his wife's report revealed a score of 65 percent. For Participation Restriction (Handicap), J.D.'s score was 30 percent, while his wife estimated his Participation Restriction (Handicap) at 100 percent— again, a much different perception.

Overall Participation Variables.   The demand on J.D.'s hearing is predictably high. He is a graduate student in biological sciences, and his classes are detailed in instruction and demanding. At home, it is important for him to be able to communicate with his wife and ease some of the stresses of being a newlywed.

Related Personal Factors.   Both J.D. and his wife indicated that he is a quiet person, somewhat introverted, but extremely intelligent. He is admittedly fascinated with technology and incorporates it in many aspects of his life, including computers, cellular phones, entertainment, and instruction.

Environmental Factors.   J.D. works part-time as a graduate assistant teaching an undergraduate biology laboratory course. The labs are taught in a large facility with poor acoustics and a substantial amount of noise for most of the class.

Rehabilitation Management

Counseling and Psychosocial Issues.   J.D. did not deny that he had a hearing problem but at the same time didn't feel like the communication difficulties that

Preparing to take an ear impression
for a new hearing aid.

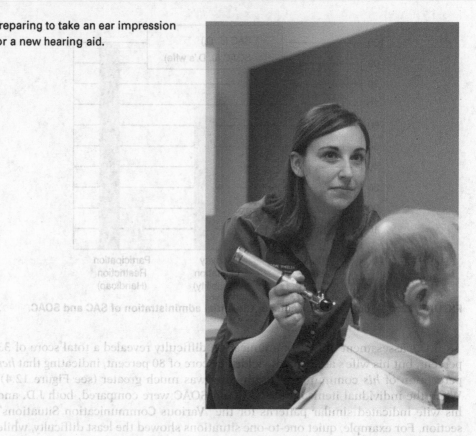

he and his wife were experiencing were as bad as *she* indicated. Regardless, he was willing to do whatever was required to maximize his communication ability both at home and at school. As a way of setting rehabilitation goals, he was asked to pick two specific communication situations that he would like to improve. For the home environment, he wanted to be able to "hear his wife better, even if she is in another room." For his school environment, he wanted to be able to hear his students' questions even if they were in the back row.

The audiologist felt it was important at this point to provide some education and informational counseling to J.D.'s wife. It was clear that she continued to feel that it was nothing more than a "listening problem." As a way of helping her understand the difficulties associated with hearing loss, she was encouraged to experience hearing loss for one day. She was given two disposable foam earplugs and instructed how to insert them correctly. Her assignment was to place the earplugs first thing in the morning and wear them throughout the day. Additionally, she was asked to write down any difficulties or frustrations she experienced.

Audibility Management

Amplification (Modifying Audibility).   Since one of J.D.'s passions was technology, it was not difficult to talk about new technology in amplification. He was intrigued with the advances and eager to get started with a trial period. The goals that he had set were translated by the audiologist into focusing on maximizing the access to soft, speech-generated sounds while minimizing the impact of any type of competing nonspeech sound, such as a running dishwasher (in the home environment) or a noisy laboratory (in his work environment). The audiologist felt that binaural hearing aids with adaptive directional microphone technology, along with aggressive nonspeech signal filtering, would help J.D. to reach his goals. J.D.'s wife felt that the BTE style was unattractive and conspicuous and wanted him to get an ITE style. However, J.D. chose a BTE because of the open-fit technology.

The hearing aids were current state of the art and featured adaptive directional microphone technology that was coupled with a speech/nonspeech detector. The result allowed the hearing aids not only to reduce nonspeech generated noise but also to track and enhance sound that appeared to be speech. The intent was to provide J.D. with as much access to speech information as possible while reducing any potential competing noise.

The hearing aids were preprogrammed prior to his fitting appointment with his threshold and suprathreshold (uncomfortable levels) information, and an initial amplification target was set using the Desired Sensation Level (DSL) I/O fitting formula (Seewald, 1992, 2000). The hearing aids were equipped with multiple listening-situation memories. The first memory was set to adaptive processing, which allowed the hearing aid to manage the sound environment. The second memory was set to force the directional microphones to receive only from the front (the direction he would be facing). The third memory was optimized to use with his cellular phone.

When the appointment for the hearing aid fitting and orientation was set, he was encouraged to bring his wife. The hearing aids were placed in his ears, and the actual fit of the hearing aids was inspected. The earmolds slipped in easily and seemed stable once in place. The BTE portions of the hearing aids fit nicely behind his ear and for the most part were covered by his hair. He reported that the hearing aids felt comfortable, and the circuits were then activated. He immediately had a look of disappointment because he expected that the hearing aids would sound louder. The audiologist explained to him that since his hearing loss was limited to just the high frequencies and that high frequencies carried more "clarity" information than "sound power" information, he would not get a large sensation of volume. Rather, he would just notice that sound was clearer and easier to understand. His wife mumbled something softly, and he immediately responded appropriately.

Using both formal and informal measures, the hearing aids were set in such a way that soft sounds were audible but soft, average sounds (like the human voice) sounded appropriate, and loud sounds seemed loud, but not uncomfortable.

Speech mapping using probe-microphone measures was used as an acoustic way of evaluating not only *how* the hearing aids were providing him with amplification but also *what* (in terms of speech or noise) type of signal the hearing aids were processing. The speech mapping indicated that not only did he have access to more of the clarity aspects of speech, but the hearing aids dynamically (using the directional microphones) followed the speech signal without having to move his head.

Finally, a formal functional assessment was performed under unaided and aided listening conditions using Gardner's High Frequency Words. Unaided, binaural testing at 50 dB HL resulted in a score of 68 percent correct. Word recognition in the aided condition showed a score of 96 percent correct.

Hearing Aid Orientation.   As a new user, it was important to cover the orientation topics (HIO BASICS) thoroughly, not only with J.D. but his wife as well:

Hearing expectations: Realistic (some situations will continue to be difficult and that the function of the hearing aids will be more "clarity" than power)

Instrument operation: On/off, telecoil, telephone use, memory button

Occlusion effect: User's voice with hearing aids in place

Batteries: Tabs, how long they will last, removal, replacement, dangers

Acoustic feedback: What causes it; when is it OK, not OK?

System troubleshooting: What to do when there are problems?

Insertion/removal: Identifying left, right, insertion, and removal

Cleaning and maintenance: Wax/debris cleaning, hair spray, excessive heat, etc.

Summarize warranty, repairs, follow-up process, etc.

Both he and his wife were encouraged to write down situations where the hearing aids seem to be helping and situations that continue to be difficult. Additionally, a HIO BASICS DVD, produced at Idaho State University, was provided to them so that they could review the topics for clarification.

Remediate Communication Activity. Prior to proceeding with the first follow-up, his wife was asked to share her experience using the earplugs for a day. Initially (early in the morning), she felt that it wouldn't affect her at all, but as the day went on, she began to understand why J.D. seemed to ignore certain communication from her. By the end of the day, she was exhausted with having to strain to understand and constantly manipulate the situation (e.g., getting closer to the talker) to hear. Her experience simulating a hearing loss occurred at the same time J.D. was experiencing *better* access to sound through his new hearing aids. The communication difficulties, for a day, traded places.

Some minor adjustments were made to address some of the concerns that were written in both J.D.'s and his wife's journals, but overall, the hearing aids seemed to be giving him access to information that improved the clarity of speech and reduced the frustration for both of them.

The audiologist shared two types of communication strategy information: one for the talker and one for the receiver. For the receiver, the acronym CLEAR was used to represent five strategies: Control the communication situation; Look at the talker, Expect realistic performance, Assert yourself, and Repair communication breakdown. For the talker, the acronym SPEECH was used to represent six similar strategies: Spotlight your face, Pause slightly between phrases, Empathize with the person, Ease his or her listening by gaining his or her attention; Control the listening situation, and Have a plan for difficult listening situations.

Environmental/Coordination: Participation Improvement. At J.D.'s one-month follow-up, the audiologist focused on improving specific situations that continued to be difficult. Additionally, the audiologist asked both J.D. and his wife to complete SAC and SOAC forms based on his experiences using amplification and the strategies offered in the AR session. One situation that continued to be difficult was his teaching environment. The background noise produced in the lab was a mix of nonspeech sounds and speech-generated noise. This often resulted in J.D.'s turning off and removing his hearing aids. A number of environmental control suggestions were made. For example, it was suggested that the class be restructured so that instruction prior to the lab activity was done by having the entire class gather in the front of the lab. This increased the signal (students' questions and comments) as compared to the background noise. Then the students would return to their lab tables and begin the activity. Another modification of the environment was to have the students signal J.D. when they needed to talk to him. J.D. would go to the student with the question, and because of the close proximity, the adaptive directional microphones on the hearing aids maximized the signal (student's voice) as compared to the background noise.

J.D. and his wife were asked to complete the SAC and SOAC forms again to estimate the residual communication difficulties following rehabilitation. The results are shown in Figure 12.5 and indicated that the use of amplification and the strategies offered in the rehabilitation process had resulted in benefits with an impact on both disability and handicap. The residual disability reported by J.D. was 20 percent (compared to an initial disability of 45 percent), resulting in a 25 percent benefit. His wife's assessment was more dramatic. The residual disability was 28 percent (compared to 65 percent initial disability), resulting in a 37 percent benefit. The residual handicap reported by J.D. was 12 percent (compared to an initial handicap of 30 percent), resulting in an 18 percent benefit. Again his wife's assessment showed greater benefit. Her residual handicap was 50 percent (compared to 100 percent initial handicap), resulting in a 50 percent benefit.

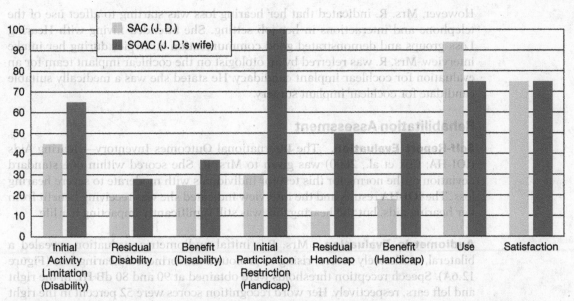

FIGURE 12.5 Summary of SAC and SOAC results (in percent), comparing results from the initial and follow-up administrations.

Both J.D. and his wife reported use and satisfaction scores of 75+ percent (see the textbook website).

Summary

Hearing loss can result in communication difficulty, and since "communication" implies both a sender and a receiver, it stands to reason that the hearing loss *also* affects those people who interact with the person with hearing loss. In the rehabilitative process, it is easy to focus on the individual with the hearing loss and forget about involving the significant other.

This case provides two examples of how the significant other can participate in the AR process. The first example is about *perception*. J.D. and his wife had very different feelings about his communication difficulties. This information helped the audiologist outline the rehabilitation process to include J.D.'s wife to a greater extent. The second example was using the rehabilitation process to work directly with the significant other. Having J.D.'s wife simulate a day with hearing loss helped her better understand the problem and move her from thinking that it was just a "listening" problem.

CASE 4: MRS. R.:—COCHLEAR IMPLANT USER

First Evaluation

Mrs. R. was a 42-year-old caseworker who presented with a bilateral fluctuating sensorineural hearing loss. She reported that her parents first noticed a hearing loss when she was 8 years old. She noted a history of chronic ear infections as a child and felt that these resulted in her hearing loss. She was fitted with her first set of hearing aids at age 10. She reported a history of dizziness and ringing in her ears that were triggered by loud noises and being in any noisy backgrounds. She stated she had constant tinnitus bilaterally; however, when she experienced episodes of dizziness, she reported that the tinnitus is very loud, similar to a car horn. She had been followed by an otolaryngologist for number of years and had three surgeries for fistulas. She denied any history of family hearing loss, and, other than the vestibular and otologic complaints, she reported being in excellent general health. She wore binaural BTE digital hearing aids, which she stated helped her immensely.

However, Mrs. R. indicated that her hearing loss was starting to affect use of the telephone and interactions in her job setting. She attended Living with Hearing Loss groups and demonstrated good communication strategies during her intake interview. Mrs. R. was referred by an otologist on the cochlear implant team for an evaluation for cochlear implant candidacy. He stated she was a medically suitable candidate for cochlear implant surgery.

Rehabilitation Assessment

Self-Report Evaluation. The International Outcomes Inventory—Hearing Aids (IOI-HA; Cox et al., 2000) was given to Mrs. R. She scored within one standard deviation of the norms for this test for individuals with moderate to severe hearing loss. The IOI-HA results and the interview indicated she was receiving benefit from her hearing aids, but the hearing loss was still significantly impacting her life.

Audiometric Evaluation. Mrs. R.'s initial audiometric evaluation revealed a bilateral, moderately severe, rising to profound sensorineural hearing loss (Figure 12.6A). Speech reception thresholds were obtained at 90 and 80 dB HL in the right and left ears, respectively. Her word recognition scores were 52 percent in the right ear and 58 percent in the left ear using the NU-6 word recognition test at her most comfortable loudness levels.

Aided frequency specific thresholds were obtained while Mrs. R. used her binaural amplification. These were obtained using pulsed narrow bands of noise from 250 to 6000 Hz. Aided thresholds fell between the mild to moderate range across the frequencies mentioned. Aided speech recognition scores with binaural amplification were obtained at 35 dB HL. Aided word recognition scores were 68 percent

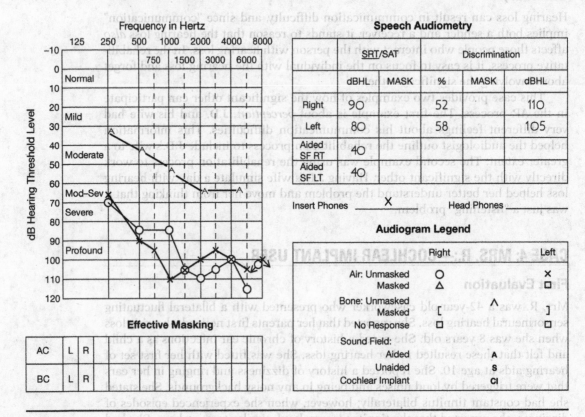

Comments:

No bone conduction scores could be obtained; Aided bilaterally

FIGURE 12.6A   Results of unaided and aided testing for Mrs. R.: audiogram of initial candidacy evaluation.

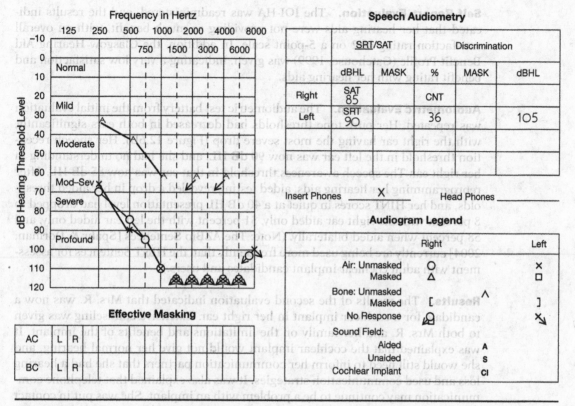

Speech Audiometry

	SRT/SAT		Discrimination		
	dBHL	MASK	%	MASK	dBHL
Right	SAT 85		CNT		
Left	SRT 90		36		105

Insert Phones ____X____ Head Phones _____

Audiogram Legend

	Right	Left
Air: Unmasked	O	×
Masked	△	□
Bone: Unmasked		∧
Masked	[	]
No Response	⚲	⤬
Sound Field:		
Aided	A	
Unaided	S	
Cochlear Implant	CI	

Comments: No bone conduction scores could be obtained; Aided bilaterally

FIGURE 12.6B Results of unaided and aided testing for Mrs. R.: audiogram of second candidacy evaluation.

when presented at 50 dB HL and 52 percent when presented at 40 dB HL. The HINT (Hearing in Noise Test; Nilsson, Soli, & Sullivan, 1994) was presented at 40 dB HL in quiet in three aided conditions, yielding the following results: right hearing aid only = 54 percent, left hearing only = 68 percent, and bilaterally aided = 78 percent. When speechreading was added, the binaural score was 99 percent.

From the results of this evaluation, Mrs. R. was not deemed a candidate for cochlear implantation at that time. Counseling included information that with her hearing aids, she was functioning at a level of many cochlear implant users. For her telephone listening issues, an amplified phone was recommended for her office. In addition, it was recommended that she try a different cell phone with a higher telecoil rating so that she could better couple her cell phone with her hearing aids. The LACE AR computer program was also recommended for home use.

Second Rehabilitation Assessment

Two and a half years later, Mrs. R. returned to the clinic after noticing a decline in her hearing. She stated she had been doing better on the telephone with the amplifier and with a new cell phone, and she felt the LACE program had been helpful, but in the past two months, she noted having difficulty again. She indicated that her understanding abilities had declined with the hearing aid in the right ear and that she was wearing her hearing aid only in her left ear. She reported that even with this hearing aid in, she still had difficulty in her working environment and may have to apply for disability due to this fact. She also noted that her tinnitus had gotten worse and that she had had several bouts of dizziness. She was seen by the otologist on the team who had given her medication that helped the vertigo and tinnitus, but her hearing had not returned to the level it had been previously.

Self-Report Evaluation. The IOI-HA was readministered, and the results indicated that her hearing aids were not providing as much benefit, with an overall satisfaction rating of 2 on a 5-point scale. In addition, the Glasgow Hearing Aid Benefit Profile (Gatehouse, 1999) was given, indicating a very low satisfaction and benefit rating with her hearing aids.

Audiometric Evaluation. The audiometric test battery from the initial evaluation was repeated. Her pure tone thresholds had decreased in both ears significantly, with the right ear having the most severe drop (Figure 12.6B). Her speech reception threshold in the left ear was now 90 dB HL, and she had no understanding in her right ear. The speech awareness threshold in that ear was now 85 dB HL. After reprogramming her hearing aids, aided testing revealed a drop in her aided thresholds, and her HINT scores in quiet at a 40 dB HL presentation level had dropped to 8 percent with the right ear aided only, 51 percent with the left ear aided only, and 58 percent when aided bilaterally. (Note: The AZBio Sentences [Spahr & Dorman, 2004] currently are being used more frequently than the HINT Sentences for assessment with adult cochlear implant candidates and users.)

Results. The results of the second evaluation indicated that Mrs. R. was now a candidate for a cochlear implant in her right ear. Extensive counseling was given to both Mrs. R. and her family on the limitations and benefits of the implant. It was explained that the cochlear implant would not give her normal hearing, and she would still need to inform her communication partners that she had a hearing loss and used communication strategies. It was also explained that telephone communication may continue to be a problem with an implant. She was put in contact with three current cochlear implant users who answered many of her questions. After consultation with the cochlear implant team, she was scheduled for surgery.

Post–Cochlear Implant Rehabilitation Management

Three weeks after surgery, Mrs. R. returned for electrical stimulation of her cochlear implant and follow-up therapy. Initially, Mrs. R. was seen on two consecutive days to program the cochlear implant processor and then for 10 more visits spread out over a three-month interval for therapy and fine-tuning of her speech processor. Threshold and maximum comfort levels were obtained for each of her active electrodes. Mrs. R. was instructed on the care and use of the cochlear implant and how to change programs. Recommendations for different programs in different listening situations were made. After the first week of cochlear implant use, it was recommended that Mrs. R. begin wearing her left ear hearing aid concurrently with her right ear cochlear implant. She reported immediately experiencing great improvements in her word-recognition ability when using both devices. Continued monitoring of her threshold and comfort levels and subsequent MAP modifications were made throughout her therapy sessions.

It is common for a cochlear implant recipient to also utilize a conventional hearing aid in the non-implanted ear.

Communication Remediation Sessions. Therapy sessions consisted of training Mrs. R. how to listen with her new device. Various exercises, including speech tracking (DeFilippo & Scott, 1978) in the implant-only and bimodal modes, were used. Homework consisted of using books on tape to increase her word-recognition abilities. Within a three-week period, Mrs. R. reported she could function on the telephone at work using her cochlear implant.

Throughout the therapy sessions, Mrs. R. kept an ongoing diary of her experiences with the cochlear implant. She listed wearing times, environmental sounds heard, and communication situations. The diary served as a focal point of behavioral counseling. Specific problems were discussed, pointing out both the benefits and the limitations of the cochlear implant, along with possible strategies she might use in each situation.

At her three-month evaluation, Mrs. R. scored 92 percent on the HINT sentences in quiet at a 40 dB HL presentation level. To evaluate her abilities in noise, the HINT sentences were given at a 40 dB HL presentation level, and a noise background was varied to determine the most difficult signal-to-noise ratio (SNR) where she could repeat 50 percent of the sentences. She was able to discriminate 50 percent of the items at a +10 SNR when the test was given in a noisy background with the cochlear implant alone and at a 0 SNR in the bimodal condition. Her IOI-CI scores were in line with normative data for hearing aid users with a mild hearing loss. Her overall satisfaction was 4.5/5.0. She continued to improve over the next two years.

Three-Year Post–Cochlear Implant Assessment.   At her three-year evaluation, Mrs. R. reported that she was not noticing any benefit from the hearing aid in her left ear. Reevaluation of the left ear indicated a significant change in thresholds and word-recognition abilities. In evaluating her abilities with the HINT test, similar results were obtained in the bimodal and cochlear implant–only conditions. At this point, the possibility of a cochlear implant for the left ear was discussed. Mrs. R. was very interested in this possibility, and the results of this evaluation were presented to the cochlear implant team, who were in agreement that a second cochlear implant may provide additional benefit. She received her left cochlear implant three months later.

Post–Bilateral Cochlear Implant.   Two weeks after surgery, Mrs. R. had her initial stimulation of the left cochlear implant using the same procedures as her right cochlear implant. Initially, it was recommended that she spend at least two to three hours a day using only the left cochlear implant so she might become adjusted to the device. She very rapidly adjusted to bilateral cochlear implantation, and at her three-month evaluation, her sound field thresholds with both cochlear implants were 15 dB HL or better from 250 through 6000 HZ, her monosyllabic words were 80 percent when scored by words correct and 91 percent when scored by phonemes correct, and her HINT scores were 98 percent in quiet. When the HINT was given in a noisy background, she was able to discriminate 64 percent of the words at a 0 dB SNR when the stimulus was presented at 40 dB HL. Her IOI-CI indicated she is perceiving great benefit from her cochlear implants, with an overall satisfaction of 4.5 on a 5-point scale. She continues to do extremely well with bilateral cochlear implants.

Summary

Cochlear implants offer an excellent opportunity for postlingually deafened adults to receive beneficial auditory information. Many cochlear implant benefits can be seen across patients, from those who have good open-set understanding, even on the telephone, to those who receive minimal auditory cues. Bilateral hearing can be obtained for cochlear implant users with either bimodal or bilateral cochlear implant stimulation. The determination of which is best for a particular patient depends on his or her residual hearing and may change over time. Mrs. R. is representative of this. Initially, she received significant benefit from the use of both a cochlear implant and a hearing aid, but with changes in her hearing, she was unable to get meaningful benefit from the hearing aid in the opposite ear. At that point, she became a bilateral cochlear implant candidate and subsequently a successful bilateral user. She represents an average postlingually hearing-impaired cochlear implant patient. She is an excellent user who can use the telephone with her devices. She does continue to use communication strategies and speechreading whenever possible. With appropriate training, a cochlear implant has the potential to improve the quality of life significantly for an individual with profound hearing loss.

CASE 5: MRS. E.—NURSING HOME HEARING AID USER

Case History

Mrs. E. was a 75-year-old resident of a local nursing home. She had been living in the facility for over two years and was quite alert mentally and able to move about the facility without any special assistance. Mrs. E. was using a BTE hearing aid in her right ear at the time she was first seen by an audiologist. It was later determined that she had been a longtime hearing aid user, having had four other instruments over a period of many years. Her present hearing aid was five years old and, according to Mrs. E., did not seem to be working as well as it once had.

Diagnostic Information

Initial efforts with Mrs. E. involved air-conduction pure tone testing and tympanometry in a quiet room within the nursing home. As seen in Figure 12.7, the client had a moderate hearing loss, which was bilaterally symmetrical. Type A tympanograms were traced bilaterally, suggesting the presence of a sensorineural disorder in each ear.

AR

Mrs. E. was concerned about the condition of her hearing aid, complaining that it did not seem to help her as much as it had in the past. She also appeared to be experiencing an excessive amount of acoustic feedback and reported having difficulty getting the earmold into her ear properly.

The hearing aid was analyzed electroacoustically by the audiologist, who found it to have a reduced gain and an abnormal amount of distortion. In discussing the feasibility of purchasing a new hearing aid, it became clear that Mrs. E. was not financially able to consider such a purchase. She was, therefore, advised to have her hearing aid serviced and reconditioned by the manufacturer. She was agreeable to this recommendation, and arrangements were made for this to occur.

In the course of working with Mrs. E., it became apparent that she needed a new earmold. In discussing this, Mrs. E. recalled that her current mold had

It is possible (and sometimes necessary) to gather basic, relevant audiometric information outside the traditional audiologic test booth if certain measures are taken to ensure the validity of the results obtained.

The repair and reconditioning of a hearing aid can be viable alternatives if the instrument is not too old and is still appropriate for the user's hearing loss.

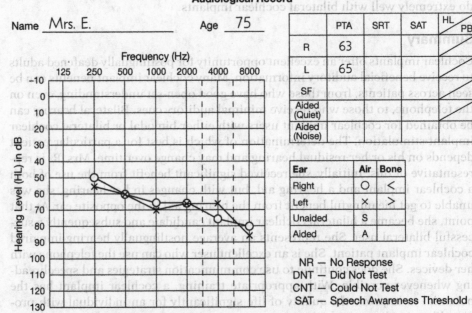

Audiological Record

	PTA	SRT	SAT	HL / PB
R	63			
L	65			
SF				
Aided (Quiet)				
Aided (Noise)				

Ear	Air	Bone
Right	O	<
Left	×	>
Unaided	S	
Aided	A	

NR — No Response
DNT — Did Not Test
CNT — Could Not Test
SAT — Speech Awareness Threshold

FIGURE 12.7   Case 5: Audiometric results for Mrs. E.

also been used with her previous hearing aid. The mold was very discolored and did not appear to fit Mrs. E.'s ear canal and pinna adequately. The audiologist took an ear impression, which was sent to a laboratory for production of a new earmold.

In approximately two weeks, both the earmold and the hearing aid were returned. Mrs. E. was then fitted with the reconditioned aid, and her initial reaction was quite positive. She was instructed to use the aid as much as possible in the following days. A subsequent electroacoustic analysis of the instrument revealed an increase in gain and a significant decrease in the amount of distortion. Real-ear measures, taken at the nursing home with portable equipment, revealed satisfactory gain. When she was seen again, Mrs. E. was still pleased with the help she was receiving from her hearing aid, but she indicated that she was still having difficulty inserting the earmold. Watching her attempt to do this by herself made it apparent that Mrs. E. was not able to manipulate her hands sufficiently to allow her to insert the earmold without great effort. It was also apparent that she was not using an efficient method when inserting the mold. To assist her, Mrs. E. was given some basic instructions on how to best insert and remove the earmold. She was encouraged to practice the procedure and was visited by the audiologist several times during the next two weeks to review the procedure and to answer any questions she might have. During these visits, it became apparent that Mrs. E.'s facility in placement of the earmold had improved.

Along with the work done with Mrs. E. to improve the way she inserted her earmold, several of the nursing home staff members working with Mrs. E. were also provided with information on how to insert the earmold properly. This allowed them to assist Mrs. E. in doing so each day. Both Mrs. E. and the staff also received helpful information on how to clean her earmold and basic instruction on the operation and use of her hearing aid.

More frequent monitoring of the status of some patients is important to facilitate success with AR.

Summary

Attempts to help Mrs. E. were successful. This is not always the case when working in a rehabilitative capacity with nursing home residents (Schow, 1982). Mrs. E.'s case illustrates one of the ways in which an audiologist can make a valuable contribution to a number of residents in a given nursing home. It is important first to identify those individuals within the facility for whom AR may be beneficial. Once this is done, the audiologist will generally work with each person individually, identifying those areas of AR that should be worked on. Individual needs must be considered, and the audiologist must be willing to devote the time necessary to accomplish the desired ends.

CASE 6: ASHLEY—NEW TECHNOLOGY FOR AN EXPERIENCED USER

Introduction

Ashley was a 20-year-old college student in her sophomore year at a small university. She had a hearing loss and wore hearing aids for as long as she could remember. She was very aware of her hearing limitations but, like many young adults, preferred that others not know of these limitations, much less that she wore hearing aids. Her close friends and family were understanding and developed strategies for communicating with her.

After struggling academically in her freshman year, she decided that part of her problem might be hearing well in the classroom. Her current hearing aids were purchased eight years ago and might not be giving her all the help she needs. However, she felt like she was in a difficult situation because with her school expenses, purchasing new hearing aids would be difficult financially.

Hearing in a classroom can be especially challenging for those with hearing loss.

Informational Counseling

Given her long history of hearing loss, the outcome of a complete hearing evaluation was not a surprise. Ashley's previous audiometric records were requested for comparison purposes from the audiologist in her home town to see if there was any change in her hearing. Her last audiogram was four years prior, and the findings from the recent evaluation showed little or no change. This came as a relief to Ashley and reinforced her suspicion that it was her hearing *aids*, not her hearing, that may not be working well.

The audiologist determined that the current hearing aids were now eight years old and explained to Ashley that hearing instrument technology had improved a great deal in that time. With Ashley's increased demand on her hearing, the new hearing aids could potentially provide a great deal of benefit.

Rehabilitation Assessment

Communication Status: Hearing Loss/Activity Limitations

Audiometry and Communication Assessment. The results of a comprehensive hearing evaluation (see Figure 12.8) showed a symmetrical, moderate sensorineural hearing loss with a very gradual slope configuration. Her word-recognition scores were 80 percent in the right ear and 76 percent in the left ear using the Northwestern NU-6 word lists. When visual cues were allowed, Ashley's word recognition scores improved to 100 percent for both ears.

Loudness discomfort levels were established for all frequencies and compared with her pure tone thresholds to establish a dynamic range (DR). In the low frequencies, her DR was 34 to 45 dB. The DR in the high frequencies was slightly less at 25 to 35 dB.

Ashley's speech recognition in the presence of competing background noise was assessed using the QuickSIN (Etymotic Research, 2001) and revealed a moderate signal-to-noise ratio loss (SNR loss) of 11 dB.

Communication Assessment. Ashley was asked to complete the SAC (Schow & Nerbonne, 1982) as a way of measuring her perceived communication difficulty. The audiologist asked her to complete the form based on her difficulty when she was *not* wearing her hearing aids. Ashley found this quite difficult because it was so rare that she didn't wear her hearing aids. The audiologist decided to have Ashley complete two forms: one representing no hearing aid use (unaided) and one representing

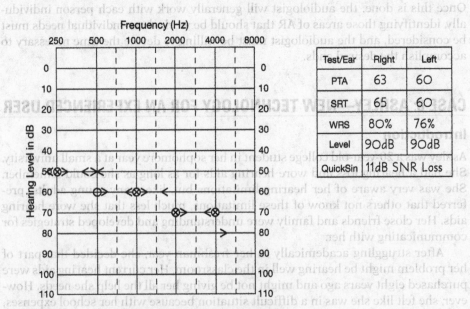

Test/Ear	Right	Left
PTA	63	60
SRT	65	60
WRS	80%	76%
Level	90dB	90dB
QuickSin	11dB SNR Loss	

FIGURE 12.8 Case 6: Audiometric results for Ashley.

using her hearing aids (aided). Her raw score for the SAC in the unaided condition was 40, indicating a substantial amount of difficulty. Her perception of communication difficulty while wearing the hearing aid was much lower with a raw score of 27, with the poorest rating for "unfavorable communication situations."

Overall Participation Variables.   Psychologically, Ashley had long accepted her hearing loss, with the exception of a rough time in middle school, where having hearing aids was a source for teasing. Since that time, however, she had developed a healthy mind-set that her hearing loss was just part of who she was. Her biggest challenge now was her participation in the college classroom.

Related Personal Factors.   Ashley was a very social individual, and, while certain social situations were more difficult, she refused to let her hearing loss interfere. Ashley grew up with technologies such as texting, instant messaging, and e-mail that enabled her to communicate effectively outside of the acoustic environment. Much of her social interaction was done using these technologies and to some extent decreased the stress of communication.

Environmental Factors.   As is often the case, freshmen and sophomore classes were large and usually in rooms with poor acoustics. Even when sitting in the front row, Ashley would find it difficult to ignore the classroom noise and focus on the instructor. Any time she would have to take her eyes off the instructor, she would struggle to hear all of what was being said.

Rehabilitation Management

Counseling and Psychosocial Issues.   Ashley never really had to deal with *losing* her hearing. Her hearing and receptive communication were the same now as she had always remembered. So, dealing with the loss of her hearing really wasn't a problem for Ashley; it was more dealing with the increased difficulty she was experiencing in the college classroom. Secondarily, she was worried about the cost of upgrading her hearing aids at a time when she was spending so much on her education. Her expectations were perhaps value driven by a seemingly inconvenient expense.

Amplification (Modifying Audibility).   Ashley's current hearing aids were programmable, single-channel BTE style with large, full-shell custom earmolds. When she and the audiologist were discussing the different hearing aid styles, Ashley was intrigued by the completely-in-the-canal (CIC) style because of how discreet they looked. She had always worn her hair long to cover the hearing aids, and the thought of being able to change that was exciting. However, the excitement was soon lost when she noticed that the cost of the CIC hearing aid was much more than that of the BTE style. The audiologist explained that while the BTE style may be more noticeable, the technology available in the BTE style could potentially provide her with more benefit in the classroom environment.

Ashley's QuickSIN score was in the moderate category, indicating that her ability to correctly process a speech signal in the presence of a competing noise was only fair. This, and the fact that Ashley was in unfavorable listening situations most of the time, led the audiologist to recommend a specific hearing aid. This particular hearing aid had multiple channels, an adaptive directional microphone, and a cutting-edge signal processor capability designed to adaptively maximize speech understanding in the presence of background noise. Additionally, the hearing aid had exceptional telephone compatibility ratings and had integrated bluetooth technology for wirelessly communicating with devices such as personal music devices, television, and theater sound systems.

When Ashley arrived for her fitting, she was reminded by the audiologist that her new hearing aids would sound much different than her current eight-year-old hearing aids. The hearing aids were programmed based on her audiogram and dynamic range findings. When the hearing aids were placed on Ashley and turned on, she was immediately concerned that there wasn't enough gain because the background noise in the room seemed too soft. As soon as she spoke and then listened to the audiologist's reply, it was clear what had happened. Ashley was used to her old hearing aids amplifying everything, including background noise. The technology in her new hearing aids was minimally amplifying the background noise and enhancing the speech, making the overall volume seem abnormally soft.

The audiologist went through a series of informal, functional adjustments to ensure that sounds were appropriately audible. As an objective measure of verification, speech mapping using probe-microphone measurements was used to further evaluate the appropriateness of the fitting and make necessary adjustments.

Ashley's hearing aids had the capability of storing alternate settings in program memories that could be changed by her, depending on the listening situation. One of the additional memory settings was programmed for extreme noise situations, such as basketball games, and the other was set for use with her cellphone .

Hearing Aid Orientation. Ashley was well acquainted with hearing aid use, and since the new hearing aids were the same style as her old ones, many of the hearing aid orientation topics seemed too basic. However, the audiologist covered each of the following topics at the level that seemed appropriate for Ashley.

Hearing Expectations. This topic was an important one to cover for Ashley because she was concerned about the expense and the tendency to inflate the expectations when something is expensive. Realistic examples of how the technology could help Ashley were presented, and she was encouraged not to become disappointed if she couldn't hear perfectly in every environment.

Instrument Operations. The operation of the hearing aids was different than Ashley's old hearing aids in that there was no manual volume control. The adaptive technology in the new hearing aids ensured that soft sounds were audible and loud sounds were still comfortable. In addition, the hearing aids constantly monitored the incoming sound and adjusted a wide range of parameters to maximize speech intelligibility. The only control on the hearing aids was a program button for Ashley to select for different listening situations, including using the telephone. Ashley was used to having a T-coil on the hearing aid to use with the telephone; however, her new hearing aids used wireless Bluetooth technology. When the audiologist demonstrated how to use the phone, Ashley was surprised at the clarity of the sound.

Occlusion Effect. Ashley wasn't bothered by the way her own voice sounded—because she had been amplified at such a young age, her voice had always sounded the same way to her.

Batteries. Ashley knew most of the battery information but was delighted to find out that the newer technology was much more efficient, and instead of getting only a few days on a battery, she could now expect a week or more.

Acoustic Feedback. Given the amount of gain necessary to address Ashley's hearing loss, she was fully aware of the concept of feedback and the annoying squealing that could sometimes occur. What was exciting to Ashley was the fact that the new technology now had a feedback management circuit and would substantially reduce those occurrences. The audiologist simulated a situation where feedback might occur by cupping her hand over Ashley's hearing aid. Only a brief chirp was heard as the feedback manager squelched the problem.

System Troubleshooting. Ashley was skilled at troubleshooting problems with her hearing aid, and there was little new that the audiologist could offer.

Insertion and Removal. Since the styles of the new hearing aids and the custom earmold were the same, Ashley had no problem inserting and removing her new hearing aids.

Cleaning and Maintenance. Ashley's new hearing aids had directional microphones and required that a special screen be changed periodically. Her good eyesight and dexterity made this a simple task.

Service and Warranty. The audiologist helped Ashley complete the warranty information and reminded her how she could obtain service not only in her college town but when she went back home as well.

After the hearing aid orientation, the audiologist suggested that Ashley keep a journal of her experiences not only for situations where she experienced problems but also for the situations where she felt the hearing aids were working well. This would allow her hearing aids to be adjusted more precisely to provide the maximum amount of benefit. The audiologist suggested that she categorize her entries into "fit" and "function" categories. The "fit" category would be anything that had to do with how the hearing aids felt on her ears, like soreness, irritation, or even how she was able to access the controls on the hearing aid. The "function" category was for anything related to how the hearing aids were helping her with communication. Ashley was very technologically oriented and immediately found an application for her smartphone that allowed her to quickly make journal entries. These entries were e-mailed directly to her audiologist so that when Ashley arrived for her first follow-up, the audiologist had a detailed picture of Ashley's experiences.

In the "fit" category, Ashley was very pleased. The hearing aids were comfortable, and she was able to access all of the controls easily.

In the "function" category, Ashley targeted her main AR goal established by her and her audiologist: to hear better in the classroom situation. The journal entries indicated that in some classroom situations, Ashley noticed improvement beyond her expectations. In other classroom situations, she almost felt that her old hearing aids did better. The audiologist asked her what was different about each of these classroom situations, and it was discovered that the classes with a smaller number and quieter students were better. The larger classes with students talking constantly while the instructor was talking were the most difficult. The audiologist explained that the hearing aids had an adaptive program to identify and amplify speech signals while attempting to reduce nonspeech signals. In the classroom environment, the hearing aids were trying to amplify *all* speech, and that was probably why the larger, noisier classrooms were so difficult. Since the instructor was usually in front of Ashley, the audiologist made an adjustment to the program that would restrict the amplification of the speech signals to what is only in front of her rather than all around her.

The journal entries described how much she enjoyed not having to worry about acoustic feedback when, for example, she bumped her hearing aid mold or put a hat on her head. With her old hearing aids she would anticipate potential feedback situations and turn the volume down. However, that usually led to communication problems because the gain was too low. Her new hearing aids did not require this strategy, and she felt that she was getting more out of every conversation.

At her six-month follow-up, Ashley was doing very well. The adjustments made to her hearing aid program had made a big difference, and even hearing in large classrooms was much less frustrating than before. She was particularly happy with the fact that she could listen and take notes at the same time and not have to rely quite so much on visual cues.

Remediate Communication Activity. Over the course of her follow-up visits, the audiologist reviewed communication strategies that included topics such as controlling the communication situation, looking at the speaker, and using communication repair strategies. For the most part, Ashley was well versed at communication strategies with the exception of being assertive. Ashley struggled with letting others know of her limitations and would often bluff her way through a difficult communication situation. When the audiologist pointed out that sometimes an inaccurate or inappropriate bluff would be more embarrassing than being assertive, Ashley agreed to work on this particular skill.

Environment and Coordination

Participation Improvement. Ashley was already outgoing and involved in many different types of social situations. The audiologist, however, asked Ashley if there were any communication environments that she avoided because it was too difficult to hear. Ashley pointed out that when she travels in a car, she prefers not to drive because she can't control the listening situation. When she is a passenger, she can get visual cues and turn her head to maximize communication. The audiologist informed her that the new technology in her hearing aids would likely be better in that situation and that, if necessary, one of the alternate programs could be specifically adjusted for that situation.

Vocational Rehabilitation Assistance.

The audiologist recognized that Ashley was very concerned about the cost of the hearing aids and the impact it would have on her school finances. The audiologist suggested that Ashley contact a vocational rehabilitation counselor to see if he or she could offer some assistance.

Ashley contacted vocational rehabilitation and completed the eligibility documentation. When she met with her vocational rehabilitation counselor, it was explained that the agency was concerned primarily with helping people with disabilities gain employment. However, the agency recognizes that helping someone be successful in school will help him or her gain employment after graduation. Ashley qualified for assistance for the purchase of her new hearing aids. While vocational rehabilitation did not pay the entire amount, the financial assistance provided was a relief to Ashley.

Summary

This case is interesting for several reasons. The first is that it highlights a few unique features of someone who has used hearing aids for her whole life as compared to someone who had normal hearing and then acquired the hearing loss over time. For example, the occlusion effect wasn't a problem for Ashley because she had always heard her voice through amplification and occlusion. Similarly, she was very comfortable with manipulating and taking care of the hearing aids from her past experience.

Another unique feature was that her hearing expectations were being influenced by value much more than you would expect from a new user with an acquired hearing loss. When Ashley was under the impression that she had to come up with money for hearing aids, her expectations were admittedly higher. Her expectations then were driven by a sense of "is the expense worth it" to have spent all this money, whereas another hearing aid user might build his or her expectations on "I want to hear like I did when I was younger." When she was able to get financial assistance from vocational rehabilitation, her expectations were less value driven and more related to specific communication situations.

Finally, Ashley had grown up with technology, and, as a result, the advanced features of her new hearing aids were intuitive for her to understand and operate. It seemed almost second nature to her, for example, to pair a Bluetooth device with her hearing aid or to understand the series of "beeps" in her hearing aid that tell her about the hearing aid status.

CASE 7: MS. C.—DIZZINESS ISSUES

Introduction

Ms. C. was a 39-year-old female referred to the Hearing and Balance Clinic for a complete evaluation of her hearing and vestibular function. Her chief complaint was intermittent, intense dizziness. These episodes began shortly after being involved in a motor vehicle accident about two weeks ago in which she hit her head on the side window.

She described the dizziness episodes as a sensation that the room is spinning around her. While each episode lasts for only a few seconds (estimates 2 to 30 seconds), it reportedly made her very unsteady on her feet, and she became nauseated for about an hour. She reported not having any advanced warning when the episodes occurred but noticed that rolling out of bed, bending over, and tipping her head back in the shower seemed to trigger an episode. She did not report any change in her hearing with the episodes but noted that she has a distant "ocean noise" in her right ear from time to time. To manage her symptoms, she reportedly held still for a few minutes, and then she could cautiously return to whatever she was doing. She was prescribed Meclizine for her dizziness but said that it really didn't help with the dizziness and just made her sleepy.

> Difficulties with dizziness can be stressful and limiting for the individual.

Rehabilitation Assessment

To address the concerns regarding the noise in her right ear, a complete hearing evaluation was performed (see Figure 12.9). The external ears, canals, and tympanic membranes appeared normal by otoscopy. Tympanometry revealed Type A tympanograms. Pure tone air and bone-conduction audiometry revealed thresholds within normal limits with a similar configuration. Speech audiometry findings were also normal with excellent word-recognition ability. To explore the noise (tinnitus) in her right ear, a comparative approach was used to get a better understanding of the perceived pitch and relative loudness. Pure tones were presented to the patient, and she was asked to judge if the tone was similar to her own tinnitus. She reported that what she was hearing in her ear was more like a noise, so narrowband masking noise was presented to her for comparison. A 250-Hz narrowband noise at 20 dB HL was found to best approximate the type and loudness of tinnitus she was experiencing.

Videonystagmography (VNG) testing was performed to evaluate the vestibular systems (see Table 12.2). The oculomotor portion of the evaluation did not provide any compelling clinical evidence that her dizziness was related to central nervous

Audiological Record

Name Ms. C.   Age 39

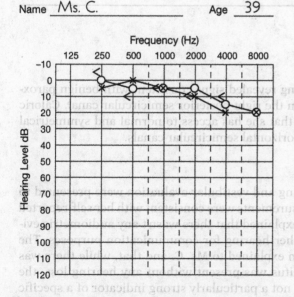

	PTA	SRT	SAT	HL / PB
R	5	5		40 / 100
L	5	10		40 / 100
SF				
Aided (Quiet)				
Aided (Noise)				

Ear	Air	Bone
Right	O	<
Left	×	>
Aided	A	

NR — No Response
DNT — Did Not Test
CNT — Could Not Test
SAT — Speech Awareness Threshold

FIGURE 12.9   Case 7: Audiometric results for Ms. C.

TABLE 12.2   Case 7: Vestibular Results for Ms. C.

VNG		
Otoscopy	Normal	External ears, canals, and tympanic membranes appeared normal.
Tympanometry	Normal	Normal pressure, volume, and compliance, bilaterally.

Oculomotor		
Gaze	Normal	No nystagmus was noted for gaze left, right, up, down, or center positions.
Horizontal random saccadic pursuit	Normal	Normal and symmetrical velocity, latency, and accuracy for all angles tested.
Horizontal smooth pursuit (tracking)	Normal	Normal and symmetrical gain, accuracy, and phase for both slow (.2 Hz) and fast (.7 Hz) targets.
Optokinetic testing	Normal	Normal and symmetrical gain for both 20 and 40 d/s targets.

Positionals		
Dynamic		
Dix Hallpike right	Positive for BPPV	After a brief latency (~10 seconds), a right, torsional upbeat nystagmus was observed. This continued for approximately one minute. Patient reported that this replicated her symptoms.
Dix Hallpike left	Negative	No nystagmus was noted; no dizziness was reported.
Roll test	Negative	No nystagmus was noted; no dizziness was reported.
Bow/lean	Negative	No nystagmus was noted; no dizziness was reported.

Static		
Sitting, head center, vision denied	Normal	No nystagmus was noted; no dizziness was reported.
Supine, head center	Normal	No nystagmus was noted; no dizziness was reported.
Supine, head right	Normal	No nystagmus was noted; no dizziness was reported.
Supine, head left	Normal	No nystagmus was noted; no dizziness was reported.
Supine, head hanging	Normal	No nystagmus was noted; no dizziness was reported.

Bithermal caloric irrigation		
	Normal	Symmetrical responses.
Fixation suppression	Normal	Normal fixation suppression.

system pathology. Positional testing revealed signs consistent with benign paroxysmal positional vertigo (BPPV) in the right posterior semicircular canal. Caloric irrigation test findings suggested that she has access to normal and symmetrical vestibular information from the horizontal semicircular canals.

Informational Counseling

The results of the complete hearing and vestibular evaluation were presented to Ms. C. The objective hearing measurements were consistent with her self-reported communication abilities. It was explained that there wasn't any audiometric evidence to suggest concern about her hearing for communication purposes. The brief tinnitus evaluation was then explained to Ms. C. and that, while there was some mild concern that the tinnitus was present without any hearing loss, the particular symptom by itself was not a particularly strong indicator of a specific cause.

The findings of the VNG evaluation were then explained. She was comforted by the fact that BPPV is the most common cause of dizziness and that it has an extremely good prognosis. She was informed that the treatment for BPPV involved a simple canalith repositioning procedure (called the Epley maneuver) in which she would be assisted through a series of body positions. This procedure was designed to relocate otolithic debris back into an area of the inner ear where it wouldn't be causing inappropriate signals to the brain. She was curious about the procedure and was interested in seeing if it would work to treat her symptoms.

Rehabilitation Management

Oculography goggles were placed on Ms. C. to allow visualization of the eyes during the Epley maneuver procedure. The procedure was performed, and the patient was allowed to relax for a few minutes prior to retesting. Ms. C. noticed an immediate sensation that "something was different." She was then retested, and the findings indicated that the BPPV had been resolved. Further information counseling was given regarding BPPV and the possibility that it would recur. She was given discharge instructions and encouraged to contact the clinic if her symptoms returned or were not completely resolved.

Summary

One of the most common sources of dizziness is a disorder called Benign Paroxysmal Positional Vertigo (BPPV). Very often, a medical provider will refer to the audiologist for a VNG, and during the evaluation, a diagnosis of BPPV is made. Audiologists are trained to remediate this condition and can effectively do so with the same equipment used for the evaluation. It can be a very satisfying form of rehabilitation for the audiologist because the person with BPPV very often leaves the facility feeling much better (less dizzy) than when he or she arrived.

Chapter Summary Points

- Hearing loss can produce a variety of difficulties for an individual, and effective AR must address these particular needs.

- Information gathering (including discussions with the patient, the use of self-report scales, hearing tests, auditory–visual skills assessment, and other relevant sources of information) is an important component of AR.

- Successful intervention depends to a large extent on the degree of motivation possessed by the individual with hearing loss.

- Today's hearing aids are complex instruments. Proper selection and fitting of these devices require extensive expertise and instrumentation in order to maximize their potential.

- The intervention process can be threatened if the person with the hearing loss has unrealistic hopes and expectations related to a component of AR (e.g., a cochlear implant) that are impossible to fulfill. Clinicians need to monitor this continuously with their patients, especially in the early stages of intervention.

- Comprehensive and effective hearing aid fitting, particularly for first-time users, should include an extensive orientation to hearing aid use and exposure to factors that facilitate communication.

- Dizziness is a common and often disruptive condition, and today's audiologist frequently can play an important role in its assessment and management.

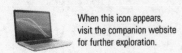

When this icon appears, visit the companion website for further exploration.

Supplementary Learning Activities

See www.isu.edu/csed/audiology/rehab to carry out these activities. We encourage you to use these to supplement your learning. Your instructor may give specific assignments that involve a particular activity.

1. CORE and CARE Worksheet and Case Study Template. To gain a better understanding of the AR process in terms of assessment and management, "take apart" a case study and place it into the CORE/CARE rehabilitation model. Step-by-step instructions are found on the website. You simply need to download the CORE/CARE template, then select an AR case from this chapter. After reading the case, type appropriate responses into the template.

2. Select an adult or elderly adult with hearing loss whom you can interview. Ideally, the person you select can meet with you, but it is possible to carry out this activity via telephone or even through e-mail exchanges. You should gather information about the person's hearing loss (degree, age at onset, type of loss, unilateral or bilateral, and any other pertinent parameters); use of hearing aids, cochlear implants, and/or HATs; how the hearing loss has affected his or her personal and social lives; as well as work and any other activities. What sorts of listening strategies, if any, does this person employ to help with communication? See the website above for further assistance as you prepare for this activity.

Recommended Reading

Busacco, D. (2010). *Audiologic interpretation.* Boston: Pearson.

Johnson, C. E., & Danhauer, J. L. (1999). *Guidebook for support programs in aural rehabilitation.* San Diego, CA: Singular Publishing.

Johnson, C. E., & Danhuer, J. L. (2002). *Handbook of outcomes measurement in audiology.* San Diego, CA: Singular Publishing.

Recommended Website

This site has a comprehensive summary on the SAC and the SOAC, including mean and range data within pure tone groups, computerized versions, comparisons with other self-reports, and critical difference (CD) scores: www2.ISU.edu/csed.

References

Cox, R., Hyde, M., Gatehouse, S., Noble, W., Dillion, H., Bentler, R., et al. (2000). Optimal outcome measures, research priorities and international cooperation. *Ear and Hearing, 21,* 1065–1155.

DeFilippo, C., & Scott, B. (1978). A method for training and evaluating the reception of ongoing speech. *Journal of the Acoustical Society of America, 63,* 1186–1192.

Etymotic Research. (2001). *Quick Speech in Noise Test (QuickSIN).* Elk Grove Village, IL: Author.

Gatehouse, S. (1999). Glasgow Hearing Aid Benefit Profile: Derivation and validation of a client-centered outcome measure for hearing aid services. *Journal of the American Academy of Audiology, 10,* 80–103.

Nilsson, M. J., Soli, S. D., & Sullivan, J. A. (1994). Development of the *Hearing in Noise Test* for the measurement of speech reception in quiet and in noise. *Journal of the Acoustical Society of America, 95,* 1085–1099.

Schow, R. L. (1982). Success of hearing aid fitting in nursing home residents. *Ear and Hearing, 3*(3), 173–177.

Schow, R. L. (1989). Self-assessment of hearing in rehabilitative audiology: Developments in the U.S.A. *British Journal of Audiology, 23*, 13–24.

Schow, R. L., & Nerbonne, M. (1982). Communication screening profile: Use with elderly clients. *Ear and Hearing, 3*(3), 133–147.

Schow, R., & Tannahill, C. (1977). Hearing handicap scores and categories for subjects with normal and impaired hearing sensitivity. *Journal of the American Audiological Society, 3*, 134–139.

Seewald, R. (1992). The desired sensation level method for fitting children. *Hearing Journal, 45*, 36–46.

Seewald, R. (2000). An update of DSL [i/o]. *Hearing Journal, 53*(4), 10–16.

Spahr, A. J., & Dorman, M. F. (2004). Performance of implant patients fit with the CII and Nucleus 3G devices. *Archives of Otolaryngology—Head and Neck Surgery, 130*, 624–628.

Stephens, D., & Kramer, S. (2010). *Living with hearing difficulties: The process of enablement*. West Sussex: Wiley.

Sturmak, M. J. (1987). *Communication handicap score interpretation for various populations and degrees of hearing impairment*. Master's thesis, Idaho State University, Pocatello.

World Health Organization. (2001). *International classification of functioning, disability, and health*. Geneva: Author.

Author Index

Subject Index